BSAVA Manual of
Canine Practice
A Foundation Manual

Editors:

Tim Hutchinson
BVSc CertSAS MRCVS
Larkmead Veterinary Group,
111–113 Park Road, Didcot OX11 8QT

Ken Robinson
BVMS CertSAD MRCVS
Rose Cottage Veterinary Centre,
Chester Road, Sutton Weaver,
Runcorn, Cheshire WA7 3EQ

Published by:

British Small Animal Veterinary Association
Woodrow House, 1 Telford Way,
Waterwells Business Park, Quedgeley,
Gloucester GL2 2AB

A Company Limited by Guarantee in England
Registered Company No. 2837793
Registered as a Charity

Illustrations for 15.14, 21.11, 21.14, 21.15, 29.6 and QRGs 25.1 and 29.2 were
drawn by S.J. Elmhurst BA Hons (www.livingart.org.uk) and are printed with
her permission.

A catalogue record for this book is available from the British Library.

ISBN 978 1 905319 48 0

The publishers, editors and contributors cannot take responsibility for
information provided on dosages and methods of application of drugs
mentioned or referred to in this publication. Details of this kind must be
verified in each case by individual users from up to date literature published
by the manufacturers or suppliers of those drugs. Veterinary surgeons are
reminded that in each case they must follow all appropriate national
legislation and regulations (for example, in the United Kingdom, the
prescribing cascade) from time to time in force.

Printed by Cambrian Printers, Aberystwyth, UK
Printed on ECF paper made from sustainable forests

Titles in the BSAVA Manuals series

Manual of Canine & Feline Abdominal Imaging
Manual of Canine & Feline Abdominal Surgery
Manual of Canine & Feline Advanced Veterinary Nursing
Manual of Canine & Feline Anaesthesia and Analgesia
Manual of Canine & Feline Behavioural Medicine
Manual of Canine & Feline Cardiorespiratory Medicine
Manual of Canine & Feline Clinical Pathology
Manual of Canine & Feline Dentistry
Manual of Canine & Feline Dermatology
Manual of Canine & Feline Emergency and Critical Care
Manual of Canine & Feline Endocrinology
Manual of Canine & Feline Endoscopy and Endosurgery
Manual of Canine & Feline Fracture Repair and Management
Manual of Canine & Feline Gastroenterology
Manual of Canine & Feline Haematology and Transfusion Medicine
Manual of Canine & Feline Head, Neck and Thoracic Surgery
Manual of Canine & Feline Musculoskeletal Disorders
Manual of Canine & Feline Musculoskeletal Imaging
Manual of Canine & Feline Nephrology and Urology
Manual of Canine & Feline Neurology
Manual of Canine & Feline Oncology
Manual of Canine & Feline Ophthalmology
Manual of Canine & Feline Radiography and Radiology: A Foundation Manual
Manual of Canine & Feline Rehabilitation, Supportive and Palliative Care:
    Case Studies in Patient Management
Manual of Canine & Feline Reproduction and Neonatology
Manual of Canine & Feline Surgical Principles: A Foundation Manual
Manual of Canine & Feline Thoracic Imaging
Manual of Canine & Feline Ultrasonography
Manual of Canine & Feline Wound Management and Reconstruction
Manual of Canine Practice: A Foundation Practice
Manual of Exotic Pet and Wildlife Nursing
Manual of Exotic Pets: A Foundation Manual
Manual of Feline Practice: A Foundation Manual
Manual of Ornamental Fish
Manual of Practical Animal Care
Manual of Practical Veterinary Nursing
Manual of Psittacine Birds
Manual of Rabbit Medicine
Manual of Rabbit Surgery, Dentistry and Imaging
Manual of Raptors, Pigeons and Passerine Birds
Manual of Reptiles
Manual of Rodents and Ferrets
Manual of Small Animal Practice Management and Development
Manual of Wildlife Casualties

For further information on these and all BSAVA publications,
please visit our website: **www.bsava.com**

Contents

Quick reference guides

Contributors

Sophie Adamantos BVSc CertVA DipACVECC DipECVECC FHEA MRCVS
Langford Veterinary Services, University of Bristol, Langford, Bristol BS40 5DU

Ross Allan BVMS PGCertSAS MRCVS
The Pets'n'Vets Family, 1478 Pollokshaws Road, Glasgow G43 1RN

Nick Bexfield BVetMed PhD DSAM DipECVIM-CA CBiol FSB MRCVS
School of Veterinary Medicine and Science, University of Nottingham, Sutton Bonington Campus, Leicestershire LE12 5RD

Marge Chandler DVM MS MANZCVSc DipACVN DipACVIM DipECVIM-CA MRCVS
The Royal (Dick) School of Veterinary Studies, University of Edinburgh, Easter Bush Campus, Midlothian EH25 9RG

Kate Chitty BVetMed MRCVS
Anton Vets, Units 11–12 Anton Mill Road, Andover, Hants SP10 2NJ

Tiny De Keuster DVM DipECAWBM
Faculty of Veterinary Medicine, Ghent University, Salisburylaan 133, 9820 Merelbeke, Belgium

Alex Gough MA VetMB CertSAM CertVC PGCert MRCVS
Bath Veterinary Referrals, Rosemary Lodge Veterinary Hospital, Wellsway, Bath BA2 5RL

Sara M. Gould BVetMed DSAM MRCVS
Vale Referrals, The Animal Hospital, Stinchcombe, Dursley, Gloucestershire GL11 6AJ

Julian Hoad BSc(Hons) BVetMed honMBVNA MRCVS
Crossways Veterinary Group, 43 School Hill, Storrington, West Sussex RH20 4NA

Alan Hughes BVSc MRCVS
The Grove Veterinary Hospital and Clinics, Holt Road, Fakenham, Norfolk NR21 8JG

Tim Hutchinson BVSc CertSAS MRCVS
Larkmead Veterinary Group, 111–113 Park Road, Didcot OX11 8QT

Scott Kilpatrick BSc(Hons) BVM&S MRCVS
The Royal (Dick) School of Veterinary Studies, University of Edinburgh, Easter Bush Campus, Midlothian EH25 9RG

Gary A. Lewin BVSc CertVOphthal CertSAS MRCVS
Veterinary Vision, Onsala Building, Haweswater Road, Penrith, Cumbria CA11 9FJ

Geoff Little MVB MRCVS
The Veterinary Defence Society Limited, 4 Haig Court, Parkgate Estate, Knutsford, Cheshire WA16 8XZ

Christine Magrath BVMS FRCVS
The Veterinary Defence Society Limited, 4 Haig Court, Parkgate Estate, Knutsford, Cheshire WA16 8XZ

Mark Maltman BVSc CertSAM CertVC MRCVS
Maltman Cosham Veterinary Clinic, Lyons Farm Estate, Slinfold, Horsham, West Sussex RH13 0QP

Lisa Milella BVSc DipEVDC MRCVS
The Veterinary Dental Surgery, 53 Parvis Road, Byfleet, Surrey KT14 7AA

Joke Monteny MSc PhD
Hond Inform, Wijtschatestraat 72, 8956 Kemmel, Belgium

Christel P.H. Moons PhD
Department of Nutrition, Genetics and Ethology, Faculty of Veterinary Medicine,
Ghent University, Heidestraat 19, 9820 Merelbeke, Belgium

Sarah Packman BVSc CertSAM MRCVS
Larkmead Veterinary Group, 111–113 Park Road, Didcot OX11 8QT

Ken Robinson BVMS CertSAD MRCVS
Rose Cottage Veterinary Centre, Chester Road, Sutton Weaver, Runcorn, Cheshire WA7 3EQ

Laura Smith RVN CA-SQP ISFM CertFN DipFN
Anton Vets, Unit 11–12 Anton Mill Road, Andover, Hants SP10 2NJ

Angelika von Heimandahl MSc BVM DipECAR MRCVS
Veterinary Reproduction Service, 27 High Street, Longstanton, Cambridge CB24 3BP

Robert Williams MVB CertSAS MRCVS
Kingston Veterinary Group, 1–2 Park Street, Anlaby Road, Hull HU3 2JF

Foreword

This brand new Foundation Manual from the BSAVA is an exciting development because it condenses the information from many important areas into a single volume. The development over the last 20 years of a range of formal specialist veterinary qualifications has produced a significant surge in the range and depth of knowledge in canine practice. Whilst we should celebrate that this range and depth now exists, it is also clear that this very range is daunting to many of us. Concise answers to common questions that occur in consulting rooms are becoming harder to find. This book swings the balance back to the practitioner.

As well as traditional systems based medicine, this Manual also provides information on the 'arts' of practice such as consultation technique and dealing with common but testing situations. In the clinical presentations section of the book, first line approaches are given in a problem-oriented setting with a significant focus on the 'nose-to-tail' physical examination, a detailed clinical history and common, readily available, diagnostic tests. This book should be the first port of call for the busy clinician faced with a range of challenging issues (not all of them medical) in the consulting room.

The editors are to be congratulated on bringing together a team of authors with such an extensive experience in a wide variety of clinical practices who were able to distil volumes of veterinary textbooks to single chapters. The quality of the illustrations and flow charts, combined with the pithy practice tips will help a generation of vets to cope with life on the front line. Inexperienced vets will benefit most, but there is something in this Manual for everyone with an interest in canine practice.

We sometimes feel that we should know everything, but in truth, after a while in clinical practice, we realise that we know nothing, but it is our ability to identify and consult appropriate authoritative sources that determines our success. This new Manual is a goldmine of information that can be consulted over and over again. It will also provide a springboard to the more detailed knowledge available in the rest of the BSAVA Manuals. I would like to thank the BSAVA for having the foresight to publish this Manual and the editors and authors for all their hard work in bringing it to life.

Professor Ian Ramsey BVSc PhD DSAM DipECVIM-CA FHEA MRCVS
University of Glasgow

Preface

The last 20 years has seen a remarkable growth in the knowledge base and skillset available in small animal practice. Publications from the BSAVA have been a useful barometer of these changes: once there was a book called *Canine Medicine and Therapeutics* which, at the time, successfully captured what practitioners needed to know on a day-to-day basis. However, with the rise of the small animal profession and the increasing depth of specialization, this volume was replaced by the hugely successful series of BSAVA Manuals – a group of publications that has itself been subject to expansion in its scope and numerous new editions. This ready-made practice library now really does provide everything the practitioner needs, whatever their speciality, but may appear daunting to the relatively inexperienced vet looking for a concise answer to one of the many common problems presented in the consulting room.

This is the niche for this new Manual. Authored by vets with many years' experience in general practice, it aims to provide the first port of call for the busy practitioner faced with uncertainty over a new case. Common sense, first line approaches are given in a problem-oriented setting, stemming from the nose-to-tail examination. We hope it will become an invaluable tool to a new generation of vets.

Tim Hutchinson
Ken Robinson
May 2015

The dog-friendly practice

Kate Chitty and Laura Smith

In recent years much has been done to make veterinary practices more 'cat-friendly', and now 'rabbit-friendly' measures are being introduced. There seems to be a feeling that all small animal practices are already 'dog-friendly' and that no further thought or research is therefore needed. Sadly, this can be far from true and a lot of dog owners do feel that more could, and should, be done for their pets too.

Many changes will help all dogs, some only certain individuals, but making the owners feel more comfortable and relaxed will help their dogs stay more calm. Changes can be time-consuming but helping both pet and owner is rewarding and can help bond clients to the practice.

The whole practice team can be involved in trying to make the environment more dog-friendly. Some clients perceive veterinary nurses as more approachable and accessible than veterinary surgeons, and providing a range of nurse clinics may therefore encourage clients to come into the practice for advice and support. Non-vets often see problems and can help devise solutions based on their knowledge of the clients and dogs, and on previous experience. They can also see how the clients and their pets respond to any changes implemented. By making clients and pets feel more relaxed, the whole working environment becomes happier and friendlier, and this ultimately helps the team to provide quality veterinary care.

Practice design considerations

Some considerations apply across the whole practice:

- Many dogs dislike walking on slippery floors. Simply using rubber mats (easily cleaned and replaced) can make a lot of difference to many dogs. The use of mats is also helpful on slippery tables and in tub-tables and sinks (Figure 1.1)
- The use of pheromone diffusers may be helpful
- Reducing certain odours, especially from anal gland secretions (a scent used when alarmed), urine and faeces, is important for clients as well as pets. Cleaning these up as quickly as possible is also important for disease control. The appropriate waste bins should be kept away from kennels, consulting and reception areas (Figure 1.2) and emptied regularly throughout the day
- Leaving doors and windows open is not helpful: they provide an obvious exit for nervous patients of all types.

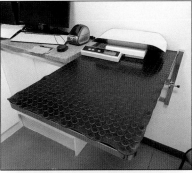

1.1
Rubber mats on consulting room tables and in baths will stop dogs slipping on the surface. (© Kate Chitty)

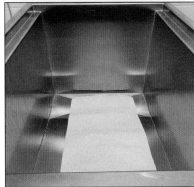

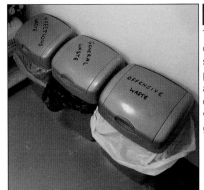

1.2
These waste bins, clearly labelled, are situated in a preparation area away from the areas of the practice where dogs usually go. (© Kate Chitty)

Entrance and outside areas

A designated area outside the practice to allow dogs to relieve themselves is ideal. Otherwise, a designated dog-waste bin situated just outside the practice is helpful (Figure 1.3). Spare 'poo bags' should be available at reception. If there is no space for a bin outside the practice, an appropriate waste bin can be provided near to the reception area.

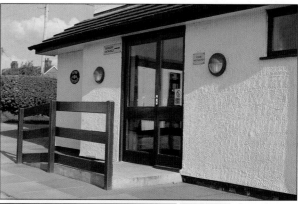

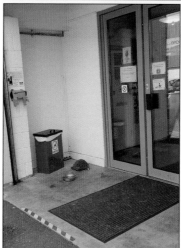

1.4 Both these practices have entrance doors that allow clients to see what is happening inside before entering the building. There is also a ramp for wheelchair access.

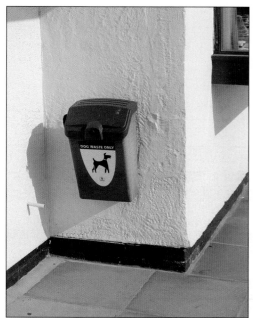

1.3 A designated dog waste bin close to the practice entrance.

A double door system provides good security, as animals trying to escape will have to negotiate two doors before they can leave the building; however, this could involve structural changes to an existing practice and so might not be practical. Where possible, room doors should always open inwards so that dogs cannot push against them to escape.

It is very helpful if at least part of the entrance door is made of glass, allowing owners of more nervous or aggressive dogs to see what is happening before they enter or leave the building (Figure 1.4).

Unfortunately, most reception areas are bottlenecks where many animals have to pass in close proximity to each other. Allowing a larger, potentially aggressive dog out of a back entrance or fire exit (in exceptional circumstances) can be much appreciated by owners.

Reception/waiting area

This is the first area within the practice that is seen by the public. Friendly staff, who are genuinely interested and helpful, are invaluable for keeping both owners and their pets comfortable. It is also worth considering facilities for children; many clients need to bring family members, and a fractious bored child can make it difficult for them and potentially cause distress to dogs in the waiting room.

Ideally, dogs should be separated from natural prey species, as both animals may be worried and/or excited by proximity. Although separate waiting areas are often advocated, this can be problematic for owners with both dogs and cats to bring them together, so other approaches can be appreciated (Figure 1.5).

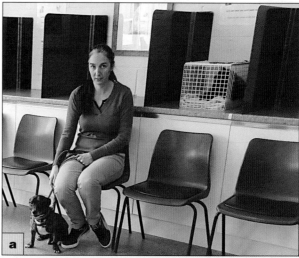

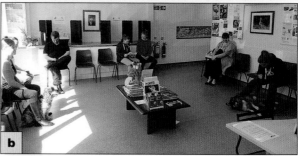

1.5 **(a)** This owner can sit with both her pets. The dog is on a lead while the cat is safely in its carrier on the shelf behind. The shelf dividers can be moved to allow for different sizes of basket and box. **(b)** The table, although low, divides the waiting room and allows dogs to sit opposite each other without feeling too threatened. (© Kate Chitty)

An alternative waiting area can be helpful for a fearful or aggressive dog; this only needs to be small (Figure 1.6). If this is not possible, owners may be asked to wait with their pets in their cars or outside, weather permitting, and be called in when their appointment is due. It is important that reception staff keep track of their appointment slot.

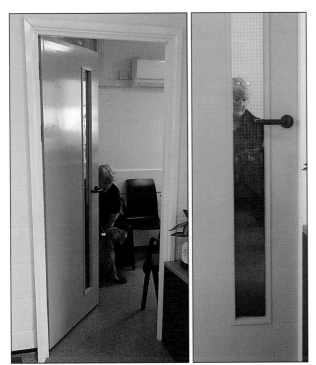

1.6 The door to this small room can be closed to provide a separate waiting area. Originally the glass panel extended the whole length of the door, but as dogs could see each other through the glass, confrontations sometimes still occurred. Reception staff realized the problem and suggested a simple solution: covering the lower part of the glass with dark plastic. This meant that a dog inside was now hidden from the sight of other dogs in the main waiting room; this proved very effective and a permanent cover is in preparation. (© Kate Chitty)

Dogs may urinate in greeting, through fear or for territorial scent marking, so all surfaces must be easily cleanable and sealed (Figure 1.7). Cleaning materials and appropriate disinfectants need to be close to hand. Although it should be discouraged, many owners will still allow their dogs to sit on seats, so these also need to be easily cleanable.

It is important that all dogs are kept under control in the waiting room; they can behave in a totally unexpected way and so need to be on a lead attached to a well fitted collar, or in a suitable container, at all times.

PRACTICAL TIPS

- It is always worth keeping a slip lead at the desk: some owners will forget their dog's lead; others will feel they do not need a lead; some may escape from a collar that is too loose
- Some practices find that a hook, placed immediately adjacent to where clients stand to pay at reception, can be helpful so that the owner can attach their dog's lead to it, leaving their hands free to deal with any paperwork, etc. while remaining in control of the dog

---

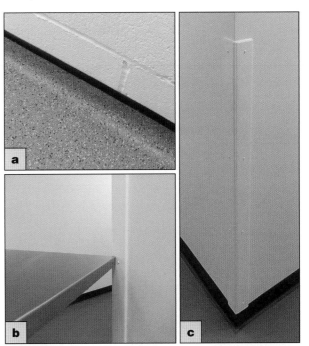

1.7 **(a)** This flooring has coved and sealed edges to aid cleaning. **(b,c)** Covering corners also protects against damage to the fabric of the building. (© Kate Chitty)

Useful information for reception staff

- A list of boarding kennels, puppy classes, dog trainers and groomers
- A lost and found book, with the number for the local dog warden. It is also helpful to record dogs looking for homes and owners looking to rehome dogs
- A book of dog breeds and colours to assist identification
- An up-to-date list of suitable blood donors
- A list of owners willing to talk about their personal experiences of dogs with conditions such as epilepsy or diabetes. It is important to record the contact details they are willing to have given out

---

Consulting rooms

Puppies and small dogs may be presented in carriers. Most will come out quietly for the owner but it may be best to place the carrier on the floor, as some dogs will dash out and could fall off a table. If a dog is likely to be difficult to extract, a top-opening carrier should be used. Carriers are less suitable for fearful and aggressive dogs, as they give them a territory to try to defend.

Many owners are keen to let their dog off the lead in the consulting room. It is worth explaining why this gives less control, especially if someone enters the room unexpectedly: even the best behaved of dogs can seize the opportunity and make a rapid exit.

Some small and medium-sized dogs are easier to examine on a table, while others are best left on the floor (Figure 1.8). The owner can often advise which their dog would prefer; size can play a part in this, but owners may prefer to try and place large dogs on tables.

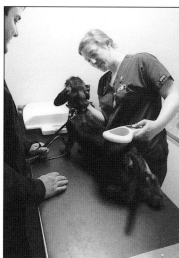

1.8 It may be appropriate to examine some dogs on a table, while others are better approached on the floor.
(© Kate Chitty)

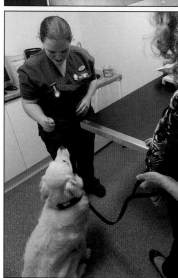

Considerations on admission

- Checking the dog's dietary requirements, and especially intolerances, is important. This applies to treat items too. Although the diet may not be the most appropriate clinically, an ill dog is less likely to appreciate a change of diet
- Ask what commands the dog responds to (e.g. Down! Stay!) and especially what commands the owner uses to encourage urination/defecation and the surface the dog prefers to use. Some dogs prefer to eliminate when they are off the lead; this may not be possible unless an enclosed area is accessible, but sometimes a secure loose lead will help
- When hospitalizing a dog, ensure that all ongoing medication for that individual is brought in and is used and stored correctly
- Always ensure any items left by the owners are clearly labelled and accounted for when the dog goes home
- It is useful to have a formal care plan recording the above

Having a chair in the consulting room can be helpful, as some owners are more comfortable if they can sit down. It can also provide some security for an anxious dog, although it may cause problems if a fearful dog hides under the chair and is hard to access safely. Should this happen, it may be best for the owner to get the dog out from under the chair, but only if this can be done safely (see Handling). It may be worth removing the chair from the room in advance if it is felt that it may cause a problem.

Offering a dog treats can help in many situations, and containers of dog biscuits can be placed in consulting rooms. A treat before an injection can often distract a dog enough so that it hardly notices what has happened. A dog may be unwilling to take a treat from the vet, but may take it from the floor or from the owner. It is surprising how many dogs will happily enter the practice after a few visits where treats are used. *Always ask before using treats, as some dogs have dietary problems and some owners disapprove or would rather bring their own treat items.*

Ward areas

Whether for day surgery or treatment over a longer period, hospitalization can be distressing for both the owner and pet. Many of the following measures will help the owner as well as the dog, and keeping the owner relaxed will stop them worrying the dog inadvertently during admission.

Housing

Metal kennels and cages can be noisy, though soft bedding can help, as can placing plastic or rubber covers for door catches to avoid clanging doors. Many dogs are affected by their reflection, either in metal surfaces, under tables/metal kennel walls or in glass doors; trying to keep reflection to a minimum by using subdued or indirect lighting can be helpful.

Where possible, cages should not face each other (Figure 1.9a). If this is not achievable, placing a towel or blanket over the door can give some privacy (Figure 1.9b). When examining an inpatient it is best to use a separate consulting room, out of sight of all other animals.

Some dogs are more comfortable in smaller kennels with a roof rather than in larger walk-in kennels. Dogs are often kept in a crate at home, and might therefore prefer a smaller space than expected from their size; asking the owner what the dog is used to can help with the choice of kennel size if there is space to choose.

Fleece beddings are good as they tend to allow liquids through (if necessary, incontinence pads or newspaper can be used underneath them); they are also thick, providing patient comfort (Figure 1.10a). Cushion beds (Figure 1.10b) can be useful for incapacitated dogs. Bedding needs to be able to withstand a hot wash (at least 60°C) to ensure elimination of infective organisms and parasites. It is best to avoid using newspaper alone as cage lining: it is bulky and can stain plastic; and puppies are often trained to urinate and defecate on it (the same can apply to incontinence/puppy pads).

Many owners will bring in food, blankets, beds and toys, whether asked to or not. An item from home can help both the dog and owner, though it is best if these have not been freshly laundered as the familiar smell is important to the dog.

Ideally, an outside run allows the dog some exercise and a chance to urinate and defecate. If no run is available, taking the dog for short walks is necessary in most cases, even for day patients.

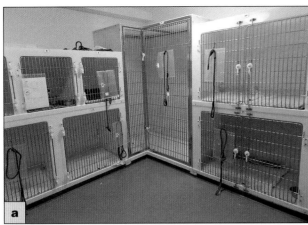
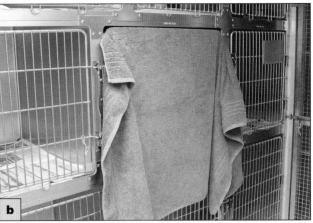

1.9 **(a)** These kennels are arranged to provide the maximum kennel space with dogs not directly facing each other. The kennels are made of moulded plastic and are easily cleaned and less noisy and bright than metal cages. Each kennel has a labelled folder for patient notes and hospital forms, and a labelled slip lead which is cleaned between patients. **(b)** If necessary, a towel or blanket can be placed over the kennel door to provide some privacy.

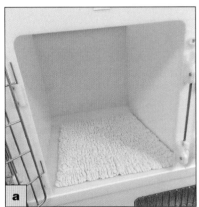

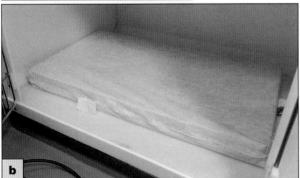

1.10 **(a)** Fleece bedding is a good cage liner. **(b)** Purpose-made cushioned beds are easily cleaned. (© Kate Chitty)

Environment

A radio (this may need a licence) in the kennel area is helpful for some dogs. Consideration needs to be given to the channel selected: dogs may be used to a certain type of music at home; a talk channel may be better for other individuals.

If an individual dog is noisy, it may be possible to house it away from the general canine ward, either in the practice's isolation area or perhaps in a collapsible crate in an otherwise uninhabited room. Sometimes reducing the lighting levels or covering the front of the cage can help. Cutting noise levels will help other patients and also the staff trying to work in that area. Although it is sometimes tempting to interact with a noisy dog, this rarely helps; in most cases the dog is

trying to get attention and interaction of any type gives the dog this attention and therefore may reinforce the unwanted behaviour. However, interactions with well behaved patients are worthwhile to reinforce good behaviour and hopefully improve the dog's experience of the visit.

Where space allows, admitting a companion dog may be helpful for calming a stressed individual (Figure 1.11). However, it is necessary to ensure that the dogs are separated during periods when there may be a chance of unexpected behaviour, such as during recovery from anaesthesia.

Owner visits: If a dog is to be hospitalized for more than a day, it is worth considering allowing the owners to visit. Consideration should be given to the timing (e.g. a quieter period when vets and nurses have time to talk to the owner) and location (e.g. a consulting room that is not in use will cause less disruption to the ward). Visits can be extremely helpful for dogs that are reluctant to eat in the hospital; having their own food/favourite items *and* being fed by their owner (Figure 1.12) can persuade many to start to eat.

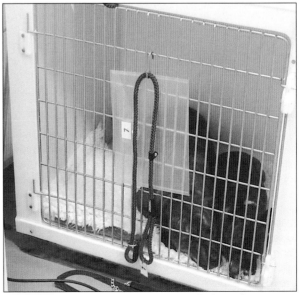

1.11 Two companion dogs kennelled together to reduce stress.

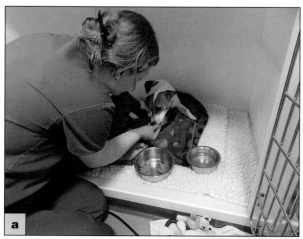

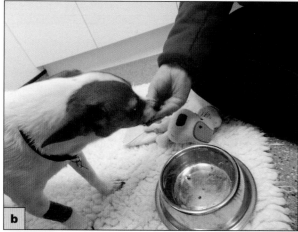

1.12 Although this dog responded to hand-feeding by the nurse **(a)**, he was more relaxed and happy when fed by his owner **(b)**. (© Kate Chitty)

Isolation

Isolation aims to separate the patient in order to protect it or prevent transfer of an infectious disease. To manage isolated patients effectively, a thorough understanding of the disease transfer mechanism is important.

Not all first-opinion practices are equipped with dedicated areas for hospitalizing patients requiring isolation, and patient isolation can be achieved in a variety of settings. Isolated patients should ideally be housed away from busy thoroughfares, ensuring that only necessary visits to the unit and patient are carried out, to keep disease transfer to a minimum. Where possible, isolated patients should be exercised away from non-isolated patients, and away from areas in use by the general public.

An independent isolation area can be very useful if managed effectively; staff training and awareness is vitally important to ensure that the isolation unit is managed appropriately. Clinics without a dedicated isolation area may choose to hospitalize isolated patients in collapsible wire crates (see Figure 1.15), utilizing an area of the practice which can be dedicated to the patient (e.g. a consulting room can be 'borrowed' for the duration of the patient's treatment). Isolation units must be clearly labelled as such, to prevent staff from entering unnecessarily (Figure 1.13). Clear signage also acts as a prompt for the use of PPE equipment.

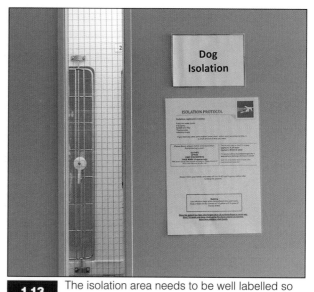

1.13 The isolation area needs to be well labelled so that appropriate people enter. The SOP is displayed on the door to ensure that anyone entering follows the correct protocol. (© Kate Chitty)

Items in the isolation unit must be kept to an absolute minimum; items not able to withstand disinfection and sterilization may require disposal.

All staff should know what equipment is present in the isolation unit. This ensures that should equipment be required that is not present in the isolation ward, it is brought in on first entering the unit, thus avoiding the risk of frequent trips in and out that would increase the risk of compromising the barrier function. It is useful to display on the entrance to the unit a list of materials found within the area, providing a visual reminder to staff and allowing any additional equipment required to be gathered prior to entering the unit.

Equipment and hygiene

- Equipment should be kept within the isolation unit. Care must be taken with bedding and food bowls: prior to removing them from the isolation unit, it is necessary to soak items in an appropriate disinfectant solution, cleaning these items separately from non-infectious items. Disposable bedding and food bowls should be considered in some cases
- Appropriate protective clothing must be worn when handling isolation patients. PPE is necessary to prevent spread of disease to other patients and also to personnel in the case of zoonotic diseases. This will include aprons or full body coveralls, shoe covers, masks, eye protection, hats and gloves (Figure 1.14). All these items should be disposable, the handler changing into and out of them at the entrance and exit of the isolation unit
- If the handler is required to care for non-isolation patients during their shift, ideally these should be dealt with first. Changes of clothing should be available for staff
- Footbaths and hand-washing facilities should be available at the entrance and exit of the unit, with an area to dispose of consumable ▶

items and PPE. Disinfectant selection for footbaths and hand washing should be based on the infectious organism present. A list of suitable products and dilutions should be readily available; a list of appropriate disinfectants can be found at www.defra.gov.uk
- Thought must be given to the removal of waste from isolation units. Double bagging of waste is appropriate in most cases, and it may be necessary to increase the frequency of waste collections during times when an isolation patient is hospitalized
- Urine, faeces and vomit should be cleaned up immediately, and the area then disinfected using an appropriate product (two staff members may be required to exercise an isolated patient, with one staff member following behind with the disinfectant solution)

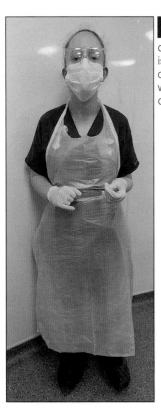

1.14 Isolation PPE in use. A hat will be donned prior to entering isolation. More extensive overalls and a mask may be warranted depending on disease risk.

Where possible, only one or two team members should be involved in the care of an isolated patient, having no involvement with other patients during their shift. Some practices may be unable to dedicate staff to isolated patients; in these cases staff caring for isolated patients should be restricted to caring also only for those with a low risk of contracting the disease. High-risk patients, including very young patients and the immunocompromised (such as those undergoing chemotherapy treatment), must be cared for by separate staff.

> **PRACTICAL TIP**
>
> Where staff are involved in the care of both isolated and non-isolated patients, efforts should be made to attend to non-infectious patients first

Owner visits to isolation patients: While it is clear that visits from owners usually have a positive influence on the patient (and are also of great benefit to the owner), it is essential to look at the pros and cons of a visit to an isolation patient. The disease present will have an influence on the health risk for the owner, but it is important also to consider risks to other pets the owner may have and the risk associated with the wider environment. If a visit is planned, owners must be fully briefed regarding the importance of wearing necessary PPE. This is ideally done prior to their attending the clinic (preferably via telephone) as once the owner is at the clinic they may be overcome by a mixture of emotions and they are unlikely to listen as intently to any instructions given.

> **PRACTICAL TIP**
>
> Videos of the pet can be emailed to owners where it is necessary to avoid visiting for biosecurity reasons

Practice equipment

Common items required are listed below. When purchasing equipment it is important to remember that canine patients come in a wide variety of shapes and sizes.

- Slip leads: for reception and kennel areas. These should be cleaned and checked for damage between use.
- Collapsible cages/crates: can be useful for providing temporary additional kennelling and can be easily stored (Figure 1.15).

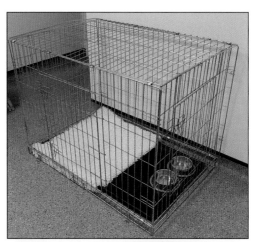

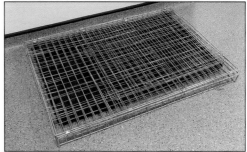

1.15 Collapsible crates can be very useful for providing additional kennelling and isolation facilities. Even the large crates take up little room when collapsed.

- Food and water bowls: variety of types and sizes, including raised bowls for dogs with spinal problems or used to eating from these at home (Figure 1.16).
- Food: different types and brands as well as treat items. It may also be helpful to get owners to bring favourite items from home.
- Handling aids: e.g. dog and cat catchers (Figure 1.17).

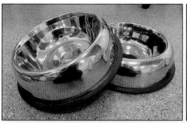
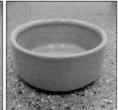
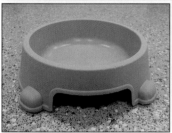
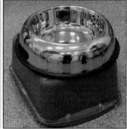

1.16 Food bowls may be made of metal, ceramic or plastic. An upturned washing-up bowl can be used to raise a bowl for a dog used to feeding at height, if a bowl designed for the purpose is not available. (© Kate Chitty)

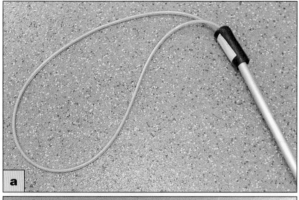
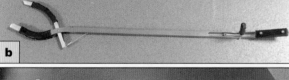
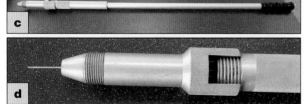

1.17 **(a)** A dog catcher. It is important that relevant staff know where to find this quickly when faced with an aggressive dog. **(b)** A cat grabber can be used to pick up the lead of an aggressive dog. **(c,d)** A pole syringe may be helpful in some cases. This is rarely required but is invaluable when faced with an extremely dangerous dog, allowing drugs to be injected from a safe distance and from behind a suitable barrier. (© Kate Chitty)

- A 'dog park' (Figure 1.18) can be really useful, e.g. for safely holding the dog whilst its kennel is cleaned.
- Stretchers: fabric stretchers work well in small confined spaces and can be easily cleaned; a sturdy towel or blanket of the appropriate size will also work well (Figure 1.19).

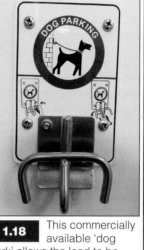
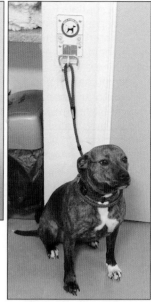

1.18 This commercially available 'dog park' allows the lead to be hooked over it without having to remove it from the dog. (© Kate Chitty)

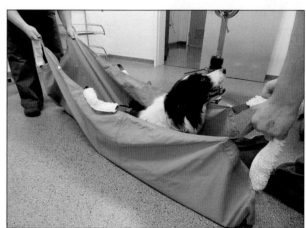
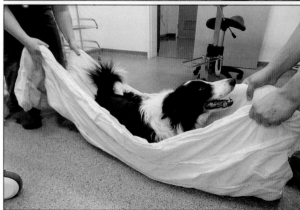

1.19 Dogs may be lifted using a purpose-made stretcher or alternatives such as a blanket or duvet, as long as the material is capable of supporting the dog's bodyweight. It is important to ensure there are enough staff to restrain the dog safely as it is lifted; in this case it would need more than the two nurses shown to ensure that the dog stayed on the stretcher. (© Kate Chitty)

- Sandbags and ropes: useful for positioning for certain procedures and can be bought or handmade (Figure 1.20).
- Tables: wheeled tables of adjustable height are helpful for moving large dogs and can help extend a work surface such as for radiography (Figure 1.21).

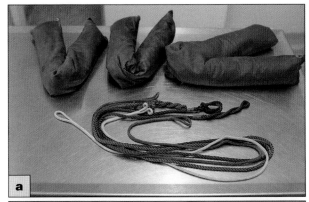

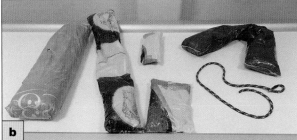

1.20 (a) A range of commercially available animal ties and sandbags for animal positioning. (b) A variety of shapes, sizes and weights of sandbag can be made from play sand, plastic bags of differing sizes and tape. These can be cleaned and disinfected between patients and are easily replaceable. (b, © Kate Chitty)

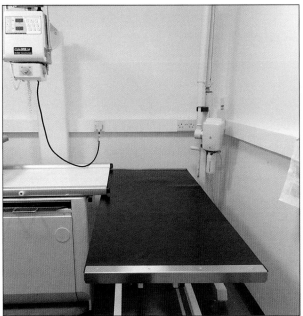

1.21 The table on the right can be used as an operating table. Its height can be adjusted and it can be wheeled around. The radiography table can be unstable if a very large dog has to be positioned near the end. Placing the trolley table under the end of the radiography table provides greater stability as well as a larger area to help with positioning the dog. (© Kate Chitty)

- Tub-tables are useful for bathing dogs (Figure 1.22) and for dental procedures.
  - Some owners are unable to carry out bathing at home for topical treatment of dermatoses.
  - Returning a dog clean and comfortable after a spell in the clinic is essential and being able to bathe the patient relatively easily greatly facilitates this.
- Mats:
  - Bath mats or towels help prevent slipping in tub-tables or baths (see Figure 1.1)
  - Non-slip radiolucent mats can be useful for radiography.
- Scales: capable of recording accurately over a range of weights (Figure 1.23).
- Nail clippers: small, medium and large.
- Blood pressure cuffs: in a range of sizes.

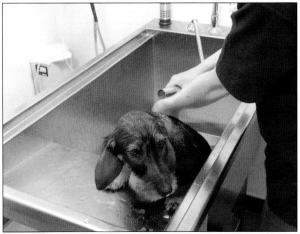

1.22 A bathing area is important for therapy and for cleaning prior to going home. (© Kate Chitty)

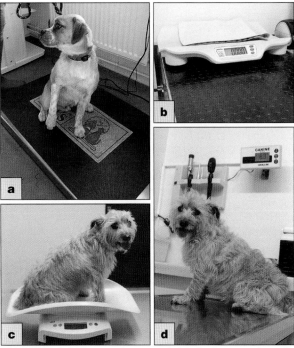

1.23 (a) Floor scales are suitable for large and small dogs. (b,c) These scales can be used for smaller dogs; the mat stops the dog slipping. (d) Scales are built into this consulting table; note the read-out on the wall above. (b, © Kate Chitty)

- Infusion pump and paediatric burettes: although an infusion pump is ideal, paediatric burettes should be used for small patients if an infusion pump is not available (some burettes can be kept in stock in case of infusion pump failure).
- Warming devices: e.g. warm air blower, heat pads, reflective blankets (Figure 1.24).

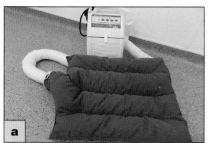
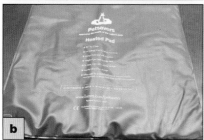
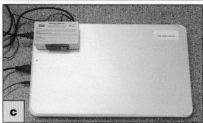
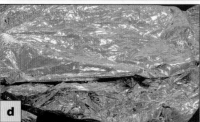

1.24   **(a)** A warm air blower. The attached 'blanket' can be used underneath anaesthetized or recumbent patients. The unit can also be used to blow warm air through wire cage fronts. **(b)** An example of a heat pad that can be used under bedding to provide extra warmth. All heat pads must be used as per the manufacturer's directions. **(c)** Solid heat pads must be used with extreme care, as they have a tendency to overheat, even when fitted with a thermostat. **(d)** Reflective heat blankets are very economical and work well placed over collapsed individuals. (© Kate Chitty)

PRACTICAL TIP

Pre-prepared kits can be very useful, especially for stressful situations such as anaesthetic emergencies (Figure 1.25), caesarean sections (Figure 1.26) or euthanasia (Figure 1.27; see also Chapter 7). Dose charts in kits – and also within the pharmacy – are especially useful for liquids, with an idea of how long an amount will last for in a patient of a set weight (e.g. meloxicam)

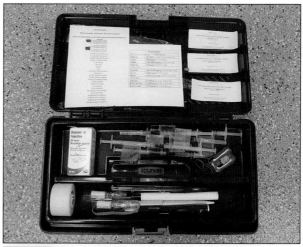

1.25   This 'crash box' is kept in the operating theatre in case of anaesthetic emergencies. The contents are labelled and are regularly checked and changed. Drug charts are on the lid of the box to avoid delay in checking doses. (© Kate Chitty)

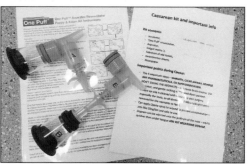

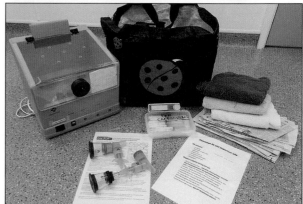

1.26   This caesarean section kit is stored with the incubator. (© Kate Chitty)

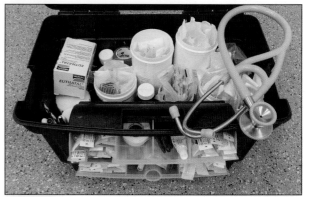

1.27   This euthanasia kit contains all that is needed for a home visit, requiring only the addition of pentobarbital and a sedative. (© Kate Chitty)

Handling and restraint

It is helpful to be aware of canine body language (see Chapter 12 and the *BSAVA Manual of Canine and Feline Behavioural Medicine*). However, many dogs can react unexpectedly, especially if they are scared or in pain. It is best to offer help from a veterinary nurse or assistant; some owners will not ask for help but will accept gratefully if it is offered. If the owner wishes to hold their pet themselves, staff need to ensure that they are able to do so safely.

WARNING

It is important to remember that the veterinary professional is responsible for the safety of the owner and the dog throughout the consultation

Some dogs are better held by their owner or handler, e.g. military or guard dogs. Others behave very differently without the owner present; just taking these animals to a quiet area with suitable assistance can help. It can also be very useful to have trained help for certain procedures; e.g. ear examination is much easier and less painful if the dog is held still. Some owners are good at learning to hold their dogs, once shown, but many worry that they will hurt the dog or compromise their bond with the pet, and so prefer to have a nurse hold it. It is important to assess each case individually.

Muzzles

Occasionally a dog will need to be restrained or muzzled for a procedure to be carried out safely. The dog should be examined and treated as quickly as possible, and the muzzle removed as soon as it is safe to do so. If a dog is likely to need muzzling for most visits, the owner can be advised on purchasing a muzzle and training the dog to accept it (see the *BSAVA Manual of Canine and Feline Behavioural Medicine*).

PRACTICAL TIP

Some owners tend to be distracted and not to listen as well whilst their pet is muzzled. If possible, it is better to talk to them after removing the muzzle or before putting it on the dog

A good range of muzzle sizes is necessary, as certain breeds may be safer in muzzles specifically designed for them, e.g. brachycephalic breeds such as bulldogs. Common types of muzzle are shown in Figure 1.28. The muzzle must be able to be cleaned and disinfected easily between dogs.

Tying a rope muzzle

If a suitable muzzle is not available, or it is not possible to put a normal muzzle on the dog, a rope tie or length of bandage can be used to create one.

1. A loose knot is placed in the rope tie or bandage
2. This is placed over the dog's nose and tightened
3. The rope/bandage is crossed under the dog's chin
4. The rope/bandage is finally tied behind the dog's ears

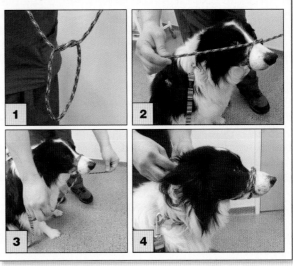

Chemical restraint

Where an animal behaves in such a way that it is unsafe to muzzle or treat it without sedation, it may be appropriate to provide the owner with appropriate medication to administer at home. The choice of medication will depend on both the health of the animal and the owner's ability to administer the medication safely. Any risks to the animal or owner should be fully discussed with the owner during the process of gaining informed consent.

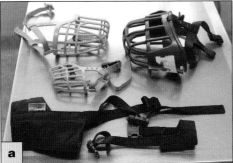
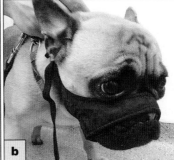
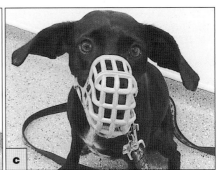

1.28 **(a)** A range of muzzles and sizes. Choice will depend on several factors, including comfort for the dog, security for the handler and access to various parts of the face. Both fabric and basket-type muzzles are easily cleaned and disinfected between patients. **(b)** A fabric muzzle can be used during a consultation, as it will only be worn for a short time. **(c)** Basket-type muzzles allow the dog to pant and to drink, and so are better if the dog needs to spend a longer time wearing the muzzle. (b,c © Kate Chitty)

Managing difficult situations

It is important to remain calm at all times, especially when presented with a challenging patient. Most owners know their dog is likely to be difficult and can become very defensive, further upsetting the situation. In many cases, just getting the owner to relax and become calmer will help; it is obvious the dog is relaxing as the owner calms down. Time spent talking to the owner allows the dog to become more settled in the new environment, gives the vet time to observe the dog and allows the owner to suggest the best way to deal with their dog, especially its likes/dislikes and the things that are likely to upset it. Some owners appear to praise bad or poor behaviour. For example, 'Good dog' may be said by an owner when a dog is growling and snapping; it can be helpful for the vet to explain quietly that although they understand this is intended to reassure the dog, the owner is actually praising poor behaviour. It is important to take care in deciding when to say this, however, as the owner may be understandably surprised, upset and defensive. Some owners will appear to laugh, although this may show embarrassment rather than amusement.

During the examination

Certain procedures will be more unsettling and confrontational to the dog, for example, sore ears can be very painful, as can lame legs. Many dogs dislike being stared at, so eye examinations can cause more problems than expected. Kneeling during the examination can help to reassure the patient (Figure 1.29); it is important not to loom over the dog. Occasionally it is better to stop the examination and use pain relief or sedation, or to explain to the owner why it is necessary to proceed even though it appears to be painful. After a painful or frightening experience, it is helpful to try to have a dog brought back to the practice for a socialization visit.

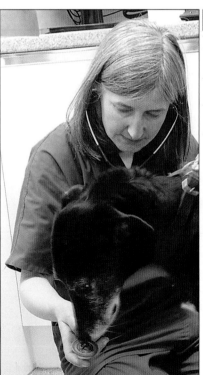

1.29
With the vet kneeling, the dog does not feel threatened and can investigate the stethoscope before it is placed on its chest.
(© Kate Chitty)

Tips for improving experiences

- It is worth spending time during puppy consultations showing and encouraging owners how to handle their puppy's ears, mouths and paws in a non-threatening way. It helps the dog become used to this handling while there is no pain or discomfort
- It is also useful to offer help if it becomes apparent that a client is struggling with a procedure such as applying ear or eye drops or cleaning the dog's ears. Nurse clinics (see below) may be useful for this, especially if the guidance can be given straight away, as owners are often busy people and may be unable to come back at a later date. A video of common procedures uploaded to the practice website can also be useful for this
- Once a dog is already fearful of attending the veterinary practice, more will need to be done to try and build good associations. It may help if the owner comes and discusses their individual needs with an allocated nurse – without their dog
- If owners have more than one dog, bringing a calm companion may help a nervous dog
- Bringing a nervous dog in to the practice for a visit without treatment may help them. Owners should be encouraged to bring dogs in for socialization at quieter times, so that they can see nurses and receptionists with treats
- If a routine procedure is being considered it may help to offer to place the dog in a kennel for several occasions prior to admission; feeding the dog in the kennel can help
- Several trips when calm and controlled will help owners, pets and staff. A more confident owner makes a huge difference to the dog's demeanour

---

Nurse clinics

Dog-friendly practices need to be appealing to owners of dogs, as well as being friendly to the patients themselves (Figure 1.30). Canine-specific nursing clinics can encourage clients, who may otherwise have sought advice elsewhere, into the practice to discuss concerns (e.g. fireworks phobia). Nurse clinics can greatly improve owner compliance and how the practice is perceived by the wider community.

Potential areas for nurse clinics

- Weight management
- Pregnancy and parturition care and advice
- Dental hygiene
- Puppy selection, care and socialization (see Chapter 12)
- Post-neutering checks
- Noise phobias and fireworks phobias
- Arthritis care and management
- Diabetic management
- Senior healthcare
- Parasite control

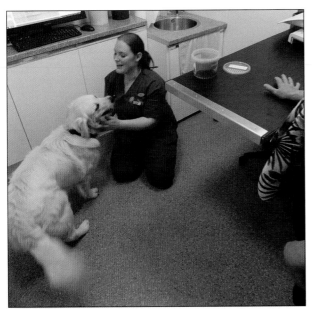

1.30 Nurse clinics tend to be less formal and often involve trying to make dogs feel more happy about visits to the practice. (© Kate Chitty)

Often, providing a named veterinary nurse to contact as a liaison between client and veterinary surgeon can encourage the client to ask questions which they may have not felt comfortable asking their vet, helping to identify potential issues before they arise. For example, the client may mention to their vet nurse concern regarding the use of tablet medication. Providing training and support to the owner or an alternative preparation of the medication can greatly improve the chance of a successful treatment outcome.

Nurses also provide a good contact point for owners when dogs are hospitalized. Owners appreciate updates on inpatients, especially if they are unable to visit. It is also important that the owners are informed as soon as the dog is safely recovered from surgery and that all postoperative instructions are completely understood and followed. Indeed, talking through postoperative care *before* admitting the dog will help owners prepare for the return of their pet. It is also useful to follow up on postoperative care with a phone call a day or two after the dog has been discharged, before the planned postoperative check. This will help with any minor fears that the owner feels are too trivial to mention to the vet.

It is essential that all team members are trained and kept well informed regarding nursing clinics and the additional services that veterinary nurses can provide. Reception staff need to be aware of the role of the veterinary nurse in the clinic, and what services veterinary nurses can provide. Veterinary nurses need to be trained and experienced in the type of clinics they are expected to run. It may be necessary for veterinary nurses to undertake the Suitably Qualified Person qualification (the SQP qualification is regulated by the Animal Medicines Training Regulatory Authority or AMTRA) in order for them to prescribe and dispense appropriate medicines (POM-VPS and NFA-VPS anthelmintics).

References and further reading

Clarke C and Chapman M (2012) *BSAVA Manual of Small Animal Practice Management and Development*. BSAVA Publications, Gloucester

Horwitz D and Mills D (2009) *BSAVA Manual of Canine and Feline Behavioural Medicine, 2nd edn*. BSAVA Publications, Gloucester

Consultation technique

Christine Magrath and Geoff Little

Most interactions between the vet and the client start and end in the consulting room, and developing a good consulting technique is essential if all other clinical and surgical efforts are not to be wasted.

A proficient consulting technique can lead to:

- Improved satisfaction for both the vet and the client
- Improved compliance and concordance
- Reduced complaints
- Enhanced relationship building
- Improved clinical performance and outcomes of care.

The consultation can be categorized into three distinct areas (Figure 2.1), which are interdependent and not to be considered in isolation:

- Perceptual
- Content
- Process.

PERCEPTUAL
What you are thinking/ feeling (e.g. clinical reasoning, attitudes, assumptions, emotions) and what you do with these thoughts/ feelings

CONTENT
What is said (questions and responses, information gathered and given, treatments discussed)

PROCESS
How you communicate, structure the interaction, relate to clients; use of non-verbal skills

2.1 Categorization of communication skills. These are interdependent and should not be considered in isolation.

The veterinary consultation guide

Traditional methods for history taking and the delivery of information can end up as a direct transmission of information between vet and client rather than an interaction, and can result in some medical information or concerns not being elicited. To amend this problem a veterinary consultation guide (Radford *et al.*, 2006) has been developed, based on the medical Calgary–Cambridge Guide, and is now used at each of the UK veterinary schools. This guide delineates the communication process skills that are needed to carry out an effective consultation. The number of skills described in the guide can seem overwhelming but not every skill is needed for every eventuality, and familiarity with this structured process strengthens the ability of the vet to obtain accurate content and deliver information that is understood by the client. To differentiate the skills, the guide is divided into six main headings (Figure 2.2).

Preparation
Even if the consultation is routine for the vet, it may be a very significant, novel and important event for the client. Adequate preparation is crucial or the smooth running of the consultation may be jeopardized. The consultation may be one small part of the vet's working day, but it may be the sole chance that the client has to interact with the practice; so every effort should be made to ensure that it is a positive experience for the client.

- It is essential to be familiar with the clinical records, taking time to study results and past history while at the same time anticipating any individual demands that the client might have.
- The consultation room and table should be clean and tidy.
- Any necessary equipment should be checked and the room should be escape-proof.
- The last consultation or task should not impinge on the next one if, for example, examining a new puppy after breaking bad news. Problems with a difficult case must not be allowed to disrupt the one in hand.
- Personal issues and physical comfort, such as hunger or lack of sleep, can affect concentration.

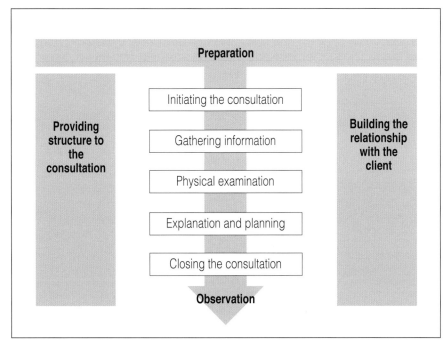

2.2 The guide to the veterinary consultation has been developed based on the medical Calgary–Cambridge Guide and is now used at all UK Veterinary schools. (Adapted from Radford *et al.*, 2006)

These should be dealt with prior to embarking on the consultation.

- If there is adequate space in the consulting room it may be helpful to have two chairs in the room. This is obviously beneficial for less able clients, but it also has advantages for all clients; if the vet and client are both sitting that helps to build two-way communication (Figure 2.3).

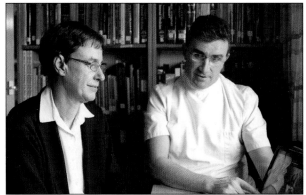

2.3 Sitting down with a client may well be appropriate when discussing results or breaking bad news.

Initiating the consultation

Getting it right at the beginning of the consultation is crucial. This is when first impressions are made, an initial rapport is established, the client's emotional state is gauged and the course of the consultation is planned. This whole process may take only a small amount of time but it has a huge impact on all that follows. The key skills needed at this juncture are not just social pleasantries, and although some of them are obvious, they can be forgotten if individuals are following a tight schedule. They have an important impact on the accuracy and efficiency of the consultation and on the relationship which is established with the client and their pet. This is a key opportunity for establishing a bond of trust with the client.

- The client and patient should be **greeted by name**.
- Individuals should **introduce themselves and explain their role** in the practice. Since many clients are regular attendees at the practice it is easy to assume that they will remember those who have looked after their pet, but not knowing the role or name of the professional can be unsettling for clients and can even be a barrier to ensuring that communication is a two-way process. During the introduction it is vital to use a combination of skills such as good eye contact, a smile or suitable facial expression depending on the case, and – if appropriate – a handshake. It is worth noting that shaking hands is a personal decision and can convey a confident, trusting and professional approach. If it does not feel comfortable, however, it may convey disinterest and apathy, and if this is the case it may be more natural not to do it.
- **Acknowledging the pet** is an important facet in building the relationship with both the patient and client, and time spent in this way can sometimes reveal information that would otherwise be undisclosed.
- **Identifying the reason for the consultation** depends on an initial 'open' question (see below) such as "How can I help?" or "What can I do for Max today?". This line of questioning should still take place even if the clinical notes appear to contain the answers, as the information there may not be correct. In follow-up visits it is easy to assume that the client's attendance is a follow-on from the previous one (which can sometimes not be the case), thereby preventing new concerns being elicited.
- Once an open question has been asked, it is important to **give the client time and space to respond**. A student elective project at Liverpool Veterinary School suggested that the average time vets take to interrupt a client is 18 seconds (Gray *et al.*, 2005), which mirrors extensive studies carried out in the medical profession. Later

research at Nottingham suggested that it took only 13.5 seconds before the client was interrupted (Brightmore, 2009). Often the client is interrupted with closed or clarifying questions, but even minimal utterances or echoing the client's words during this initial flow of information can inadvertently direct the client away from disclosing all their concerns. In contrast, active listening is a skilled process and can result in more concerns being elicited and a reduction in late-arising concerns (Figure 2.4).

- Do not concentrate on preparing the next question: instead, focus on what the client is saying
- Provide the client with enough 'wait time' to complete their story. Getting all the information out at an early stage can actually speed up the consultation
- Remember that clients will often present problems in an order that is not necessarily related to their clinical importance, so avoid being drawn into believing that the first complaint is the major one
- Encourage the client's responses with paraverbal expressions such as "hmm", "uh-huh", "yes", "I see"
- Repeating the client's expressions and paraphrasing, although useful skills to demonstrate listening later in the consultation, can often act as an interruption during the opening stage
- Don't forget the importance of non-verbal skills such as eye contact, facial expressions, proximity and direction of gaze in demonstrating interest at this early juncture
- Do not be tempted to make a premature diagnosis, as this may prevent you from genuinely listening to the client's full story
- Pick up verbal and non-verbal cues, as this shows genuine interest. A verbal cue may be something like "I don't think I could go through that again". Non-verbal cues may include, for example, a frown, the breaking of eye contact, or a shrug of the shoulders. A suitable response could be along the lines of, "I sense you are not quite happy with..." or "Am I right in thinking that...?"
- Listening and observing at this stage will enable the client's ideas, concerns and expectations (ICE) to be expressed. According to medical research these cues often appear early on in the consultation and are expressed as non-verbal cues and indirect comments rather than overt statements. Not checking out these cues with the client can result in assumptions being made

2.4 Tips to improve active listening after the opening question.

- **Screening** is a very specific skill that allows the vet to discover all of the problems that the client wishes to discuss. Often the client will present with an initial complaint; exploring this avenue without making an attempt to discover if they are worried about more than one thing can lead to additional concerns arising near the end of the consultation. This can easily add time, which can mean further pressure in a tightly managed appointment schedule. Screening also helps to keep an open mind and provides a method of finding out the client's ideas, concerns and expectations in addition to gleaning extra clinical information. Repeating each point prior to screening can be useful in establishing that all the facts have been taken on board, and allows the client to correct any information that has been misinterpreted. "As I understand it, Rex has had diarrhoea and vomiting for 2 days and has been off his food since yesterday, as well as being more tired than normal. Is there anything else you've noticed?".
- Successful screening until the client has nothing more to reveal should elicit a number of problems, making this an ideal time to **organize thoughts and share them with the client**. This 'agenda

setting' or structuring of the consultation prevents aimless and unnecessary questioning and allows the client to feel more involved. "Shall we start with the coughing and sneezing, and then move on to Buster's anal glands?"

Gathering information

Good history taking and the information it yields contributes a major percentage of the data needed for diagnosis. Understanding the process of gathering information is therefore key for an effective consultation. The rationale behind this component of the consultation includes:

- Making sure that any information gathered is accurate, complete and understood, and agreed by both parties. This information can be categorized into:
  - Background information
  - Clinical content (biomedical perspective)
  - The owner's ideas, concerns and expectations
- Exploring any information gathered in a structured manner while at the same time ensuring that the client is involved and understands where the consultation is going, and why
- Ensuring that the client feels valued and listened to.

To achieve these aims, an in-depth analysis of the problems outlined in the initiation stage is needed. Several process skills provide guidance towards achieving this goal and at the same time give an opportunity for personal style and individual personality to be used.

- **Knowing when to use open and closed questions.** Both open and closed questions are valuable in obtaining information from clients (Figure 2.5). It is important to start with an open question, moving to closed questions to achieve more focus. One may then need to return to an open question to explore other avenues before asking further closed questions. This is known as 'Open to closed coning' (Figure 2.6). Both types of questioning are valuable, but starting with an open technique introduces an enquiry without shaping the client's response. For example: "Tell me more about Ben's cough" or "Tell me more about Ben's problems from the beginning". Although using closed questions is important to investigate specific details and give more control over the dialogue, it can limit the amount and type of information if used too early. Using open questions early in the discourse encourages clients to tell their whole story and provides the vet with time to listen and think. In contrast, if closed questioning is used prematurely, the responsibility of what the next question will be lies with the vet, narrowing the field of enquiry with the possibility of missing information. Once individuals embark on closed-ended enquiries there is a tendency to follow each one with another, and thinking about the next closed question can result in the vet not listening or thinking about the client's responses. As the consultation continues it is important to become more focused, initially using more focused open questions such as, "What makes Ben's cough

Open questions

- Invite the client to respond in an open manner without unduly focusing or directing their response
- Direct the client, but invite them to elaborate
- Allow the vet more thinking time to better direct the consultation
- Contribute to more effective and efficient diagnostic reasoning
- Examples of open questions include:
  - "What can we do for Lilly today?"
  - "What have you noticed about Ben's cough since it started three weeks ago?"

Closed questions

- Usually elicit a one-word answer, often "Yes" or "No"
- Benefits of closed questions include:
  - Clarification of a situation, e.g. "What I understand is that his diarrhoea contains blood; is that correct?"
  - Summarizing a situation, e.g. "So, he has been vomiting for a week, has had diarrhoea for the last 2 days and there is some blood in his motions; is that correct?"
- Other examples of closed questions include:
  - "Lilly has come in today because she is vomiting; is that correct?"
  - "Does Ben cough only during exercise?"

2.5 'Open' and 'closed' questions.

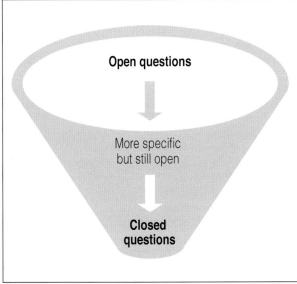

2.6 Open to closed 'cone'. Starting with open questions and moving towards more specific points is an efficient way of gathering information.

worse or better?". The gathering information stage should end with closed questions to ascertain fine detail and analyse clinical signs in detail. For example, "As I understand it, Ben's cough is worse after exercise; is that correct?"

- **Attentive listening and facilitating the client's responses.** This enables clients to tell the full story. This is equally important at this part of the consultation as it is at the initiation stage. Active listening at this juncture brings several advantages, such as appearing interested and supportive while picking up cues to the client's concerns and emotional state. This skill may appear straightforward but in reality, especially under the pressure of a busy consulting schedule, requires a very skilled technique that actively encourages clients to continue with their account. All the skills used in active listening at the initiation

phase apply to this section, and those that could be counterproductive at the earlier stage, such as paraphrasing and repetition, now come into their own. Often, repeating the last few words (echoing) a client has said helps them to keep talking, while paraphrasing goes one step further, as it also helps to check the vet's interpretation of what the client has said. Other facilitation skills, such as pauses to allow the client to provide more information, and comments such as "go on" can also encourage the client to divulge more.

- **Understanding verbal and non-verbal cues.** Clients may continue, either intentionally or unintentionally, to provide cues at this stage, particularly if they have been encouraged to continue the dialogue. By this stage it is easy to miss these messages by appearing to listen but not actually registering the information or watching the body language. Often clients will repeat these cues and if they are not picked up and checked out it can give the impression of disinterest and poor client care. Research from human medicine (Levinson *et al.*, 2000) has shown that if cues are picked up and acknowledged it shortens the consultation.

- **Ensuring accuracy and facilitating further dialogue with the use of internal summarizing.** Using this skill clearly conveys that the vet is listening. More importantly, it allows the client to confirm or alter the vet's understanding. Not summarizing periodically can result in an inaccurate interpretation of the client's statements. Summarizing also invites the client to expand on their problems. There are also advantages for the individual gathering the information, as it allows them to check the accuracy of what the client has said and rectify any misconceptions. It also provides an opportunity for the vet to order their own thought process, recall information at a later stage and help differentiate between the clinical aspects and the client's perspective.

- **Using easily understood language.** Using highly technical language can overwhelm clients, and even simple day-to-day medical terminology can be ambiguous. Many clients are reluctant to ask for clarification in case they appear stupid. It is important, however, to gauge the client's educational level at an early stage to avoid patronising comments if the client has a medical background or first-hand knowledge of the disease in question.

Using these process skills should tease out all the information the client needs to impart relevant to the patient. This may, however, be delivered in a 'random' manner, with the client switching between the clinical perspective (biomedical history), background information (long-term history) and their ideas, concerns and expectations (client's perspective) (Figure 2.7).

The onus is therefore on the vet to weave back and forth and explore each contrasting perspective as it arises, and then to process it for the purpose of recording and presenting a history. Including and exploring the client's perspective as part of this history-taking framework provides certain advantages such as:

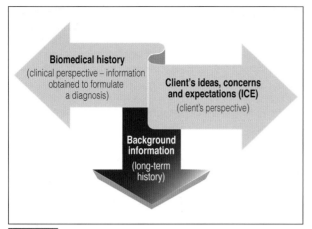

2.7   Grouping of gathered information.

- Helping to support the client and build the relationship
- Providing additional clues that relate directly to the clinical perspective; using more traditional history-taking methods can deter clients from divulging their ideas and concerns, even when the information could prove useful
- Ensuring the information imparted during the explanation and planning phase addresses the client's unique perspective; otherwise recall, understanding, satisfaction and compliance may be reduced.

Physical examination

Physical examination is discussed in detail in Chapter 3. The skilled clinician will be able to overlap the physical examination with the information gathering stage, using the time spent listening to the initial responses to open questions to set the animal at ease with a gentle, tactile approach, whilst still conveying the verbal and non-verbal encouragement to the client to confirm that their responses are being listened to. The more specific closed questions can accompany the physical examination of specific areas. For example, "She was in season two months ago; is that correct?"

Explanation and planning

Sharing information

An essential part of every consultation is the sharing of information with the client. As already discussed, a good starting point is to ascertain the client's own 'starting point': a Mr or Mrs may be a surgeon; a Dr may be a doctor of divinity! If in doubt, it is better to stick to lay terms. To remove doubt, a question can be asked such as, "The blood test results indicate that Pepe is diabetic; is that something you are acquainted with?". Even if they are not medically minded they may well have a diabetic in the family and as such will have some knowledge of the condition. Once the vet has ascertained the level of the client's understanding, this will enable them to structure the way in which they impart information and advice. As a rule, it is better to err on the cautious side and to explain things in lay terms as opposed to using medical jargon. However, if it has been established that the client is an orthopaedic surgeon, for example, it is better to refer to an 'osteosarcoma' than a 'nasty growth'.

It is also important to appreciate that some clients will want to know all there is about their pet's condition, whereas others will want to know the bare minimum: "What is the problem, can you sort it and how much will it cost?". The client may indicate by what they say, or by their body language, just how much they want to know (Figure 2.8). If that is not clear, the vet should not be afraid of asking the client just how much detail they would like.

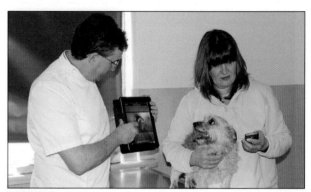

2.8   It is important to maintain the client's interest and not to let your enthusiasm for the subject dominate the consultation.

Some people are better at absorbing information through the spoken word, some through the written word, and yet others through pictures or anatomical models. It is best to have all such media available when imparting information. For example, words may be quite sufficient when explaining the benefits of kennel cough vaccine to a client whose dog is due to go into kennels. But what about trying to explain a ruptured cruciate ligament and its proposed repair to a client who wants to know chapter and verse? Here, words alone are not the best medium: a simple hand-drawn diagram in conjunction with an anatomical model, or indeed a video, can be used to explain both the injury and the proposed surgical procedure.

It may be that the individual taking part in the consultation is the only person who needs to be informed, but more likely there will be others who need to know and who will be receiving the information second hand. What are the chances of that client retaining all the information they have been given if they are not provided with appropriate information to take away? And what are the chances of their relaying the information in an accurate way to other family members at home? Concordance is likely to be less than optimum unless all those concerned in the decision making feel they have been fully informed. Another concern is that family members may well seek to fill the gaps in their knowledge by referring to the Internet (see later). However, the emergence of digital multimedia atlases will bring an exciting new dimension to the clinician's consultation technique, along with the ability to email details to the client to share subsequently with other members of the family who may not have been present during the consultation.

When imparting any information it is important to provide it in small, bite-size pieces that the client can take in and digest, although the size of those chunks will depend on the level of understanding of the client. It is also important to ascertain whether the information is being digested by the client, so-called 'chunking and checking'.

The information should be provided in a logical order. 'Signposting' will help in taking the client on that journey. For example, "Before Helen, the nurse who has been looking after Zac, brings him through, I just want to go through what we have done today in terms of investigating the cause of his cough. As we agreed, when you left him with us this morning, we were going to X-ray his chest and, if we thought necessary, give him an anaesthetic to look down his windpipe. Well, starting with the results of the X-rays, let me show you what we found…". The other thing about the order in which the information is imparted is that clients are more likely to remember the first information they hear. This memory can be enhanced by repeating the same information at the end of the dialogue.

What is the best way of finding out whether a client has taken in the information or not? The vet could ask them the direct question "Do you understand what it is you have to do?". However, this does sound a little intimidating and is likely to be met with a curt response such as "Yes!". Many of those clients, on the way out, may well ask the receptionist for a translation of what it is the vet was trying to convey. Much more effective, and more client-friendly, is to take a different approach, such as, "Just to make sure I've explained it fully, would you like to go through what it is we have to do for Pepe between now and the next consultation in 10 days?"

> ### WARNING
>
> Clients often present their pets because they are concerned, and one of the things they are looking for is reassurance that whatever is worrying them can be resolved. *It is important not to give premature reassurances.* Saying things along the lines of "I'm sure he will be alright" or "I'm sure we'll be able to cure him" can backfire and may, in extreme cases, lead to clients taking action against the practice when things turn out differently. Rather than reassuring the client about the disease, the vet can reassure the client about their intent to do the best for the patient

Planning

Within most consultations there will be a course of action, or alternatives, that need to be put to the client for their consideration. In some cases the course of action the vet wishes to take will, in his/her mind anyway, be clear cut with no reasonable alternatives. In other situations there may well be no obvious way forward: the vet may wish to suggest further tests to help clinch a diagnosis; or there may well be a number of justifiable options, each with its own set of merits. Planning should be about shared decision making or 'concordance' and one way forward (and indeed a way to encourage concordance) is to involve the client. This can be done by sharing thoughts with them, by allowing them to contribute to the discussion, and by answering their ancillary questions that have been stimulated by the further light shed on the case during the consultation. When there are alternative ways forward, it is important to outline the whys and wherefores and the differing costs associated with each alternative.

> ### PRACTICAL TIP
>
> It can be useful to refer to the way forward as the 'preferred plan' because plans can always be altered if necessary as the case progresses and a change of plan is something that is accepted by most

Consent

It is vitally important to obtain informed consent for any procedure the vet wishes to carry out on a client's pet. Having a signature on a consent form is not sufficient. Flemming and Scott (2004) outlined what the veterinary consent process should encompass (Figure 2.9).

- The diagnosis or nature of the patient's ailment
- The general nature of the proposed treatment and any other alternatives
- Proposed treatments and the purpose or reason for each treatment
- The risk or dangers involved in the proposed treatments
- The probability or prospects of success with each alternative treatment
- The prognosis or risk if the client refuses treatment
- The costs of the various alternative treatments
- The name of the individual who will actually perform that surgery if it is somebody else other than the person obtaining the informed consent
- The location and method of transportation to that location if the treatment is to be administered at another site

2.9   Elements of the veterinary consent process (Flemming and Scott, 2004).

Informed consent: The client must, to the best of the veterinary surgeon's knowledge, understand just what they are consenting to. And this can only be the case if the vet, or some other member of the team, has gone through the proposed procedure and the form with them, prior to obtaining their signature. Unfortunately, even after signing a consent form many clients still do not understand basic information about the fees, risks, benefits and alternatives of their proposed treatment options. There are many reasons for this failure of truly informed consent and the ongoing lack of understanding (Figure 2.10).

Client factors

- Time or stress pressure
- Feelings of intimidation
- Learning disabilities
- Hearing or visual disabilities
- Limited proficiency in English
- Poor literacy
- Poor educational level
- Perception that the consent form is just a legal procedure

Clinical factors

- Lack of time from the viewpoint of the clinician and other healthcare professionals
- Overly complex or overly broad written materials
- Poor explanation of risk
- Wrong assumptions about client's comprehension
- Poor quality consent forms and lack of associated written material

2.10   Factors that impede truly informed consent.

Verbal consent: It is not always necessary to obtain written consent before going ahead. In certain cases verbal consent can be sufficient, although it still must be 'informed'. For example, seeking verbal permission over the phone, to perform euthanasia of a patient that is under anaesthetic is perfectly acceptable. However, a written record must be made, in the clinical notes, of obtaining verbal consent.

Financial considerations
The question of cost normally comes into the decision-making process and it is something that should initially be broached in the consulting room. Apart from routine procedures with a fixed fee (e.g. routine castration), this is not something that should be left to the receptionist to discuss. For example, if there are alternatives and/or the possibility of ongoing costs associated with investigative work, hospitalization, etc., who better than the veterinary surgeon to pull the estimates together and discuss it with the clients? Terms such as 'significant costs' or 'not too expensive' should be avoided: these are relative terms and what you may consider 'not too expensive' may to some appear to be extortionate and to others very cheap.

It should always be borne in mind that when cases are hospitalized and/or where further tests become recommended, the ongoing costs can be significant for the client and the final, or indeed the interim bill, can bear little resemblance to the sum that was discussed initially. Even after careful discussion a client may still have felt pressured into proceeding down a line of therapy, with a specific cost in mind, only to find themselves involved in a course of treatment of indeterminate length, outcome and cost; complaints and claims are often born out of such a mix.

Pressure may not necessarily be due to the influence of the vet, but it could be the client themselves who may well feel it is their responsibility to come to the aid of their pet in its time of need. They may even feel a sense of guilt for having let their pet get into its current situation. The role of the veterinary surgeon is not to be judgmental but to provide balanced advice, to provide all the facts at his/her disposal and to offer alternatives that are in the best interest of the pet and the owner – and in that order.

Estimate or quote?
- The bill can often be the trigger for a complaint, especially if the client's expectations have not been met, for example in terms of the clinical outcome. Add to this disappointment a bill that is double or three times the original sum discussed with the client, and that is a potentially very volatile situation
- For most procedures it is not possible to provide the client with a quote, which by definition is a 'fixed price' for work undertaken. In the main, the veterinary practice will be providing clients with estimates, and this needs to be made clear to the client – both verbally, when discussing fees, and when obtaining informed consent

Concordance and compliance
Concordance is all about shared decision making and *compliance* is concerned with whether the client, or indeed the practice, adheres to the agreed course of action (Figure 2.11). It is important to bring clients along during the consultation process. It is then much more likely that they will adhere to the proposed treatment plan.

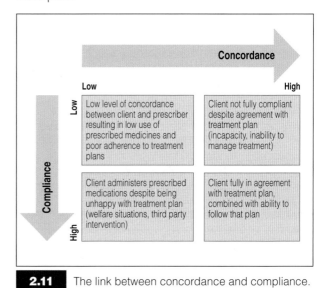

2.11   The link between concordance and compliance.

Although very few practices actually measure compliancy rates, where they have been measured there are some common findings:

- There are differing compliance rates between practices and between different team members in the same practice
- Compliance rates are higher when the practitioner has carried out a comprehensive consultation with the client
- Compliance rates are higher when the client has been offered alternatives (where appropriate to do so)
- Compliance rates are higher where conditions are perceived by the client as serious
- Practitioners often overestimate their clients' compliance rates.

It should never be forgotten that compliancy works both ways. In other words, when the vet has agreed on a way forward with a client, there is an onus on him/her and on the practice to adhere to the plan. However, it should have been explained to the client that the proposed plan may need to be altered as the case progresses. It is vitally important, if the treatment plan has to be altered, that the practice does its utmost to inform the client of the proposed changes, along with the financial implications, before the change is implemented. Of course there may be a need to take immediate action when a case requires it, but to embark on another set of blood tests or another series of radiographs without first discussing this with the client may well result in an unhappy outcome.

Referring cases
No matter how much information is gathered and retained, and which skills are developed, there will always be gaps in the individual veterinary surgeon's

repertoire. Fortunately there will be others, either in the same practice or elsewhere, who will be able to fill those gaps. It is important to offer clients a referral if that is in the best interests of the patient. With experience it can be possible to sense when a client is unhappy with the way a case is progressing; in those circumstances it may be prudent to suggest that somebody else's opinion would be valuable at that point in time, rather than learning that the client has gone elsewhere.

When a decision is made to refer a case, it is important to provide the other veterinary surgeon with as much relevant information as possible. In addition to providing all the paperwork, radiographs, laboratory test results, etc., it is advisable to speak with that individual, to fill them in on both the case history and the relationship with the client. This communication works both ways, and it is vitally important to ensure being brought up to speed by the referral practice as soon as practicable and certainly before seeing or speaking with the client again following the referral visit.

Closing the consultation

This is the vet's opportunity to summarize what has gone on during the preceding part of the consultation, in terms of the clinical concerns raised by the client, the results of the examination and any proposed treatment or investigative plans.

Should there be any further action required as a result of the consultation, e.g. a further appointment or the need to admit the pet, either now or at some point in the future, this should be discussed with the client if it hasn't already been covered. This may be the time to complete a consent form, or to go through instructions and directions if the client is to be referred.

PRACTICAL TIP

The client should be provided with a 'safety net', i.e. what action they should take if they have concerns about their pet after they have left the practice. It may well be that the practice will arrange a follow-up consultation or phone call, but irrespective of that it is a good idea to provide clients with details of what to do should they have any concerns. Something along the lines of, "If you have any concerns about Pepe, you mustn't sit there and worry. We would much prefer you phone, even if you think it's something trivial. There is always somebody here to help; give us a call any time"

Arranging a repeat consultation has many benefits for the patient, the owner and the clinician:

- It facilitates any necessary changes to the original treatment plan
- By keeping a better eye on the patient's progress, it enhances healthcare
- It demonstrates to the client a genuine interest in their pet's wellbeing
- It helps to build a relationship with the client
- It improves clinical skills by more closely monitoring the effects of differing treatment regimes.

Remember to say 'Goodbye' to both the client and their pet and, if appropriate to do so, walk with them back to the reception desk to help them with the next steps in the treatment plan, whether that be to book their pet in for another consultation or to be admitted as an inpatient for surgery or further investigative work.

Troubleshooting: what to do when things don't go according to plan

The consultation is getting bogged down and not flowing smoothly

Everybody who has been in practice for some time will recognize that there are times when things appear to be getting out of control. The perfectly planned consultation, for whatever reason, appears to be heading off the tracks: the client has for some reason suddenly become angry; or the client has appeared to 'switch off'. Being aware of body language, such as sudden loss of eye contact, can help a great deal in detecting a problem.

- The first thing to remember is that the internal turmoil you may be experiencing will probably not be apparent to the client; what to you seems like an eternity, when you are desperately trying to think of a way forward, will, to the client probably seem to be only a moment's aberration.
- The consultation, like all other procedures we carry out in practice has an underlying format that we follow for maximum efficiency and effectiveness. Keeping the structure in mind gives us something safe we can fall back on, if we find ourselves off course. Where are we in the process? Can we go back a step to regain our footing?
- If you are really struggling you can always 'take time out' by, for example, using the stethoscope to listen to the patient's chest, or finding a justifiable reason to leave the room.
- Other coping strategies include showing empathy with the client, describing where either you or a colleague has faced this difficult clinical problem and how you coped. Using stories about personal pets helps build a non-existent rapport or repair a broken or damaged one.

Dealing with difficult situations

Breaking bad news

The vet is often faced with the challenge of having to break bad news to a client. For example:

- Biopsy results indicate that their pet has cancer; the vet may wish to persuade a client that it would be kinder to perform euthanasia rather than to continue with treatment
- A cat that was rushed into the practice following a road traffic accident has just died in the 'prep' room and the vet has to go back into the waiting room to tell the client.

Although there will be subtle differences in the approaches to each of the above, there are common factors in the approach to breaking bad news.

- The waiting room should never be the place in which to impart such news. Face-to-face, in a quiet, private room is far preferable. Creating as comfortable an environment as possible for the client is very important and providing seats is one way of seeking to achieve this.
- When breaking bad news, it is always a good idea, where appropriate, to 'fire a warning shot' initially. Use can often be made of previous discussions, or notes on the clinical record. For example: "You will recall when we sent the biopsy off to the lab, I said I was concerned it may be something serious; well, unfortunately it has come back and the news isn't good"; or "As you know, when you brought Chloe in following the traffic accident she was in a very bad way. Three of us have been working on her ever since in an attempt to save her, but despite our best efforts her heart stopped twice and unfortunately we were unable to bring her back a third time". Once you have fired the warning shot, pause for a short while to allow the news to sink in and to allow the client to respond before adding anything further. They may well come back with a comment such as, "So it is cancer?" or, in Chloe's case, "You mean she's died?". You can respond by saying something along the following lines: "Yes it's come back as a form of lymphoma; is this something you have heard of?"; or "Yes, I'm awfully sorry, but Chloe has passed away. She will not have suffered as she never really regained consciousness."
- It is not uncommon for clients to go through a whole range of emotions following the loss of a pet. One of the more common emotions is guilt; a feeling that they could have done more. There is really nothing to be gained from subjecting clients to more anguish and grief by reinforcing their feelings of guilt. To a certain extent the client's welfare is our concern too, and we should do all we can to help them through the grieving process.

Apologizing

In these litigious times, people are often encouraged never to admit liability. All too often, however, this is linked with a fear of apologizing or saying 'sorry' for what has happened. There is a distinction between admitting liability and saying sorry. Professional indemnity insurance providers would never want the practice to admit liability, but clients all too often are quoted as saying, after a complaint or a claim has been resolved, "If only somebody had said 'sorry', we would never have taken our complaint to our solicitor". To square this conundrum, there is a need to appreciate that there is a big difference between telling a client that "The whole practice team is devastated that Sam died unexpectedly under the anaesthetic" and "I'm very sorry, but I've killed Sam!"

The triple As

- **Acknowledge:** Clients want their feelings and their situation acknowledged. They also want it acknowledged if a problem has occurred, even if that problem was something as simple as a misunderstanding. Effective communicators locked in a difficult conversation learn to acknowledge that an event has occurred ▶

that the client is unhappy about. However, one should never admit liability before contacting one's professional indemnity insurer
- **Apologize:** Ineffective communicators fail to apologize, either because of their egos or because they fail to understand that they can apologize without admitting guilt. Effective communicators learn to apologize for *what* happened and apologize for the fact *that* it happened without admitting to any personal contribution
- **Assure:** Complainants want assurances that what they or their animal experienced will never be repeated. Effective communicators learn to give assurances that they will take steps to prevent the problem's recurring and outline any steps already taken

Dealing with emotions

When dealing with difficult situations the veterinary surgeon may not only be faced with trying to resolve the situation clinically, but he/she may often be in a situation where he/she has to deal with clients' emotions. These emotions can include sorrow, guilt and anger. Although these are often presented as stand-alone emotions, they can sometimes present as a cascade, with one following on from another. For example: A client brings their chronically ill pet into the practice, only to be told the only kind option is euthanasia. In this situation the client may feel guilty, followed by angry, and then sad.

The best way of dealing with clients' emotions is to express *empathy*. Empathy is not the same as sympathy, which is more a feeling or an expression of pity or sorrow for the individual. Empathy is the understanding and sensitive appreciation of another person's predicament, and the communication of that understanding back to that person.

- The key to empathy is overt communication to the client, so that they appreciate your understanding and support. We do this not only by inwardly naming the client's emotion, but also considering the intensity of that emotion and vocalizing that back. For example, "I see you are extremely upset by what has happened" or "I feel you have a sense of guilt over what has happened."
- Avoid falling into the trap of telling a client you understand why they are feeling the way they do by saying something like "I can understand why you are finding this bill difficult to pay". This is very likely to receive a response from a disgruntled client along the lines of "How can you possibly understand; have you just been made redundant?; you have absolutely no idea how I feel or what I am going through!". However, showing empathy for a lost pet by sharing genuine, personal feelings of loss can be very helpful if done sensitively.
- When empathizing with a client it is very important, not only to identify the correct emotion, but to reflect the intensity of that emotion. For example, if a client is very angry, telling them that you can see they are a 'little upset' is likely to aggravate the situation; it is better to say something like, "I can see that you are extremely angry about the way things have evolved."

After you have reflected the emotion, wait for a response from the client. Allowing the client time will often throw further light on why they are angry or why they are feeling guilty. Do not interrupt in an attempt either to hurry the process or to help the client; this is very likely to achieve neither. The process then mirrors the consultation model:

- You need to gather information and by using skills such as 'screening', you need to get to the bottom of what is causing the client's anxiety
- By summarizing, you not only demonstrate that you have been listening, but you have created a list that needs to be addressed
- You can then move to the imparting information and planning stages, where you tell the client what you propose to do, checking with them that this is a mutually agreed plan
- Finally, close the process and provide a safety net.

The constant threads

Three elements are constant throughout the consultation, from the initiating stage to closing it. These continuous threads ensure that all other tasks are carried out effectively:

- Providing structure to the consultation
- Building the relationship with the client and patient
- Observation of both client and animal.

Providing structure to the consultation

Without structure the consultation can meander in an aimless fashion. Used in the right way this process can speed up the consultation but clinicians need to be aware that this is a two-way process and not a case of exerting absolute control, otherwise it may limit the client's responses and ability genuinely to listen to the vet. It is also worth noting that these skills allow a flexible approach and are not written in tablets of stone. Key points to consider are as follows:

- The vet should ensure that the client is kept abreast of where the consultation is going; otherwise they may not be aware of why the questioning or explanation is moving in a particular direction or why the examination is proceeding in a particular fashion. For example, it is worth explaining to a client who has presented their pet, concerned about a small lump they have discovered on its flank, why you are performing a complete examination of the patient
- Summarizing has an important role in ensuring the structure of the consultation remains overt. Using the skills employed in the gathering information stage will probably result in information being delivered in a less ordered form, and there may be a tendency to revert to closed questioning prematurely to try and control the direction of the consultation
- Internal summarizing and signposting provides an alternative approach to gaining order and control without foregoing the benefits of using an open-to-closed cone. It allows the vet to draw and review simultaneously any information gathered to date. This information can then be streamed into a coherent pattern, providing the vet with time to

consider where to go next and to be clear in his/her own mind what information is still needed or requires clarification. Summarizing without signposting is less likely to establish a structured way forward
- Signposting initiates and gains the client's attention to what the vet is about to say. This can be used in two different ways:
  - To draw the client's attention to the introduction of the first summary: "Can I check that I've understood you? Please let me know if I've missed anything"
  - To make the client aware of the progression from one section to another, or explain the rationale for the next part of the consultation: "You mentioned three important areas: first the cough; secondly, you said Baxter was scratching excessively; and thirdly you said his booster was out of date. Initally I would like to ask a few questions about the cough and then we can come back to the two other concerns. Is that OK?"

Once a clear plan of how the consultation should proceed has been agreed, the vet should be able to carry out the rest of the consultation in a logical sequence. Following a structure like this provides the vet with an opportunity to consider what has and hasn't been achieved, thereby providing flexibility to cover missed opportunities. There is no doubt that veterinary practitioners find themselves under constant pressure and time constraints, and the time taken over each section of the consultation needs to be balanced. However, following a structure and getting all the issues out at an early juncture can actually make the time spent on the consultation quicker and more efficient.

Building the relationship with the client and patient

This starts from the moment the consultation begins and does not end until the client leaves. It can often be the foundation of an ongoing relationship. In the human medical profession, relationship problems have featured highly as predictors of poor outcome, with lack of warmth and friendliness being one of the most important variables relating to poor levels of patient satisfaction and compliance (Korsch *et al.*, 1968).

The main advantages to building the relationship with the client and pet include:

- The establishment of trust between client, pet and vet
- The creation of an atmosphere that aids the main stages of the consultation (initiation; gathering information; physical examination; explanation and planning; closing)
- The development of a rapport where the client feels at ease, respected and understood
- The reduction of potential complaints and claims
- An increased satisfaction for both the vet and the client.

An array of skills is needed for dealing with feelings and attitudes when building the relationship, and in this context the importance of non-verbal communication cannot be underestimated. What is actually said accounts for 7% of the message and how the words are said (tonality) accounts for 38% of the message; body language (Figures 2.12 and 2.13) accounts for the remaining 55% of the overall message (Mehrabian, 1971). Used simultaneously, non-verbal cues can strengthen and allow verbal messages to be delivered more accurately; without appropriate non-verbal signals it is easy to misunderstand the verbal message. Being able to recognize non-verbal cues is essential but unless they can be checked out verbally with the client it may lead to misinterpretation or in some cases inhibit relationship building. Equally, understanding and paying attention to one's own non-verbal skills may prevent misunderstandings and contradictory messages being relayed.

- It is important that the amount of space between individuals is comfortable. Many factors such as prior relationships, age, sex and culture can influence this
- Many head movements such as nodding and shaking can give opposing messages. Nodding tends to strengthen listening and conveys interest. However, if it is too vigorous it may signal to the listener that the speaker has made their point or taken up enough time. Shaking the head in most cultures demonstrates disagreement
- Folded arms may act as barriers. Conversely, open positions, particularly if combined with open palms, indicate openness and security
- A slumped posture can indicate disinterest, while a relaxed posture and leaning slightly forward can establish rapport by giving the impression of calmness and interest
- Genuine interest and concern can be demonstrated with good eye contact
- Frowning, surprise and smiling can alter facial expressions and indicate how someone is genuinely feeling
- Hand shaking can demonstrate a confident, trusting and professional approach. However it may convey disinterest if it does not feel comfortable and if this is the case it may be better not to do it. A weak hand shake can have a negative effect

2.12 Non-verbal signals.

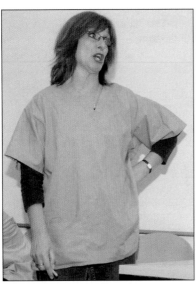

2.13

This photograph, taken in a training environment, shows an aggressive posture.

The vet may have elicited the client's ideas, concerns and expectations during the gathering information stage of the consultation, but having discovered these feelings it is important to act on them. Not only could these thoughts have a direct bearing on the clinical perspective but, unless they are acknowledged and addressed, they may interfere with the whole process of developing rapport. This 'acknowledging

response' (Figure 2.14) ensures that the client's emotions and thoughts are accepted and valued, yet does not necessarily mean that the vet agrees with the client. This supportive measure can be very effective in building the relationship.

- Use genuine comments such as, "I can see why that would cause you concern"
- Acknowledge the client's feelings and uneasiness by naming, restating or summarizing the sentiment. For example: "So you are worried that we might have to put Buster to sleep?"
- Use attentive silences and appropriate non-verbal behaviour to make room for the client to say more
- Try not to answer with "Yes, but…"

2.14 Tips for improving the acknowledging response.

Building a rapport with the client also relies heavily on the ability to be empathic – hearing or seeing what the client is feeling and being able to communicate that understanding back to the client: "I can appreciate how angry this is making you feel…"; "I can see how upset you are about Baxter's condition… ". Some individuals have an innate ability to empathize but many of the skills needed in this situation can be learnt. It is not necessary to have shared an experience or feel that the experience would be difficult in order to empathize. However, it is necessary to see the problem from the client's perspective.

Observation
Again, this should commence from the moment the vet comes into contact with the client and the patient. The vet should observe both parties, and the interaction between them. He/she is looking not only for clinical signs, but to gauge the relationship between the owner and their pet. It may also afford an idea as to how the patient, or indeed the owner, is going to react as the consultation progresses.

References and further reading

Abood SK (2007) Increasing adherence in practice: making your clients partners in care. *Veterinary Clinics of North America: Small Animal Practice* **37**, 151–164

Brightmore H (2009) *Solicitation of agenda and interruption of the opening statement in veterinary consultations: a preliminary study.* BVMedSci dissertation, University of Nottingham

Flemming DD and Scott JF (2004) The informed consent doctrine: what veterinarians should tell their clients. *Journal of the American Veterinary Medical Association* **224**, 1436–1439

Gray C and Moffett J (2010) *Handbook of Veterinary Communication Skills.* Wiley-Blackwell, Oxford

Gray CA, Eves RE, Walsh SJ and Wilson CJ (2005) A final year special study module in veterinary communication skills. *AMEE conference abstracts.* Available at www.amee.org

Hadlow J and Pitts M (1991) The understanding of common terms by doctors, nurses and patients. *Social Science and Medicine* **32**, 193–196

Korsch BM, Gozzi EK and Francis V (1968) Gaps in doctor-patient communication. *Paediatrics* **42**, 855–871

Kurtz S, Silverman J, Benson J and Draper J (2003) Marrying content and process in clinical method teaching: enhancing the Calgary–Cambridge guides. *Academic Medicine* **78**, 802–809

Levinson W, Gorawara-Bhat R and Lamb J (2000) A study of patient clues and physician responses in primary care and surgical settings. *Journal of the American Medical Association* **284**, 1021–1027

McGrath C and Little G (2012) Communication. In: *BSAVA Manual of Small Animal Practice Management and Development*, ed. C Clarke and M Chapman, pp.285–304. BSAVA Publications, Gloucester

Mehrabian A (1971) *Silent Message.* Wadsworth, Belmont, CA

Mossop L and Gray C (2008) Teaching communication skills. *In Practice* **30**, 340–343

Radford A, Stockley P, Silverman J *et al.* (2006) Development, teaching, and evaluation of a consultation structure model for use in veterinary education. *Journal of Veterinary Medical Education* 22, 38–44

Silverman J, Kurtz SA and Draper J (2005) *Skills for Communicating with Patients, 2nd edn.* Radcliffe Medical Press, Oxford

Preventive healthcare: a life-stage approach

Alan Hughes

Canine consultations can be divided into two main groups:

- 'Routine' health checks of generally healthy dogs, equivalent to the 'wellness' clinics that a medical practice may organize for its human patients. For dogs, these are often linked to a vaccination programme. Some practices also offer interim health checks between the annual vaccinations, particularly for senior dogs, so that they are routinely checked every 6 months
- Consultations for dogs with injuries, illness or undergoing an inpatient procedure such as surgery. These are covered in the relevant chapters of this Manual.

The content and emphasis of a routine consultation will vary according to the life stage of the dog concerned.

Examinations for life stages

- Neonates: 1–3 days after birth
- Puppies:
  - Pre-sale checks: 6–8 weeks
  - First vaccination and health check: 6–8 weeks
  - Second vaccination and health check: 10–12 weeks
- Juveniles/adolescents: 5–8 months
- Adults: 1–7 years of age
- Pregnant and pre-whelping bitches: 3–4 weeks after mating
- Postparturient bitch: 1–3 days after giving birth
- Seniors: >7 years old (age varies with breed, see later)

Pregnancy and pre-whelping health checks

A check performed 3–4 weeks after mating can include pregnancy diagnosis, by abdominal palpation or ultrasonography (see Chapter 5).

Pre-whelping health checks have three main purposes:

- To ensure that the bitch is healthy and able to proceed with the pregnancy and the subsequent nursing of a litter of puppies (Figure 3.1)
- To check, as far as possible, that the fetuses are healthy and developing normally. Abdominal palpation of the bitch and auscultation of fetal heartbeats provides minimal information on the health of the litter. For more detailed examination, including fetal heartbeats and approximate litter size, ultrasonography is the ideal tool
- To provide advice to the owners of the bitch (Figure 3.2), especially if they are relatively inexperienced in dog breeding.

Examination and assessment	Acceptable findings	Findings that may cause concern
General condition and health	Good general health and condition with no evidence of significant disease. BCS 4/9 to 5/9	Any significant departure from good health is likely to be more serious in a pregnant bitch BCS 1/9 to 3/9: If underweight the nursing bitch may not lactate effectively and is likely to lose even more weight BCS 6/9 to 9/9: Obesity is a risk factor for dystocia, and over-feeding during pregnancy should be discouraged
Risk of dystocia	The risk of dystocia is lower for some breeds (e.g. dolichocephalic breeds) especially if they have a reasonably sized litter and the stud dog is of comparable size and conformation	Some breeds (e.g. brachycephalic breeds) are particularly prone to dystocia, especially if the litter is small in number and/or the puppies are relatively large
Mammary glands	Normally 5 pairs, each with a functional teat	Some teats may be absent, non-functional or deformed, affecting the bitch's ability to feed puppies

3.1 Health checks for a pregnant bitch. BCS = body condition score (see Chapter 4).

- **Gestation period:** Due to the longevity of viable canine sperm after mating, and some variation associated with differing litter sizes (larger litters tend to be born earlier), the apparent gestation period of the bitch is not fixed at 63 days (the time from ovulation to birth) but may range in practice from 58 to 72 days after mating
- **Giving birth:** Describe the normal process of parturition, including the three stages of labour (see Chapter 5) and advise the owner as to when veterinary help should be sought. This advice should ideally be simple and clear-cut, and therefore easy to remember. For example the owner should phone the veterinary practice if:
  - A green vulval discharge is present but no puppies have been expelled
  - The first puppy is still not expelled after 2 hours of active straining
  - The subsequent puppies are not expelled after a further hour of active straining
  - The bitch does not settle within 1–2 hours and feed the pups after a number have been delivered
- **Management of the pregnant bitch:** Discuss, with particular regard to correct feeding, exercise, preventive healthcare (e.g. safe, effective parasite control)
- **Follow-up:** Explain the value of a post-whelping examination of the bitch and puppies

3.2 Advice that can be given to owners of a pregnant bitch.

Post-parturition and neonatal health checks

This consultation usually takes place 1–3 days after a bitch gives birth, and serves three main functions:

- To ensure that the bitch is healthy, has not suffered any complications associated with parturition, and is able to nurse her litter successfully (Figure 3.3)
- To examine the neonatal puppies (Figure 3.4). While they are so young, a detailed clinical examination of the puppies is not possible but gross abnormalities (e.g. cleft lip and/or palate (see Figure 5.12), polydactyly, umbilical hernia, atresia ani) can be identified
- This is another opportunity to advise the inexperienced breeder on the care and management of the bitch and her litter (Figure 3.5).

More detailed information on reproduction can be found in Chapter 5.

Examination and assessment	Acceptable findings	Findings that may cause concern
General health and condition	Good general condition BCS 4/9 to 5/9 Early to mid adulthood (1–6 years old) Body temperature may be moderately raised during lactation	Poor general condition or a significant pre-existing condition BCS 1/9 to 3/9 Younger (<1 year) or older (>7 years) than ideal Subnormal body temperature (<37.8°C) or pyrexia (>39.5°C)
Behaviour	Adjusted well to nursing puppies; settled and allowing the puppies to feed Concerned but not over-protective Prepared to attend to her own needs, e.g. feeding, drinking, toileting	Some bitches appear to be frightened of, or even aggressive towards, their litter, especially if it is their first (some breeds, e.g. Bull Terriers, seem to be more prone to this aberrant behaviour) Bitch may be unsettled, restless and not allow the puppies to feed
Abdominal palpation	Comfortable, relaxed abdomen. The involuting uterus is usually easily palpable and must not be mistaken for a retained fetus (in the latter, one can usually palpate an indentation between the head and the thorax)	Painful abdomen One or more retained fetuses palpable
Vulval discharge	A small volume of blood-stained discharge may be lost from the vulva for several days	Frank vulval haemorrhage may indicate significant uterine trauma during parturition A foul-smelling discharge may indicate metritis, possibly associated with putrefaction of a retained fetus
Mammary glands	10 functional teats The glands should be warm, moderately distended and comfortable	Agalactia is uncommon but may be secondary to another condition or the result of a difficult parturition (e.g. caesarean section) One or more mammary glands that is hot, firm, swollen, painful and reddened may indicate mastitis

3.3 Examination of the periparturient bitch.

Examination and assessment	Acceptable findings	Findings that may cause concern
General behaviour	Sleepy (especially if recently fed), but can be roused Often wriggle and vocalize during examination	Not interested in feeding Unable to rouse on handling Crying constantly or repeatedly, not settling to feed
Size	Even-sized puppies	A relatively small puppy may indicate other congenital problems
General condition	The abdomen should be soft, comfortable and moderately full after feeding The skin tone should be elastic The mucous membranes are pink	The abdomen is distended, tense and painful or empty Inelastic skin suggests dehydration Pale or cyanosed membranes
Sucking reflex	Strong, vigorous	Weak or absent
Gross anatomy and conformation		If abnormal this may indicate a congenital abnormality, and this may necessitate humane euthanasia (e.g. cleft lip/palate, cyclopegia, atresia ani, hydrocephalus)

3.4 Examination of neonatal puppies.

- Correct feeding of the bitch to ensure adequate lactation without excessive loss of condition throughout the period of nursing (see Chapter 4)
- Recognition and avoidance of eclampsia, especially in relatively small breeds with large vigorous litters of 7–21 days of age
- Adequate endoparasite control. Safe and effective elimination of roundworms (mainly *Toxocara canis*) in the puppies usually begins with worming the pregnant bitch and continues with the litter a few days after birth
- Monitoring the health and development of the litter. Identical puppies should be marked (e.g. with nail varnish) to allow identification of different individuals. The puppies should be weighed every 1–2 days on accurate scales – a steady increase in weight (while remaining at a BCS of 4/9 to 5/9) should reassure owners that the puppies are thriving. Any loss of weight should alert the owners to a possible problem

3.5 Important considerations in the care of a bitch and her litter.

PRACTICAL TIPS

- To avoid the dam becoming too anxious or distressed while her puppies are examined, it is sometimes helpful for her to be taken out of the consulting room or to be restrained and comforted by a veterinary nurse or by one of the owners, provided they are able to do so safely and have been informed of the potential risks involved
- Alternatively, the consultation may take place in the bitch's home, providing an opportunity to observe her and the puppies in a more natural environment

Pre-sale examination

This consultation may be requested by a breeder, usually when the puppies are 6–8 weeks of age, to identify any congenital or developmental abnormalities or disease that may affect the value of the puppy and its suitability for its new home. In the absence of problems, the breeder may ask for written certification that the puppy has been examined by a veterinary surgeon and found to be free of evidence of abnormality or disease. This document can then be shown or passed on to the new owner. An example is given in Figure 3.6.

Puppy health checks

There are usually two (sometimes three) routine consultations for new puppies, often arranged to coincide with the puppy's primary vaccination course (see later). The first will often be shortly after acquisition by the new owner.

PRACTICAL TIP

Unless the owner has any concerns about the health of the new puppy, it is advisable that the first consultation is booked for a few days after arrival in the new home. Bringing the new puppy to the veterinary practice on the day of collection from the breeder only adds further to its physiological stress, and this is not a suitable time for its primary vaccination course to be started. A few days at home, however, allows the puppy and owners to become familiar with each other, and for any problems to be identified. For example, a reliable assessment of the puppy's appetite can not be made whilst it is still very unsettled in its new home

The first puppy health check (6–8 weeks of age)

This first health check (Figure 3.7) has a number of important aims.

- Any serious congenital or developmental problems should be identified and consideration given as to whether the puppy should be returned to the breeder.
- This may be the first visit to the veterinary surgery for both the puppy and its owner. Positive, constructive relationships between the veterinary practice as a whole, the individual veterinary surgeons, the puppy's owners and their puppy may be determined at this very first consultation.
- This is an ideal opportunity to provide helpful advice on many aspects of preventive healthcare and the routine care of the new puppy. Whilst the new owner is likely to be enthusiastic and receptive to advice, it is important to avoid information overload. Many practices provide some written information (e.g. puppy booklets; Figure 3.8) for owners to take home. In some

---

12th June 2013
Anytown Veterinary Clinic

Re: A black male puppy of 6 weeks of age born to the Cocker Spaniel bitch 'Fido' belonging to:
Mr and Mrs Smith of 1 High Street, Anytown

This is to certify that on the 10th June 2013 I examined the above-mentioned puppy and found no evidence of serious congenital or developmental abnormalities, or other disease or illness. I therefore judge him to be fit for sale.

Signed...
[Name of veterinary surgeon]

3.6 An example of a certificate of pre-sale examination for a puppy.

1. **Before the client is called into the consultation room,** check that certain essential items of information have been recorded in the patient's records, and note any that need to be requested:
   – The owner: Name and address, contact telephone numbers, email address, any other pets
   – The puppy: Breed (knowing this beforehand may avoid embarrassing mistakes in misidentifying the puppy's breed!), age, gender (clients may be quite upset by the simple mistake of referring to a male puppy as 'she')
2. **Greeting.** Calling the owners by name, and the puppy too, immediately sets a positive tone to the consultation and reassures the client that you are interested in them and their new puppy as individuals
3. **Building rapport.** Even a brief comment, such as referring to the sad loss of a previous pet, or a flattering remark about their new puppy, will help a great deal in establishing a positive relationship
4. **History taking.** See below for guidelines
5. **Clinical examination.** A systematic general clinical examination should now be performed, tailored to be appropriate for a new puppy. See below for guidelines
6. **Weigh the puppy**
7. **Preventive healthcare**
   – *Vaccination.* Provided the puppy is judged to be in good general health, it is usual to administer the first stage of the primary vaccination course (see later). Taking into account any vaccinations given whilst with the breeder, the first dose will usually incorporate all of the core vaccines, and any of the non-core vaccines deemed advisable depending on the puppy's lifestyle and location (see Figure 3.18)
   – *Parasite control.* Regard should be given to any antiparasite treatments administered prior to this consultation. The veterinary surgeon should emphasize the importance of regular treatment
   – *Diet recommendations.* A puppy will often arrive in its new home with advice on diets from its breeder, and sometimes a small supply of the recommended food. Unless this is judged unsuitable, or the puppy requires a special diet (e.g. a light diet to manage a gastrointestinal problem), the author's usual advice is to continue to feed the breeder's choice of diet for 1–2 weeks after acquisition, and only then to switch to the owner's preferred diet if desired, but taking 1–2 weeks to accomplish this change. There are many good quality proprietary diets carefully formulated for puppies that are readily available

   – *Neutering.* If there is no intention to breed from the puppy in the future, the advantages (and any disadvantages) of neutering (see Figure 3.11) should be introduced for the owner to consider, and details given of timing and costs
   – *Tooth brushing.* Owners should be shown how to brush the puppy's teeth correctly, and encouraged to do so every day as an important element of dental homecare
8. **Other advice for new owners.** Some of this may be presented by the practice nurse:
   – *Pet insurance*
   – *Microchipping.* It is recommended that all new patients should be checked for the presence of a microchip and, if found, the new owner asked for the registration documents as proof of their legitimate ownership. If they are not able to provide them, or if the details do not correspond with those of the client, the database company should be contacted and the situation reported
   – *Health schemes.* There are a variety of these, from those in a single-site practice, to those across large corporate groups. They generally offer a programme of preventive healthcare for a fixed fee, sometimes linked to other potential benefits such as discounts or special offers; if these are operated by the practice, they should be explained to the new owner
   – *New clients.* If the client is new to the practice, services such as out-of-hours emergency provision, requests for prescriptions, home visits, etc. can be described. Some practices take this opportunity to provide a guided tour of the practice
9. **Closing remarks.** The owner should be advised when the puppy needs to return for the next part of its vaccination course (usually 2–4 weeks later and at least 10 weeks of age when maternally derived antibodies will no longer be present to affect vaccine efficacy). It is usually practice policy to advise that the puppy is not adequately protected to mix with other potentially disease-carrying dogs, or to walk them where they may have been, until a certain time (usually 1–2 weeks) after the second vaccination. However, the importance of socialization should be discussed and tips given on how to do this safely (see Chapter 1). Some practices offer 'puppy parties' to the owners of new dogs, often run by veterinary nurses, where the puppies have an opportunity to socialize under controlled conditions, whilst their owners can learn about various aspects of their care
10. **Provide summary sheets** of all recommended advice (possibly in the form of a booklet), as there will be too much information presented for the new owner to take on board in one go

3.7   The first puppy consultation. Following a modified version of the Calgary–Cambridge Guide (see also Chapter 2), a number of stages can be identified.

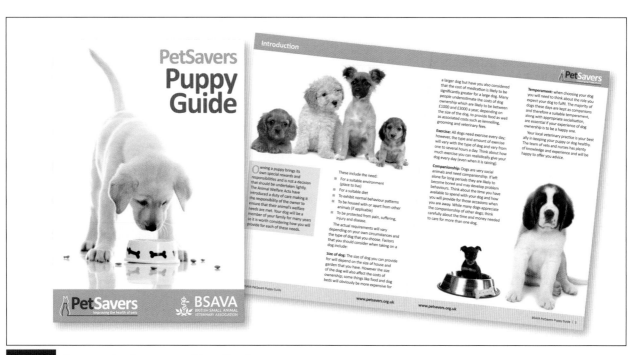

3.8   An example of a puppy guide written for owners.

practices the time available is shared with a practice nurse, allowing some of the healthcare messages to be reinforced. In any event, significant time must be allowed for this all-important consultation.

History taking

There are a number of essential questions to ask the owner of a new puppy:

- How long have you owned the puppy?
- What was the source of the puppy – a breeder, rescue shelter, dealer, pet shop or private home?
- Have you owned a dog before?
- Are there any health issues with this puppy that you are concerned about?
- If so, were these apparent immediately after acquisition or were they mentioned by the breeder?
- If possible problems are identified, specific questions relating to these should be asked. For example, if the owner complains that the puppy has diarrhoea: What is the nature of the diarrhoea? Has there been any vomiting? Is the puppy eating? What diet is being fed?
- If the owner reports that the puppy has been given any vaccinations or other preventive healthcare measures (e.g. worming treatments) prior to acquisition, are there any written details to clarify and support this (e.g. vaccine records)?
- If the puppy has had its tail docked, does the new owner have the correct documentation certifying that the breeder had this performed in the correct circumstances?

Tail docking regulations in England

NB Regulations vary in other parts of the UK

An exemption from the ban on the tail docking of puppies is allowed for those puppies intended for certain working uses such as gun-dogs. The owner of the puppy should have documentation to demonstrate that:

- The procedure was performed by a veterinary surgeon
- The puppy was less than 5 days old
- The veterinary surgeon performing the procedure had seen evidence that the puppy is likely to be used for working in the future
- The puppy has been microchipped (or is to be microchipped by a certain age)

These are correct at time of going to press; further information and up-to-date regulations are available at www.rcvs.org.uk. There is also a leaflet available from the BVA Animal Welfare Foundation (www.bva-awf.org.uk)

Clinical examination

The systematic head-to-tail approach to clinical examination (see QRG 3.1) should be tailored for a new puppy to look for common abnormalities and conditions such as those noted below:

- Head and neck:
  - Teeth: Deciduous dentition. Check that the correct complement of teeth is present and correctly erupted. Check for malocclusion, especially prognathia or brachygnathia
  - Oral cavity: Cleft palate
  - Eyes: Congenital abnormalities of the eyelids (e.g. entropion, coloboma). Congenital ocular abnormalities (e.g. persistent pupillary membranes, microphthalmia)
  - Ears: Parasitic otitis
- Forelimbs: Congenital deformities (e.g. carpal valgus or varus)
- Hindlimbs: Congenital deformities (e.g. hip dysplasia, patellar instability)
- Thorax:
  - Congenital deformities of the sternum or ribs
  - Congenital heart murmurs
- Abdomen:
  - Inguinal or umbilical hernias
  - Females: Intersex variations
  - Males: Cryptorchidism
- Anal area: Anal gland impaction
- Skin and coat: Skin parasites (e.g. fleas (Figure 3.9), lice, mites).

The second puppy health check (10–12 weeks of age)

The main purpose of this check is to administer the second (and usually final) part of the puppy's primary vaccination course (see later). This is a good opportunity to check on the puppy's progress and development (including weight gain) with a brief clinical examination, and to address any concerns that the owner may raise. There may be items from the first consultation (e.g. microchipping) that the practice or the owner has chosen to delay until this consultation.

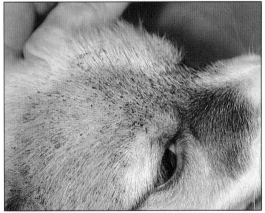
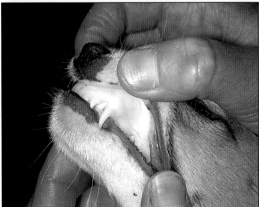

3.9 This Jack Russell Terrier puppy had a severe flea infestation with resultant severe anaemia. (© Susan Paterson)

Juvenile/adolescent health checks

It is recommended that adolescent dogs are examined at approximately 6 months of age. As well as a thorough physical examination (see later) and addressing any clinical concerns, this allows the veterinary surgeon to discuss a range of issues, some of which may also have been raised when the puppy was first presented.

- **Vaccination.** The veterinary surgeon should check that the course of recommended core vaccines has been completed correctly, and discuss any non-core vaccines. Owners should be reminded that a booster vaccination will be required annually, with the first due 12 months after completion of the puppy's primary course.
- **Parasite control.** Six months is often the age at which the dog is switched from a puppy worming programme (e.g. monthly) to an adult programme (e.g. every 3 months). It is important to discuss the ongoing requirement for regular, routine ectoparasite control (see later).
- **Diet.** Feeding appropriate to the growing dog's age and breed is important to ensure correct development.
- **Other services.** This is an ideal time to promote valuable services such as microchipping (Figure 3.10) and pet insurance if not taken up when a puppy.
- **Travel abroad.** Owners may be planning to take their dog abroad in the future and this may be a suitable time to explain the PETS Travel Scheme (see Figure 3.13), as some forward planning may be required.
- **Neutering *versus* breeding.** Now that the dog is approaching puberty (usually occurs at 6–10 months of age) this is an ideal time to discuss neutering, or ambitions to breed. Most practices advocate the routine neutering of dogs if there is no intention to breed. Advantages of neutering are listed in Figure 3.11. Some clients still believe that allowing a bitch to have one litter confers some physical or behavioural benefits on her but this has not been proven. It is important to inform clients about the commitment and responsibility required in breeding dogs, which should not be undertaken lightly.

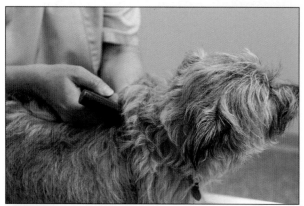

| 3.10 | This 3-year-old terrier is having a microchip inserted. |

Male dogs
▪ Reduces the risk of aggression especially towards other (male) dogs
▪ Prevents testicular neoplasia
▪ Prevents some prostatic disease
▪ Reduces the risk of perineal hernias
▪ Reduces 'antisocial behaviour', e.g. territorial urination
▪ May facilitate training and behaviour control
▪ Prevents unwanted pregnancies

Bitches
▪ Prevents pyometra
▪ Prevents neoplasia of the uterus and ovaries
▪ May prevent or reduce the incidence of mammary gland neoplasia, particularly if performed before the second 'season'
▪ Prevents unwanted pregnancies
▪ Prevents the bloody vulval discharge during oestrus
▪ Prevents pseudopregnancy

| 3.11 | Arguments in favour of routine neutering (see also Chapter 5). |

A thorough examination, again using a systematic approach to avoid omissions (see later and QRG 3.1), should be performed during this consultation. There are a number of aspects of the adolescent dog's health to be considered:

- **Growth and development.** Large breeds may still be growing rapidly at 6 months of age, whereas small breeds may be approaching their adult size. Apart from checking for normal general development, congenital or developmental conditions not apparent in the puppy may now be identified, e.g. orthopaedic conditions such as hip dysplasia
- **Weight and condition.** Incorrect weight or poor body condition, possibly associated with inappropriate nutrition, may be apparent at this time. Steps should be taken to remedy this
- **Specific concerns** raised by the owner, or conditions identified during the examination.

Routine health checks for adult dogs

These consultations are usually timed to coincide with the dog's annual booster vaccinations.

A clinical examination employing a systematic approach (see below and QRG 3.1) should be employed during this consultation. It is important that an accurate weight is measured (Figure 3.12) and recorded in the dog's clinical notes. Any health problems identified at this time, raised by the owner, or possibly ongoing from the dog's previous medical history, should prompt a closer examination of relevant areas. This is a good time to 'catch up' with a dog's progress if it has a chronic, ongoing or recurrent problem. Should a specific problem require deeper investigation, it may be advisable to book the dog in for a further appointment.

Other matters that might be addressed at the routine annual examination include:

- **Vaccination.** Core vaccination should be administered as outlined in Figure 3.18 to maintain protection against these important diseases. Non-core vaccinations may be given in

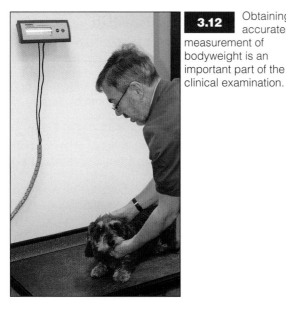

3.12 Obtaining an accurate measurement of bodyweight is an important part of the clinical examination.

addition, depending on the owners' requirements, the dog's lifestyle and regional considerations
- **Parasite control.** This is an ideal opportunity to check that a parasite control programme is in place and that it is appropriate for the dog in question. Dogs travelling abroad may have specific parasite control requirements which can be addressed at this examination, and the requirements of the PETS Travel Scheme for dogs intended to be returned to the UK should also be borne in mind (Figure 3.13)
- **Blood screening tests.** Some veterinary practices recommend an annual blood screen, usually comprising haematology and biochemistry panels, with the intention of identifying problems not found during the clinical examination. In an otherwise healthy dog in which the owner does not raise any concerns, and no problems are identified during the clinical examination, the value of this is questionable. Conscientious owners may, however, be reassured by this being offered as a service.

Under the current scheme (modified in January 2012) dogs may return to the UK after travel to an EU or one of the listed non-EU countries provided that the following apply:

- They are microchipped. This must be performed before any other travel-related procedures, to ensure correct identification of the pet concerned
- They are vaccinated against rabies and given their rabies boosters at the intervals required by the data sheets of the vaccine used. There must be a time interval of 21 days between the first rabies vaccination and return to the UK
- They have the correct accompanying documentation. For pets travelling from within the EU, this will be the EU Pet Passport completed and signed, and issued by a veterinary surgeon licensed by Defra (i.e. an LVI)
- They have been treated for tapeworm 1–5 days prior to arrival in the UK

Dogs returning to the UK after travel to an unlisted non-EU country should have a blood test taken at least 30 days after vaccination to demonstrate satisfactory protection from rabies, and there is then a 3-month wait from the date the blood was taken before entry is permitted

3.13 A brief overview of the PETS Travel Scheme. This information was correct at time of going to press, but it is advisable to check with the appropriate authorities for the most up-to-date information and for more details (see www.defra.gov.uk).

Routine health checks for senior dogs

Depending on the dog's general condition and the presence of any specific clinical problems, the veterinary surgeon may decide to increase the frequency of health checks to every 6 months for some senior dogs.

> Dogs over 7 years of age should be classed as 'senior', as the problems associated with ageing may begin to develop in this group. It should be remembered, however, that this process may begin 1–2 years earlier in giant breeds, and 3–5 years later in smaller breeds

A thorough clinical examination using a systematic approach (see QRG 3.1) is important. A large number of problems associated with ageing may be identified more commonly now. These include:

- Eyes – cataracts
- Skin – seborrhoea
- Heart – valvular disease
- Kidneys – renal dysfunction
- Limbs – osteoarthritis.

If suspected, attention can then be focused on these specific problems to enable accurate diagnosis, and correct treatment and management as appropriate.

Other matters that might be addressed at the routine annual examination include:

- **Preventive healthcare:**
  - The annual core vaccination programme (plus any non-core vaccines required) (see later) should continue. Clients often ask whether it is necessary to continue with booster vaccinations in older dogs. It is important to remind them that protection cannot be assured beyond the time intervals described in the vaccine's data sheets, and that if the dog is still active and socializing with other dogs then it is still susceptible to infectious disease, probably more so with the reduced innate immunity of older pets
  - A parasite prevention programme appropriate to the dog's lifestyle should continue for life
- **Diet:**
  - Even in the absence of specific disease conditions being identified, consideration should be given to whether the dog's diet should be modified
  - Just as with people, the most common diet-related problem is obesity; this can affect (Figure 3.14), or predispose to, a number of clinical conditions seen especially commonly in

- Osteoarthritis
- Other orthopaedic conditions (e.g. patellar luxation)
- Skin disease (e.g. seborrhoea, skin fold dermatitis)
- Cardiac disease (e.g. congestive heart failure)
- Respiratory disease (e.g. chronic pulmonary airway disease)
- Endocrine disorders (e.g. diabetes mellitus)

3.14 Types of disease that may be exacerbated by obesity.

older dogs. If not addressed at previous health checks, it now becomes even more important that dietary modification is instituted in the older obese dog. Senior diets, sold as part of the proprietary life-stage diet ranges, will usually have a lower calorie content to help tackle this problem. Sometimes, however, a diet with even fewer calories is required to address a significant obesity problem. It is important that advice and support from a veterinary surgeon or veterinary nurse with experience in pet nutrition is available to manage and monitor the more significant weight loss intended in these cases Return to the maintenance diet is only advisable once the target weight is achieved

- Senior proprietary diets will often have other modifications designed to help manage specific age-related problems (e.g. joint supplements for osteoarthritis, reduced protein content for renal dysfunction). Sometimes specific clinical diets may be recommended, as in other life stages, to address specific diseases

■ **Laboratory screening:** Although it was argued above that routine blood screens in otherwise apparently healthy adult dogs may be of limited value, there may be greater clinical advantage to be gained from these in senior dogs, as many of the problems associated with abnormal blood results may present initially with no signs, or with non-specific or subtle signs. A routine blood screen for senior dogs may be recommended at the time of their annual health check. This is of most use if also combined with urinalysis (Figure 3.15), and clients may be asked to bring a fresh urine sample from their dog at this time. As at other times, any abnormalities detected in these may prompt further diagnostic investigation.

Blood biochemistry	
■ Total protein	■ Cholesterol
■ Albumin	■ Bile acids
■ Globulin	■ Creatine kinase
■ Urea	■ Phosphorus
■ Creatinine	■ Calcium
■ Alkaline phosphatase (ALP)	■ Sodium
■ Alanine aminotransferase (ALT)	■ Potassium
■ Glucose	■ Chloride
■ Bilirubin	■ Total T4

Haematology	
■ Red blood cells (RBC)	■ Differential white blood cell
■ Haemoglobin	count
■ Haematocrit	■ Segmented neutrophil count
■ Mean cell volume (MCV)	■ Lymphocytes
■ Mean cell haemoglobin (MCH)	■ Monocytes
■ Mean cell haemoglobin	■ Eosinophils
concentration (MCHC)	■ Basophils
■ Platelets	■ Atypical cells
■ Absolute white blood cell	
count (WBC)	

Urinalysis	
■ Glucose	■ Nitrites
■ Ketones	■ Leucocytes
■ Blood	■ Specific gravity
■ Protein	■ pH

3.15   A routine blood and urine test panel for senior dogs.

End-of-life examinations

Veterinary surgeons are frequently asked to advise on whether euthanasia is appropriate for an older dog. Whilst any individual clinical condition must be considered, often it is the dog's overall health, condition, comfort and apparent enjoyment (its 'quality of life') that is being assessed at this time.

Old age is not a disease and of itself is no justification for euthanasia of a pet (although often owners feel under some pressure from friends or family to act at this time). Due consideration also needs to be given to the owner's welfare, however. For example, an elderly dog that regularly toilets indoors may be quite content in itself but could cause the owner considerable distress. It should also be borne in mind that most significant chronic disorders (e.g. neurological deterioration with age) are usually only likely to worsen with time, and whilst elderly animals should not be euthanased prematurely, it should be considered that in these cases, if the owner is initially dissuaded from losing their pet, they often express regret when presenting the dog again a short time later when the condition has deteriorated further.

Quality of life is clearly a very subjective concept but one that veterinary surgeons are often asked to judge. They are usually well placed to do so, provided this is after careful questioning of the owner who will be familiar with the dog's normal habits. If an elderly dog has deteriorated beyond the point at which its comfort and wellbeing can be assured, the veterinary surgeon should discuss euthanasia with the owner. Hopefully this can be performed whilst the dog retains some dignity, and such that the owners' final memories of their pet are not dominated by a protracted and miserable end of their companion's life. Euthanasia is discussed in more detail in Chapter 7.

General clinical examination

It is important to develop a routine and systematic approach to this, so that the examination can be completed in the limited time available during a consultation, but without overlooking anything (see QRG 3.1). The clinical examination may be varied depending on three factors:

■ The signalment of the dog – age, breed, gender
■ Any previous clinical history which may be relevant to the dog's current health status. For example, in a dog with a previous history of chronic skin disease, special attention should be devoted to examining the skin at each routine health check, as a means of monitoring this problem
■ Any clinical abnormalities that are identified during the examination. For example, if enlarged submandibular lymph nodes are identified, a more careful examination of the other superficial and internal lymph nodes would be appropriate to assess their size.

Adopting and practising a systematic approach (see QRG 3.1 and Figure 3.16) will ensure that all available parts of the body are assessed. If an abnormality is identified, further information can be gained by focusing on this body system.

Head and neck

- Nares, planum nasale, nasal bones
- Lips: external surfaces, mucous membranes, mucocutaneous junctions, commissures
- Gums
- Teeth: buccal, lingual and occlusal surfaces
- Oral cavity: tongue, hard and soft palates, oropharynx
- Temporomandibular joints
- Eyelids: external and conjunctival surfaces, canthi, margins, nictitating membranes
- Eyes: conjunctivae, sclerae, corneas, pupils, irises, anterior chambers
- Cranial bones
- Ears: pinnae, opening of external canals and vertical canals
- Submandibular lymph nodes
- Salivary glands
- Larynx and trachea

Forelimbs

- Scapula and associated muscles
- Prescapular lymph nodes
- Axilla
- Shoulder, elbow and carpal joints
- Humerus and associated muscles
- Antebrachium
- Feet: metacarpals, digits, pads, claws, interdigital skin

Thorax

- Thoracic spine, sternum, ribs, intercostal spaces
- Auscultation of lungs
- Auscultation of heart

Abdomen

- Lumbar spine, abdominal wall
- Inguinae
- Umbilicus
- Costal arch, caudal border of liver, kidneys, spleen, bladder, abdominal lymph nodes, stomach, small and large intestines

Hindlimbs

- Pelvis and associated muscles
- Popliteal lymph nodes
- Femur and associated muscles
- Tibia, fibula and associated muscles
- Hip, stifle and hock joints
- Feet: metatarsals, digits, pads, claws, interdigital skin

Perineum and tail

- Anal sphincter
- Anal glands
- Tail

Female features

- Vulva
- Teats
- Mammary glands
- Uterus

Male features

- Penis and prepuce
- Scrotum and testes

Skin and haircoat

3.16 A 'head-to-tail' approach to a systematic clinical examination. See also QRG 3.1.

With a gentle, tactile approach to the examination (Figure 3.17), as well as gaining an overall assessment of the health status of the dog, the examination can be used to help the patient relax before proceeding to concentrate on a specific area. Handling and restraint is discussed in Chapter 1.

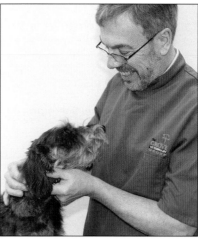

3.17 A short time spent trying to reassure and relax the patient is not wasted, and may actually save time later in the examination.

Body temperature, heart and pulse rate, and respiratory rate (the 'TPR') are often considered the baseline parameters to measure in a clinical examination.

- Body temperature is most rapidly and accurately measured using a digital thermometer (see Figure 18.3), preferably with a disposable cover for hygienic reasons, inserted into the rectum.
- Heart rate is measured during auscultation (counting in groups of ten for 15 seconds).
- Pulse rate (rhythm and quality) is assessed most easily by palpation of the femoral artery on the inside of the thigh.
- Respiratory rate is counted over a 15-second period, preferably before the dog becomes stressed by the examination (i.e. a resting rate).

Vaccination

The regular (annual) health check for dogs often coincides with routine vaccination. It is essential that a full clinical examination (see above) is performed whenever a dog attends for vaccination.

- It is important to ensure that the dog is healthy. *Vaccines should never be administered to a patient that may be immunocompromised, either through a significant illness or treatment such as ciclosporin.*
- This is an ideal opportunity to provide a general health check for a canine patient that often would not arise otherwise. Indeed, it could be argued that one of the principal benefits of annual booster vaccinations is the chance to perform a health check (see above).
- This examination is an essential element in reassuring the client that the practice is providing good value for money. It should be made clear that the fee charged for vaccination includes that for a clinical examination.

As a result of changing patterns of disease, improvements in vaccine design, and concerns expressed by a minority of dog owners about problems perceived to be associated with 'over-vaccination', canine vaccination programmes have undergone considerable debate and scrutiny in recent years. From this controversial topic has emerged the notion of 'core' and 'non-core' vaccines.

Core vaccines

In discussing a suitable vaccination programme for a dog with their owner, it is important to remember that a core vaccine:

- Is highly effective at providing protection
- Is safe
- Protects against diseases that have high mortality and/or are highly infectious
- May protect against zoonotic disease.

Thus, core vaccines are considered essential to protect ALL dogs against a number of serious, often potentially fatal, infections:

- Canine distemper
- Canine parvovirus
- Infectious canine hepatitis
- Canine leptospirosis.

These vaccines should be boosted as required to maintain an adequate level of immunity against these diseases at all times (although it should be remembered that no vaccine provides 100% protection). Due to improvements in vaccine design, and studies evaluating the immunity they achieve, it is now not always considered necessary to boost all of these vaccines every year (Figure 3.18). Generally, leptospiral vaccines are required annually to maintain immunity but vaccines against parvovirus, distemper and hepatitis can be administered less frequently to the adult dog, often every 3 years. **It is important that a new graduate seeks advice from a senior member of the practice as to what is that practice's protocol for vaccination programmes.** The strain(s) of organism used to produce a particular vaccine may vary from one manufacturer to another, and it is important to know which is in use in a practice so that any recent or local variation is taken into account, and so that dogs which have previously been vaccinated elsewhere are given the correct booster.

The role of serological testing

Theoretically, serological testing would be used as an integral part of designing a suitable vaccination programme for an individual dog, as it would provide information regarding the diseases that the dog could be susceptible to, and those that it appears still to be adequately protected against. The practical reality is, however, that such testing is far from reliable, overlooks the role of cell-mediated immunity and completely uneconomical for most owners. Thus, the veterinary surgeon should use their knowledge and experience, the available data on vaccines, and the disease risks for that individual dog, to devise and recommend a suitable programme of vaccination

---

Non-core vaccines

These are to protect against diseases that:

- Have a low mortality or can be treated effectively (e.g. kennel cough)
- Only affect specific populations as a result of their lifestyle or geographical location.

Thus, these may be considered less essential for every dog.

Examples of non-core vaccines available in the UK include:

- Rabies: usually only essential for dogs travelling abroad to countries where rabies is endemic, either in the dog population or in a wildlife reservoir. The vaccine protects individual dogs and reduces the risk of importing this serious and zoonotic disease into the UK. This vaccine is compulsory for dogs requiring a passport under the PETS Travel Scheme (see earlier)
- *Bordetella bronchiseptica*: protects dogs against a major cause of kennel cough; this intranasal vaccine is often administered to dogs that are regularly in contact with others, and especially prior to entry to boarding kennels
  - Immunocompromised owners (e.g. transplant patients, chemotherapy patients) should avoid contact with vaccinated dogs for 6 weeks, as stated on the data sheet
  - Concurrent use of antibacterial drugs should be avoided
- Parainfluenza virus: protects against another cause of the kennel cough syndrome
- *Leishmania*: provides some protection for dogs travelling to hot climates where leishmaniosis is endemic, and should be used alongside protection from biting insects that transmit the disease
- Herpesvirus: administered to breeding bitches where there is a risk of losing puppies to 'fading puppy syndrome', one cause of which is believed to be canine herpesvirus.

Age of dog	Core vaccinations required
6–10 weeks	Distemper, parvovirus, leptospirosis and hepatitis
At least 10 weeks	Repeat of the above 2–4 weeks later (depending on data sheet recommendations). This second puppy vaccination must be given at an age of at least 10 weeks to ensure that all maternally derived antibodies have been exhausted. The new Lepto4 vaccine designed to protect against newly emerging serovariants in Europe and the USA requires a 4-week gap between the first and second doses
15 months	First adult booster, including distemper, parvovirus, leptospirosis and hepatitis
2 years	Leptospirosis
3 years	Leptospirosis
4 years	Distemper, parvovirus, leptospirosis and hepatitis
5 years	Leptospirosis
6 years	Leptospirosis
7 years	Distemper, parvovirus, leptospirosis and hepatitis
Older	Leptospirosis every year; distemper, parvovirus and hepatitis every 3 years

3.18   A typical programme of core vaccinations. The programme should maximize a dog's protection against these diseases, whilst minimizing any accusations of 'over-vaccination'.

Common parasites

Ecto- and endoparasites are a common cause of clinical problems in dogs, varying from the relatively trivial nuisance (e.g. harvest mites) to the severe, even life-threatening (e.g. lungworm). Owners often express distaste at their pet's harbouring a visible parasite burden, and some infections carry a zoonotic risk. Safe and effective parasite control therefore forms an important component of the routine healthcare programme for all dogs, although requirements may vary according to the dog's age, lifestyle and role. Common ectoparasites and helminth endoparasites of dogs are discussed in Figures 3.19 and 3.20.

Species (most common in bold)	Transmission	Clinical signs and health risks	Diagnostics	Treatment and control
Fleas				
Ctenocephalides felis (cat flea) – most common flea found on dogs **Ctenocephalides canis** (dog flea) *Archeopsylla erinacei* (hedgehog flea)	Life cycle 14–140 days depending on environmental conditions; most rapid in warm moist surroundings. Pupae relatively resistant; can survive for months until suitable conditions develop. Vibrations, heat and exhaled carbon dioxide from the dog stimulate adult fleas to jump aboard	Pruritus and self-traumatic dermatitis. Allergic dermatitis. Very severe infestations in young puppies may cause anaemia (see Figure 3.9). The flea is the intermediate host to *Dipylidium* tapeworm larvae, transmitted via ingestion (zoonotic)	Fleas found on dog. Use a fine comb through the coat; identify fleas, eggs and flea faeces (containing host's blood; dissolve in drop of water or on damp cotton wool)	Treat infested dog and all in-contact animals in household with appropriate adulticides, ideally combined with treating all animals in household with insect growth inhibitors (IGRs). Apply ovicidal/larvicidal drugs to dog that are then shed into immediate environment; usually combined with adulticides. Treat environment with appropriate insecticides/IGR combinations. Thorough cleaning, especially soft furnishings and bedding, and careful disposal of infected materials. Avoid contact with potentially infested animals (e.g. cats, hedgehogs). Owner education paramount to ensure adequate preventive control
Ticks				
Ixodes ricinus (castor bean or European sheep tick) *Ixodes canisuga* (dog tick) *Ixodes hexagonus* (hedgehog tick) *Haemaphysalis Dermacentor* spp. – much less common, found in UK only in certain regions	Life cycle up to 12 months. Dogs infested by walking through long grass, rough grazing. Some regions of UK (e.g. East Anglia, Scotland) have a far greater prevalence of ticks	Skin irritation and pain at attachment site. Heavy infestations in young or debilitated dogs may cause anaemia. Transmission of infectious diseases: Lyme disease (*Borrelia burgdorferi*) uncommon in UK but potentially serious (and zoonotic). Ticks on dogs that have travelled abroad, including Europe, may transmit ehrlichiosis, babesiosis (both zoonotic) and *Mycoplasma haemocanis*	Close inspection of dog may enable ticks to be found	Treat dog with appropriate acaricides; some have tick-repellent activity. None is completely effective. Frequent inspection and careful removal of ticks: preferably use proprietary device to ensure mouthparts are extracted from skin (note *slight risk of zoonotic borreliosis and ensure device does not squeeze ingested blood from tick back into dog*). Avoid exercising dogs in tick-prevalent areas
Lice				
Trichodectes canis (biting louse) *Linognathus setosus* (sucking louse)	Life cycle entirely on dog host; survival off host short lived. Transmission by direct contact with infected host or via shared grooming equipment	Very young, old or debilitated dogs are at greater risk of infestation, suffering marked pruritus and resultant self-trauma	Finding lice and eggs in the dog's coat 	Regular examination and grooming. Apply suitable insecticides
Ear mites				
Otodectes cynotis 	Entire life cycle (approx. 3 weeks) in external ear canal of host. Transmission by direct contact with infected host. Mite commonly found on cats, ferrets and foxes	Marked aural pruritus and an accumulation of dark wax in the external ear canals, leading to otitis externa	Otoscopic examination will reveal the mites, seen as small white parasites moving about in the canal	Systemic acaricide, including all in-contact animals even if asymptomatic. Topical medication to clean external ear canals and treat any inflammation or secondary infection (some cleaning preparations also have acaricidal action)

3.19   Common ectoparasites of dogs. See also Chapters 27 and 29. (Illustrations © Susan Paterson) (continues)   ▶

Species (most common in bold)	Transmission	Clinical signs and health risks	Diagnostics	Treatment and control
Skin/fur mites				
Sarcoptes scabiei	Life cycle 10–21 days, entirely on host. Adults can survive up to 2 weeks off host in ideal conditions. Transmission by direct contact. Highly contagious	Causes scabies, an intensely pruritic dermatitis, initially in less hairy parts such as pinna margins (see Figure 27.8). Zoonotic: *S. scabiei* var. *canis* will not breed on humans but causes pruritus	Microscopic examination of multiple deep skin scrapes. Mites often present in small numbers, risking false negative results. Serology	Appropriate acaricidal treatment, including in-contact animals
Demodex canis	Adults live in hair follicles and sebaceous glands. Life cycle approximately 3 weeks, entirely on host. Transmission from nursing bitch to puppies by direct contact within first few days after birth	Small number of mites usual, producing no clinical signs. On some individual hosts (possible genetic predisposition or immunocompromised) mites multiply and cause disease. Can be localized or generalized, and latter either juvenile-onset or adult-onset	Squeeze affected skin to expel mites from follicles, and then make deep skin scrapes (see QRG 27.2). These and hair pluckings examined microscopically for adult mites and immature stages	Localized disease may resolve spontaneously. Generalized forms may require prolonged and extensive treatment. Treat secondary bacterial infections. Investigate and treat underlying conditions in adult-onset demodicosis
Cheyletiella parasitovorax (rabbit fur mite)	Obligate parasites with life cycle on a single individual. Transmission is direct or via fomites such as grooming equipment	Dry scaly pruritic dermatitis. Can be zoonotic	Identification of mites on tape strips examined microscopically (see QRG 27.1)	No authorized product but insecticides such as fipronil and selenium sulphide may be effective. Treat environment with insecticidal spray and wash bedding
Trombicula (subgen. *Neotrombicula*) *autumnalis* (harvest mite)	Adults live in soil. Parasitic larvae produced in late summer and autumn. Clusters of mites seen as bright orange specks, frequently on interdigital skin and around the base of the pinnae	Can be associated with localized pruritus	Visible to the naked eye	Fipronil may be effective, although infestation is self-limiting

3.19   (continued) Common ectoparasites of dogs. See also Chapters 27 and 29. (Illustrations © Susan Paterson) ▶

Species (most common in bold)	Transmission	Clinical signs and health risks	Diagnostics	Treatment and control
Intestinal nematodes				
Toxocara canis (dog roundworm)	Transmission to adult dogs through ingestion of infective embryonated eggs from the environment. Puppies are infected via placenta or milk or from mother's faeces	Heavy infestation in puppies may lead to poor growth and typical pot-bellied appearance. GI disturbances often occur. Transtracheal migration of many larvae in puppies may cause respiratory signs. Zoonotic: especially in children through ingestion of eggs from environment. In aberrant human host, visceral larva migrans may develop – larvae travel to organs such as brain or retina where they encyst and may cause disease	Identify eggs microscopically after faecal flotation	Ubiquitous: all adult dogs should be treated regularly without recourse to a specific diagnosis. Give anthelmintics at regular intervals (3, 6 or 12 months depending on lifestyle) throughout life. Treat pregnant bitches with fenbendazole from day 40 of pregnancy to 2 days postpartum. Treat puppies from 2 weeks of age, monthly until 6 months old. Client education: encourage owners to collect and hygienically dispose of dog faeces promptly, to prevent environmental contamination
Toxascaris leonina	Transmission to adults is through ingestion of infective embryonated eggs from the environment	More likely to infect older puppies and adults. Zoonotic risk lower than for *T. canis*	Identify eggs microscopically after faecal flotation	Regular anthelmintic treatment. Prompt hygienic disposal of faeces

3.20   Common helminth parasites of dogs. (continues) ▶

Species (most common in bold)	Transmission	Clinical signs and health risks	Diagnostics	Treatment and control
Intestinal nematodes contd				
Ancylostoma caninum, Uncinaria stenocephala (hookworms)	Infective larvae enter host by direct ingestion, via paratenic host, or by passage through pedal skin. Transmission may be common in kennelled dogs	Anaemia: may be severe and acute, especially in heavy infestations in young puppies. Intestinal or respiratory disease. Pedal dermatitis. Zoonotic: larval migration through skin causes dermatitis; adult worms in bowel may cause enteritis	Identify eggs microscopically after faecal flotation	Regular anthelmintic treatment. Prompt hygienic disposal of faeces
Trichuris vulpis (whipworm)	Transmission through ingestion of eggs from contaminated environment. As with hookworms, grass paddocks on which dogs have been kept for years may become very heavily infected	Heavy infestations may cause haemorrhagic colitis, anaemia, and stunted growth of puppies	Identify eggs microscopically after faecal flotation	Regular anthelmintic treatment. Prompt hygienic disposal of faeces
Lungworms				
Angiostrongylus vasorum (dog lungworm)	Life cycle approximately 50 days. Transmision via ingestion of infected intermediate host; these slugs and snails are often quite small and can be ingested accidentally when dog eats vegetation, plays with toys or drinks from bowls kept outside. Until recent years was confined to restricted areas of UK (e.g. SW England, South Wales, Surrey) but now reported in most counties, possibly partly due to increasing urbanization of fox (also a definitive host)	Potentially very serious, even fatal: respiratory signs; bleeding diatheses; neurological signs. Non-specific signs (e.g. inappetence, vomiting, diarrhoea, weight loss)	Identify L1 larvae in faeces (Baermann technique). Egg shedding intermittent; examine separately faecal samples collected on 3 consecutive days to reduce risk of false negatives. L1 larvae may also be detected in bronchoalveolar lavage (BAL) samples	Treat with an appropriate systemic anthelmintic authorized for use against this parasite, e.g. products containing milbemycin or moxidectin
Oslerus osleri	Life cycle 10–18 weeks. Transmission via ingestion of larvae in contaminated environment. Associated with grass paddocks used regularly to exercise dogs for many years	Inflammatory nodules formed around worms in airways cause respiratory signs, especially a persistent cough	Visualization of airway nodules by bronchoscopy or radiography. Detection of L1 larvae in a BAL sample	Avoid keeping dogs on 'stale' grass paddocks where contamination levels are high. Appropriate anthelmintic treatment
Crenosoma vulpis (fox lungworm)	Transmission via ingestion of larvae in mollusc intermediate host. Main definitive host is the fox: increasing urbanization of this species may have led to parasite becoming increasingly common	Mild to moderate respiratory signs	Baermann faecal analysis technique	Treat with an appropriate systemic anthelmintic authorized for use against this parasite or against *A. vasorum*
Tapeworms				
Dipylidium caninum, Taenia pisiformis, Taenia multiceps, Echinococcus granulosus, Echinococcus multilocularis	Transmission via ingestion of intermediate host. *D. caninum*: fleas ingested accidentally when dog grooms. *Taenia, Echinococcus*: infected cysts eaten by dog through hunting or scavenging activities, or in raw/undercooked meat. *E. multilocularis* mainly confined to Continental Europe	Motile proglottids may cause minor irritation to perianal area. Heavy infestations may lead to GI disturbance and weight loss. *Echinococcus* carry serious zoonotic risk	Proglottids may be detected in faeces, in environment or adherent to coat around anal area	Treat with appropriate cestocides. Treatment for fleas is an integral part of *Dipylidium* control. *Taenia, Echinococcus*: prevent dogs hunting and scavenging; do not feed raw or undercooked meat. For animals whose lifestyle potentially brings them into contact with infected intermediate hosts (e.g. farm dogs in Welsh hill farms) cestocide treatment should be repeated regularly (monthly) to limit reinfection. NB PETS travel scheme (see Figure 3.13)

3.20 (continued) Common helminth parasites of dogs.

References and further reading

BSAVA (2013) *PetSavers Puppy Guide.* [available from www.petsavers.org.uk]

Evans J and White K (2002) *The Book of the Bitch, 2nd edn.* Interpet, Dorking

Soulsby E (1983) *Helminths, Arthropods and Protozoa of Domesticated Animals, 7th edn.* Lea & Febiger, London

QUICK REFERENCE GUIDES

QRG 3.1 Head-to-tail general examination

See also Figure 3.16. More detailed ocular, neurological and oral examinations are described in Chapters 21, 11, 16 and 20.

1 Examine the cornea, sclera, anterior chamber, pupil and iris in both eyes, the external surfaces and margins of the upper and lower eyelids, the nictitating membranes, the conjunctivae and the periorbital skin.

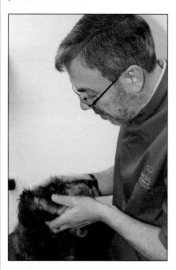

2 Examine the buccal surfaces of all the teeth, the gums and the lips. The external nares are also inspected.

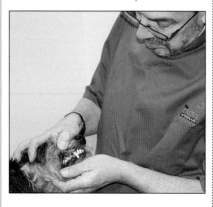

3 Open the mouth and examine the lingual and occlusal surfaces of the teeth, the oral mucosal membranes, the oropharynx and the hard and soft palate. The range and ease of movement of the temporomandibular joints can also be assessed.

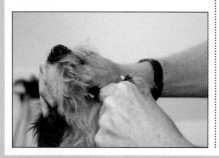

4 Examine both surfaces of the pinnae and the dorsal aspects of the external auditory canals, as well as the skin and coat of the face in that area.

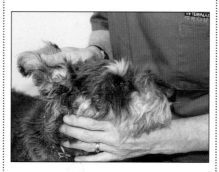

5 Palpate around the head and face on both sides, particularly caudal to the angles of the jaw to assess the submandibular lymph nodes. Also palpate around the ventral neck and throat, and assess tracheal sensitivity.

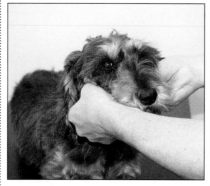

6 Gently palpate the abdomen to assess size and shape of the abdominal organs (liver, kidneys, gastrointestinal tract, bladder, uterus) and for the presence of abnormal structures, fluid or gas. Any apparent pain on palpation should be noted. The spine, ribs and sternum are also palpated.

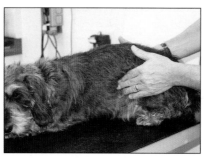

7 Inspect the skin and haircoat for skin lesions, coat abnormalities, cutaneous/subcutaneous masses and evidence of ectoparasites (grooming with a flea comb may assist this).

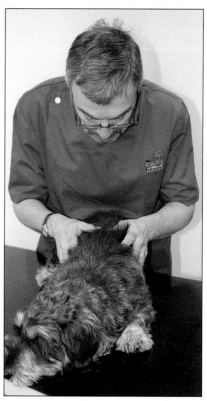

8 Palpate and inspect the structures on the ventral body surface (mammary glands in the bitch; scrotum, testes and prepuce in the dog). The femoral pulse is also palpated at this time.

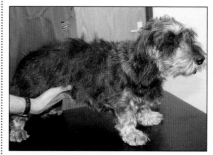

9 Lift the tail to examine the anal sphincter, perianal skin (and the vulva in the bitch). The anal gland area should also be palpated externally.

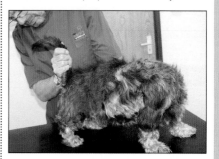

▶

QRG 3.1 *continued*

10 Palpate each leg in turn along its length and then gently manipulate it to assess movement. The superficial lymph nodes (popliteal and prescapular) are also assessed at this stage.

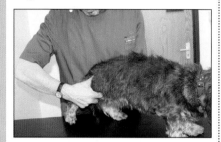

11 Examine each foot, including the pads, toes and claws.

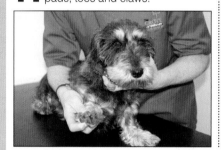

12 The heart, and then the lung fields, are carefully auscultated on each side.

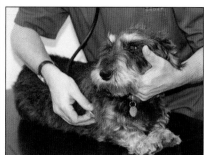

The clinical examination may be varied depending on signalment, previous clinical history and clinical abnormalities identified.

■ If indicated by the history or by the initial external examination, the external auditory canal and the tympanic membrane are examined using an otoscope with a clean speculum of the correct size (see also QRG 22.2).

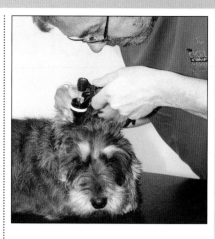

■ If the history or initial examination indicate, the eyes, including their internal structures, are examined in a darkened room with magnification from a direct ophthalmoscope (see also Chapter 21).

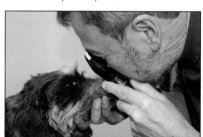

Nutrition

Marge Chandler

Dogs are often considered to be omnivores, meaning that they will eat both plants and animals; however, they do have some nutritional limitations. Like cats, dogs conjugate bile acids only with taurine, cannot synthesize vitamin D, and require dietary arginine. Unlike cats, however, dogs can live on a balanced and complete vegetarian diet. If food is available *ad libitum*, dogs will eat larger and fewer meals (four to eight per day) than cats. Obesity and weight management are mentioned below; see Chapter 14 for consideration of polyphagia and unintended weight loss.

Nutritional assessment

The World Small Animal Veterinary Association (WSAVA) has established an initiative to establish nutritional assessment as the fifth vital assessment (5VA) after temperature, pulse, respiration and pain; and the WSAVA has set up guidelines and tools for assessing nutritional status (www.wsava.org/educational/global-nutrition-committee).

Nutritional assessment includes consideration of animal-specific, diet-specific, feeding management and environmental factors.

- Animal-specific factors include age, life stage, activity, and disorders requiring specific dietary management.
- Diet-specific factors include diet safety and appropriateness (considerations include balance, quality, spoilage, contamination).
- Feeding factors include feeding frequency, timing, location and method (considerations include over- or underfeeding, treats, scavenging).
- Environmental factors include housing, other pets, access to the outdoors, and environmental enrichment.

The nutritional assessment has two parts: a screening evaluation and, when needed, an extended evaluation.

Screening evaluation
The screening evaluation should be performed for every pet at every visit, together with routine history-taking and physical examination. It includes:

- Dietary history
- Bodyweight
- Body condition score (BCS)
- Muscle condition assessment
- Evaluation of the haircoat.

Methods for assessing body condition score use either a 9- or a 5-point scale (Figure 4.1), with 4/9–5/9 or 3/5 ideal for dogs. Body condition is determined using visual appearance (e.g. is a waist apparent) and palpation of the amount of fat over the ribs. A body fat index (BFI) has also been developed, which is especially useful for overweight dogs (Figure 4.2).

The BCS and BFI evaluate body fat, but muscle loss can occur separately from fat loss, especially during illness (Figure 4.3). Disease may cause loss of muscle mass due to cytokine and neurohormonal effects on metabolism. Muscle mass scoring systems are based on palpation of skeletal muscle over the skull, scapulae, spine and pelvis (Figure 4.4).

If abnormalities are found during the screening evaluation of the dog, or an unconventional diet is being fed, an extended evaluation may be indicated.

Extended evaluation
Additional animal-specific factors include changes in food intake or eating behaviour.

The diagnostic investigation usually includes a minimum database (haematology, serum chemistry, urinalysis, possibly blood pressure) and other indicated tests, e.g. faecal tests, serum folate, vitamin B12, thyroxine, canine-specific pancreatic lipase, and imaging. The effects of nutrient wasting diseases such as diabetes mellitus or protein-losing enteropathies should be considered. Serum electrolyte concentrations or appetite may be affected by medications.

Diet-specific factors include the caloric density of the food. Any additional foods, e.g. treats, scavenging and food given to administer medication, should be evaluated for their effect on the overall diet balance and caloric intake. If contamination of the food is suspected, testing should be performed (e.g. for aflatoxins, *Salmonella*). The diet should also be assessed to determine whether it is complete and

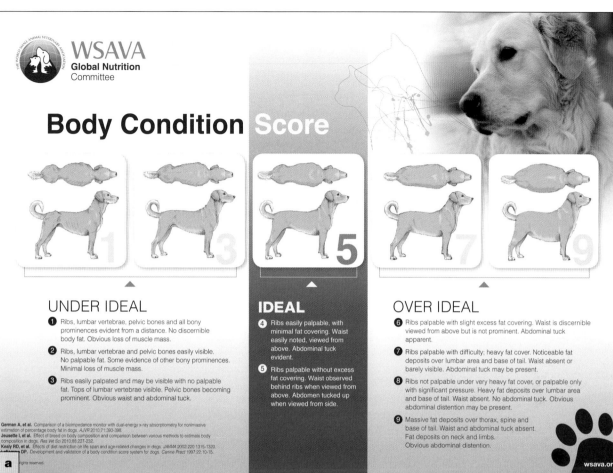

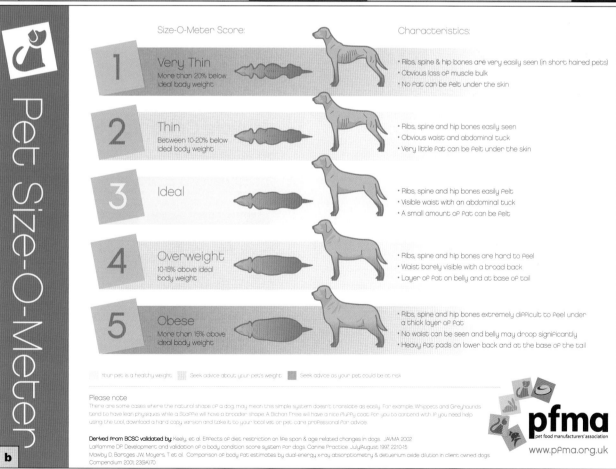

4.1 All dogs should be assigned a body condition score (BCS). **(a)** This WSAVA chart scores body condition out of 9. (Courtesy of WSAVA Global Nutrition Committee) **(b)** A 5-point scale may also be used for body condition scoring. (© Pet Food Manufacturers Association)

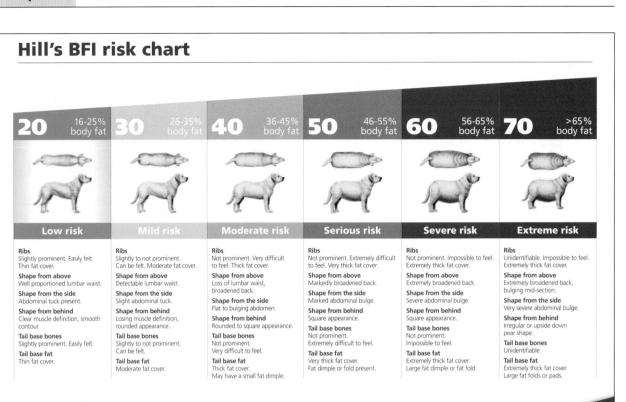

Hill's BFI risk chart

20 16-25% body fat	30 26-35% body fat	40 36-45% body fat	50 46-55% body fat	60 56-65% body fat	70 >65% body fat
Low risk	**Mild risk**	**Moderate risk**	**Serious risk**	**Severe risk**	**Extreme risk**

Low risk

Ribs Slightly prominent. Easily felt. Thin fat cover.
Shape from above Well proportioned lumbar waist.
Shape from the side Abdominal tuck present.
Shape from behind Clear muscle definition, smooth contour.
Tail base bones Slightly prominent. Easily felt.
Tail base fat Thin fat cover.

Mild risk

Ribs Slightly to not prominent. Can be felt. Moderate fat cover.
Shape from above Detectable lumbar waist.
Shape from the side Slight abdominal tuck.
Shape from behind Losing muscle definition, rounded appearance.
Tail base bones Slightly to not prominent. Can be felt.
Tail base fat Moderate fat cover.

Moderate risk

Ribs Not prominent. Very difficult to feel. Thick fat cover.
Shape from above Loss of lumbar waist, broadened back.
Shape from the side Flat to bulging abdomen.
Shape from behind Rounded to square appearance.
Tail base bones Not prominent. Very difficult to feel.
Tail base fat Thick fat cover. May have a small fat dimple.

Serious risk

Ribs Not prominent. Extremely difficult to feel. Very thick fat cover.
Shape from above Markedly broadened back.
Shape from the side Marked abdominal bulge.
Shape from behind Square appearance.
Tail base bones Not prominent. Extremely difficult to feel.
Tail base fat Very thick fat cover. Fat dimple or fold present.

Severe risk

Ribs Not prominent. Impossible to feel. Extremely thick fat cover.
Shape from above Extremely broadened back.
Shape from the side Severe abdominal bulge.
Shape from behind Square appearance.
Tail base bones Not prominent. Impossible to feel.
Tail base fat Extremely thick fat cover. Large fat dimple or fat fold.

Extreme risk

Ribs Unidentifiable. Impossible to feel. Extremely thick fat cover.
Shape from above Extremely broadened back, bulging mid-section.
Shape from the side Very severe abdominal bulge.
Shape from behind Irregular or upside down pear shape.
Tail base bones Unidentifiable.
Tail base fat Extremely thick fat cover. Large fat folds or pads.

PRESCRIPTION DIET

www.HillsWeightLoss.co.uk   www.HillsWeightLoss.ie

4.2 The body fat index (BFI) is especially useful for overweight dogs (© Reprinted with permission by the copyright owner, Hill's Pet Nutrition, Inc.)

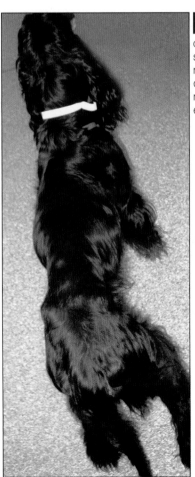

4.3 This 2-year-old Gordon Setter is showing severe muscle loss. The dog had a thoracic mass and was eating poorly.

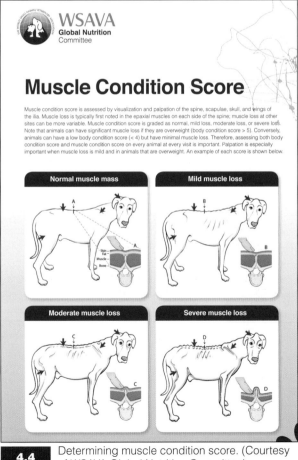

WSAVA Global Nutrition Committee

Muscle Condition Score

Muscle condition score is assessed by visualization and palpation of the spine, scapulae, skull, and wings of the ilia. Muscle loss is typically first noted in the epaxial muscles on each side of the spine; muscle loss at other sites can be more variable. Muscle condition score is graded as normal, mild loss, moderate loss, or severe loss. Note that animals can have significant muscle loss if they are overweight (body condition score > 5). Conversely, animals can have a low body condition score (< 4) but have minimal muscle loss. Therefore, assessing both body condition score and muscle condition score on every animal at every visit is important. Palpation is especially important when muscle loss is mild and in animals that are overweight. An example of each score is shown below.

Normal muscle mass | Mild muscle loss
Moderate muscle loss | Severe muscle loss

4.4 Determining muscle condition score. (Courtesy of WSAVA Global Nutrition Committee)

balanced. Many homemade diets are not balanced, including many published in books or online. Some commercial diets are incomplete treats and should be labelled as 'complementary' food. Pet foods that are complete and balanced will state this on the label.

Dietary recommendations

Ideally, every dog should have a dietary recommendation on its discharge sheet. If no change is recommended, the owners should be advised that the current diet is adequate.

Therapeutic diets may be indicated; however, not all patients with a disease (e.g. hepatic, renal, cardiac) need a commercial therapeutic diet labelled as being for such disease. A concurrent disease may take precedence for diet recommendations, or a specific commercial diet may not be appropriate for the individual dog because of the disease stage or manifestation. For example, some diets for liver disease are protein-restricted, which is most appropriate when hepatic encephalopathy is present. In early (e.g. International Renal Interest Society (IRIS) Stage 1) chronic kidney disease however, a senior diet may initially be better than a severely protein-restricted diet. While the use of therapeutic diets for specific disorders is beyond the scope of this chapter, Figure 4.5 notes the features of some of the available diets that may be appropriate for a range of conditions. For more detail on clinical nutrition the reader is directed to the *BSAVA Manual of Canine and Feline Rehabilitation, Supportive and Palliative Care*.

Disorder	Potentially beneficial dietary attributes
Chronic kidney disease	Restricted phosphorus, moderate protein restriction, increased vitamins, high palatability, omega-3 fatty acids, medium-chain triglycerides
Cognitive dysfunction	Antioxidants, omega-3 fatty acids
Chronic small intestinal diarrhoea	Hydrolysed protein or novel protein, high digestibility, moderate to low fat
Colitis (chronic, idiopathic)	Increased mixed fibres (soluble and insoluble)
Constipation	Increased mixed fibres (soluble and insoluble)
Food hypersensitivity	Hydrolysed protein or novel protein
Hyperlipidaemia	Low fat (not necessarily low in calories unless weight loss is needed)
Liver disorders with hepatic encephalopathy	Vegetable proteins and moderate to restricted protein level, high palatability
Obesity	Low fat, low calories, ± high fibre, increased protein, possibly L-carnitine
Osteoarthritis	Omega-3 fatty acids
Pancreatitis	Low fat (not necessarily low in calories unless weight loss is needed)
Urolithiasis	Exact diet depends upon type of stone; generally decrease urine concentration, may adjust urine pH and decrease constituent stone minerals

4.5 Beneficial dietary attributes for dogs with selected disorders.

Life-stage feeding

Life-stage feeding means feeding to suit the needs of a dog of a specific age or physiological state, e.g. maintenance, reproduction, growth, old age. Requirements are summarized in Figure 4.6 and discussed further below.

Adult maintenance

Healthy adult dogs not doing hard work or exercise and neither pregnant nor lactating have 'maintenance' nutritional requirements. Further division is sometimes made into young adult or junior dogs, and mature or middle-aged dogs. One definition of 'junior' dogs includes those still growing but sexually mature; while young adults may be up to 5 years old.

> **PRACTICAL TIP**
>
> For nutritional purposes, feeding a dog as an individual is more important than the definitions of age brackets

Energy requirements

As healthy adult dogs vary in bodyweight from about 1 kg to 115 kg, energy requirements are often determined by the *metabolic weight*, which reflects actively metabolizing tissues. Various calculations are proposed for estimating metabolic weight; the most commonly used is bodyweight in kg to the power of 0.75. This, in turn, is used to calculate the *resting energy requirement* (RER), the calories needed at rest in a thermoneutral environment.

> **Resting energy requirement**
>
> RER is usually estimated as:
>
> RER (kcal) = $70 \times$ bodyweight (kg)$^{0.75}$
>
> For dogs between 2 kg and 30 kg, an alternative linear equation may be used:
>
> RER (kcal) = (bodyweight (kg) $\times$ 30) + 70

Healthy, non-working, pet dogs require 1.4–1.8 x RER for *maintenance energy requirements* (MER), also called *daily energy requirements* (DER). This is not an exact science, however, and the DER should be used as a starting guide only. As individual requirements vary greatly, dogs should be fed in order to achieve their ideal (not necessarily current) bodyweight and BCS. Variation occurs due to differences in activity, neutering status, individual metabolism and sometimes environmental temperatures. Due to this variation, owners may find that their dog gains or loses weight if fed according to the package label, and should be advised accordingly. Adjustments are made by estimation until the desired BCS is achieved. There is no magic formula for this, so consistency and patience are required. Owners should be encouraged to bring their dogs for regular weight checks and assessment of BCS until the ideal is reached.

Protein

Protein requirements are dependent upon the quality (amino acid profile) and digestibility of the food. The

Life stage	Energy (kcal)	Protein	Fat	Carbohydrates
Adult	1.4–1.8 x RER	18–23% DMB	10–15% DMB	No specific requirement
Work	2.0–5 x RER	22–34 % DMB 18–25% calories	15 to >50% DMB 20–75% calories	15–65% DMB <10 to 60% calories
Growth (after weaning):				
▪ <50% adult weight	3 x RER	22–32% DMB	10–25% DMB	20% DMB
▪ 50–80% adult weight	2.5 x RER	22–32% DMB	10–25% DMB	20% DMB
▪ >80% adult weight	1.8–2.0 x RER	22–32% DMB	10–25% DMB	20% DMB
Gestation	1.8–2.0 x RER in first 4 weeks 2.2–3.5 x RER in last 5 weeks	20–25% DMB	>8.5% DMB	>20% DMB
Lactation	2–4 x DER	25–35% DMB	>20% DMB	>23% DMB

4.6 Approximate macronutrient guidelines for canine life stages. Always feed calories to ideal body condition as there is great individual variation in requirements. Amounts required by working dogs will depend upon the type and duration of the work.

absolute minimum allowance for crude protein on a dry matter basis (DMB) for adult dogs is 10%, with a recommended range of 15–30%.

Feeding frequency
Adult dogs may be fed once or twice a day, though feeding only once a day may increase the risks of gastric dilatation–volvulus in deep-chested dogs and of hypoglycaemia in toy breeds.

Puppies and feeding for growth
Most commercial puppy foods are higher in calories than adult maintenance foods. After weaning, puppies should be fed for an *optimal* growth rate for bone development and maintenance of appropriate BCS (Figure 4.7), rather than at maximal growth. Excessively rapid growth, especially in large-breed dogs, increases the risk of orthopaedic disorders. If puppies are fat during growth, they are more likely to become over-weight adults. Feeding for a slower growth rate does not decrease the final adult size of the dog, although that size will be achieved at a greater age.

Energy requirements for puppy growth

Per kilogram of bodyweight:

- From weaning to 50% of mature bodyweight, estimated DER = 3 x RER
- For 50–80% adult weight, estimated DER = 2.5 x RER
- During the remaining growth period, estimated DER = 1.8–2.0 x RER

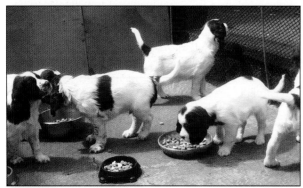

4.7 These growing English Springer Spaniel puppies are showing good body condition (BCS 5/9). (Courtesy of Jimmy Simpson)

Protein and other nutrients
Protein requirements of puppies are highest at weaning and decrease until maturity. For puppies 14 weeks and older, minimum protein requirements are estimated to be 17.5% DMB, with a recommended range of 22–32% DMB, consistent with most commercial puppy foods.

Calculating DMB

To convert from an 'as fed' to a dry matter basis

1. Subtract the percentage of moisture (water) from 100% to determine the percentage of dry matter:
   - If the moisture is >14% it will be stated on the label
   - For dry foods, either obtain the figure from the manufacturer or, less accurately, estimate it at 10%
   - For example, for a canned food this might be: 100%–83% water = 17% dry matter

2. Divide the percentage of the 'as fed' nutrient by the percentage of dry matter (as a fraction)
   - For example, for the same canned food diet with 20% protein on an 'as fed' basis: 7.5% as fed protein (on the label) ÷ 0.17 = 44.1% protein DMB

Notes:

- *When calculating using percentages, first divide the percentage by 100: e.g. 17% becomes 0.17*
- *The amount of a nutrient on a dry matter basis will always be larger than it is on the 'as fed' basis*
- *Remember to use the percentage dry matter, not the percentage moisture.*

To convert from a dry matter basis to an 'as fed' basis

Multiply the 'as fed' figure by the percentage dry matter:

- For example: 44.1% (DM) x 0.17 = 7.5% as fed

Growing puppies also have a requirement for the omega-3 fatty acid docosahexanoic acid (DHA) for normal neural, retinal and auditory development. Fish oils containing omega-3 fatty acids have been shown to improve trainability in puppies.

Growing dogs require more dietary calcium and phosphorus than do adults. However, if puppies are fed a correctly formulated puppy food these minerals should not be supplemented, especially in large breeds, as this can result in orthopaedic developmental disorders. Supplements may contain an incorrect ratio of calcium to phosphorus, and maintaining the correct Ca:P ratio of 1:1 to 1.8:1 in the diet is also important for correct bone growth. It is important to emphasize this to owners.

Feeding frequency

After weaning, most puppies should be fed a measured or weighed amount of food, as free choice or timed feeding are more likely to result in too rapid growth. From 6 weeks to 6 months, puppies should be fed two or three times a day. NB: Toy or other small-breed puppies can become hypoglycaemic if not fed at least this frequently.

Feeding during reproduction and lactation

Prior to breeding, bitches should be in ideal body condition. Most bitches gain 15–25% bodyweight during pregnancy. Most canine fetal growth occurs in the last trimester (about 3 weeks) of gestation.

Energy requirements during pregnancy

- In early pregnancy, energy requirements are only about 18 kcal/kg more than maintenance DER
- After day 40 of gestation, energy needs increase to about 36 kcal/kg more than DER (i.e. an increase of 30–60% of DER), depending upon litter size. After whelping, the energy requirements increase even further and peak between 3 and 5 weeks of lactation. Requirements during this time are 2–4 times maintenance DER

As food intake may be limited by the size of the uterus during pregnancy, a food of higher energy density (>4 kcal per kg of food) may be necessary. Similarly, as the energy requirements of lactation are high, dietary energy density should continue to be high.

PRACTICAL TIP

The energy density of a diet is not always obvious from the packaging. In order to be able to give good advice, it may be necessary to contact the manufacturer

---

Protein and other nutrients

During late pregnancy, protein requirement also increases by 40–70% above maintenance, which requires a diet with 20–25% crude protein DMB. The protein quality should be good, as deficiencies may decrease birth rates and increase early puppy mortality. During lactation, the protein requirement increases more than the energy requirement, so diets should contain high-quality protein at 25–35% DMB. As commercial diets for gestation and lactation are uncommon, a good puppy food, which should be adequate in energy and protein, is often fed during gestation and lactation.

During late pregnancy, dogs may have a requirement for dietary carbohydrates, as >50% of the energy for fetal development comes from glucose. Feeding a diet with 20% carbohydrate calories or >23% carbohydrate DMB should help prevent hypoglycaemia and ketosis in the dam. Sufficient carbohydrate intake also provides for adequate production of milk lactose (Figure 4.8).

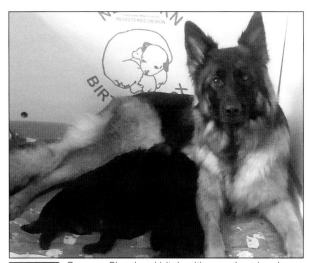

4.8 German Shepherd bitch with puppies showing good growth from adequate lactation. (Courtesy of Nicki Redpath)

Providing fat as at least 20% DMB and including all essential fatty acids is important during late pregnancy and lactation. Increased dietary fat increases caloric density. Inclusion of fish oils in the diet of pregnant and lactating bitches may aid fetal neurological and retinal development (Bauer *et al.* 2006).

Feeding older dogs

Dogs are considered older when they reach about half their life expectancy, e.g. 7 years for small dogs, 5 years for large dogs, and even earlier for some giant breeds. Changes with ageing may include weight gain, arthritis and behavioural changes, as well as increased risk for many other diseases.

Energy requirements

At around 7 years of age there is often a decrease in energy expenditure, and a DER of about 1.4 x RER or less may be appropriate. This is very individual and the diet should be appropriate for body condition and any concurrent disorders. An increase in dietary fibre may help prevent constipation and usually decreases the caloric density.

Protein and other nutrients

Recommendations for protein intake for older dogs are controversial. As muscle mass loss (sarcopenia) is common with ageing, more protein may be needed; however, as the incidence of renal insufficiency increases with age, this must be addressed carefully. High-protein diets have not been shown to increase the risk of kidney disease, but if renal function is already impaired they may or may not affect disease progression (Elliott, 2006). High-quality protein at 15–25% DMB is appropriate for many older dogs.

Phosphorus should be adequate but not excessive, with recommended concentrations of 0.3–0.7% DMB.

The use of diets containing omega-3 fatty acids and antioxidants, such as vitamins E and C, has been researched in older dogs. Oxidative metabolism creating free radicals has been associated with the signs of ageing, and some antioxidant combinations have been shown to decrease oxidative stress and improve cognition. Increased dietary concentrations of omega-3 fatty acids can improve the signs of osteoarthritis. The use of medium-chain triglycerides has also been recommended as an energy source for brain tissue in older dogs and to improve age-related cognitive decline (Taya *et al.*, 2009; Pan *et al.*, 2010).

Feeding for exercise and work

Dietary recommendations for exercise or work depend upon the intensity and duration of the work. Sprinting dogs such as racing Greyhounds have more type II (fast-twitch) muscle fibres, which have more glycolytic capability than type I (slow-twitch) fibres. Dogs performing endurance tasks, e.g. sledge dogs, have more muscle oxidative capacity and type I fibres. Agility dogs, hunting dogs, and dogs doing similar exercise are intermediate athletes; they are more similar to endurance dogs than to sprinting dogs in energy use and muscle type. The determination of fibre type is mostly genetic, although it can be influenced by training.

Muscles need adenosine triphosphate (ATP) for energy. In the first seconds of exercise the source is muscle creatine phosphate. Glucose from muscle and then liver glycogen stores is then metabolized anaerobically by glycolysis. After several minutes the body shifts towards aerobic glucose oxidation. With prolonged exercise, fatty acid oxidation begins, first from fatty acids stored in muscles, and then from lipid stores.

As sprinters depend on anaerobic carbohydrate metabolism and endurance athletes rely on oxidative metabolism, their dietary and caloric requirements differ.

Energy requirements for working dogs

- In dogs sprinting for short periods DER may be 1.6–2 x RER
- For intermediate athletes DER ranges from 2 to 5 x RER
- Dogs doing extremely high levels of work may need >5 x RER

Protein and other nutrients

Sprinting dogs may require a high-carbohydrate diet, although research results are conflicting on the effects on speed of high-carbohydrate *versus* high-fat diets. The more endurance that is required, the more dietary fat may be needed to delay fatigue, although increased fat should be introduced slowly and the diet should remain balanced. Many sporting dogs benefit from the increased caloric density of commercial performance diets, although they should not be allowed to become overweight.

Protein requirements increase slightly with increased work, to maintain protein synthesis. Protein is used as an energy source during work, although for only 5–15% of energy. Generally, fat and carbohydrates should provide energy, and protein should be used for muscle anabolism. High-protein diets (37% of calories) decrease the performance of sprinting dogs compared with a diet containing 24% calories as protein. Intermediate athletes should have at least 24% of calories in the form of protein, which may not be met by some commercial diets.

There is some evidence that vitamin E, at 500 IU/kg DM, can improve performance in endurance dogs through its antioxidant properties improving resistance to muscle fatigue. Selenium may also have beneficial antioxidant effects, but no good evidence exists in dogs.

Choosing a food

The food chosen should be appropriate for the life stage and have appropriate caloric density for the dog's activity and body condition (see above).

Commercial petfoods

The label of a commercial petfood should state that it is a 'complete' food for the life stage, as some are 'complementary' treats. Supplementing with complementary foods, human foods, or treats can cause dietary imbalance, especially if these represent >10% of calorie intake. Ideally, petfood companies should do controlled feeding trials, employ veterinary or animal nutritionists and have good quality control. Top petfood companies support and publish good evidence-based pet nutrition research.

PRACTICAL TIP

Packaging may state 'premium', 'human grade products' or 'hypoallergenic'; these terms have no legal labelling definition and should not be taken into consideration when choosing a food

---

Homemade and raw diets

If an owner wishes to feed homemade or raw diets, the veterinary surgeon should inform them of the potential benefits and risks. The lack of preservatives or additives is appealing to some owners, but means the diets may spoil or become rancid more quickly. Owners should also be aware that a properly balanced homemade diet is not necessarily cheaper than a commercial diet.

The feeding programme for some homemade diets is meant to balance over weeks rather than per meal; however, in a study of such feeding programmes none was found to be balanced and complete (Stockman *et al.*, 2013). A study of a bones and raw food (BARF) diet showed deficiencies in calcium, phosphorus, potassium and zinc (Dillitzer *et al.*, 2011). When human vitamin supplements are used there is a risk of excessively high vitamin D content. Similarly, diets published in books or on websites are often unbalanced or incomplete. Some adult dogs may be able to cope with dietary imbalances, but these may negatively affect the bones, coat, faecal quality, skin and immune system of growing dogs.

Studies on bacterial contamination of canine raw food diets have shown that 80% of diets tested positive for *Salmonella* and many were also positive for *Escherichia coli* and *Yersinia enterocolitica* (Weese *et al*., 2005). Thirty per cent of stool samples from dogs fed raw diets were positive for *Salmonella*. Healthy dogs may cope with ingestion of pathogenic bacteria, but very young, old or immunocompromised dogs may not. Parasites potentially present in raw meat include *Toxoplasma gondii, Sarcocystis, Neospora caninum, Toxocara canis, Taenia* and *Echinococcus*.

> **WARNING**
>
> When handling raw foods, hygiene is very important. Raw meat should not be handled by small children, the elderly or the immunocompromised

Eating bones is sometimes claimed to benefit oral and dental health. However, a study in wild dogs found that although only 2% had dental tartar, 41% had periodontitis (Steenkamp and Gorrel, 1999). Thus, while teeth may appear cleaner, the gums are not necessarily healthier. Bones are sometimes fed as a calcium source; however, analysis of the BARF diet has not confirmed that feeding bones provides adequate calcium. There is also a risk of bones obstructing the oesophagus, stomach or intestines with potential fatal complications. There is no objective evidence that feeding raw bones is safer than feeding cooked bones. If an owner wishes to feed a homemade diet, they should be made fully aware of the risks of inducing malnutrition; any homemade diet should be checked or formulated by a veterinary nutritionist.

Obesity

Overweight or obesity is the most common canine nutritional disorder in many countries, and there has been an estimated 400% increase in the last 25 years in Britain. A survey by Courcier *et al*. (2010b) of prevalence in different countries reported rates of between 24% and 59% in adult dogs.

Severely obese dogs with body fat >40% (Figure 4.9) are at greater risk for anaesthetic and surgical complications, heat or exercise intolerance, cardiorespiratory disorders, dermatopathies, neoplasia, urogenital disorders, abnormal glucose tolerance,

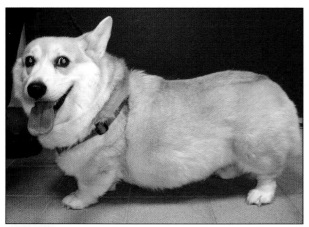

4.9 This 5-year-old male neutered Corgi had a BCS of 9/9 and almost 50% body fat. He was at serious risk of obesity-related disease and a weight loss programme was instigated.

and early mortality. Obesity also exacerbates signs of tracheal collapse and laryngeal paralysis. In a study of obese dogs with osteoarthritis, clinical signs of lameness improved when they lost 6–9% of their bodyweight (Marshall *et al*., 2010). A lifelong feeding trial in Labradors showed that lean dogs on restricted feeding lived almost 2.5 years longer and had less chronic diseases (e.g. arthritis) than those fed *ad libitum* (Kealy *et al*., 2002). Feeding highly palatable diets *ad libitum* is one of the most important factors influencing obesity. Giving table scraps and treats to dogs also contributes. In some adult dogs, up to 50% of calorie intake may be table scraps or human foods, particularly in toy breeds.

Feeding frequency may affect food intake and metabolic efficiency. Increased frequency of meals results in more energy loss due to meal-induced thermogenesis; however, in a small study (Bland *et al*., 2009) the number of meals fed was not linearly associated with canine body condition. Smaller food bowls can help regulate portion size (Murphy *et al*., 2012). Many dogs increase their food intake in the presence of other animals, but being a sole dog in a household has also been associated with increased risk of obesity. Low activity levels are a predictor of obesity in both dogs and cats (Courcier *et al*., 2010ab).

Weight management

Many obesity management programmes exist, and options should be discussed with owners of overweight dogs. Referral to a veterinary nutritionist or a weight loss clinic may help. Losing weight is more difficult than preventing obesity, as the metabolic rate is lowered during calorie restriction. As weight gain often starts after neutering if calorie intake is not adjusted, owners should be advised of the risks at that time. If weight gain and an increase in BCS is noted during the nutritional assessment, an intervention should occur. Further details on obesity and weight management can be found in the *BSAVA Manual of Canine and Feline Rehabilitation, Supportive and Palliative Care*.

References and further reading

Bauer JE, Heinemann KM, Lees G and Waldron MK (2006) Retinal functions of young dogs are improved and maternal plasma phospholipids are altered with diets containing long-chain *n*-3 polyunsaturated fatty acids during gestation, lactation, and after weaning. *Journal of Nutrition* **136**, 1991–1994S

Bland IM, Guthrie-Jones A, Taylor RD and Hill J (2009) Dog obesity: owner attitudes and behaviour. *Preventive Veterinary Medicine* **92**, 333–340

Courcier EA, O'Higgins R, Mellow DJ and Yam PS (2010a) Prevalence and risk factors for feline obesity in a first opinion practice in Glasgow, Scotland. *Journal of Feline Medicine and Surgery* **12**, 746–753

Courcier EA, Thomson RM, Mellor DJ and Yam PS (2010b) An epidemiological study of environmental factors associated with canine obesity. *Journal of Small Animal Practice* **51**, 362–367

Debraekeleer J, Gross K and Zicker S (2010) Feeding growing puppies: post weaning to adulthood. In: *Small Animal Clinical Nutrition, 5th edn*, ed. MS Hand *et al*., pp. 311–320. Mark Morris Institute, Topeka, KS

Dillitzer N, Becker N and Kienzle E (2011) Intake of minerals, trace elements and vitamins in bone and raw food rations in adult dogs. *British Journal of Nutrition* **106**, S53–S56

Elliott D (2006) Nutritional management of chronic renal disease in dogs and cats. *Veterinary Clinics of North America: Small Animal Practice* **36**, 1377–1384

Fascetti AJ and Delaney SJ (2012) Feeding the healthy dog and cat. In: *Applied Veterinary Clinical Nutrition*, ed. AJ Fascetti and SJ Delaney, pp.75–94. Wiley Blackwell, Oxford

Kealy RD, Lawler D, Ballam J *et al*. (2002) Effects of diet restriction on life span and age-related changes in dogs. *Journal of the American Veterinary Medical Association* **220**, 1315–1320

Laflamme DP (1997) Development and validation of a body condition score system for dogs: a clinical tool. *Canine Practice* **22**, 10–15

Laflamme DP (2008) Pet food safety: dietary protein. *Topics in Companion Animal Medicine* **23**(3), 154–157

Lindley S and Watson P (2010) *BSAVA Manual of Canine and Feline Rehabilitation, Supportive and Palliative Care: Case Studies in Patient Management.* BSAVA Publications, Gloucester

Marshall WG, Hazewinkel HAW, Mullen D *et al.* (2010) The effect of weight loss on lameness in obese dogs with osteoarthritis. *Veterinary Research Communications* **34**, 241–253

Murphy M, Lusby AL, Bartges JW and Kirk CA (2012) Size of food bowl and scoop affects amount of food owners feed their dogs. *Animal Physiology and Nutrition* **96**, 237–241

National Research Council (NRC) (2006) Feeding behaviour of dogs and cats. In: *Nutrient Requirements of Dogs and Cats*, pp.22–27. National Academies Press, Washington DC

Pan Y, Larson B, Araujo JA *et al.* (2010) Dietary supplementation with medium-chain TAG has long-lasting cognition-enhancing effects in aged dogs. *British Journal of Nutrition* **103**, 1746–1754

Steenkamp G and Gorrel C (1999) Oral and dental conditions in adult African wild dog skulls: a preliminary report. *Journal of Veterinary Dentistry* **16**(2), 65–68

Stockman J, Fascetti AJ, Kass PH and Larsen JA (2013) Evaluation of recipes of home-prepared maintenance diets for dogs. *Journal of the American Veterinary Medical Association* **242**, 1500–1505

Taya AM, Henderson ST and Burnham WM (2009) Dietary enrichment with medium chain triglycerides (AC-1203) elevates polyunsaturated fatty acids in the parietal cortex of aged dogs: implications for treating age-related cognitive decline. *Neurochemistry Research* **34**, 1619–1625

Weese JS, Rousseau J, and Arroyo L (2005) Bacteriological evaluation of commercial canine and feline raw diets. *Canadian Veterinary Journal* **46**, 513–516

Useful websites

American Academy of Veterinary Nutrition: www.aavn.org
American College of Veterinary Nutrition: www.acvn.org
Pet Food Manufacturers Association: www.pfma.org.uk
WSAVA: www.wsava.org/educational/global-nutrition-committee

Reproductive management

Angelika von Heimendahl

This chapter considers the management of canine reproduction: how to prevent unwanted pregnancies; pre-breeding advice; and normal whelping. It also discusses common neonatal problems. Details of reproductive physiology can be found in the *BSAVA Manual of Canine and Feline Reproduction and Neonatology*. A clinical approach to some disorders of the reproductive tract is given in Chapter 26.

Prevention of breeding in the bitch

Prevention of breeding in the bitch is one of the most common requests in general practice. Neutering advice varies greatly throughout the world, depending very much on welfare views of managing canine populations and the rights of the individual. In the UK most practices recommend spaying at 6 months of age or waiting until the bitch has had one season. In the USA many puppies are neutered before 12 weeks of age while in the possession of the breeder or a rescue centre. At the other end of the spectrum, in Norway ovariohysterectomy is considered mutilation and prohibited under an animal welfare act, as it is defined as invasive elective surgery on a healthy animal.

There are temporary and permanent, invasive and non-invasive methods to choose from. When advising on which method to choose to prevent oestrus in the female, or whether to leave them entire, it is important to inform the owner of the different options and also to take known factors (e.g. previous accidental matings, entire dog cohabiting) into consideration.

Non-invasive, temporary approach
Drugs can be used for the temporary suppression of oestrus (Figure 5.1).

Progestogens
Synthetic analogues of progesterone are often used for the short-term postponement (given in early pro-oestrus) or prolonged delay (given in anoestrus) of oestrus. Care should be taken if administering progesterone analogues during pro-oestrus as the combination of oestrogen and progesterone may induce uterine disease and subsequent pyometra. Progesterone also

Drug	Example of commercial product	Comments
Proligestone	Delvosteron	Injectable
Medroxyprogesterone	Promone-E	Injectable
Megestrol	Ovarid	Daily tablet
Testosterone	Durateston	Injectable
Norethisterone [a]	Many products	Short-acting

5.1 Drugs used for the temporary suppression of oestrus. [a] = not authorized for use in dogs.

alters behaviour, libido and appetite, leading to decreased activity and weight gain. Progestogens have also been reported to lead to mammary gland tumours, diabetes mellitus and Cushing's syndrome.

GnRH superagonist
In some countries implants of the gonadotrophin-releasing hormone (GnRH) superagonist deslorelin are inserted during oestrus and then subsequently every 12 months to suppress oestrus. This has far fewer side effects than progestogens as it works at the pituitary level to suppress GnRH receptors. The drug is not yet authorized for this use.

Invasive, permanent approach
The most common technique used is ovariohysterectomy (OHE; see QRG 5.1). As the removal of the ovaries and uterus is irreversible, it is important to be aware of the advantages and disadvantages of the procedure for each individual.

> **Advantages of neutering**
> - Decreased incidence of mammary gland neoplasia
> - No uterine or ovarian disease
> - No oestrus and associated problems (male attention, roaming, pseudopregnancy, vaginal hyperplasia)
> - No pregnancy-related problems

- Early neutering decreases the incidence of mammary gland neoplasia. Bitches that have been neutered before puberty have an incidence of mammary gland neoplasia of <0.5%. This increases with each season and there seems to be no benefit after three seasons (Egenvall *et al.*, 2002).

- Pyometra is a common problem in entire females and about 15% will develop it during their lifetime. With the removal of the gonads and uterus, the occurrence of any diseases of these organs is eliminated.
- Problems with oestrus range from difficulties of giving bitches their usual walk, through not wanting to have an animal with sanguineous discharge in the house twice a year, to not being able to avoid accidental matings. The practicalities of non-surgical options should be discussed with the owners.

The disadvantages of neutering are often not discussed, as spaying is presented as the 'responsible pet ownership' option. There are, however, certain problems that may arise with neutering.

Disadvantages of neutering

- Surgical procedure and potential complications
- Risk of urinary incontinence
- Increased risk of obesity

- Short-term surgical complications range from haemorrhage of the ovarian and/or uterine pedicles, to postoperative infections and the breakdown of sutures. Long-term problems are mostly ovarian remnants and granulomas.
- Urinary incontinence is caused by the lack of stimulation of the external urethral sphincter by oestrogen. Incontinence can start from 6 months to many years after removal of the gonads, but on average, if it does occur, onset is about 2.5 years after neutering. Leaving bitches entire for longer has no preventive benefit. Urinary incontinence is much more common in breeds with an adult bodyweight >30 kg and in some breeds in particular, such as Boxers. Neutering before 3 months of age also increases the likelihood of developing urinary incontinence later in life.
- The decrease in mammary gland tumours is a well known advantage of early neutering. It is less well known that certain uncommon high-morbidity tumours (e.g. haemangiosarcoma, osteosarcoma and transitional cell carcinoma; Society of Theriogenology (2009)) may occur after early neutering, which in the UK is carried out at 6 months or, more recently, at 6–8 weeks of age.
- A decrease in activity and a lowered metabolism may lead to obesity and associated problems such as diabetes mellitus, cranial crucial ligament injury and osteoarthritis.

Ovariectomy *versus* ovariohysterectomy

The use of OHE is based on the belief that the removal of the uterus will prevent any future disease of the organ. Another concern of many practitioners is the occurrence of so-called 'stump pyometras'. In fact, once the ovaries are removed, the uterus atrophies and becomes totally inactive. **Stump pyometra only occurs in combination with an ovarian remnant and never on its own.**

Extensive trials in Utrecht (Okkens *et al.*, 1997) compared two groups of bitches, one group ovariectomized and the other ovariohysterectomized, for 8–11 years after surgery. There was no difference in the degree of pyometra or any uterine disease, or in urinary incontinence. Although surgeons that have performed OHE for many years are very skilled and fast, ovariectomy is a less invasive procedure, requiring smaller incisions and less surgical time. It can also be performed endoscopically.

Pregnancy termination

Before embarking on any treatment to terminate a possible pregnancy, the likelihood of conception at the time of mating should be established. This is possible without any risk to the outcome as the drug used, aglepristone, may be used throughout pregnancy.

Aglepristone is a synthetic steroid that has a strong binding affinity for progesterone receptors in the uterus of the bitch. It has a short half-life of around 4 days. As it blocks progesterone, it is important to administer during late pro-oestrus or oestrus, as there is a danger of sperm 'outliving' the treatment or further later matings, still achieving fertilization. Another approach is to wait for 3–4 weeks to establish whether the bitch has become pregnant, and then treat.

Using aglepristone (Alizin) in the bitch

- Inject 10 mg/kg s.c.: two injections over 24 hours
- Accurate bodyweight required for correct dose
- Can be used on days 0 to 45 of pregnancy
  - Prior to day 22 = ~100% efficacy
  - After day 22 = 95% efficacy
- Use at the end of oestrus

Prevention of breeding in the male dog

Routine neutering of male dogs is increasing in the UK. Many practices will recommend castration at 6 months of age. The reasons given are a reduction in testicular and prostate gland disease, and the prevention of unwanted male sexual behaviour such as marking and aggression. Most testicular neoplasia is benign, however, and the common prostatic hyperplasia is very treatable. It is also worth mentioning that castration delays physeal closure and may affect the circumference of long bones. This can be a problem in large breeds prone to osteoarthritis, as there is the tendency for weight gain, giving a fat body on a longer limb and greater leverage on susceptible joints. Dogs are very trainable and unwanted behaviour can easily be avoided. In the case of aggression, in particular fear aggression, castration neither helps nor aggravates the problem. If the dog lives in a controlled responsible pet ownership situation there is no compelling medical reason why the animal should be castrated at a young age.

Non-invasive, temporary approach

There have been several approaches using progestogens, androgens and prolactin, but the drug of choice is the deslorelin implant. Deslorelin is a GnRH superagonist that reduces the production of follicle-stimulating hormone (FSH) and luteinizing hormone (LH) from the pituitary gland, preventing spermatogenesis (Figure 5.2) and testosterone production. Serum testosterone drops to <1 ng/ml within 2–3 weeks and sterility should be achieved by 4–6 weeks post-implantation. Implants are available in different strengths: 4.7 mg and 9.7 mg, one lasting 6 months and the other for 12 months, although individual response may vary greatly. One of the side effects is that testicles shrink markedly but increase in size again when the deslorelin wears off.

> ### WARNING
>
> Care should be taken when valuable stud dogs are presented for implantation, as return to fertility cannot be guaranteed

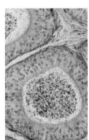 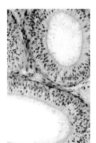 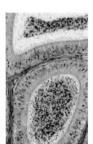

| 15 days prior to 4.7 mg deslorelin implant | 15 days after 4.7 mg deslorelin implant | Recovery |

5.2 Histology of seminiferous tubules before and after deslorelin implant, showing complete absence of sperm while the implant is active.

Immunosterilization is a technique that promises to become available in the future. Several targets of immunocontraception have been identified, such as GnRH, LH and sperm antigens.

Invasive, permanent approach

Castration using an open surgical approach is described in QRG 5.2. Ease of surgical sterilization depends on age (paediatric, adult, geriatric) and the location of the testes (descended, monorchid, cryptorchid). Males castrated before 7 weeks of age have smaller penile and preputial development, with a higher incidence of paraphimosis.

> ### Advantages of neutering
>
> - No testicular neoplasia
> - Reduced incidence of benign prostatic hyperplasia
> - Reduced incidence of marking, roaming and overt male sexual behaviour

> ### Disadvantages of neutering
>
> - Potential complications during surgery
> - Increased risk of certain cancers, e.g. prostatic carcinoma
> - Increased risk of obesity

Breeding advice

There are four main groups of breeders:

- Show and pedigree breeders (organized through the Kennel Club in the UK)
- Breeders of working dogs, mainly Border Collies
- Breeders of racing Greyhounds
- Pet owners, who may wish to have just one litter from their pet.

It is usually the owner of the bitch who approaches the owner of the stud dog to ask for use of the male.

Pet owners should be advised on health testing prior to breeding, the demands of a litter on space and time, and possible complications during pregnancy, birth and lactation. Owners who believe that every bitch should have one litter before she is neutered should be informed that this is not the case. First whelpings have a higher complication rate, and subsequent neutering could then mean a second surgery.

> ### BVA Health Schemes
>
> Canine health schemes provide dog breeders with the option of testing for certain inherited diseases. The following schemes are available and a list of breeds and conditions are attached to each one. Latest information can be found at www.bva.co.uk
>
> - Hip scheme
> - Elbow scheme
> - Eye scheme
> - Chiari malformation/syringomyelia scheme

Most general practices will also deal with Kennel Club (KC) members. The KC has subgroups of breed societies, which are very knowledgeable about their specific breed, its characteristics, problems and any health testing they will recommend before choosing a breeding animal. Many people are not aware of the fact that even when the animals fail testing the offspring can still be registered through the KC as long as the pedigree proves that they are pure-bred. The KC will register puppies born to a dam over 12 months of age, although most breed societies recommend waiting until 2 years of age for a first litter.

Some physiological considerations
Puberty

- The age of puberty (i.e. first oestrus, sperm production) varies greatly between individuals and also between breeds.
  - Bitches usually 'come into season' for the first time aged 6–12 months, but for some this may be as late as 24–30 months of age.
  - Dogs usually produce some sperm by the age of 6 months, but should not be used for breeding until they are at least 12 months of age, in order to produce sufficient numbers of mature fertile spermatozoa.
- Puberty is affected by age, weight and body condition. The bitch or dog needs to have reached about 80% of its adult bodyweight, with some accessory fat deposits. Larger breeds tend to reach that weight later and therefore start puberty later.

- The first oestrus of a bitch is sometimes unovulatory, with long periods of sanguineous vulval discharge and low progesterone levels. The next oestrus will usually follow shortly afterwards and follow through normally with ovulation occurring; this is sometimes referred to by breeders as a 'split season'. This has no bearing on her future fertility.

The canine oestrous cycle

The normal bitch cycle is unique in the world of mammals, having the following characteristics.

- Long inter-oestrus interval, which is non-seasonal: bitches will cycle on average every 7 months, although inter-oestrus intervals of 5–12 months are normal. Some more 'primitive' breeds (e.g. Basenji) will have only one oestrous cycle a year.
- Long duration of pro-oestrus/oestrus: up to 30 days.
  - Outward signs of pro-oestrus are a serosanguineous vulval discharge and an enlargement of the vulval lips. 'Days in season' are counted from then on. Increased interest from male dogs and frequent urination are further signs.
  - During early oestrus, oestrogen declines and cells inside the unovulated follicles begin to produce progesterone, so that mating technically takes place in the early luteal phase (Figure 5.3). The change from oestrogen to progesterone also causes characteristic changes in vaginal cytology (see later) and visible shrinkage of the vulval mucosa, resulting in small wrinkles.
  - A bitch is said to be 'in season' when she will accept mating. Behavioural changes include standing, turning of the tail, and spinal lordosis. Bitches in oestrus produce pheromones that can be detected by male dogs and also seem to stimulate GnRH release in other females. However, mating behaviour is not a good indicator of the fertile period.
- Bitches are spontaneous multiple ovulators. Ovulation may occur as early as 5 days into pro-oestrus/oestrus or as late as 25 days, although most bitches will ovulate between 10 and 15 days after the onset of pro-oestrus.
- Unlike in other mammals, the oocytes produced are immature and cannot be fertilized for at least 48 hours after ovulation, even if sperm are present.
  - After maturation is completed, the oocyte remains viable for up to 3 days, which is defined as the 'fertilization period' (Figure 5.4).
  - The combination of long oocyte survival and long sperm survival time means that matings that occur over a long period during oestrus can result in pregnancies.
- Non-pregnant and pregnant females undergo similar physiological changes.
  - Progesterone influences the transport time of the ova/embryos through the oviduct and encourages the closure of the cervix. The progesterone phase of the cycle lasts for 61–65 days regardless of whether the bitch is pregnant or not. In pregnant bitches, the progesterone phase ends at parturition (see Figure 5.11).
  - The luteal phase in the pregnant and non-pregnant bitch is almost identical. The fall in progesterone level at the end of 2 months induces a rise in prolactin and, with it, lactation. The changes caused by the long progesterone phase and the subsequent prolactin phase in the non-pregnant female, such as increased appetite, change in character, mammary gland development, lactation and nesting, have been described as 'pseudopregnancy'. In other species this refers to females that have had sterile matings or have uterine contents that will keep them in a 'state of pregnancy'. In the bitch this phase is physiological and only sometimes causes problems, which are easily treated with 5–7 days of anti-prolactins such as cabergoline.
  - The influence of oestrogen followed by progesterone may lead to cystic endometrial hyperplasia and/or pyometra. Fertility in the bitch will deteriorate over successive seasons if she does not become pregnant.

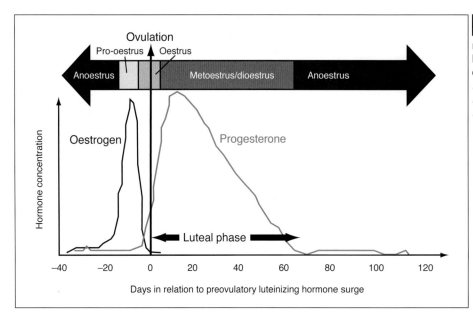

5.3 Different stages of the oestrous cycle in relation to changes in plasma hormone concentrations and ovulation. (Reproduced from *BSAVA Manual of Canine and Feline Reproduction and Neonatology, 2nd edn*)

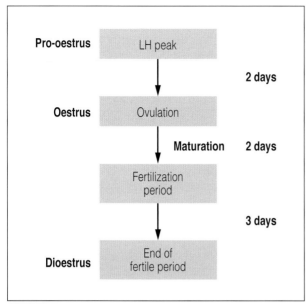

5.4 Timing of ovulation and fertilization. LH = luteinizing hormone.

Inducing oestrus

Predicting the start of a season is impossible because of the variation in inter-oestrus intervals between bitches, and even within one individual. Oestrus can sometimes be brought on by the presence of other bitches in oestrus, by changes of environment or by the introduction of an unknown male. This great variation makes planning the year ahead very difficult for breeders, especially when they want to use a stud dog from overseas.

Drugs that have been used to induce oestrus in the bitch

- Prolactin antagonists, e.g. cabergoline
- GnRH agonists, e.g. deslorelin

Note that these drugs are not specifically authorized for this use

---

Pre-breeding examination

Bitches and dogs presented for breeding purposes should be examined for general health and possible previous breeding history.

- Animals with known conditions such as epilepsy, diabetes mellitus, disc prolapses, hip dysplasia or degenerative eye diseases should be excluded from breeding.
- Although many registered breeds have specific health problems, there is also over-optimism that 'crosses' are always healthy.
- Vaccinations and worming should be up to date before the bitch comes into season, if at all possible.
- Some breeders still request swabbing dogs or bitches for possible infections. These swabs have no clinical relevance, as they tend to grow a mixture of staphylococci, streptococci and *Escherichia coli* that will not be a problem. Only if there is an unusually copious amount of

malodorous discharge is an investigation useful. Routine use of antibiotics is detrimental to the commensal bacterial flora of the mucosa and counterproductive, as well as potentially creating resistance in the long term.

Assessing fertility in the male dog

Fertility in the male dog can be evaluated by collecting and assessing semen. Testosterone production and Leydig cell maturation starts at about 5 months of age and most dogs will produce viable sperm by the time they are 10–12 months old, with smaller breeds maturing slightly earlier than larger breeds. Total sperm output increases from then on until about 2 years of age, when it plateaus.

Spermatogenesis

- Spermatogenesis in the dog follows the same path as in other species
- Spermatogenesis and final maturation take about 60 days
- Dogs will store large numbers of spermatozoa (400–1200 million) depending on body size and testicular volume
- Daily production of sperm in a frequently ejaculated dog will reach about 400 million per day

---

Semen collection: There are several collection kits available commercially. A dog handler or familiar person should be present. It is usually best to have a teaser bitch in season available in order to achieve ejaculation.

1. Once the bulbous part of the penis begins to swell, the prepuce is pushed backwards over the bulbus penis.
2. The base of the penis is held by the person collecting and turned backwards, so that collection takes place between the hindlegs of the dog.
3. Dogs ejaculate in three fractions. In a medium-sized dog the following volumes may be produced:
   i. A small amount of prostatic fluid (0.5–1.0 ml)
   ii. Sperm-rich fraction (0.5–3.0 ml)
   iii. Prostatic fluid (5–20 ml).
4. Once ejaculation occurs, the first and second fractions are collected (Figure 5.5).
5. The semen is kept at room temperature for evaluation.

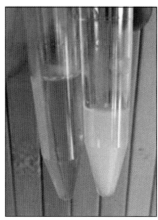

5.5 Collection tubes with different fractions of the ejaculate. The prostatic fluid is clear whereas the sperm-rich fraction is a cloudy white.

Semen evaluation: The following parameters can be assessed.

- Volume: can be measured easily using calibrated collection tubes.
- Colour: should be assessed to record possible contamination with urine or blood.
- Sperm concentration: can be determined using specialist equipment or a haemocytometer counting chamber. Total sperm output (TSO) can be calculated by multiplying volume by concentration.
- Motility: assessed subjectively by placing a small amount of sperm on a warmed slide under the microscope. Sperm motility is extremely temperature-dependent and care must be taken to achieve and maintain body temperature on the slide during assessment. In a normal fertile dog, >80% of the sperm will show forwardly progressive motility.
- Morphology: requires vital staining of spermatozoa, which will kill them and allow assessment under high magnification (Figure 5.6). Spermatozoa are made up of the head (containing the nucleus and acrosome), the midpiece (containing the mitochondria) and the tail. A normal fertile dog will have 80% normal live spermatozoa.

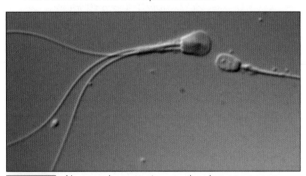

5.6 Abnormal spermatozoa, showing one sperm with three tails and another with a swollen midpiece. Both heads also have several vacuoles on the surface.

Optimum mating time

Breeders have determined optimum mating times for dogs over thousands of years. They use behavioural changes and outward signs of the drop in oestrogen and rise in progesterone to find the right time for mating:

- Bitch standing and receptive
- Dog showing mounting and mating behaviour
- Mating on set days (e.g. days 11 and 13 when ovulation is likely)
- Colour change of vulval discharge from sanguineous to serum colour
- Decrease of vulval swelling and wrinkling of the inner vulval mucosa.

When these parameters are recorded carefully and accurately, and animals are of a reasonable breeding age (2–6 years), pregnancy rates are remarkably high, at between 70 and 80%.

Veterinary surgeons are often contacted when a bitch has been mated several times and not become pregnant, or when breeders have used progesterone testing successfully before. Stud dog owners find it particularly useful to have bitches tested before the

stud is brought over as they often have no other control over the suitability of mating dates. It is also useful to emphasize to breeders that once the ovulation date is determined, whelping dates can be predicted accurately as well.

Once ovulation has taken place, matings may be attempted from +1 to + 4 days from then. Usually two matings are booked with the stud dog within this period.

Veterinary techniques that can be used to determine optimal mating time are:

- Vaginal cytology
- Plasma progesterone assay
- Endoscopy
- Ultrasonography.

Vaginal cytology

Vaginal cytology is used routinely to determine different stages during pro-oestrus and oestrus in the bitch. It is cheap and easy and requires just a little experience. Samples are collected by aspiration with a plastic catheter and 1 ml syringe, or using a cotton bud. The cells (not too many) are transferred on to a microscope slide and spread into a thin film. Smears are then stained using Wright–Giemsa (or Diff-Quik) in the usual way.

The cells found will indicate whether there is any hormonal influence:

- With the increase of oestrogen, the cells become larger and rounded, with a small nucleus (Figure 5.7a)
- A rise in progesterone causes the cells to keratinize (Figure 5.7b); the percentage of anuclear cells usually increases to >80% during the fertilization period
- Once large numbers of polymorphonuclear leucocytes are found, the fertile period has ended.

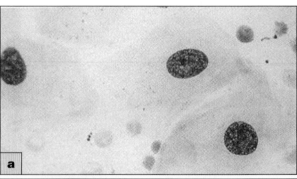

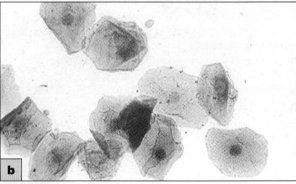

5.7 Vaginal cytology. **(a)** Large rounded cells with small nuclei are typical of the oestrogen phase. **(b)** Keratinized squamous cells are typical of the fertile phase. (Diff-Quik; original magnification X400)

Plasma progesterone assay

Progesterone is produced in the bitch by pre-ovulatory follicles and corpora lutea. Plasma levels accurately reflect stages in the oestrous cycle (see Figure 5.3). They can be used to:

- Predict ovulation
- Confirm ovulation has taken place
- Monitor 'silent seasons'
- Determine the end of the fertile period
- Monitor the luteal phase during pregnancy
- Predict parturition.

Progesterone can be measured in house, using semi-quantitative ELISA kits (Figure 5.8), or sent to commercial laboratories.

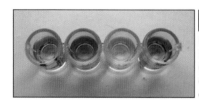

5.8

ELISA wells from an in-house testing kit (Premate), showing different concentrations of progesterone.

PRACTICAL TIP

Plasma progesterone levels are measured in either ng/ml or nmol/l: 1 ng/ml = 3.14 nmol/l

Interpretation of progesterone levels

- Luteinizing hormone (LH) release: progesterone 4.5–7.5 nmol/l (1.5–2.5 ng/ml) 36–48 hours before ovulation
- Ovulation: progesterone 15–20 nmol/l (5–7 ng/ml)
- Fertile period: progesterone 25–75 nmol/l (10–25 ng/ml)

Once progesterone starts to rise, it roughly doubles every 2 days, and testing should be spaced accordingly so as to limit expense to the breeder. Given the 2 days' maturation time for canine oocytes and the long fertilization period, testing should not be more frequent than every 48 hours.

Endoscopy

Endoscopy reveals the changes in the vaginal mucosa relating to the different stages in the cycle (Figure 5.9). Unlike in other species, the mucosa changes from being moist, pink and oedematous during pro-oestrus to a shrinking and wrinkly appearance with a pale colour during peak oestrus. As the bitch moves into metoestrus the mucosa takes on a patchy thin-walled appearance.

Endoscopy is a helpful tool, if available, and most bitches will not require sedation, but it cannot be used alone to determine optimum mating time.

Ultrasonography

Using real-time B-mode ultrasonography and 5 MHz, 7.5 MHz and 10 MHz probes it is possible to visualize the ovaries of the bitch. Follicular growth can then be monitored on a daily basis to detect ovulation. However, the corpus haemorrhagicum, which follows ovulation, has a very similar appearance to pre-ovulatory follicles. In most animals some clipping of the flank area is required; this is very unpopular with breeders as it can take many months for the hair to grow back and excludes them from showing the dog.

Mating

The act of mating takes longer in dogs than in most other animals. The dog and bitch will display courting behaviour when they first meet but it is usually the bitch who decides whether she will accept the

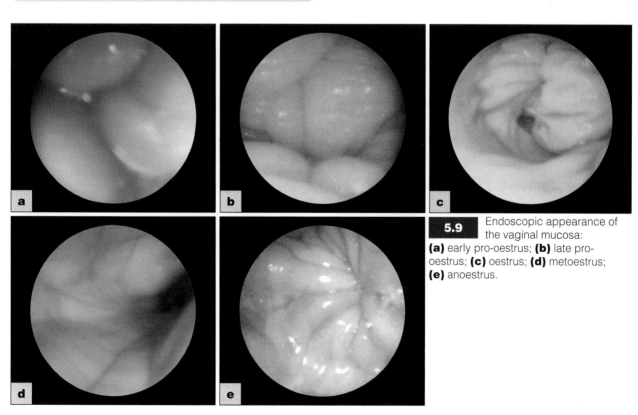

5.9 Endoscopic appearance of the vaginal mucosa: **(a)** early pro-oestrus; **(b)** late pro-oestrus; **(c)** oestrus; **(d)** metoestrus; **(e)** anoestrus.

male, unless he is very experienced and dominant. The dog will then mount the bitch and try to achieve intromission, with a partially erect penis, helped by the penile bone. Once intromission has been achieved, the bulbous part of the penis will extend fully inside the vagina and thus 'tie' the male to the female. This is followed by ejaculation. The tie can last for 5–60 minutes. Breeders refer to matings where a tie is not achieved and the dog ejaculates as 'slip matings'; they can still lead to pregnancies but pregnancy rates are lower and fewer puppies are usually born.

Sperm survival in the female tract is particularly long: good-quality semen can survive and fertilize for up to 7 days.

Pregnancy diagnosis

Early pregnancy diagnosis in the bitch is difficult and unreliable. Owners will sometimes notice a persistent swelling of the vulva, change in behaviour, swelling of the nipples and occasional malaise. A small amount of white sticky non-odorous discharge can sometimes be observed in mid-pregnancy.

Manual palpation

Depending on the size of the bitch and the experience of the veterinary surgeon, the pregnant uterus can be palpated at around 3 weeks of gestation. Each conceptus has a circumference of around 15 mm and they are well separated from each other. At 4 weeks they have grown to around 25 mm; they then start to become soft, and the uterus extends overall.

Ultrasonography

B-mode real-time scanners using a 5–10 MHz probe can be used to detect pregnancy from about 17 days onwards, although given the long sperm survival time it is better to wait until about 25–28 days. As well as establishing an estimate of the number of puppies, viability through imaging heart beats can also be assessed. Figure 5.10 shows an ultrasound image of a 4-week pregnancy.

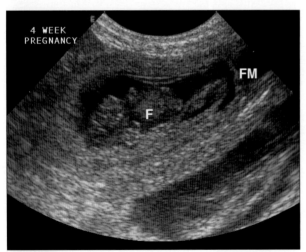

5.10 A 4-week pregnancy in a Jack Russell Terrier. The fetus (F) is clearly visible, surrounded by fetal fluids and fetal membranes (FM), within the uterus. (Reproduced from *BSAVA Manual of Canine and Feline Ultrasonography*)

Relaxin assay

Relaxin is the only pregnancy-specific hormone in the bitch and is produced in measurable amounts from about 25 days of pregnancy. It can be assessed using whole blood and an in-house ELISA kit or by a commercial laboratory. Persistence of relaxin for a few days after possible fetal reabsorption sometimes leads to false-positive results.

Radiography

Radiography is a very useful tool in later pregnancy, from about 42 days onwards. It is also helpful close to birth to establish accurate numbers and positioning of the puppies.

Normal pregnancy

Physiological changes in the bitch

The bitch has to undergo certain changes to accommodate a pregnancy.

- Blood volumes are increased by about 40%, which is achieved mainly through haemodilution.
- Cardiac output and oxygen demand increase by 20%.
- Pregnancy may induce transient type 2 diabetes. Calcium demand increases with fetal growth and mineralization and with initiation of lactation. Supplementation with calcium should be avoided, however, as it hinders the secretion of parathyroid hormone.
- Food intake increases to around 125% of the normal ration, depending on the number of puppies, during the last trimester of pregnancy. Changing bitches on to puppy food at this stage of the pregnancy will give them a higher concentration of nutrients and sufficient calcium intake. Puppy food is also useful during lactation when food intake has to increase still further.

Gestation length

The range in time from mating to parturition in the bitch is not down to a varying length of gestation, but rather to the long survival time of the sperm. **Gestation length is consistent at 63 days from ovulation or 61 days from fertilization**. It is, however, influenced by litter size, with larger litters inducing birth slightly earlier. As a rule of thumb, every puppy over the breed average will decrease gestation length by 0.25 days (Bobic Gavrilovic *et al.*, 2008).

WARNING

If ovulation has been monitored, bitches should not be allowed to go over the due date for more than 24 hours. Primary inertia is a very common condition in the bitch and care must be taken not to miss it due to the mistaken belief that pregnancy may be extended without any problem

---

Pre-whelping health checks are advised (see Chapter 3).

Parturition

Determining the day of parturition

As noted above, the easiest way is to determine when ovulation occurred and count 63 days from then. Other indicators that can be used are listed below.

- **Behavioural changes:** including nesting, panting, separation from other animals and sometimes vomiting and diarrhoea.
- **Outward signs of impending birth:** including marked relaxation of the pelvic, abdominal and perineal musculature, due to elevated relaxin levels.
- **Drop in body temperature:** body temperature fluctuates in the last week before parturition, but drops markedly 12 hours before birth, induced by the drop in progesterone. This does not always happen in single puppy pregnancies.
  - Rectal temperature drops from 38.5°C to:
    - 35°C in small breeds
    - 36°C in medium-sized breeds
    - 37°C in large breeds
    - This difference is due to changes in the ratio between body surface area and volume (bodyweight).
  - Owners should measure body temperature, using the same thermometer, three times a day.
- **Drop in plasma progesterone to base levels** (Figure 5.11)**:** veterinary surgeons can confirm the end of gestation by measuring plasma progesterone levels, which drop from 12–15 nmol/l (4–5 ng/ml) to <6 nmol/l (<2 ng/ml) 24 hours before birth. The in-house ELISA tests are fast and reliable for these measurements.

Initiation of parturition

As in other species the release of adrenocorticosteroid hormone by the puppies stimulates the production of prostaglandin F2α, which in turn leads to a rapid decrease in progesterone. The change in the progesterone:oestrogen ratio is the major cause for placental separation, receptor sensitivity to oxytocin and the dilation of the cervix.

> **PRACTICAL TIP**
>
> It is not possible for the veterinary surgeon to palpate the cervix in a bitch as it is too cranial to reach digitally

Stages of parturition

- **First-stage labour** usually lasts for 6–12 hours, but may take as long as 36 hours in primiparous bitches. Signs are panting, shivering and occasional vomiting, although it may not be obvious in some bitches.
- **Second-stage labour** is marked by the first puppy engaging in the pelvis and subsequent strong uterine contraction expelling the puppy. Rectal temperature returns to normal.
  - Each puppy is usually born inside an intact amniotic membrane and the mother has to turn and remove it quickly by licking after the birth.
  - 60–70% of puppies are born in anterior and 30–40% in posterior position.
  - A breech birth presents with only the tail protruding and both hindlegs forward.

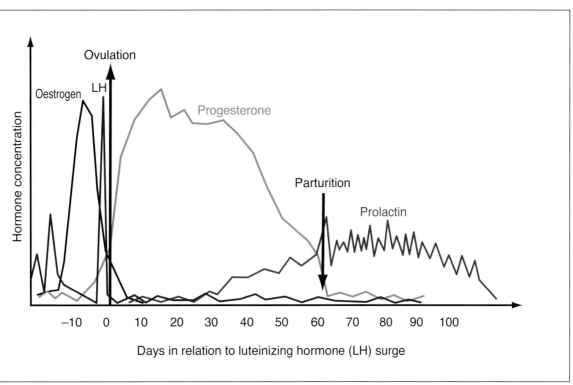

5.11 Endocrinological changes during pregnancy and lactation in the bitch. (Reproduced from *BSAVA Manual of Canine and Feline Reproduction and Neonatology, 2nd edn*)

- **Third-stage labour** is not easily distinguishable in bitches, as placentas are delivered at different times during the birth and do not always immediately follow the birth of a puppy.
  - Retained placentas are extremely rare in the dog and not too much emphasis should be placed on 'missing' placentas.
  - Bitches should be discouraged from eating the placenta, as it leads to vomiting and diarrhoea. In nature eating the placenta cleans the nest and keeps predators away, rather than having any nutritional value.

Normal time parameters around birth

- First-stage labour: around 6–12 hours (longer for first litter)
- Active pushing in second stage: around 30 minutes
- Time between puppies: not more than 3 hours
- Birth from first to last puppy: never more than 24 hours

Birth complications

Manipulation and treatment of inertia and dystocia are successful in less than one third of cases and early decision-making towards caesarean section is often life-saving for puppies and sometimes the dam.

Indicators for caesarean section

- Greenish-black vaginal discharge at full term, without second-stage labour
- More than 61 days after mating, body temperature <37°C and serum progesterone <2 ng/ml (primary inertia)
- >24 hours first-stage labour with no puppies
- >3 hours since last puppy born, and majority of litter still *in utero*
- Three administrations of oxytocin have not resulted in all puppies being delivered

---

The caesarean operation is described in QRG 5.3.

Postpartum care of the dam

Once the last puppy has been delivered, the bitch will usually settle down and make sure the puppies are clean and settled, then have a drink and possibly something to eat.

Lochia (vaginal discharge after giving birth) will be brownish-black and it is normal for the bitch to pass the occasional blood clot. Discharge usually occurs after feeding the puppies, as the release of oxytocin for milk let-down will also induce uterine contractions, helping involution.

It is important to make sure that all the mammary glands look normal in colour and are not hardening. Bitches that do not clean themselves may need some help to make sure the perineal area stays clean and does not become odorous and dirty, especially in long-haired breeds.

Postpartum complications are relatively rare in bitches, compared with many other species.

Neonatal care

The most important contribution towards the wellbeing of puppies is a warm environment. Room temperature in the first week should be between 26 and 28°C, possibly uncomfortable to the lactating bitch but vital to the puppies. Heat lamps and heat pads are of limited use.

It is important that the bitch has enough milk for the number of puppies she has given birth to (puppies are content and putting on weight) and that she cares for them (bitch will clean puppies meticulously, including all urine and faeces). Well fed puppies will only cry for a short time at the start of feeding (squabbling over the best place) and then settle down to drink. Neonates that are fed sufficiently will have a well rounded abdomen, which is soft and shows no pain reaction on palpation. Puppies will feed every 2–4 hours and sleep most of the time between feeding.

Post-parturition and neonatal health checks are also discussed in Chapter 3.

Physical examination

- Neonates have no thermoregulation in the first 2 weeks of life and need to be examined in a warm environment (28–32°C). Heart rate in the first week is 200–250 beats/min and body temperature 36–37°C, well below the adult temperature.
- Checking oral mucous membranes will help to assess hydration, with tacky to dry mucous membranes indicating 5–7% dehydration. When puppies reach 10% dehydration they also have a noticeable decrease in skin elasticity.
- Neonates presented to the veterinary surgeon or born at the surgery (oxytocin, caesarean section) should always be checked for cleft palate (Figure 5.12), atresia ani and any other obvious abnormalities.
- Haircoat (covering of the paws and tips of the ears) can give some indication of prematurity or heavy ectoparasite infestation.
- Any discharge from eyes or nose, urine staining or diarrhoea should be noted.
- The abdomen should be well rounded without tension or pain response during palpation.
- The sucking reflex should be present.

Clinical signs of any problems are often unusual or non-specific, and a comprehensive history from the owners and comparisons with littermates may be needed.

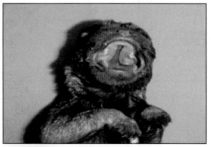

5.12 A newborn puppy with a severe cleft palate. Treatment of such a case would be very difficult, and euthanasia should be advised.

Common paediatric emergencies

Neonatal mortality in puppies in the UK is around 10–20% in the first 3 months of life, with most deaths occurring at birth or in the first week. This is high compared with other veterinary species. In most cases one or two puppies in the litter will die, but it is not unusual to lose whole litters.

It is important to stress to owners that early intervention in neonatal disease can make a significant difference to the outcome of treatment. One should also be realistic about the support that can be provided and explain the different possible outcomes as well as the costs involved.

Hypothermia

Puppies have little subcutaneous fat at birth and use non-shivering thermogenesis for heat regulation. Due to the high surface area to volume ratio in newborns, heat loss is much greater than in older animals.

Hypothermia in newborns

- <34°C at birth
- 35.5°C days 1–3
- <37°C at 1 week of age

Mild hypothermia is expressed through restlessness, crying, reddened mucous membranes and the skin feeling cold to the touch. In more severe cases the neonates become lethargic and uncoordinated. Moisture appears around their lips, and heart and respiratory rates start to fall. Hypothermia in the neonate decreases gut motility, which eventually leads to ileus.

WARNING

Owners will often try and treat 'cold puppies' by encouraging food intake in whichever way possible. Tube-fed or syringe-fed hypothermic neonates will either regurgitate and aspirate food – resulting in pneumonia, or will become bloated – resulting in respiratory distress

---

It is important to rewarm neonates slowly. If outside heat sources (lamps, heat pads, hot water bottles) are used the patient must be checked frequently and its position relative to the heat source changed at regular intervals. In severe cases warm fluids can be given intravenously, intraperitoneally or intraosseously. The temperature of the fluids should never be more than 2 degrees warmer than the body temperature of the patient; otherwise they may develop cyanosis, diarrhoea and fitting. **Only when the neonate has reached its normal body temperature should feeding be attempted.**

Trauma

Unfortunately, dropping or stepping on young puppies is a common occurrence, with owners becoming very distressed. If the puppy has survived the fall and shows no obvious sign of injury it is best to send it home under close observation. In cases of fractures, prognosis in young animals is very positive. Internal organ damage or bleeding are very difficult to treat.

Infectious diseases

More than 90% of the passive immunity of the neonate is provided through colostrum intake and thus depends on the immune status of the dam, who should therefore not be moved to another environment during pregnancy. Permeability of the gut to immunoglobulins starts to decline after 8 hours and is no longer possible after about 48 hours. Passive immunity can last for 6–16 weeks and may interfere with vaccinations.

Canine herpes has been much discussed by breeders recently, although the number of confirmed cases is low. The virus is acquired *in utero* or at birth and causes neurological signs. Puppies cry continually and die within 24–48 hours. Treatment is usually unsuccessful and mortality is close to 100%. The most useful diagnostic tool is post-mortem examination of the puppies, as there are classic changes (small white ischaemic dots) on the liver and kidneys. There is now a vaccine available that is given to the bitch after mating and before parturition.

'Fading puppy' is a general term used to describe the loss of neonates through lack of suckling and weight loss. The onset can be sudden and can start from 24 hours to 2 weeks of age. Clinical signs are not specific and causes may be as varied as bacterial infections, poor mothering, inadequate whelping facilities and congenital abnormalities. Treatment needs to be immediate, with antibiotics, fluids and glucose; the still healthy puppies in the litter also need to be treated.

Diarrhoea in neonates is very common and is usually caused by overfeeding. The puppies should be removed from the dam for 12 hours so that they cannot feed, followed by small frequent meals and oral rehydration. Antibiotics should be avoided in these cases as they further upset the gut flora.

Hypovolaemia

The neonate is particularly susceptible to dehydration, as water makes up >80% of its bodyweight, and water turnover is double that of an adult. Due to the neonate's limited ability to conserve fluids and the immaturity of the kidneys, fluid requirements are high (13–22 ml/100 g bodyweight per day), but total volumes that can be given are low. Maintenance dose is 6 ml/kg/h with an addition of 50% of the deficit over 6 hours. Fluids may be given intravenously, intraosseously, intraperitoneally or subcutaneously, the latter two routes not having very high absorption rates. In most cases lactated Ringer's solution with 20 mmol/l maintenance potassium is sufficient. In severely acidotic patients (on blood sampling) bicarbonate should be added.

Hypoglycaemia

Clinical signs of hypoglycaemia are tremors, excessive crying and irritability, followed by more severe signs of lethargy and coma. Puppies are born with very little stored glycogen and a poor gluconeogenic response of the liver but in a warm healthy environment will survive 24 hours without feeding before blood glucose levels fall below normal levels. Other common causes of hypoglycaemia, besides starvation, are congenital metabolic diseases (e.g. glycogen storage disease and hepatic shunts). Most hypoglycaemic puppies will respond to feeding (making sure also that body temperature is adequate). In severe cases, dextrose at 0.5–1 g/kg i.v. as part of a 5–10% Ringer's or normal saline solution can be administered.

References and further reading

Barr F and Gaschen L (2011) *BSAVA Manual of Canine and Feline Ultrasonography*. BSAVA Publications, Gloucester
Bobic Gavrilovic B, Andersson K and Linde Forsberg C (2008) Reproductive patterns in the domestic dog: a retrospective study of the Drever breed. *Theriogenology* **70**, 783–794
Egenvall A, Bonnett P, Ohagen P *et al.* (2002) Incidence of and survival after mammary tumours in a population of over 80,000 insured female dogs in Sweden from 1995–2002. *Preventive Veterinary Medicine* **69**, 109–127
England G and von Heimendahl A (2010) *BSAVA Manual of Canine and Feline Reproduction and Neonatology, 2nd edn*. BSAVA Publications, Gloucester
Okkens AC, Kooistra HS and Nickel RF (1997) Comparison of long-term effects of ovariectomy versus ovariohysterectomy in bitches. *Journal of Reproduction and Fertility* **51**(Suppl), 227–231
Society of Theriogenology (2009) Position statement on mandatory spay–neuter: Basis for position on mandatory spay–neuter in the canine and feline [available at www.therio.org]

QRG 5.1 Ovariohysterectomy: hints and tips
by Tim Hutchinson

Positioning and preparation

- The bitch is placed in dorsal recumbency. It is preferable to support the thorax with sandbags or a rolled towel rather than using a trough to maintain position: troughs may interfere with access and tend to compress the abdomen, making exteriorization of the ovaries more difficult.

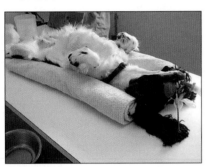

- Hair is clipped and the skin prepared aseptically from the costal arch to the pubis and to 5 cm lateral to the line of the nipples. This may seem excessive to many surgeons, but will facilitate extension of the incision should difficulties be encountered. Most practices will use a single fenestrated drape rather than a four-quadrant technique.
- An assistant is not usually required. However, inexperienced surgeons may value a scrubbed assistant to help with exteriorizing the ovary and ligating the ovarian pedicle, or for obese bitches.

Technique

- A right-handed surgeon will usually stand on the bitch's right flank, as this facilitates manipulation of the intra-abdominal structures (especially the ovarian pedicles). A left-handed surgeon may prefer to stand on the bitch's left flank.

Note: The dog's head is to the right in all the photographs here and the surgeon is right-handed.

1 With the right hand holding the scalpel, the surgeon uses the left hand to tense the skin away from the midline, so that the skin and subcutaneous tissue part easily with a confident scalpel cut.

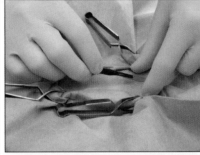

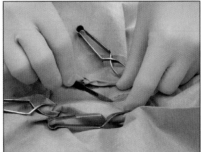

Tension is applied to the skin with the thumb and forefinger of the left hand, whilst the scalpel incision is made from cranial to caudal with the right hand.

- The incision should be as long as is required to access the relevant intra-abdominal structures without compromise. There are no prizes for short incisions and healing time is the same regardless. In fact, it may be argued that an incision that is too short may be more uncomfortable postoperatively, due to increased stretching required intraoperatively, and may delay healing due to bruising caused by that increased stretching.

- As a rule of thumb, a useful starting incision is one that is half the length of the distance between the umbilicus and the pubic brim and centred midway between those two landmarks.

2 In lean animals the linea alba may be visible at this stage, but if there is significant fat coverage a thin connective tissue line between the left and right subcutaneous abdominal fat can usually be seen, and separated with the scalpel to expose the linea alba. Subcutaneous vessels will ooze gently, which can frustrate the surgeon, but there is no need for active haemostasis; they will stop oozing by themselves with simple pressure once the wound is closed at the end of the procedure.

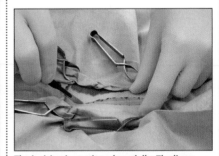

The incision is continued caudally. The linea alba is now visible through the subcutaneous fat. Small amounts of cutaneous haemorrhage can be ignored.

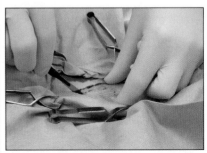

Tension is applied to the fat with the left hand as it is incised, to expose the linea alba. NB The connective tissue is not cleared from the underlying muscle. ▶

QRG 5.1 *continued*

■ Contrary to advice given in many surgical texts, the author prefers not to elevate the fatty tissue from the body wall: this creates a dead space that cannot be closed easily and will often lead to seroma formation. A seroma beneath the midline laparotomy wound can often be erroneously mistaken for herniation, prompting unnecessary surgical intervention at a later stage.

3 The linea alba is grasped with thumb forceps and elevated.

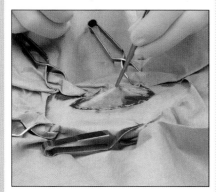

4 With sufficient elevation the linea alba can be penetrated by a stab of the scalpel (with the scalpel held horizontally, cutting edge away from the body) without fear of damage to the viscera.

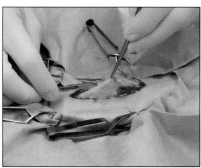

5 The abdomen can then be opened along the linea alba using scissors; the lower blade is introduced through the stab incision and used to elevate the linea alba so that it can be cut confidently without fear of visceral damage.

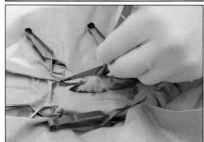

■ Whether the bladder has been emptied prior to surgery or not, it is usually readily apparent and is a useful landmark for locating the uterus: the bladder is reflected to reveal the uterus beneath, which is obvious from its unique bifurcated shape and pink colour that is distinct from the surrounding bowel.

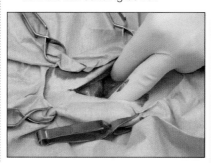

6 One horn of the uterus is grasped and elevated, then followed cranially to locate the attached ovary.

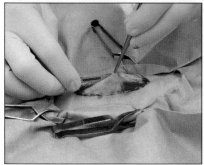

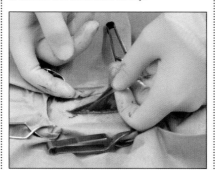

7 The ovary is exteriorized.

■ Exteriorization of the ovary is the part of the procedure that most surgeons find difficult; it is a skill that must be honed through repetition.

■ For a right-handed surgeon the ovary is held firmly in the right hand and traction is applied caudally and away from the body. The ovarian ligament can be palpated as a tight band running cranially from the ovary and the ovarian pedicle will course directly down into the body. The ovarian ligament should be snapped without placing undue tension on the pedicle. This can be achieved by breaking down the ligament with the nail of the index finger of the left hand until it is felt suddenly to give.

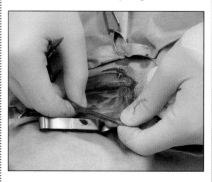

■ Alternatively, the ovarian ligament can be isolated from the surrounding connective tissue and cut with scissors. There is a small vessel that runs alongside the ovarian ligament, which does not require ligation, but a small clamp may be applied at the ovarian end if necessary to stem haemorrhage to improve visibility.

■ With the ovarian ligament sectioned, the ovary should easily be exteriorized from the abdomen and the pedicle can be seen through the fat of the broad ligament.

■ A window is created in the broad ligament to isolate the pedicle.

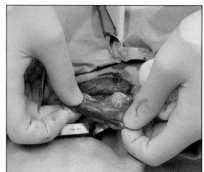

The broad ligament is exposed and a window created using a finger.

8 Paired artery forceps are placed across the pedicle. Placement of the forceps can be made easier by holding the ovary between the first finger and thumb and using the other three fingers to depress the abdominal wall. ▶

QRG 5.1 *continued*

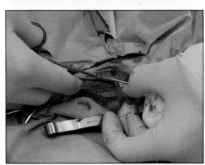

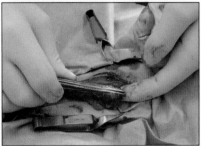

The ovarian pedicle is clamped.

- The pedicle is ligated 1 cm below these clamps. This may be facilitated by first placing a third pair of artery forceps to crush the fat at the desired location for ligation.

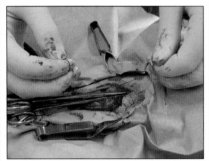

The third pair of clamps has been removed and the area of crushed tissue is ligated.

- Most absorbable suture materials that provide short- to medium-term support are suitable but inexperienced surgeons might prefer the security of a 3 metric (2/0 USP) braided synthetic absorbable suture material such as polyglactin 910 (e.g. Vicryl) or lactomer 9–1 (e.g. Polysorb).

9 With the pedicle ligated, the clamps can be twisted apart to tear through the tissue, or the tissue can simply be cut between the clamps.

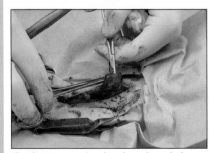

The clamps are twisted to shear through the pedicle.

- One forceps is left attached to the ovarian end of the pedicle to control haemorrhage and the other released from the ligated stump.
- It is helpful to hold the stump with thumb forceps prior to release, to ensure that the ligature is firm and there is no haemorrhage.

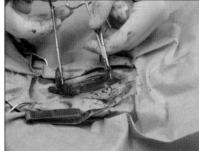

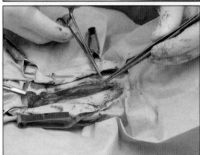

The ligated pedicle is checked for haemorrhage before it is released into the abdomen.

10 The procedure is then repeated for the other ovary.

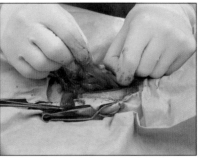

The ovary has been elevated and retracted caudally to allow the ovarian ligament to be broken down using the digits of the left hand.

11 The broad ligament of each uterine horn should be sectioned (with scissors) from the level of the ovary to the cervix, through the least vascular portion, to allow the whole uterus to be elevated from the body. Paired clamps are then placed across the cervix or the body of the uterus.

- The two uterine vessels can be ligated together with the body of the uterus (or cervix) in small dogs, but in larger dogs it may be helpful (and give peace of mind to the inexperienced surgeon) to place transfixing ligatures through the uterine body and around each vessel separately.
- Once ligated the uterus can be sectioned between the clamps and removed.

- The uterine stump is inspected for haemorrhage before it is released into the abdomen.

12 The procedure is then repeated for the other uterine horn.

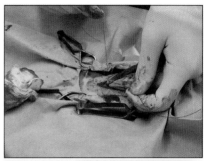

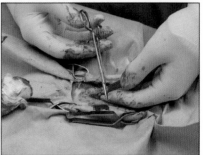

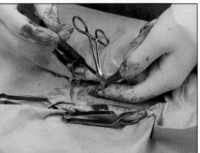

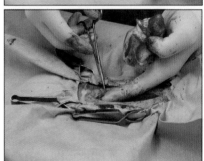

The cervix is ligated, clamped, sectioned and checked for haemorrhage before being released into the abdomen.

- It is likely that every surgeon will experience, at least once, an ovarian or uterine stump that is inadequately ligated and haemorrhages after release into the abdomen. In such circumstances the following steps should be taken:

1. Don't panic – you are not the first surgeon to experience this!
2. Alert a colleague that you might require their assistance.
3. Provide adequate exposure of the bleeding stump:
   i. The uterine stump can be exposed by retraction of the bladder ▶

QRG 5.1 *continued*

ii. The left ovarian pedicle can be exposed by elevating the descending colon and pulling it to the right to use the mesocolon to separate the abdominal viscera from the bleeding vessel

iii. The right ovarian pedicle can be similarly exposed by elevating the duodenum and pulling it to the left.

4. Use a swab to remove the accumulated blood to allow examination of the stump or pedicle – it may be helpful to have the abdominal wall retracted with gusset retractors and use a scrubbed assistant to hold the abdominal viscera away.

5. Place forceps on the vessel and ligate below the tip of the forceps. NB Bleeding ovarian pedicles are often quite friable and attempts to elevate them by pulling on the forceps may lead to further tearing and bleeding. It is better to have an assistant maintain exposure and for you to work with two hands to ligate the vessel intra-abdominally.

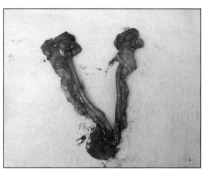

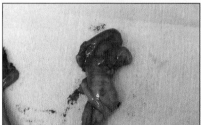

The uterus and ovaries after removal. Both ovaries can be seen to have been removed completely.

13 Whilst it may seem a bold step for an inexperienced surgeon, it is preferable to close the linea alba with a simple continuous suture pattern, so that tension is dissipated along the entire wound.

- A monofilament suture material suitable for tendons should be used, such as polydioxanone (e.g. PDS II) or polyglyconate (e.g. Maxon).
- 3 metric suture (2/0 USP) is suitable for small to medium-large dogs (up to 30 kg), with 4 metric suture (1 USP) used for larger dogs.
- Good knot security is essential, with at least six throws on the first knot and seven on the last.

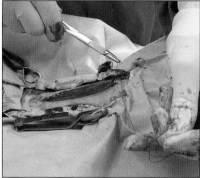

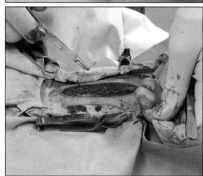

The linea alba is closed using a continuous suture pattern.

- Dead space within the fat is closed using continuous absorbable suture material. Again, it is preferable to use monofilament suture material to avoid tracking of infection should the bitch interfere with the wound postoperatively.

14 The skin can be closed either subcutaneously or with non-absorbable sutures, which are usually removed 10 days after surgery.

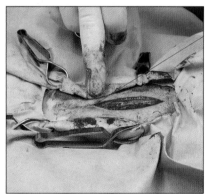

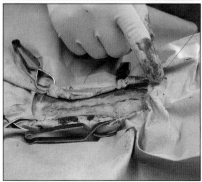

The skin is closed, here using a subcuticular continuous pattern.

- The practice might have a preferred policy for suture choice and closure pattern, so this should be discussed with the practice principal.
- It is a common mistake to place skin sutures too tightly, especially on the ventral midline. When the bitch is placed in an upright position the skin will naturally fall together, so relatively loose sutures are preferable, which will allow for the anticipated postoperative swelling along the line of the incision without inducing cheese-wiring! Sutures that are placed too tightly will be uncomfortable and lead to self-trauma. This may introduce infection and is the commonest cause of wound problems after ovariohysterectomy.

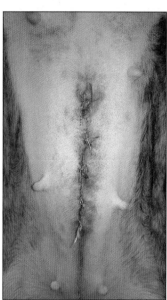

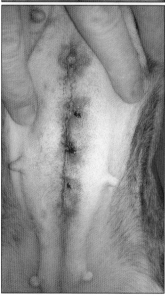

This wound was closed with cruciate mattress sutures. Whilst this is a popular pattern amongst inexperienced surgeons, there is a tendency to tie the sutures too tightly, with the result that the wound tends to invert. This causes discomfort and leads to self-mutilation. Following removal of these sutures it can be seen that the wound is healing poorly where the sutures have been placed. ▶

QRG 5.1 *continued*

Postoperative care

- Postoperatively the wound should be covered for at least 24 hours with a sterile adhesive dressing (e.g. Primapore). After this, provided there is no discharge, the wound may be left uncovered.

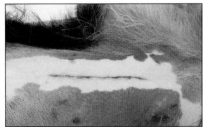

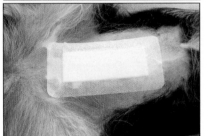

The closed wound is covered by a sterile adhesive dressing.

- It is vital that the bitch does not lick the wound, so use of a barrier collar or T-shirt should be advised.
- Whilst neutering is often considered routine, the client should be advised that their bitch has had major abdominal surgery. She should be taken for short toilet walks only (on a lead) for the first few days and kept restricted to gentle lead exercise for at least 10 days postoperatively.
- Analgesia requirements will vary from bitch to bitch and each should be assessed as an individual.
- The client should be encouraged to contact the practice at any point if they are concerned. However, a routine examination should be arranged 48 hours after surgery. The bitch should be checked for adequate pain control and for any obvious post-anaesthetic complications (ensure eating and drinking, urinating and defecating are normal). The wound should be checked to ensure there is no abnormal swelling or discharge.

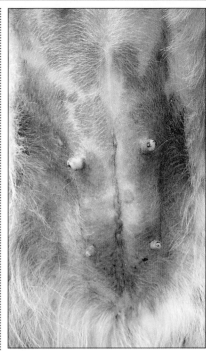

A normally healing ventral midline incision, viewed at the 48-hour postoperative check.

- A further examination is usually booked for a week later and the bitch should be kept to short lead walks in the intervening period.

QRG 5.2 Castration (Orchidectomy): hints and tips

by Tim Hutchinson

It is this author's firm opinion that castration should be performed using an open rather than a closed technique. Closed castration relies on indirect occlusion of the spermatic vessels by ligation of the soft tissues around them. Ligatures that at the time of surgery may appear to have been placed well may subsequently prove to be inadequate, with the result that the vessels may slip through the tunic and haemorrhage intra-abdominally. With open castration, ligatures are placed directly on to the vessels and afford greater security from haemorrhage.

Positioning and preparation

- The dog should be positioned in dorsal recumbency. If castration is routine, with both testicles descended into the scrotum, a trough may be used for positioning, but if either of the testicles is undescended then it is preferable to use a rolled towel or sandbags to avoid the edges of the trough compromising access.

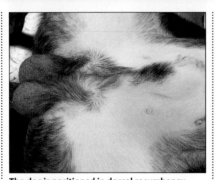

The dog is positioned in dorsal recumbency, with the legs splayed.

- Whilst it is good practice – and part of standard aseptic technique – to remove hair from a wide area around the site of the incision, prescrotal castration is one procedure where the author prefers to keep hair removal to a minimum. Many male dogs become profoundly irritated by excessive hair removal in the inguinal region, especially if there is clipper rash. Postoperative licking can be intense, leading to wound infection,

dehiscence and often a massively swollen and oedematous scrotum. The author's preference is to remove a small strip of hair from directly in front of the scrotum, but to ensure that a wide area of surrounding hairy skin has been scrubbed.

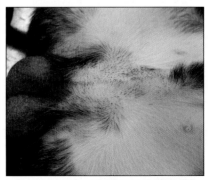

Hair has been removed only over the site of the incision. A broad border, including the inguinal region and scrotum, has been prepared with skin disinfectant.

- A small fenestration in the surgical drape is used. ▶

QRG 5.2 *continued*

Technique

- The author's preference, as a right-handed surgeon, is to stand on the dog's right flank.

Note: The surgeon is right-handed in all the photographs here.

1 The first testicle is squeezed cranially out of the scrotum into the prescrotal region and the left hand used to tense the skin over it and hold firmly. A scalpel is used to cut through the skin (at the midline) and subcutaneous tissues directly down to the spermatic sac, with the left hand continuing to squeeze the testicle through the incision.

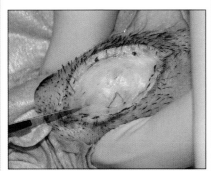

The left hand is used to squeeze the testicle cranially to the scrotum, and the skin is incised in the midline directly over the displaced testicle. The dog's head is to the right.

2 The scalpel is used to incise the spermatic sac, so that the testicle can be squeezed through the incision and the sac pulled down around the cord.

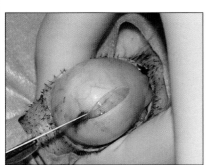

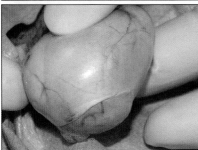

The left hand maintains pressure on the skin over the testicle, so that the spermatic sac bulges through the incision. The dog's head is to the right.

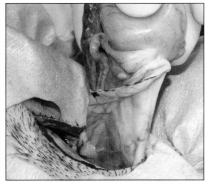

The testicle is exposed and the sac everted. The dog's head is to the left.

3 The sac must be detached from the caudal pole of the testicle by tearing, to free the testicle completely from its soft tissue attachments.

- With gentle traction a large portion of the spermatic cord can be exteriorized, so that paired forceps can be placed proximal to the pampiniform plexus.

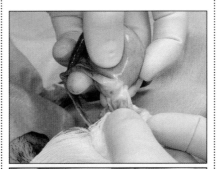

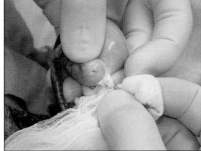

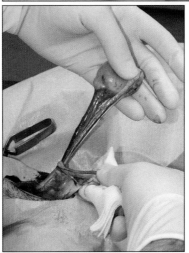

The tunic is separated from the spermatic cord by traction. It is helpful to use a swab to aid grip. The dog's head is to the left.

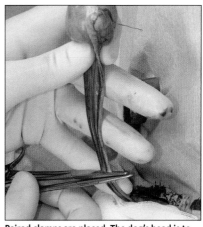

Paired clamps are placed. The dog's head is to the left.

4 The spermatic cord is ligated 1 cm proximal to the forceps. Ligatures may also be transfixed through the vas deferens for greater security if required.

- Most absorbable suture materials giving short- to medium-term support are suitable for these ligatures, but inexperienced surgeons might prefer the security of a 3 metric (2/0 USP) braided synthetic absorbable suture material such as polyglactin 910 (e.g. Vicryl) or lactomer 9–1 (e.g. Polysorb).

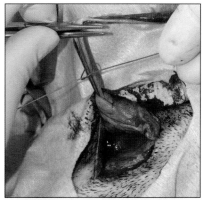

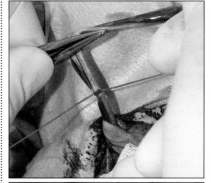

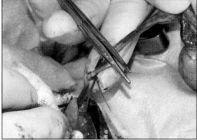

The ligature is placed proximal to the clamps. The dog's head is to the left.   ▶

QRG 5.2 *continued*

5 The spermatic cord is then cut between the forceps. The ligated pedicle should be held after release of the forceps, to ensure that there is no haemorrhage or slippage of the ligature.

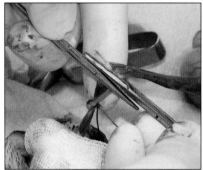

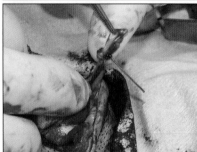

The clamps are sheared apart and the pedicle inspected for haemorrhage before it is released. The dog's head is to the left.

6 The process is then repeated for the second testicle.

■ The scrotum is not routinely ablated, as it will shrink by itself in time to a vestigial structure and this avoids the complications associated with scrotal ablation. Clients should be prepared for this, especially as immediate postoperative swelling may give the appearance that nothing has been removed.

7 There is no need to suture the spermatic sac, so closure consists of suturing the subcuticular tissues and the skin.

■ There may be a preferred practice policy for whether absorbable sutures or skin sutures are placed, so this should be discussed with the practice principal.

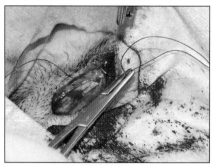
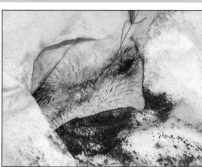

The skin is closed with two layers of sutures, here placed subcutaneously. The dog's head is to the right.

Inguinally retained testicles

■ When testicles have descended through the inguinal ring but not into the scrotum, they are usually palpable within the inguinal region as firm rounded structures that are usually smaller than a fully descended testicle. Occasionally they may be pushed into a pre-scrotal incision; if this is not possible, they are accessed by grasping between the fingers and thumb of the non-dominant hand, tensing up to the overlying skin and incising directly on to them with a scalpel
■ Ligation and closure is then performed as for a fully descended testicle

Abdominally retained testicles

■ If either (or both) testicles cannot be palpated, it should be assumed that they have not passed through the inguinal ring and are still within the abdominal cavity. The dog should be prepared for a caudal abdominal approach, with hair clipped to 5 cm cranial to the umbilicus, lateral to the nipples and around the penis. The skin incision is made parallel to the penis and continued through the subcutaneous fat (ligating vessels as required). By retracting the penis away from the surgeon the ventral midline is exposed, allowing routine entry into the abdominal cavity via the linea alba
■ Locating the testicle is then straightforward: the vas deferens is identified between the bladder and colon. Tracing the path of the vas deferens will lead to the testicle, which will often be considerably smaller than a descended counterpart
■ Ligation is routine, as is closure of the abdomen
■ There will be a pocket of dead space that is difficult, if not impossible, to close between the penis and body wall. Seroma formation at this site is not uncommon

Postoperative care

■ Analgesia should be tailored to the individual patient. Antibiosis is unnecessary for a short clean surgical procedure such as routine castration.
■ As castration wounds can often be irritating to the dog, a barrier collar should be offered in all cases. Owners should be alerted to the fact that the scrotum has not been removed but will shrink gradually over the coming weeks.
■ Owners should be instructed to contact the surgery at any time if

they are concerned; however, a routine re-examination should be scheduled for 48 hours after the surgery. The dog should be checked for adequate pain control and for any obvious post-anaesthetic complications (ensure eating and drinking, urinating and defecating are normal). The wound should be checked to ensure there is no abnormal swelling or discharge. A further examination is usually booked a week later and the dog should be kept to short lead walks in the intervening period.

QRG 5.3 Caesarean section: hints and tips
by Tim Hutchinson

Preoperative preparation

Preparation for a caesarean section will differ from that for a routine bitch ovariohysterectomy because preparation must take into account the delivery of (hopefully) a litter of live puppies.

The following should be available:

- Extra personnel to assist with reviving puppies
- An incubator for the puppies – this can be purpose-made or consist of an enclosed box with hot water bottles and blankets
- Access to doxapram to stimulate breathing in neonates
- Intravenous fluids for the bitch
- Towels: there will be a large volume of fluid from the uterus; towels placed around the animal and the operating table will be necessary to absorb this.

Patient preparation

- Consider withholding standard premedication agents and not administering opiate drugs until after all the puppies have been delivered, to avoid respiratory suppression in the puppies.
- Give careful consideration to the use of other analgesics, as it is unlikely that any will be authorized for use in pregnant or lactating bitches. Analgesia needs to be assessed on an individual basis and 'off-licence' permission granted by the owner of the bitch.

- Positioning the bitch on her back for surgery may compromise her respiration due to the pressure of the distended abdomen on the diaphragm. It may be necessary to elevate the head end of the table.
- Skin preparation, draping and the surgical approach to the abdominal cavity are as for ovariohysterectomy (see QRG 5.1).

Technique

With any caesarean section there is the need to deliver puppies quickly and return the bitch to consciousness promptly, to facilitate suckling and promote puppy survival. It is therefore necessary to work swiftly.

1 Create a longer abdominal incision than is usually required for ovariohysterectomy, so that the uterine horn can be exteriorized on to the surgical drape.

2 Incise the antimesenteric surface of the uterus between two puppies, to allow removal of at least two (and sometimes three or four puppies) from the same incision.

3 Break the membranes from around the puppy. Clamp the umbilical cord approximately 3 cm from the puppy. Cut the cord at the placental side of the forceps and pass the puppy immediately to a nurse to begin reviving it with vigorous towel rubbing. The placenta can then be removed from the uterus by gentle traction.

4 Repeat the procedure for the other uterine horn and create additional incisions in the uterus if required to facilitate rapid access to the puppies.

- There is no need for active haemostasis of vessels in the uterine wall; bleeding will stop quickly as the uterus contracts and involutes.
- Complicated suture patterns are not required for the uterine incisions. A simple inverting continuous pattern can be placed quickly and it should be appreciated that the rapid contraction and involution of the uterus will render any incision a fraction of its original size within a few hours.
- There will be contamination of the abdominal wound by uterine fluids. However, this is likely to be sterile, so quickly sluicing with sterile saline is sufficient prior to routine closure, using continuous suture patterns for the abdominal wall, subcutaneous tissues and skin.

Postoperative care

The puppies should be encouraged to suck from the bitch as soon as she is returned to her kennel, but she should be supervised at all times. As soon as she is able to walk she should be discharged to allow her to settle more readily back into her home environment.

Caesarian section should be considered to be relatively clean surgery of short duration and there is rarely indication for the use of antibiotics.

Considerations for surgical cases

Julian Hoad

The vast majority of pet dogs will, at some stage or another, require some form of surgical intervention. This may be a 'routine' elective procedure, such as neutering, or a non-routine non-elective procedure, such as removal of a foreign body or tumour, or repair of a fracture or traumatic wound. In all but a very few cases this will entail the patient undergoing general anaesthesia. Whilst with modern anaesthetics and monitoring equipment the risk of mortality has reduced dramatically over recent years, the perioperative period is still associated with appreciable morbidity and mortality. Although the surgeon may have clear ideas about what this means and what precautions to take, it is important to realize that the owner may have very different concerns (Figure 6.1). Addressing these concerns adequately will undoubtedly reduce client anxiety

and will also reduce the veterinary surgeon's level of stress and minimize the risk of client complaints or financial disputes.

Proper planning of the perioperative requirements of the patient will reduce the risks of surgery and anaesthesia, and also improve the chances of a successful outcome. Details of specific surgical procedures can be found in the appropriate chapters of this Manual. Further information on anaesthesia and on surgical principles may be found in the *BSAVA Manual of Canine and Feline Anaesthesia and Analgesia* and the *BSAVA Manual of Canine and Feline Surgical Principles: A Foundation Manual*.

Informed consent and client preparation

Written consent should always be obtained from an owner prior to any surgical procedure. In some circumstances it may be necessary to obtain oral consent, for example if, during the course of an investigation, an alternative procedure becomes necessary and the client is phoned for permission. In such cases it is important to make a clear record in the patient's notes of the advice given, in particular that any risks were made clear. The written consent should be in the structure of a consent form, an example of which may be found on the Veterinary Defence Society website (www.veterinarydefence.co.uk). It is important to ensure the client has actually read and understood the form.

For consent to be valid, it must be voluntary and informed.

- **Voluntary:** An owner has the right to decline or refuse consent for a procedure. Generally, where there is refusal, explaining the benefits and risks of the technique compared with alternative techniques may change the client's mind. However, it is never acceptable to try to force a client to consent to any procedure, nor would it be wise to do so, as this will only cause more anger (and potentially legal problems) should complications occur.

Economic considerations

- Cost
- How quickly does money need to be made available?
- Will insurance cover it?
- Will further costs be likely (follow-up radiographs, etc.)?
- Are there different options (lesser procedure, fewer associated tests, reduced hospital time)?

Patient considerations

- How likely is the procedure to succeed?
- How risky is the procedure?
- Is it painful?
- Will it impact on the pet's temperament?
- Is the procedure 'worth it' with regards to age or health?

Practical considerations

- When can it be done (will it interfere with a family holiday or a business trip)?
- Can the owner cope with any aftercare (bandage changes, aiding mobility)?

Moral/personal considerations

- Has a relative had a similar procedure or condition?
- Has the owner had an unfortunate experience before?
- Is there disagreement or dispute in the owner's household which could affect whether the procedure is carried out?
- Does the owner have confidence in the veterinary surgeon performing the procedure?

6.1 Owner/client considerations for surgical procedures.

■ **Informed:** It is the duty of the veterinary surgeon to explain the procedure in terms that the client may understand. This must include any known risks associated with the technique or the anaesthetic (information should not be withheld just because it may upset or worry the client). The costs should be discussed: not only of the procedure itself, but also of any likely follow-up consultations, radiographs or bandage changes. In any non-routine surgical case the option of referral should be made available if the procedure is not usually performed at the practice. Clearly, to give this due attention can take some considerable time and it may not easily be fitted into a consultation period at the time of diagnosis. It may be preferable to make a separate appointment to discuss the surgery, ideally the day before the planned procedure.

Many disputes in veterinary practice are caused by a failure to provide fully informed consent. This may be a failure to provide an adequate estimate of costs, or it may be that the owner's expectations of recovery were unrealistic due to being misinformed. Time spent explaining the procedure to the client should improve client satisfaction and reduce any incidence of reprisals.

PRACTICAL TIPS

■ The client should be made aware that the dog's hair will need to be shaved for the surgical procedure. Some owners may find this more alarming than the procedure itself, so it is worth preparing them. Additionally, some owners, especially those breeding or showing dogs, may be reluctant to have their animals shaved. These concerns must be addressed prior to admission, as shaving the dog against the owner's wishes may constitute 'surgical trespass', rendering the vet liable to legal proceedings
■ It is also worth describing the likely size of the surgical wound, or any disfigurement

---

Preoperative assessment

Patient assessment prior to surgery provides the most important means of increasing patient safety and reducing perioperative complications. An overview of pre-anaesthetic assessment is provided here: the reader is directed to the *BSAVA Manual of Canine and Feline Anaesthesia and Analgesia* for more detailed information.

ASA classification

It is helpful to categorize patients as being at 'low' or 'high' risk from procedures and to take further precautions as appropriate. A scale of patient physical condition has been developed by the American Society for Anesthesiologists (ASA) that enables the user to predict the level of risk for individual patients (Figure 6.2). A thorough preoperative assessment on the day of admission allows the clinician to assign an ASA score to the patient.

Patient class	Physical condition	Examples
I	Normal healthy patient	No disease detectable
II	Mild systemic disease	Mild compensated cardiac valvular disease, well controlled diabetes, uncomplicated fracture
III	Severe systemic disease	Mild congestive heart failure, poorly controlled diabetes mellitus, hyperadrenocorticism, pyrexia, mild to moderate dehydration
IV	Severe systemic disease that is a constant threat to life	Heart failure, severe dehydration, anaemia, toxaemia, uraemia, cachexia
V	Moribund, unlikely to survive beyond 24 hours without surgery	Severe trauma, shock, severe infection, terminal malignancy

6.2 American Society of Anesthesiologists (ASA) physical condition scale.

Signalment

Breed and age are relevant factors to be considered prior to general anaesthesia.

■ **Breed:** Not all dogs have the same tolerances to anaesthetic or sedative agents. For example, Boxers and many giant breeds have a low tolerance of acepromazine. Additionally, brachycephalic dogs often have mild hypoxia prior to anaesthesia (it is not unusual to find a P_aO_2 of <70% in a British Bulldog breathing room air) and may benefit from preoxygenation or may require relatively small endotracheal tubes.
■ **Age:** Immature or elderly patients may have relatively inefficient liver metabolism, resulting in a lower tolerance of anaesthetic or sedative agents. Additionally, elderly patients are more likely to be suffering from systemic illness.

Medical history

Details of the patient's history that may be relevant include any difficulties or problems associated with previous surgery, or the presence of any other condition.

It is important to confirm the presenting complaint: for example, to check which limb is to be radiographed. If removing multiple lumps, it is important to make sure that all lumps to be removed are documented and marked with indelible marker if appropriate. It may be worth discussing with the owner what course of action should be taken if further lumps are found intraoperatively, as occasionally an incidental finding can turn out to be clinically important (Figure 6.3).

Clinical examination

Where possible, the patient should have been given a full clinical examination (see Chapter 3) no more than one week prior to surgery. Any significant problems noted on auscultation should be followed up by radiography, electrocardiography or echocardiography as indicated.

In addition, special considerations on the morning of surgery should include the following:

■ **General health:** This should take in hydration status (it is worthwhile asking whether there has been any diarrhoea or vomiting in the week prior to

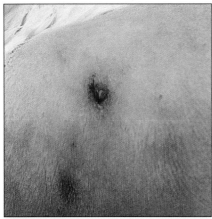

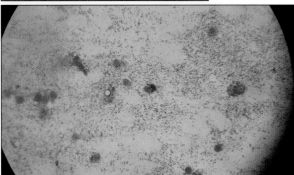

6.3 A skin mass 3 mm in diameter was noted during routine ovariectomy of a 3-year-old Golden Retriever. Fine-needle aspiration suggested that this was a mast cell tumour (MCT). The mass was removed using 2 cm margins; subsequent histopathology (original magnification X400) confirmed a grade II MCT with clear margins.

surgery) and body condition score (see Chapter 4). Obese dogs may have cardiorespiratory compromise; dogs with cachexia may be prone to hypoglycaemia whilst anaesthetized
- **Thoracic auscultation:** Murmurs or arrhythmias may require further investigation prior to anaesthesia. Clients should be asked whether there have been any coughing or breathing problems in the last few weeks. A cough may indicate airway disease (see Chapter 24) and should always be investigated prior to anaesthesia
- **Skin:** In particular, any skin changes that may indicate a chronic disease such as hyperadrenocorticism; also any damaged or infected skin that may interfere with aseptic catheter placement or increase the risk of postoperative infection at the surgical site
- **Nervous system:** Mentation should be assessed, as central nervous system depression may reduce tolerance to anaesthetic agents. *Ensure that any epileptic patients have been given their medication that morning, and adjust the anaesthetic protocol by avoiding acepromazine premedication and tapering the anaesthetic dose.*

Pre-anaesthetic testing

Most practices have in-house laboratories that enable relatively inexpensive biochemistry and haematology tests to be run. However, it is important to balance what *can* be tested with what *should* be tested. It is pointless running a 12-point biochemistry panel on every patient, regardless of age, breed and clinical condition. Indeed, since normal variations in blood

parameters occur, it is likely that a proportion of 'normal' animals could have surgery delayed, and the owners incur further costs, on the basis of an outlying blood result. It is far better to adapt screening protocols specifically to identify 'at-risk' patients. Studies have shown that preoperative blood tests in young healthy animals have little or no benefit.

The decision to perform pre-anaesthetic laboratory testing should be based on the findings of the clinical examination. The tests should preferably be carried out in advance (though ideally no longer than one week in advance), rather than on the day of surgery, so that steps can be taken where appropriate, based on the findings (Figure 6.4).

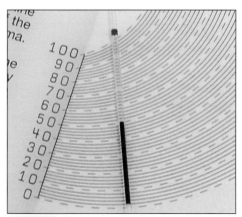

6.4 This 5-year-old neutered female Dobermann was admitted for exploratory laparotomy. Coagulation tests had been performed in the week preceding surgery, in order to rule out von Willebrand's disease.

A good basic panel of tests would include:

- Packed cell volume (PCV; Figure 6.5)
- Total protein (TP)
- Albumin
- Blood glucose
- Urea.

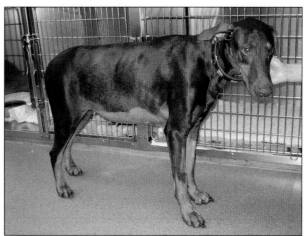

6.5 Haematocrit tube used to assess PCV. The PCV reading in this case was 50% and was within the normal range for a Greyhound.

As a general rule, any pre-anaesthetic test is only valuable if the results will direct a change in anaesthetic protocol. Figure 6.6 provides suggestions for 'tailor-made' pre-anaesthetic protocols.

Patient group	Tests	Rationale	Response if abnormalities found
1. Younger dogs (<7 years) with concerns raised on clinical examination (e.g. weight loss, polyuria/polydipsia malaise, weakness)	PCV, TP/albumin, blood glucose, urea	PCV will give an indication of anaemia and hydration status (together with TP). Low albumin may lead to poor/delayed healing and may indicate cachexia or neoplasia. Hypoglycaemia may occur in juvenile starved patients, in cachexic patients, or over-controlled diabetics. High urea may indicate poor renal function	Full haematology, including evaluation of a fresh blood smear. Ultrasonography and/or radiography. Diabetics: check fructosamine levels, commence glucose therapy. Check urine specific gravity, measure creatinine
2. Older dogs (≥8 years) showing no sign of disease	As above, but consider full haematology and more comprehensive biochemistry panel, full urinalysis	Occult disease may be present	Further tests (e.g. radiography, ultrasonography, bile acid function) as directed by abnormal results
3. Older dogs (≥8 years) showing signs of disease (e.g. weight loss/gain, hair loss, coat/skin changes, lethargy)	As for group 2, but consider thyroid testing in overweight dogs	Hypothyroid dogs may be at increased risk of haemorrhage and anaesthetic complications	Stabilize on thyroid medication prior to surgery, if possible
4. Dogs with bruising; certain breeds (e.g. Dobermann); dogs in lungworm endemic areas; dogs undergoing spleen, liver or kidney biopsy	As for groups 1–3, depending on age and signalment, plus coagulation tests	Any abnormal coagulation results should be investigated. Any underlying cause (neoplastic, hepatic) should be controlled if possible	With von Willebrand's disease, no treatment may be needed provided strict attention is paid to haemostasis. However, fresh blood (or at least fresh-frozen plasma) should be on hand if required. If lungworm is suspected, a Baermann test should be performed on faeces prior to surgery and treatment instigated as required
5. Dogs with neoplastic disease	As for group 3, but include calcium in biochemistry profile. Ultrasonography of the pelvis and abdomen. Thoracic and abdominal radiography	Some tumours (e.g. anal sac adenocarcinoma) cause a paraneoplastic syndrome resulting in hypercalcaemia which dramatically increases the risk of fatal cardiac arrhythmia during anaesthesia. Imaging is necessary to detect metastatic or contemporaneous disease and to stage the tumour	Plan for additional treatment, such as chemotherapy, or consider referral, palliative care or euthanasia
6. Dogs with urinary tract disease	As for groups 1–3, depending on age and signalment, plus electrolytes, blood urea nitrogen and creatinine, full urinalysis (including specific gravity, microscopy and urine culture), haematology	Urine culture is frequently negative, even when there are obvious signs of infection. However, it is important to try to obtain a culture if possible to direct antibiotic selection. Azotaemia together with hyposthenuric urine suggests chronic renal failure and indicates ASA grade III and above. Chronic renal failure is frequently associated with non-regenerative anaemia	Mild azotaemia may be improved by 24–48 hours of intravenous fluid therapy prior to surgery. The pros and cons of performing surgery on patients with a poor ASA score should be discussed with the owner

6.6 Suggested pre-anaesthetic tests for specific patient categories and procedures.

Preoperative preparation

Starvation

Since the presence of food in the stomach is associated with an increased risk of aspiration should vomiting occur whilst the dog is anaesthetized, a period of starvation is advised. Generally speaking, food need only be withheld for 5–6 hours prior to surgery, and water need not be withheld. Very young animals and those suffering from malnutrition may be at risk of hypoglycaemia with prolonged starvation. There is an increased risk in some dogs of postoperative gastritis if food is withheld for more then 8–10 hours.

Voiding

Owners should be asked to take the dog for a short walk on the morning of surgery to give the patient an opportunity to empty its bowel and bladder, as some dogs do not like to void in unfamiliar territory. It is not just unpleasant to have leakage during a procedure but it may be uncomfortable for the patient and compromise aseptic technique.

Bathing

A heavily soiled or muddy coat may be a source of postoperative infection, so owners should be instructed to bathe any particularly soiled pets. Care should be taken, particularly in long-coated breeds, to ensure the dog is completely dry as this could predispose to hypothermia.

Special considerations

■ Intravenous fluid therapy is recommended for all procedures involving anaesthetic: not only does the administration of fluid help to guard against hypotensive episodes, but it is reassuring to have immediate access to a vein in the event of an emergency. Elderly patients, particularly those with mild renal insufficiency, must have intravenous fluid therapy to try to instigate mild diuresis perioperatively.

■ It is worthwhile planning the surgical caseload to allow special cases to be treated early in the day, in order that recovery occurs while there is a full complement of staff. This also gives patients longer to recover from the anaesthetic if discharge is planned for the same day. Another reason for scheduling elderly, cachectic and immature dogs early in the day is that these animals have low glycogen reserves and may be prone to hypoglycaemia.

■ Diabetic dogs should be well monitored in the days leading up to surgery, and a pre-anaesthetic blood glucose sample should be assessed. Recommended protocols for administering insulin to these patients may be found elsewhere (see *BSAVA Manual of Canine and Feline Anaesthesia and Analgesia*).

■ Aggressive or nervous dogs should be treated with care, not only from the view of personal safety (and that of others), but also because the release of catecholamines due to stress sensitizes the cardiovascular system to the effects of anaesthetic agents and can precipitate hypovolaemic shock or cardiac disturbances. It may be advisable in most cases to sedate aggressive dogs away from their owners, as they may relax when not in their owner's presence. In some circumstances, however, the owner may be the only person capable of safely handling an aggressive dog, e.g. guard dogs, military dogs, police dogs.

■ Dogs with cardiovascular compromise or traumatized patients are similarly at risk of sudden decompensation or vascular compromise. Attempts should be made to stabilize these patients as well as possible prior to anaesthesia (see Chapters 8 and 10) and to modify the anaesthetic protocol accordingly.

■ Any animals falling into category III or above on the ASA scale (see Figure 6.3) have a 3–4 times increased morbidity rate compared with those in groups I and II, and have a commensurately higher mortality rate. Special attention should be paid to these dogs (Figure 6.7) and the anaesthetic protocol should be adjusted accordingly (Figure 6.8). The owners should be informed of the higher risks, and the potential risk:benefit balance should be assessed. Dogs with respiratory or cardiac disease may benefit from 5–10 minutes of preoxygenation prior to induction of anaesthesia (Figure 6.9).

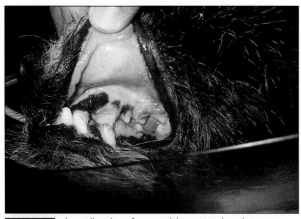

6.7 Jaundice in a 9-year-old neutered male crossbreed terrier. His ASA class was considered to be III. An oesophagostomy feeding tube had been placed 3 days prior to general anaesthesia (for liver biopsy).

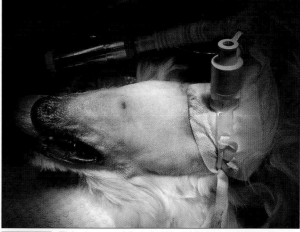

6.8 This 4-year-old male West Highland White Terrier had advanced temporomandibular osteopathy. Intubation was not possible orally and so a temporary tracheostomy was performed. This is a high-risk procedure.

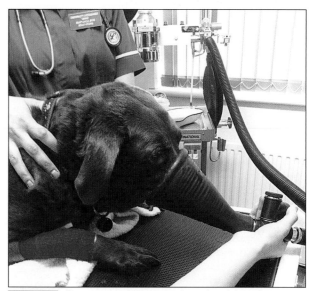

6.9 Preoxygenation can reduce the risk and respiratory stress of anaesthesia, as with this 10-year-old Labrador Retriever with laryngeal paralysis.

Postoperative care

The patient should be monitored continuously post-operatively until the endotracheal tube has been removed and the patient is able to support itself in sternal recumbency. At this stage a little water may be offered and, as soon as the patient is fully conscious, food may be given. It is important to try to encourage the patient to urinate prior to discharge, as this implies reasonable hydration and kidney function.

The surgical wound should be checked period-ically to ensure that there is no sign of haemorrhage or self-mutilation. In most cases, self-mutilation is a sign of poor theatre technique (e.g. clipper rash, over-tight sutures) or inadequate analgesia, so consider-ation should be given to improving theatre protocols and pain relief. The patient should be assessed for pain using an objective pain scoring system, and analgesia balanced to effect. The author's preference is to use the Colorado State University Pain Scale (see www.vasg.org/pdfs/CSU_Acute_Pain_Scale_Canine.pdf), although there are several other very good pain scales available (e.g. Glasgow Composite Measure Pain Score (short-form version); www.gla.ac.uk/faculties/vet).

Any postoperative medication should be made ready, and postoperative rehabilitation or physiotherapy plans discussed with the nursing team. For further information the reader is encouraged to consult the *BSAVA Manual of Canine and Feline Anaesthesia and Analgesia* and the *BSAVA Manual of Canine and Feline Rehabilitation, Supportive and Palliative Care: Case Studies in Patient Management.*

Discharging the patient

It is vital that the patient is not discharged until fully recovered from anaesthesia.

WARNING

It is never acceptable to allow a dog to leave the surgery prior to full recovery from anaesthesia; this may be tantamount to negligence

Dogs should be ambulatory and able to eat a little food, and ideally should have urinated before going home. Prior to discharge, wounds should be examined to ensure there has been no further bleeding and any bandages assessed for slippage. The perineal and urinary regions should be checked: it is very poor practice to discharge a patient that has soiled itself.

The client should be informed as to the specific surgical procedure performed and the success or otherwise of that procedure. If any tests are outstanding, or if biopsy samples have been taken, the client should be made aware of when to expect the results.

PRACTICAL TIP

It is a good idea to clarify whether the client should contact the practice or the practice will contact the client. Not receiving results can be an understandable cause for complaint

Finally, it is worth remembering that most owners are unused to surgical wounds, and some may be quite 'squeamish'. If a wound is left uncovered, it may be wise to mention the size and position of the wound to the owner before discharging the dog, just to prepare them (Figure 6.10). On occasion, it may be necessary to place a bandage or dressing to spare the owner's feelings.

Postoperative advice to clients

In addition to the general advice above, specific advice should be given to the owner concerning the following:

- **Feeding:** Generally, unless there is specific reason not to, dogs should be allowed a little food once they have recovered enough to maintain sternal recumbency or stand. Clients should be advised to feed a small amount of food shortly after returning home: there is no reason not to give the patient's normal food, but a tinned 'recovery diet' may be given if preferred and is usually appreciated by the owner. The dog should be given free access to drinking water

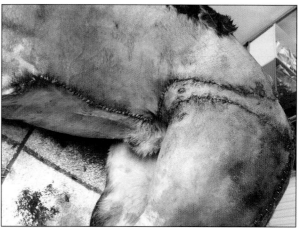

6.10 Extensive wound reconstruction following removal of a mast cell tumour from a 7-year-old cross-breed dog. The owners had been counselled on the likely appearance of the wound prior to surgery and knew what to expect.

- **Wound care:**
  - A sutured wound should be left dry for 2–3 days: any dried blood around the wound may be gently cleaned off after that time
  - The owner should be encouraged to check the wound twice daily (unless covered by a bandage or dressing) to check for any premature loosening of sutures or discharge. The wound and surrounding areas should be examined for swelling or redness, and gently pressed to see whether any pain is developing that might indicate the presence of infection (Figure 6.11)
  - Any self-mutilation should be dealt with promptly, either using an Elizabethan collar, or by applying a bandage or dressing
  - Bandages should be checked at least twice daily for signs of slippage, soiling or strike-through. Limb bandages especially should be checked to ensure there is no rubbing at the proximal edge. If left exposed, the toes should be carefully checked for signs of swelling or poor circulation (most owners can be taught to check capillary refill time in the toes of a light-skinned dog). If lameness of a bandaged limb develops or worsens, the dog should be seen by the vet at the earliest opportunity. Bandage disease, such as pressure sores or hypoxic tissue damage, can cause extremely severe problems and may become very painful. In rare instances it can lead to loss of a digit or limb
- **Exercise:** Regardless of the procedure, exercise should be kept to a minimum for 24–48 hours following anaesthesia. Provided there are no specific contraindications, such as after fracture repair or cruciate surgery, there is no reason why exercise cannot be increased in the following days, although on-lead exercise may be more appropriate for 10–14 days, or until the sutures are removed
- **Medicines:** The client must be given clear instructions for any medicine dispensed: in particular, when they should be started or whether any side effects may be seen. In some cases slow recoveries from anaesthesia or surgery are perceived by clients to be side effects of medication and this can adversely affect compliance

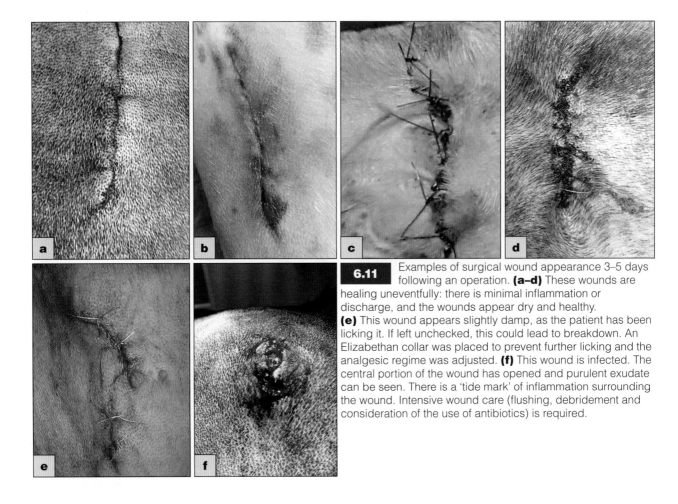

6.11 Examples of surgical wound appearance 3–5 days following an operation. **(a–d)** These wounds are healing uneventfully: there is minimal inflammation or discharge, and the wounds appear dry and healthy. **(e)** This wound appears slightly damp, as the patient has been licking it. If left unchecked, this could lead to breakdown. An Elizabethan collar was placed to prevent further licking and the analgesic regime was adjusted. **(f)** This wound is infected. The central portion of the wound has opened and purulent exudate can be seen. There is a 'tide mark' of inflammation surrounding the wound. Intensive wound care (flushing, debridement and consideration of the use of antibiotics) is required.

■ **Pain:** Although pain assessment in dogs is reasonably subjective, the owner should be made aware of the expected pain this type of procedure may cause. Clear guidance should be given to enable the owner to monitor for pain (Figure 6.12); client handouts can be sourced online at www. aahanet.org
- Restlessness and vocalization may be signs of pain, but are occasionally seen as post-anaesthetic phenomena when no invasive procedure has been carried out, suggesting that they may be anaesthetic 'hangover' responses. Instructing the owner to touch gently around a wound may elicit whether there is post-surgical pain present
- Postoperative pain is always pathological and serves no useful function. It is never acceptable to use pain as a method of reducing patient activity. Consideration should be given to using combinations of analgesic agents if a single one proves insufficient. Analgesic drug dosages may be found in the *BSAVA Small Animal Formulary*, or in the *BSAVA Manual of Canine and Feline Anaesthesia and Analgesia*

■ **Postoperative check-up:** A date should be made for the postoperative check-up (see below). The client should be made aware of the importance and role of this check, and whether any charge will be made for it.

Postoperative check-up

Postoperative check-ups fulfil several functions (Figure 6.13). It may be a matter of practice policy whether every routine and non-routine surgical procedure is subject to a postoperative check-up, but generally speaking it is advisable to check every patient following general anaesthesia to ensure that no complications have arisen as a result either of the anaesthetic or of the surgical procedure itself. Timing of the postoperative check will depend on the patient's signalment and the nature of the operation; as a general guideline, the author tends to see most cases again between 48 and 72 hours postoperatively.

In some instances it may be acceptable to allow the owner to make the decision as to whether they are happy with progress following a routine neutering, although the author would urge inexperienced

- Vocalizing
- Restlessness or shivering
- Hunched posture
- Reluctance to exercise or interact
- Hiding
- Demanding increased attention/affection
- Changes in sleep (unable to sleep or sleeps more than usual)
- Licking or chewing at wound
- Vacant stare or glazed eyes
- Lameness
- Panting
- Acting out of character (aggression or nervousness)
- Loss of appetite and water intake
- Lethargy or weakness

6.12 Signs of postoperative pain in dogs.

Function	Examples
Allows assessment of the patient – to look for any anaesthetic morbidity	Acute kidney injury, dehydration, inappetence, vomition, exacerbation of occult illness
To check for complications after surgery	Wound infection or breakdown, self-mutilation, blood loss
To improve surgeon satisfaction, or to learn from complications	A good outcome may boost confidence. A poor outcome should be used as a learning exercise
Allows the client to voice any concerns or queries	Changes in behaviour or mobility may prompt concerns. The aims and treatment targets should be reinforced at this point and appointments made for further follow-up
To reinforce postoperative care requirements	Improve medicine compliance or emphasize importance of physiotherapy techniques (see *BSAVA Manual of Canine and Feline Rehabilitation, Supportive and Palliative Care*)
To discuss results of investigations	Present radiographic findings or indicate the next level of treatment, and discuss prognosis

6.13 Functions of the postoperative check-up.

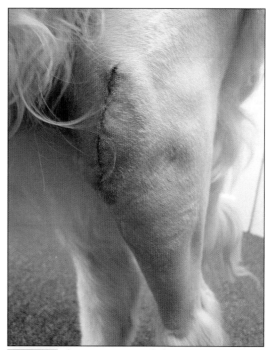

6.14 Appearance at a 3-day postoperative check-up following cranial cruciate ligament repair. The wound looks comfortable, with no sign of infection. The owner should be fully informed about ongoing exercise and physiotherapy requirements.

surgeons to re-check every case: this will not only improve surgical satisfaction at seeing 'completed tasks' but will also improve recognition of stages of wound healing by building up a mental database of post-surgical cases. Certainly, any non-routine surgical case (e.g. tumour resections, orthopaedic cases) should receive at least one postoperative check.

What to check for will depend to some extent on the nature of the surgery; however, all post-surgical patients should be examined for general health, including temperature, pulse and respiration. Lack of urination may indicate renal failure (acute or an exacerbation of occult chronic) or dehydration and should be investigated thoroughly. Vomiting or diarrhoea may be transient and should be investigated as suggested in Chapter 13. Wounds should be carefully checked for signs of infection, suture failure or other complication; for example, failure to close dead space adequately may result in seroma formation – these are generally non-painful, but a scrotal seroma or haematoma can be extremely painful and is a relatively common complication of castration when performed by inexperienced surgeons.

When rechecking non-routine cases, it is important to tailor the postoperative check-up to cover specific points. In these circumstances it is advisable to consult a book, or a more experienced colleague, for more precise guidance for that procedure. In this way the most appropriate advice can be given with regard to, for example: levels or types of exercise; at what stage physiotherapy is recommended; when repeat radiographs should be scheduled (Figure 6.14).

References and further reading

Baines S, Lipscomb V and Hutchinson T (2012) *BSAVA Manual of Canine and Feline Surgical Principles: A Foundation Manual*. BSAVA Publications, Gloucester

Fossum TW (2012) Preoperative assessment of the surgical patient. In: *Small Animal Surgery, 2nd edn*, ed. TW Fossum, pp.18–22. Mosby, St. Louis

Jones RS (2007) Legal and ethical aspects of anaesthesia. In: *BSAVA Manual of Canine and Feline Anaesthesia and Analgesia, 2nd edn*, ed. C Seymour and T Duke-Novakovski, pp.1–5. BSAVA Publications, Gloucester

Lindley S and Watson P (2010) *BSAVA Manual of Canine and Feline Rehabilitation, Supportive and Palliative Care: Case Studies in Patient Management*. BSAVA Publications, Gloucester.

Muir WW (2007) Considerations for general anaesthesia. In: *Lumb and Jones' Veterinary Anaesthesia and Analgesia, 4th edn*, ed. WJ Tranquilli *et al.*, pp.7–30. Blackwell, Ames, Iowa

Posner LP (2007) Pre-anaesthetic assessment. In: *BSAVA Manual of Canine and Feline Anaesthesia and Analgesia, 2nd edn*, ed. C Seymour and T Duke-Novakovski, pp.6–11. BSAVA Publications, Gloucester

Ramsey I (2014) *BSAVA Small Animal Formulary, 8th edn*. BSAVA Publications, Gloucester

Schmon C (1993) Assessment and preparation of the surgical patient and the operating team. In: *Textbook of Small Animal Surgery, 2nd edn*, ed. DS Slatter, pp.162–178. Saunders, Philadelphia

Euthanasia: considerations for canine practice

Ross Allan

As a vocation, the drive for those entering the veterinary profession is to diagnose illness in animals, successfully treat them and make them well. However, in the course of their training, students become increasingly aware that this is not always possible, nor always practical for the owner. For the recent graduate working in general practice, the reality becomes even starker. Since it is not always possible to maintain the animal's health and quality of life, euthanasia and the decisions surrounding it are part and parcel of the working day of the veterinary surgeon. As a profession, vets owe it to their patients, their clients and themselves to evaluate the factors influencing the decision to perform euthanasia, and to examine how stress can be minimized for both the owner and the pet, and how mishaps can be prevented. Euthanasia is not, nor ever should be, considered as clinical failure or automatically the only option for those with restricted funds.

Decision-making and consent

Rapid progress in veterinary medicine, coupled with increasing clinical ability, means that most conditions presenting in practice have scope for further treatment. Clients rely on vets for information and advice on the condition that their pet has and on the treatment options available. The advice given should be impartial and should not pre-empt the clients' thoughts. It is wrong to prejudge their decisions or choice of treatment.

Approach to the client

Although we know that all life will inevitably end at some point, the loss of a pet may be exceptionally hard. For many owners, especially those that are young, it may be the first time they have been faced with decisions concerning a loved one. In some instances the decisions they have to make are more complicated than when a relative is unwell. Many discussions with clients will be over clinical options, but as a pet ages the treatment choices will gradually become intertwined with the possibility of euthanasia.

At the time of euthanasia, clients' emotions can be heightened to a level that they may experience only a few times in their lives. Emotions last experienced at the loss of a close family member often arise, as do memories of the relationships the client had with their pet and family member in the past. What is said, and the way the vet behaves in front of the client at this time is crucial. Whilst empathy comes naturally to many within the veterinary profession, there are also pointers to learn that can help to ensure the client feels that the vet cares about them and, most importantly, their pet:

- Ensure that you know the client's name, as well as the pet's name and sex
- If you have not met the client before, make sure to introduce yourself and the veterinary nurse
- When discussing quality of life, or at the time of the decision-making, it may help to sit down
- Remove the stethoscope from around your neck. This conveys that you are concentrating on what the client is saying – and caring about their pet, not thinking about anything else
- Do not stand on the other side of the table from the client; move around to be on the same side of the table as the owner
- Stand with an 'open' posture: hands should not be crossed or in pockets; feet should be slightly apart
- Stand in a similar posture to the one the client is taking. This shows that you are concentrating on what they have to say
- Take your time – 'silence says a thousand words'. Take care to speak slowly and give time for the owners to think about what you have said. There is a natural tendency for vets to rush the euthanasia consult; allowing time will ensure the client feels you care.

The points above are no substitute for genuine empathy and concern – clients will know if the veterinary staff genuinely care (Figure 7.1); the clients deserve this, as do their pets.

Quality of life

What determines 'quality of life' (QoL) is open to debate. The owner should have a key role in the discussion and will often begin to form an opinion of what to do; whether to continue to treat (if an option), or whether euthanasia would be the right thing.

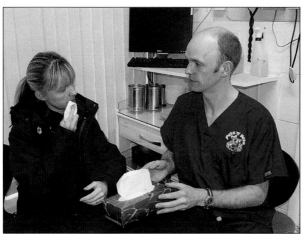

7.1 Euthanasia is performed frequently by many vets in general practice. It should be remembered, however, that it is a far from common experience for most pet owners. The vet must aim to make an empathetic connection with owners, whilst offering appropriate sympathy.

Questions that may help guide an owner to consider their pet's quality of life are listed in Figure 7.2.

- Does your pet play with you, or enjoy being petted/brushed?
- Does he/she look forward to food?
- Does he/she still want to go out for a walk?
- Does he/she suffer urinary or faecal incontinence?
- Does he/she want to interact with you and your family?

7.2 Questions that can be used to guide an owner to consider their pet's quality of life.

PRACTICAL TIP

Clients may find it helpful to compile a diary, especially if their pet has a chronic illness. Such a diary can have two columns per day: one listing the good points of the day; the other listing the bad points. This may give clients a better appreciation of the state of their pet's health and allow them to recognize when quality of life is deteriorating

Pain is often an owner's prime concern, and it is important to try to explain as well as possible whether a dog could be experiencing pain and, if so, whether the management of that pain could be improved. It is important to consider and explain the level to which pain can now be controlled. In many cases this will mean that quality of life can be increased, or managed better from day to day.

At this stage many owners will commonly ask, "What would you do if it was your pet?". While it can be appropriate to give an opinion, it is important to make clear that the final decision has to be theirs – they know their dog better than anyone else. Once the decision has been made, it is essential to support them in that decision, and reinforce that the correct choice has been made. The owner should also sign a euthanasia consent form. This serves to document that permission was given for euthanasia of the dog and that a conversation took place around the decision to euthanase. The completed form should be retained by the practice.

Acting without consent

Situations may occur when euthanasia is required without direct owner consent. The vet's overriding professional obligation is to the welfare of the animal under their care. If euthanasia is truly required it is incorrect to postpone it simply to give time for the owner to be contacted or traced. Should this situation arise, it would be wise to get a second opinion from a colleague. The details of the clinical deliberation that occurred, resulting in the decision being made without the owner being present, should be clearly put into the clinical notes. Detailing this deliberation – and the efforts that have been made to contact the owner – reduces the risk of complaint should the owner appear at a later date

Intraoperative euthanasia

In some circumstances exploratory surgery may be performed to confirm a diagnosis, or to assess whether surgery could be performed depending upon what is found. While modern diagnostic imaging means that it is rarer to have to do so, in some cases a decision regarding euthanasia may have to be made while the dog is on the operating table.

Preparation is essential to avoid a difficult situation. The client must be fully aware of what may be found during surgery, the possible merits of performing surgery, and any issues affecting surgical recovery.

- The worst situation would be to call the owner during surgery and get either an engaged tone, or an owner unable to make a decision on whether to proceed with surgery, euthanasia, or recovery from anaesthesia. In any of these circumstances, if in doubt, euthanasia should NOT be performed as long as the animal does not suffer.
- For any surgical procedure where there is the prospect that euthanasia may be required, full discussion must be held with the client prior to surgery. They should be given an anticipated time that surgery may be performed and all routes of contact must be clarified.
- In some instances it may be that a consent form is signed giving permission for euthanasia if the surgical findings are hopeless, but even in these circumstances it is prudent to attempt to contact the client to discuss the findings prior to administering the lethal dose.

The decision to perform euthanasia is one for which the client may require time to reflect and consider. With modern analgesics, recovery from anaesthesia and euthanasia later in the day is far preferable to clients feeling regret at making the decision too quickly, or feeling that they were at all pressurized into making a decision.

Preparation for euthanasia

At the practice

Sometimes the choice of euthanasia will require prompt decision-making, but in most circumstances there will be the opportunity to get to know the owner and the pet prior to the time of euthanasia. This is important. Clients will feel more open and trusting when a relationship has developed. In addition, there will be the opportunity for the clinician to plan the final euthanasia consultation. This is preferable, as it enables stress to the owner, pet and the vet to be minimized; simple things can make all the difference (Figure 7.3).

- Quiet waiting room and practice: no barking dogs or staff laughing. Arrange a consultation time for the last appointment before a break or the end of the day
- Ensure all staff members are aware
- No staff intrusion into the consult room: have a spyglass in the consulting room door, or a slide sign showing that the room is in use
- Vet who knows the pet and owner: ideally, you will have met the clients before, and have read the history
- A nurse to help: ideally one that knows the clients as well. If not, introduce them
- Turn any phones in the room to silent. Make sure no mobile phones are in pockets
- Intravenous access: use a preplaced intravenous catheter if possible. If this has not been possible, take more than one needle into the room
- Bed for the dog – on the table whenever possible
- Tissues to hand for owners

7.3   Reducing stress for pets, owners and staff during a euthanasia consultation.

The decision on whether or not to stay for the euthanasia is one the owner must make. Some owners prefer to remember their dog as it was; others would rather be with the dog until the euthanasia has been performed and the vet has said that the dog's heart has stopped beating. It is wise to offer owners both options, and let them make the decision. At this stage it is useful briefly to describe the process (see later).

Home visits

Home visits may be preferable, especially if a pet is very elderly or collapsed. In many cases this removes any suggestion of the procedure being rushed, and can result in the euthanasia event itself being one of the most rewarding many vets experience.

Suggestions to ensure that home visits are smooth and proceed without distress are given in Figure 7.4. Equipment required for euthanasia is shown in Figure 7.5.

- Ensure the vehicle is clean prior to the visit. Many owners may wish to assist transfer of their pet into the vehicle and it is important to make sure that you will not be embarrassed by the condition or contents of your vehicle. Parking facing away from the house will enable easier transfer of the pet into the vehicle
- Lay the pet on a large blanket or old duvet prior to euthanasia. Ensure that there is plenty of absorptive material, e.g. an incontinence pad. The pet can be wrapped up in the blanket afterwards. Do not transfer to a 'body bag' until back at the surgery
- A stretcher or zip-closing transportation bag can be used, but often clients may prefer their pet to be taken to the vehicle upon their bed
- Ensure the vehicle is suitably lined in case of spillages during transit
- Have a list of 'items required for euthanasia' in the home visit box, to help ensure you do not leave anything you need at the practice
- Ensure there is a veterinary nurse or other staff member to help
- Preplaced intravenous catheters are useful. These can be placed at the surgery on the day prior to euthanasia. Ensure they flush correctly prior to administering pentobarbital

7.4   Preparation for a home visit for euthanasia.

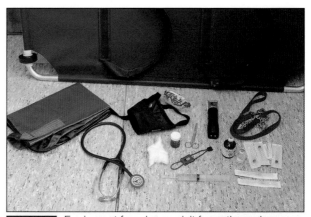

7.5   Equipment for a home visit for euthanasia, including: stretcher; pentobarbital for injection; scissors; clippers; foldable body transport carrier; muzzles; tourniquet; stethoscope; swabs with surgical spirit; sedatives; spare needles and syringes.

Explaining the process

One difficulty of euthanasia is that often clients will have misconceptions over what happens prior to the event itself, whether from TV, relatives or previous experiences. No two euthanasia events are the same, however, and it is important to take the client on the journey through the consultation to ensure that they are aware of the process and feel part of it. For this reason it is helpful to explain to the client both prior to and during the event what is happening (Figure 7.6). At this time clients will be acutely sensitive and will notice if veterinary staff speak of their pet impersonally. Using words like 'they' or 'it' should be avoided at all costs: *use the pet's name!*

Action/ occurrence	Explanation examples
Clipping	"I will need to clip a small patch of hair."
Venous access	"I will place the injection into the vein in Buster's leg."
Restraint	"The nurse, Jenny, will help to support Buster as he gets the injection."
Movement at time of injection	"There can often be a small movement as the needle goes in. This is normal".
Discomfort	"Apart from the needle going in, Buster won't feel anything."
As injection is administered	"You may notice Buster taking a few deep breaths. These are the last breaths as his body shuts down. It wouldn't be unusual for some to occur even after he's passed away".
Predict the unexpected	"Kidney problems often mean a few deep breaths can be taken after the injection has been given. This is normal".
Eyes remain open	"When Buster passes away his eyes will stay open. They do not close over."
Relaxation	"As Buster passes away his muscles will relax. This may mean that his bladder leaks a little. I will place some tissues under him just in case".
Agonal gasps and twitching	"Buster has passed away now. His body may tremble a little and take some large gasps as if he is breathing, but these are just reflexes, and settling."

7.6   Suggestions for explaining the euthanasia process to the client.

Euthanasia techniques

It is important to have a nurse available to help perform euthanasia; they should restrain the dog (Figure 7.7), but take care not to appear to be holding it too tightly as clients may find that extremely upsetting.

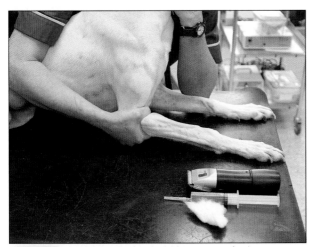

7.7 A Whippet being held by a nurse for intravenous injection.

It is often useful to have a chair available for the owner at the top of the table so that they can sit with their pet, and comfort them by stroking or talking to them as the injection is administered. This is an individual preference, and some owners may not want to do this. Clients often like to talk to the nurses at this time; in many practices the clients will have known the nurse for a great many years and find this easier than talking to the vet. Time should be allowed for this to occur so that the client does not feel that their pet's euthanasia is being rushed.

It is preferable to have a nurse that is familiar with how the vet will administer the intravenous injection. It should be borne in mind that blood pressure may be poor, and if an intravenous catheter is not being used it is important that the nurse is instructed beforehand as to when to release the pressure they have applied in order to raise the vein.

> **PRACTICAL TIPS**
> - Do not be afraid to discuss what you are going to do with your colleague prior to commencing euthanasia. You must work together to make it as smooth as possible – communication is key
> - It is better to have the dog supported in sternal rather than lateral recumbency – this makes finding a vein slightly easier by improving cephalic vein pressure

Sedation

There is debate in many practices over whether sedating the dog prior to euthanasia is appropriate. Some vets believe that owners may not wish it, as it can mean that their pet is not fully conscious when it receives the injection; others feel that sedation can reduce the risk of the dog struggling whilst restrained as the injection is administered – this may be distressing to owners and staff should it occur. The response to the administration of pentobarbital may be less predictable in a sedated animal and venous pressure may be reduced, thereby making injection administration more challenging. The use of sedation should be discussed with the individual owner, and they should be made aware of what the vet is doing – prior to doing it.

If sedation is deemed appropriate the following protocols could be considered:

- Buprenorphine (20 μg/kg) + acepromazine (20 μg/kg): suitable for older or quiet animals – and can be administered subcutaneously
- Butorphanol (0.1 mg/kg) + medetomidine (10 μg/kg): will ensure profound sedation but ideally needs to be given intramuscularly or intravenously. It may be particularly useful for aggressive or boisterous dogs, though owners should be warned that if intravenous access is not readily available (due to aggression) intramuscular administration may provoke an aggressive reaction from their pet; the owner should be counselled that this is only while the sedative is being administered, with the aim of allowing the euthanasia to be performed peacefully.

NB: The dosages above are for sedation; the actual doses used for sedation prior to euthanasia may be greater, especially in aggressive or boisterous dogs, as oversedation is not then a concern.

The time required between sedation and euthanasia is liable to variation depending on the dosages administered, the infirmity of the pet and the degree of stimulus the pet is experiencing at the time. If too much time passes, venous access may be difficult due to decreasing blood pressure. Generally 5–10 minutes is long enough.

> **PRACTICAL TIP**
> If sedation is not possible or appropriate, pre-clipping the area for injection and then applying a local anaesthetic skin cream (e.g. EMLA) is helpful for reducing the risk of the dog moving while the euthanasia injection is being administered

Following sedation, dogs may be left with owners in the consulting room. It should be remembered however that a sedated dog is under veterinary care and the veterinary surgeon is responsible for its actions. Many owners will appreciate the time to speak to someone about the memories they have of their pet. Asking questions such as "How old was Rusty when you got him?", or saying "He has been a lucky dog to have you look after him for so long", will often bring forth a torrent of emotions and memories of the times the client had with their pet.

If a dog is very fractious, oral sedation at home prior to euthanasia might be considered. Acepromazine tablets are of use, but their sedative effect is variable; there are reports that using the oral forms of acepromazine and phenobarbital in combination can be more effective. Many vets prefer not to use oral sedation, instead opting for injectable sedation as it is more reliable.

Routes of euthanasia

Intravenous injection via the cephalic or saphenous vein is the recommended method for administering pentobarbital (150 mg/kg or higher). Where venous access is anticipated to be difficult, it is preferable to preplace a venous catheter.

PRACTICAL TIP

In circumstances where pre-placement is not possible and access is difficult but euthanasia is urgently required, e.g. after a severe road traffic accident or for an emaciated animal, it can be useful to use a tourniquet around the upper limb. This often helps more than digital pressure. Rubber bands and artery forceps can suffice if there is no tourniquet available

Other routes for euthanasia are possible but have disadvantages that mean they are normally unsuitable for performing in front of an owner:

- Intraperitoneal: slow, unpredictable and can be stressful when the owner is present; doses of 200 mg/kg are required
- Intrarenal: rapid, but likely painful due to distension of the renal capsule; doses of 200 mg/kg are required
- Intrahepatic: not as rapid as renal injection, but reasonably quick and does not normally elicit pain; doses of 200 mg/kg are required
- Intracardiac: rapid and predictable, especially where venous access is not possible. Generally, if the dog is collapsed or unconscious doses of 150 mg/kg are required. *Very unsuitable for performing in front of owners, especially due to risk of the injection entering the lungs, leading to coughing and distress.*

Owing to the ready availability of pentobarbital, using overdoses of intravenous medications such as propofol, thiopental or potassium chloride for the purpose of elective euthanasia is unjustified.

What to do if something goes wrong

Situations occur where things do not go to plan: there may be no nurse available; the injection may be administered perivascularly; the dog may be aggressive; the owner may become aggressive – to name but a few. It is important not to panic. Clients will pick up nervousness shown by the vet if things go wrong.

Talk calmly to the client and explain what has happened, and what requires to be done:

- **No nurse available:** Sedation will help – "I am going to give Flossie a sedative to enable me to give her the euthanasia injection"
- **Perivascular injection:** "The needle has slipped out of the vein. This happens occasionally, especially when the blood pressure is poor. What I need to do is shave a small patch of hair from another leg to give the injection there. This will just take a few moments"
- **Aggressive or distressed dog:** "I appreciate that you are not keen for me to sedate Rex, but unfortunately I do need to give him a sedative so that I can give the injection while causing minimal distress for him, and for you and me as well."

After euthanasia

Often owners wish to stay with their dog for a time after euthanasia, though some do not. Provision for the owners to exit rapidly should be prepared prior to the event itself in case it is required.

Clients will often share memories of their pet's life at this time. It is important to share this time with them and reassure them that they gave their pet the best home they could.

Options for cremation or burial

It is necessary to discuss the options for disposal of the body. Most pet crematoria companies will offer a variety of caskets, or biodegradable containers if the client wishes to have their dog's ashes returned.

Home burial is a way of owners personalizing the loss of their pet. Dogs should be buried around a metre deep and may be wrapped in a biodegradable material – not plastic. The site chosen should not be close to water courses. It is advisable for owners to discuss home burial with their own Local Authority prior to burying, as there may be local or regional variation in the guidance provided.

Pet cemeteries have grown in popularity recently and may be the preferred choice of clients who wish to have a coffin or headstone for their dog. Clients should be aware that there may be an initial fee and an annual maintenance charge associated with this.

Options for disposal are preferably discussed with the owner pre-euthanasia, possibly at the time the decision is made on whether the owner wishes to be present during the euthanasia event itself. If this is not possible, however, the question can be raised afterwards; a phone call later that day or the next is probably most suitable. This small delay is often necessary because clients wish to discuss the options with their family. Care must be taken to ensure that the pet is not transported to a crematorium in the intervening time, as this would be embarrassing and very distressing for all involved.

The practice will have a protocol for storage of cadavers and for disposal where owners do not wish to be involved (see *BSAVA Manual of Small Animal Practice Management and Development*).

Payment

Asking for remittance at this time can be very difficult. Some owners feel this is wrong, but if the practice has no experience of the client, or if they have a poor history of settling their account it is not inappropriate to ask for the bill to be paid, especially if owners have elected for private cremation. If the client is well known, however, payment may be left for another day.

Bereavement

The death of a pet may mean that the owner experiences more heightened emotions than they have for some time.

Kübler-Ross (1969) researched the emotions experienced by people who were themselves terminally ill. As she researched these she hypothesized that the emotions experienced at this time were similar to those experienced during any catastrophic personal loss in life; such as the loss of a loved one. Kübler-Ross noted that those going through any major stressful event involving some element of loss experienced five key components (Figure 7.8). The level to which any one individual experienced these stages varied; not all people experienced all of them, they were not necessarily chronological and neither did all stages necessarily occur in all people.

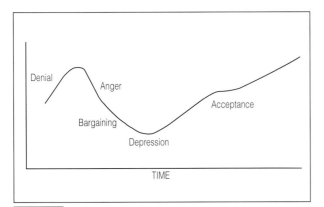

| **7.8** | Kübler-Ross emotions of loss. |

The theory might be applied to veterinary medicine as follows:

- **Denial:** This may manifest as owners being unwilling to accept that the time to make the decision to perform euthanasia has arrived
- **Anger:** Clients may become verbally abusive, or want to leave the consulting room far more quickly than anticipated
- **Bargaining:** This is often encountered in veterinary medicine where a decision to perform euthanasia is not time-critical. Often clients will wish to postpone for a few days, or try another avenue of treatment, even when it is not likely to be effective. This is normal human instinct and not necessarily a sign that the client does not trust the vet's diagnosis
- **Depression:** Clients will often be inconsolable after the euthanasia event itself, often more than they ever expected
- **Acceptance:** Clients realizing that they have made the correct decision, at the right time, and that their pet was well looked after, is what is hoped will happen before the client leaves the consulting room. The reality is, however, that it can take a while for clients to digest what has happened and arrive at this point.

Realizing that these are normal emotions, should help vets to speak to clients appropriately, and guide them through what is a stressful time.

Remembrance cards (Figure 7.9) or phone calls on the day or a few days after the event can be useful, and there are some who are strong advocates of this. Clients may often go through emotions of self-blame, feeling that they have let their pet down or else kept them alive for too long. An empathetic phone call can help resolve these feelings. It must be cautioned, however, that these contacts a few days after the event can also unearth emotions clients would rather not experience again. For this reason, any such decision should be based on knowledge of the individual client.

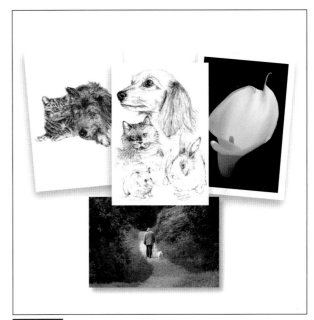

| **7.9** | Examples of pet bereavement sympathy cards. |

Client resources

- *Coping with The Loss of your Pet.* BSAVA PetSavers client leaflet [also available online to BSAVA members]
- *Coping with Pet Loss.* Society for Companion Animal Studies (SCAS) client leaflet [available from www.scas.org.uk]
- Pet Bereavement Support Service. A telephone and online service run jointly by SCAS [www.scas.org.uk] and the Blue Cross [www.bluecross.org.uk]

References and further reading

Clarke C and Chapman M (2012) *BSAVA Manual of Small Animal Practice Management and Development.* BSAVA Publications, Gloucester
Kübler-Ross E (1969) *On Death and Dying.* Macmillan, New York
Stewart MF (1999) *Companion Animal Death: A Comprehensive Guide for Veterinary Practice.* Butterworth-Heinemann, Oxford

Dealing with emergency cases

Sophie Adamantos

In most small animal practices true emergencies will be relatively uncommon, but with the increase in emergency centres within the UK there will be practices where emergency cases are in the majority. Although emergency medicine can be stressful it can also be extremely satisfying. Maintaining a calm approach is vital and makes everything easier. With a standardized, logical approach to patient management the veterinary team can make the difference between life and death. This truly is the area of practice where interventions can have an immediate effect! Common emergency presentations are listed in Figure 8.1.

■ Acute distress/pain
■ Acute gastrointestinal problems
■ Choking
■ Collapse
■ Dyspnoea
■ Heart failure
■ Seizures
■ Toxicity
■ Trauma

8.1 Common emergency presentations in canine practice.

Telephone triage

In most emergency situations the first person in contact with the owner will be the receptionist or veterinary nurse who answers the telephone. Those answering the telephone should maintain a calm and professional manner at all times. It is vitally important that staff are briefed as to how to deal with owners who may be emotional or distressed. Staff must have received appropriate training for the recognition and management of emergency situations over the telephone. Outside normal working hours it is often better for a nurse or vet (rather than a receptionist) to deal directly with owners calling in, but during the day this is not usually possible and in these circumstances having lists of what to do and when can be helpful. Identifying what constitutes an emergency can be challenging over the telephone: what constitutes an emergency in the mind of a worried owner may be

anything but; however, there are a number of situations where the dog should be seen immediately (Figure 8.2). **Where there is any doubt, the owner should always be advised that their pet is seen as soon as possible.**

The dog should be seen _immediately_
■ Loss of consciousness
■ Unable to stand or move
■ Problems breathing
■ Severe bleeding (including vomiting blood)
■ Severe trauma
■ Acute-onset fits (seizures) or 'funny turns'
■ Fainting
■ Bloating
■ Witnessed toxin ingestion
■ Trying to vomit and cannot
■ Severe pain
The owner should be advised that the dog should be seen urgently
■ Severe vomiting or diarrhoea
■ Trauma
■ Bleeding
■ Acute-onset eye problems (pain, clouding, redness)
■ Severe acute-onset lameness
■ Less serious wounds
A vet or nurse should speak to the owner
■ Problem after surgery
■ Straining
■ Not eating
■ Coughing or wheezing

8.2 Recognizing emergency situations. This list is not exclusive; there are other situations in which the dog should be seen promptly. Speaking to the owner may help to clarify the situation.

It may be useful to provide receptionists with a checklist or to have a standard operating procedure so that correct advice is given. It is useful to obtain some information about the pet and its main problems, but spending too much time doing this should be avoided.

- The owner's name and phone number must be obtained early in the call in case there is a loss of contact.
- Limited information such as signalment of the dog (to allow preparation), the pet's name and the

major problem, as well as an estimated time of arrival, is probably all that is necessary at this stage.

- If the owner requests to be seen immediately, it is better for both the dog and for client management to see the pet (and also for the vet's peace of mind). Assessment of the dog's wellbeing can be very difficult to do over the phone and it is easier when the pet has been seen.
- Staff answering the telephone should be able to inform owners how to reach the practice and provide them with a postcode if SatNav is available.

WARNING

- Owners will often ask for advice rather than coming to the practice. If there is any doubt about the clinical state of the dog this should be avoided. It is useful to remember that the majority of owners are not medical professionals and may not accurately assess the health status of their pet or the urgency of the situation
- Owners should not be asked to administer any medications unless previously advised for a known medical problem

---

Basic first aid information may be provided if necessary for situations such as bleeding, burns and seizures (Figure 8.3) but veterinary care should not be delayed due to this. Owners should be warned that dogs in pain may behave abnormally and therefore should be approached and handled with extra care.

Condition	First aid advice
Bleeding	Apply pressure using clean absorbent material, e.g. a T-shirt or sheet
Seizures	Do not attempt to restrain the dog Transport the dog carefully to the veterinary surgery Do not place blankets over the dog as this may lead to overheating
Burns	Apply cool water to the burnt area for at least 10 minutes Avoid ice packs; use a tap, bath or hose
Heat stroke	Wet the dog using cool water (tap, bath or hose)

8.3 Basic first aid advice for owners. Further information on management of these conditions is given in Chapters 10, 11 and 18.

Preparation

Following the telephone conversation, preparation should begin for the dog's arrival. This is made easier by having some idea of the main problem.

Basic equipment for any emergency case should include that necessary for placement of an intravenous catheter, blood sampling and for measuring packed cell volume, total protein, glucose and urea or creatinine. Oxygen supplementation should also be easily available. If the patient is known to be dyspnoeic or collapsed, easy access to an endotracheal tube and laryngoscope and emergency drugs, including anaesthetic agents, is advised.

Basic equipment for an emergency patient

- Materials for skin preparation (swabs, surgical spirit, antiseptic solution)
- No. 11 scalpel blade (for facilitative skin nick prior to catheter placement)
- Intravenous catheters (various sizes)
- Connector, bungs and extension set
- Adhesive tape
- Needles and syringes (various sizes)
- 5 ml saline to flush syringe after placement
- Tubes for blood collection (EDTA for haematology; heparin for plasma; plain for serum)
- Capillary tubes (for PCV measurement)
- Facemask and anaesthetic circuit connected to oxygen supply

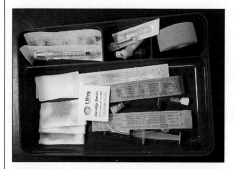

Hospital triage

Once the patient arrives it should be assessed immediately and a decision made as to the urgency of the problem. Rapid major body system assessment for identification of serious abnormalities (see Figure 8.4) allows this decision to be made. A suggested protocol for cardiopulmonary resuscitation (CPR) is provided at the end of the chapter (QRG 8.1).

If the patient is considered to be unstable, the dog should be removed from the owner and consent obtained for basic investigation and therapy. Owners are frequently distressed and someone should be made available to talk with and calm them; a cup of tea is often much appreciated. If this is not possible immediately, the owner should be reassured that their pet is in the best place and that experienced people are dealing with it and that the vet will be back as soon as possible once treatment is underway. Separating the clinical problem from the emotionally anxious owner reduces stress for the clinical team and allows them to concentrate fully on the patient.

WARNING

Under no circumstances attempt to stabilize a patient with the owner present. It induces stress and the clinician's concentration is distracted by anxious questioning; it is in no-one's best interest!

A full, complete medical history is not required at this stage. Basic information for immediate management of the case is all that is required. A full history may be obtained at a later stage when everything is under control.

Basic information for an emergency patient

- Signalment
- Husbandry information, to include vaccination status and worming history
- Previous medical history, including current medications
- Current problem; length of problem; have the owners administered anything?

Major body system assessment and stabilization

The aim of the major body system assessment is to identify problems that are immediately life-threatening, and allow initiation of therapy and instigation of an investigative plan. The major body systems are the cardiovascular, respiratory and neurological systems (Figure 8.4); once these have been assessed, significant findings should prompt interventions for stabilization. Once the patient is more stable, a complete physical examination should be performed to allow more directed therapy.

Body system	Assessment
Cardiovascular	Heart rate Pulse quality Mucous membrane colour Capillary refill time Auscultation
Respiratory	Respiratory rate Respiratory effort Observe and listen for pattern and noise Auscultation
Neurological	Mentation Posture Pain sensation

8.4   Major body system assessment.

PRACTICAL TIP

A few dogs presenting as emergencies may have no abnormalities on physical examination but this does not mean that they do not require immediate therapy. A classic example of this is toxin ingestion

---

Dogs requiring hospitalization should have intravenous access established for administration of medications. A cephalic vein catheter is most appropriate, as it is simple and quick to place and secure (see *BSAVA Guide to Procedures in Small Animal Practice*). Once the catheter is in place, a small amount of blood can be obtained for a minimum database; this is required for all dogs unwell enough to require hospitalization for medical problems, and for surgical patients requiring anaesthesia.

Wounds and open fractures should be covered with a sterile temporary dressing during initial assessment and stabilization; then managed appropriately as soon as possible.

Minimum database
This should include:

- Packed cell volume (PCV)

- Total protein (TP) measured by refractometry (sometimes termed total solids)
- Blood glucose
- Blood urea or creatinine.

Measuring electrolytes, particularly potassium, is extremely useful as many unwell emergency patients have electrolyte abnormalities.

PCV and TP: PCV and TP measurements can identify the presence of anaemia and help identify the aetiology (Figure 8.5).

PCV	TP	Possible causes	Action
Increased (>55%)	Increased (>75 g/l)	Dehydration	Rehydrate
	Normal (50–75 g/l)	Normal for breed (e.g. sight hounds) Polycythaemia	Haematology
Normal (37–55%)	Increased	Hyperglobulinaemia Artefactual	Biochemistry
	Decreased (<50 g/l)	Acute haemorrhage Hypoproteinaemia	Administer intravenous fluids if hypovolaemic Biochemistry
Decreased (<37%)	Normal	Chronic anaemia Haemolytic anaemia	Haematology
	Decreased	Haemorrhage Anaemia and hypoproteinaemia	Haematology and biochemistry

8.5   Common abnormalities of PCV and TP; suggested causes and interventions.

Glucose: Blood glucose should be measured in any **collapsed** patient, as hypoglycaemia is easy to identify and address. Furthermore, hypoglycaemic dogs will not respond to other therapies until their blood glucose is normal. In a collapsed dog, a blood glucose concentration of <3.0 mmol/l should prompt administration of glucose (0.25 g/kg i.v.) and investigation for the underlying cause (Figure 8.6).

Hypoglycaemia as a result of seizure activity is extremely rare and it is more likely that in a seizuring patient the hypoglycaemia is the cause of the seizure. Investigation should therefore be directed at the

Blood glucose concentration	Common causes	Action
<2.5 mmol/l	Insulin overdose Insulinoma Toy dog hypoglycaemia Puppy hypoglycaemia Sepsis	Consider serum insulin measurement Administer glucose 0.25 g/kg i.v. (0.5 ml of a 50% glucose solution diluted 1:1 with saline) Maintain on 2.5–5% glucose infusion
2.5–3.5 mmol/l	As above	Monitor
>14 mmol/l	Stress (rare) Diabetes mellitus	Urinalysis Fructosamine assay Rehydrate prior to considering insulin administration if ketotic

8.6   Common abnormalities of blood glucose concentrations; suggested causes and interventions. Reference level is approximately 4–6 mmol/l.

cause of hypoglycaemia. Adult dogs also very rarely have hypoglycaemia related to inappetence, although this is seen in puppies (see Chapter 5).

Hyperglycaemia is rarely seen as a result of stress in dogs, except in severe hypoperfusion and head trauma, and in these situations blood glucose is still generally <12 mmol/l. A blood glucose concentration above 14 mmol/l should therefore prompt investigation for diabetes mellitus.

Urea and creatinine: Serum urea or creatinine concentration gives an indication of kidney function (Figure 8.7). If serum concentrations are increased, a urine sample should be obtained (if easily possible) prior to starting fluid therapy, in order to allow differentiation of prerenal, renal and postrenal causes.

Urea	Creatinine	Common causes	Action
Increased	Normal	Prerenal azotaemia Gastrointestinal haemorrhage High-protein diet	Urinalysis Faecal examination Consider fluid therapy
Normal	Increased	Muscular animal/ normal for breed (e.g. Greyhound)	None
Increased	Increased	Prerenal azotaemia Renal azotaemia Postrenal azotaemia	Careful physical examination Urinalysis Consider fluid therapy

8.7 Common abnormalities of blood urea and creatinine concentrations; suggested causes and interventions. Note that reference intervals vary markedly according to the analyser used.

Cardiovascular abnormalities – assessment and management

Hypoperfusion (shock)

The main aim of the cardiovascular assessment is identification of hypoperfusion (shock). There are four common types of hypoperfusion and careful cardiovascular examination will allow differentiation between them.

- **Hypovolaemic shock.** The most common cause of hypoperfusion in dogs is hypovolaemia, typically as a result of blood loss or fluid loss into the gastrointestinal tract.
- **Cardiogenic shock** is caused by failure of the pump mechanism, as a result of either decreased myocardial function or arrhythmias.
- **Obstructive shock** is caused by interference with filling of the right side of the heart, for example as a result of cardiac tamponade or gastric dilatation–volvulus (GDV).
- **Distributive shock** is caused by excessive vasodilatation as a result of overwhelming inflammation or infection, and is also known as endotoxic or septic shock.

Hypoperfusion, whatever the cause, should be treated as a matter of urgency, as prolonged hypoperfusion is associated with organ dysfunction and increased mortality. In many forms of hypoperfusion,

fluid therapy is the primary intervention required for stabilization. This is particularly true in hypovolaemic and distributive shock, where there is either a true or relative deficit in intravascular volume. Careful cardiovascular assessment will enable the clinician to rule out underlying cardiac disease as the cause of hypoperfusion. The presence of a murmur, jugular distension or arrhythmias should prompt further examination of the heart for the presence of cardiogenic shock.

> **WARNING**
>
> **Fluid therapy is contraindicated in cardiogenic shock**

As the most common cause of hypoperfusion is hypovolaemia, assessing patients with cardiovascular compromise for this as a priority is a sensible approach. The dog should be assessed for the severity of the hypovolaemia (Figure 8.8), which will allow the clinician to titrate therapy.

Parameter	Mild (compensatory)	Moderate	Severe (decompensatory)
Heart rate (beats/min)	130–150	150–170	170–220
Mucous membrane colour	Pinker than normal	Pale pink to normal	White/muddy/grey
Capillary refill time (CRT)	Vigorous; <1 second	Reduced vigour; 1–2 seconds	>2 seconds or absent
Pulse amplitude	Increased	Normal to decreased	Decreased
Pulse duration	Short	Normal	Very short
Mentation	Normal	Slightly depressed	Obtunded
Suggested initial isotonic crystalloid dose	10 ml/kg i.v. over 20 minutes	20 ml/kg i.v. over 15–20 minutes	30–40 ml/kg i.v. over 15 minutes

8.8 Assessment of severity of hypovolaemia, with suggested initial fluid therapy.

Most dogs respond in a similar way to increasing severity of hypovolaemia (see Figure 8.8). Initially, the response to hypovolaemia results in a hyperresponsive picture on cardiovascular examination:

- Mucous membranes appear pinker than normal
- Capillary refill time (CRT) is shortened
- Pulse pressure is heightened or bounding.

As the severity of hypovolaemia worsens:

- Heart rate will increase
- Pulse quality will decrease
- Mucous membranes will become paler
- CRT will become prolonged.

Where there are deviations from the expected pattern, careful examination for other forms of hypoperfusion should be undertaken. This should include looking for signs of cardiac failure, infection/inflammation or obstruction to venous filling, e.g. jugular vein or abdominal distension. Historical information may also be useful, such as the presence of a chronic cough and heart murmur which may indicate the presence of congestive heart failure, or in entire bitches where pyometra may be a consideration leading to distributive shock.

Management

Management of hypoperfusion should be a priority if identified. Prolonged hypoperfusion increases the risk of complications including organ dysfunction.

Fluid therapy must be titrated to the individual patient. When devising a fluid therapy plan the following questions should be considered:

- What route?
- What type?
- How much?
- Over what period?

> ### WARNING
>
> **Contraindications to fluid therapy**
>
> Whilst fluid therapy is vital for successful management of many types of shock, in certain circumstances it may make the situation worse. Fluid therapy should **not** be administered in the initial stabilization period, unless there are specific indications to do so, if any of the following signs/conditions is present:
>
> - Left-sided congestive heart failure
> - Jugular distension
> - Pericardial effusion
> - Supraventricular tachycardia (heart rate >250 beats/min)

Hypovolaemic shock: Hypovolaemia is managed with intravenous fluid therapy. Despite a large volume of research in this area in human medicine, there is no evidence to suggest that there is a benefit associated with the use of another type of fluid over isotonic crystalloids. For this reason, isotonic crystalloid fluids such as 0.9% saline or lactated Ringer's solution should be used for initial resuscitation.

> ### PRACTICAL TIP
>
> Fluid therapy for hypoperfusion is an inexact science and all doses should be administered to effect; if the initial dose is not effective this should prompt re-evaluation of the patient

When using isotonic crystalloids it is helpful to think about the 'shock dose'. This is a safe volume to administer to a healthy dog without evidence of cardiovascular/respiratory or renal disease. It is also a reflection of the complete blood volume. A full shock dose is 60–90 ml/kg, but it would be unusual to administer this as a single dose. More commonly, a proportion of the shock dose is administered, depending on the severity of the signs. Suggested initial doses are listed in Figure 8.8. These initial doses should be administered rapidly, i.e. as a bolus, typically over 10–20 minutes. In large dogs this is best achieved using a pressure bag (Figure 8.9).

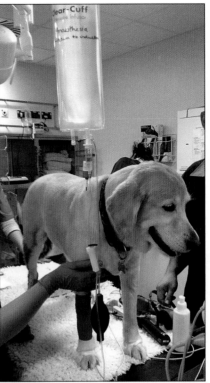

8.9   Administering a bolus of Hartmann's (lactated Ringer's) solution, using a pressure bag, to a 5-year-old female neutered Labrador Retriever with hypovolaemia as a result of severe haematuria.

Once the initial bolus has been given, the patient should be reassessed.

- If the patient is stable, fluid therapy can be stopped.
- If the dog still has signs of hypovolaemia, a further dose can be administered.
- If a full shock dose has been administered and the patient is still unstable, the dog should be carefully reassessed for ongoing haemorrhage or the presence of other forms of hypoperfusion (distributive, cardiogenic or obstructive).

Other types of hypoperfusion: Management of other forms of hypoperfusion is aimed at the underlying condition. In some circumstances more than one type of hypoperfusion can co-exist, generally in conjunction with hypovolaemia, and therefore fluid therapy may be involved in the management of these cases.

Cardiogenic hypoperfusion: This indicates myocardial dysfunction, either as a result of pump failure or arrhythmias. Management of arrhythmias requires electrocardiogram (ECG) analysis. Commonly utilized therapies include lidocaine for the management of ventricular arrhythmias and beta-blockers and calcium channel blockers for the management of supraventricular arrhythmias. If there is an underlying myocardial disease, such as dilated cardiomyopathy, therapy is aimed at improving inotropy. Ventricular arrhythmias can occur as a result of both cardiac and non-cardiac disease; if these are identified and cardiac disease is excluded, careful examination for concurrent abdominal (particularly splenic) or respiratory disease should be performed.

Obstructive hypoperfusion: This is most commonly seen as a result of GDV or pericardial effusion. In these situations therapy is aimed at the underlying cause; i.e. drainage of the pericardial effusion or gastric decompression. In GDV, gastric decompression should occur at the same time as, or after, fluid therapy. Gastric decompression is very important in stabilizing these dogs, as it removes the cause of obstruction.

Distributive hypoperfusion: This is more challenging to manage as affected dogs have widespread vascular dysfunction as a result of systemic inflammation. This results in global vasodilatation and a relative hypovolaemia and, hence, hypoperfusion. Therapy should be aimed at addressing the underlying disease. Due to the relative hypovolaemia, intravenous fluid therapy is extremely important in the management of these cases.

In infectious causes of distributive hypoperfusion, such as septic peritonitis and pneumonia, antimicrobials play a vital role in management, and the collection of samples for culture and sensitivity testing should be prioritized alongside the administration of early appropriate antimicrobials. Fluid therapy remains the mainstay of management in these cases. In some cases inotropes and vasopressors are necessary for the management of perfusion, but the use of these is beyond the scope of this Manual.

WARNING

Corticosteroids are not required for the emergency management of any type of shock and should not be given. High-dose corticosteroid administration is not indicated in any emergency

---

Other parameters
In addition to measurement of heart rate, pulse rate, pulse quality, mucous membrane colour and CRT, cardiovascular examination of the emergency patient includes venous filling, cardiac auscultation and palpation of the apex beat.

Apex beat

- Palpation of the apex beat is an often overlooked part of the cardiovascular assessment but can provide useful information
- The apex beat is quicker to palpate and easier to feel than a pulse in dogs with suspected cardiopulmonary arrest
- Absence of an apex beat, in association with weak pulses, is suggestive of a pericardial effusion

---

The findings from each of these assessments should be cross-referenced, and unexpected findings should alert the clinician to perform further investigations. The presence of injected mucous membranes with severe tachycardia may indicate sepsis or systemic inflammation. Weak pulse quality with a normal heart rate may indicate the presence of an arrhythmia or electrolyte disturbances.

Respiratory abnormalities – assessment and management
During the major body system assessment (see above) the dog should be examined for signs of dyspnoea. Dyspnoea alone rarely causes complete collapse and if a patient has signs of collapse as well as dyspnoea, then examination for the presence of cardiovascular compromise, e.g. left-sided congestive heart failure (CHF) or sepsis, should be instigated.

All patients presenting with dyspnoea should be provided with oxygen therapy (Figure 8.10) and have their stress levels reduced. This is most easily achieved through the use of an oxygen tent at a distance from human interactions. Once the patient is calmer, a more thorough examination can take place. Oxygen should be provided during this assessment, and an anaesthetic circuit (without a mask) is an easy way to do this; using this method, an inspired oxygen concentration of approximately 30–40% is possible.

Examination of the respiratory tract should include observation initially. Signs commonly associated with upper airway obstruction that can be observed include audible noise (stertor or stridor) and a prolonged inspiratory phase. Paradoxical respiration (the thoracic wall moving in during inspiration) is commonly associated with pleural space disease in dogs, and an expiratory push is often seen with lower airway disease.

Auscultation can provide valuable information, but is performed more easily when the dog is not panting. However, panting should not be prevented in dyspnoeic dogs; it can allow assessment of pleural space disease as breath sounds are amplified and so the absence of breath sounds is easier to identify. Commonly heard sounds include: fine end-inspiratory crackles that are associated with pulmonary oedema; coarse inspiratory crackles associated with airway disease; and expiratory wheezes which are associated with bronchoconstriction. It is also common to hear generalized harshness, which is non-specific and may be associated with a variety of respiratory diseases. As respiratory signs are commonly caused by left-sided heart failure, the heart should be auscultated carefully as well. An increased heart rate (>120 beats/min) or arrhythmia in association with a loud murmur should increase the suspicion of heart failure.

Useful investigative tests in the dyspnoeic patient include imaging, particularly ultrasonography, which can be used even in inexperienced hands to identify pleural effusion. Thoracic radiography for evaluation of the parenchyma can aid in diagnosis (see Chapter 24), as the distribution and pattern are typically associated with specific diseases, for example:

- Peripheral alveolar/interstitial pattern in *Angiostrongylus vasorum* infection
- Perihilar alveolar pattern in cardiogenic oedema
- Ventral alveolar pattern in aspiration pneumonia; always evaluate the lung fields overlying the cardiac silhouette if this is a concern.

Management
Management of respiratory signs should be aimed at treating the underlying cause and relieving the dyspnoea. A quiet environment can provide as much improvement in a dog as oxygen therapy, and

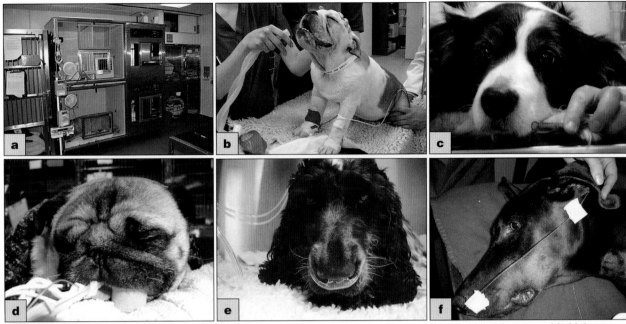

8.10 Modes of oxygen therapy. **(a)** Oxygen cages are very expensive but are well tolerated and can provide high concentrations of oxygen to dogs of a variety of sizes. **(b)** A Bulldog puppy with pneumonia. During the initial examination, flow-by oxygen was provided using a T-piece. This is a non-invasive and low stress way to provide oxygen while allowing full access to the dog. **(c)** An 8-year-old Border Collie receiving oxygen supplementation via tubing during stabilization for hypovolaemia. **(d)** Endotracheal intubation, as in this Pug, allows any upper respiratory obstructions to be bypassed and can provide 100% oxygen supplementation. **(e)** A 4-year-old Cocker Spaniel receiving oxygen using nasal prongs. These provide up to about 40% oxygen supplementation and are variably well tolerated. A bridge of tape over the nose can make keeping them in place easier. **(f)** A 5-year-old Dobermann with pulmonary thromboembolism secondary to immune-mediated haemolytic anaemia receiving oxygen via nasal catheters. If placed bilaterally, these will provide up to 70% oxygen.

minimal stress should continue. Longer-term oxygen therapy can be provided using nasal insufflation or an oxygen cage. Medium-sized and large dogs will overheat in oxygen tents and so these should be avoided for all but the smallest dogs.

In dogs with upper respiratory obstruction as a result of airway disease, judicious sedation can play an important role in management. Very low doses of sedatives such as acepromazine (0.005 mg/kg i.v.) and butorphanol (0.1 mg/kg i.v.) can be given as required. The dogs should be watched very carefully after administration as some dogs can deteriorate following sedation.

Where there is a suspicion of left-sided CHF, treatment with furosemide should be given at an initial dose of 2–4 mg/kg i.v. or i.m. This dose may be repeated if the dog does not urinate or there is no reduction in respiratory rate within an hour.

If pleural space disease is suspected, thoracocentesis should be performed as a priority as it will provide both relief of respiratory distress and diagnostic information. This technique is described in the *BSAVA Guide to Procedures in Small Animal Practice*.

Neurological assessment and management

The aim of neurological assessment of the emergency patient is to assess mentation, pain perception and ability to ambulate, i.e. function of the brain and spinal cord. This should enable the clinician to exclude significant central nervous system (CNS) disease. It is important to assess patients when they are cardiovascularly stable, as hypoperfusion has significant effects

on mentation and the ability to respond to pain due to the CNS's high metabolic requirement.

Seizures

Seizures, if present, should be managed as a priority (Figure 8.11) in order to prevent ongoing effects on the body such as hyperthermia. When presented with dogs with acute-onset seizures and no prior history, it is important to rule out metabolic causes prior to loading the dog with long-acting anti-epileptic drugs. This approach is somewhat different to a dog with epilepsy, where metabolic problems have already been ruled out (see Chapter 11).

1. Place an intravenous catheter as soon as possible
2. Provide flow-by oxygen if possible
3. Administer diazepam 0.5 mg/kg – i.v. if possible, rectally if not
4. Check blood glucose. If <3.0 mmol/l, administer 0.25 g/kg glucose i.v. as a bolus
5. Check body temperature. If >41°C begin active cooling (see Chapter 18)
6. If still seizuring, repeat diazepam intravenously up to a total of three doses
7. Perform testing for an emergency database to include electrolytes, urea and calcium if possible
8. Where there is a suspicion of hepatic encephalopathy, consider other anti-seizure medication such as propofol
9. Ongoing management will depend on the aetiology
   - Where a toxic cause is suspected, management of seizures with propofol is most appropriate as it acts rapidly
   - Where the dog is a known epileptic, or metabolic causes have been excluded and epilepsy or intracranial causes are suspected, a long-acting epileptic agent should be given (see Chapter 11)

8.11 Emergency management of seizures. It should be noted that seizures very rarely cause hypoglycaemia; if a dog is found to be hypoglycaemic during a seizure, the investigation should be aimed at identifying the cause of the hypoglycaemia.

Other conditions

Severe neurological diseases and signs often benefit from specialist intervention and may require advanced imaging such as magnetic resonance imaging (MRI), therefore, referral should be considered early in the course of the assessment.

Intracranial disease

Intracranial disease can be more immediately life-threatening to the pet than spinal disease and therefore should be prioritized. In many situations stabilization of the intracranial signs will rely on a combination of some or all of the following: seizure control; airway protection; provision of oxygen and perfusion; and exclusion of metabolic or physiological derangements, e.g. hypoglycaemia, hyperammonaemia or hyperthermia that may promote ongoing signs.

Intracranial hypertension (ICH) is a sequel of intracranial disease or trauma, which requires rapid management. It can be difficult to detect, as many of the findings relied upon for diagnosis are relatively late changes. The presence of deteriorating mentation in the face of adequate perfusion or alterations in pupillary responsiveness or symmetry should alert the clinician to the possibility of ICH. Peripheral hypertension and bradycardia (the Cushing response) may be seen. This is a protective mechanism to ensure perfusion to the brain. If ICH is suspected, management with hyperosmolar solutions (e.g. mannitol or hypertonic saline) should be used and their effect monitored. Typically they should result, at least, in improved mentation. The use of scoring systems such as the Modified Glasgow Coma Scale (MGCS) (see *BSAVA Manual of Canine and Feline Neurology*) are to be recommended; the MGCS is repeatable and provides a subjective way to monitor patients at risk of, or being treated for, ICH.

Spinal disease

Spinal disease, while usually less immediately life-threatening, should also be prioritized, as severe lesions where there is loss of pain perception respond more favourably to early intervention. Dogs with high cervical injury should also be prioritized due to the risk of respiratory compromise related to respiratory muscle paralysis.

Traumatic spinal injuries with loss of pain perception associated with palpable spinal deviation have a very poor prognosis for full recovery. It may be advisable to discuss with the owners early on, whether they would like to proceed with further emergency care with such a poor prognosis. Care should be taken in this assessment, however, and the patient should be cardiovascularly stable prior to the examination being performed. Dogs with spinal trauma should be transported strapped firmly to a flat, firm board to immobilize the spine. Immobilization while on the treatment table may also be necessary (Figure 8.12). Where there is any doubt, advice from a neurologist should be sought.

> **WARNING**
>
> High-dose corticosteroid therapy is not indicated in the emergency management of any type of neurotrauma

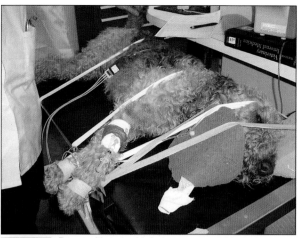

8.12 Dogs with spinal injuries may need to be strapped down to immobilize the spine and avoid further injury.

Monitoring during stabilization

The most useful method of monitoring during the stabilization period is repeated physical examination, concentrating on the major body systems. Where abnormalities have been identified in the emergency database, the tests should be repeated regularly (as frequently as every 30 minutes where they are life-threatening; up to 1–4 hours apart for others) to detect progression. Other monitoring that may be useful includes electrocardiography, blood pressure and in some cases pulse oximetry, though this is prone to errors in conscious dogs.

Secondary assessment

Once the major body system assessment is complete, and life-saving or stabilizing therapy has been administered, the patient should undergo a secondary assessment. The initial assessment will often have allowed the veterinary surgeon to create an initial problem list and the start of a diagnostic plan. The secondary assessment should include a full history and thorough physical examination of the whole dog, with repeat cardiovascular, respiratory and neurological assessments in greater detail where necessary. Once this has been completed, further diagnostic tests can be performed, or therapeutic agents administered where a diagnosis has been reached.

Useful additional diagnostic tests

■ Full haematology and biochemical testing, while useful, will rarely change the management of emergency patients immediately. It is far more useful to tailor tests and expedite those that are important for the individual case, e.g. a platelet count estimation on a blood smear in a dog with signs of haemorrhage. Full profiles can then be submitted to an external laboratory for interpretation by a clinical pathologist.

■ Common causes of emergency presentations in dogs often involve the gastrointestinal tract and therefore imaging of the abdomen, e.g. radiography or ultrasonography, is useful for diagnosis.

- Complicated echocardiographic evaluation is rarely required, although it is useful to learn how to assess left atrial size for dogs presenting with signs of heart failure (see *BSAVA Manual of Canine and Feline Cardiorespiratory Medicine*).
- Radiography of the thorax and abdomen and ultrasonography are also useful for detecting the presence of fluid in body cavities. The utilization of ultrasonography to identify small volumes of fluid within the peritoneal space (sometimes referred to as a FAST scan) in dogs presenting with an 'acute abdomen' is a particularly useful skill and can enable sampling and therefore therapeutic planning.
- When a fluid sample is obtained from a body cavity, further analysis including cytology should always be performed. Where there is a suspicion of sepsis, sampling and cytology should be performed in house, with a further sample submitted for culture and sensitivity testing.

Ongoing management

Once the patient is stable and a plan has been created, the care does not end! The patient should be monitored appropriately to ensure it is stable and remains so. Fluid therapy plans should be created, and modified depending on the progression of the patient. In many cases dogs presenting as emergencies will need ongoing care for a period of time before they are well enough to go home. Many patients will need regular monitoring and assessment, and consideration should be made as to whether this is possible within the practice.

References and further reading

Bexfield N and Lee K (2014) *BSAVA Guide to Procedures in Small Animal Practice, 2nd edn.* BSAVA Publications, Gloucester
Brown A (2012) Shock, sepsis and SIRS. In: *BSAVA Manual of Canine and Feline Surgical Principles: A Foundation Manual*, ed. S Baines et al., pp.127–141. BSAVA Publications, Gloucester
Fletcher D J, Boller m, Brainard B M et al., (2012) RECOVER evidence and Knowledge gap analysis on veterinary CPR. Part 7: Clinical guidelines. *Journal of Veterinary Emergency and Critical Care* **22** (SI), 102—131
Humm K and Adamantos S (2012) Fluid therapy and electrolyte and acid–base abnormalities. In: *BSAVA Manual of Canine and Feline Surgical Principles: A Foundation Manual*, ed. S Baines et al., pp. 104—126. BSAVA Publications, Gloucester
King L and Boag A (in production) *BSAVA Manual of Canine and Feline Emergency and Critical Care, 3rd edn.* BSAVA Publications, Gloucester
Luis Fuentes V, Johnson Le and Dennis S (2010) *BSAVA Manual of Canine and Feline Cardiorespiratory Medicine, 2nd edn.* BSAVA Publications, Gloucester
Pead M J and Langley-Hobbs S J (2007) Acute management of orthopaedic and external soft-tissue injuries. In: *BSAVA Manual of Canine and Feline Emergency and Critical Care, 2nd edn*, ed. LG King and A Boag, pp. 251–268. BSAVA Publications, Gloucester
Platt S and Olby N (2013) BSAVA Manual of Canine and Feline Neurology, 4th edn. BSAVA Publications, Gloucester
Waddell L S and King L G (2007) General approach to dyspnoea. In: *BSAVA Manual of Canine and Feline Emergency and Critical Care, 2nd edn*, ed. LG King and A Boag, pp. 85–113. BSAVA Publications, Gloucester

QRG 8.1 Cardiopulmonary resuscitation

CPR should be used:

- In a dog with confirmed cardiopulmonary arrest (CPA)
- In any unresponsive apnoeic dog (until CPA has been ruled out).

Recognition of an unresponsive apnoeic patient is all that is initially required (rapid assessment of Airway, Breathing, Circulation) as basic CPR must not be delayed.

Personnel

- Ideally, a minimum of three people are required for effective CPR: one person to perform cardiac compressions; one to ventilate; and one to monitor, administer drugs and obtain equipment. If a team is present, the team leader should give clear orders that are repeated back by the team member carrying out the task, to ensure the task is completed correctly.
- If only two people are available, they should concentrate on basic life support, ensuring that cardiac compressions and ventilation are optimized. The person administering ventilation can also monitor the effectiveness of the compressions by palpating for pulses between ventilations.
- If there is only one person available, effective CPR is almost impossible. The caregiver should shout or call for help (use bystanders if possible) and intubate the dog. Flow-by oxygen at a high rate should provide enough oxygen while the operator delivers cardiac compressions. Basic life support should be optimized in this situation, as continuous cardiac compressions are essential for a positive outcome.

PRACTICAL TIPS

- Good training and regular rehearsals will help towards a successful outcome
- When animals are at risk of cardiopulmonary arrest, a crash box should be easily accessible and ready for use

Equipment

- Organized and regularly audited crash trolley, containing:
  - Laryngoscope with a variety of blades
  - Cuffed endotracheal (ET) tubes: full range of sizes with stylets and dog urinary catheters (8 Fr recommended) with 2 mm ET tube connector for difficult intubation
  - White open weave (WOW) bandage for securing ET tube and holding upper jaw
  - Swabs
  - Ambu bag (self-reinflating bag)
  - Intravenous catheters: range of sizes
  - Intraosseous catheters
  - Dog urinary catheters for intratracheal drug administration
  - Relevant drugs

▶

QRG 8.1 *continued*

Indication	Drug and concentration	Dose
Cardiac arrest	Adrenaline (1:1000; 1 mg/ml) – Low dose	0.01 mg/kg
	Adrenaline (1:1000; 1 mg/ml) –High dose	0.1 mg/kg
	Atropine (0.6 mg/ml)	0.04 mg/kg
Ventricular fibrillation or pulseless ventricular tachycardia	Lidocaine (20 mg/ml)	2 mg/kg
Drug reversal	Naloxone (0.4 mg/ml)	0.04 mg/kg
	Flumazenil (0.1 mg/ml)	0.01 mg/kg
	Atipamezole (5 mg/ml)	100 µg/kg

- Needles and syringes to match drug doses required
- Bags of sterile fluids for intravenous administration: 0.9% saline and lactated Ringer's (Hartmann's) solution
- Intravenous fluid administration sets
- 0.9% saline to flush intravenous/intraosseous catheters
- ECG monitor, pads and gel
- End-tidal carbon dioxide ($ETCO_2$) monitor (if available)
- Oxygen saturation (S_pO_2) monitor
- Blood pressure monitor
- Thermometer
- Blood sample pots/tubes.
■ Charts – these must be clear and in the CPR area:
  - Local CPR protocol
  - Drug dosages – preferably in both mg/kg and ml for weights 5–50 kg.
■ Oxygen supply with necessary tubing/non re-breathing circuit (Bain or T-piece).

Patient preparation and positioning

The dog should be positioned in lateral recumbency.

Technique

The priority is to begin basic life support.
   If possible, advanced life support and monitoring (see below) should be started simultaneously.

Basic life support (BLS)

This consists of chest compressions and ventilation.

PRACTICAL TIPS

- Each BLS cycle lasts 2 minutes
- Begin the first cycle as soon as possible, and complete it uninterrupted
- Chest compressions and ventilation are carried out simultaneously
- If possible, change the person performing chest compressions between cycles to avoid fatigue

Chest compressions

- **Perform 100–120 compressions per minute.**
- Compress the thorax by a third to a half of its resting width and allow full chest recoil between compressions.
- Each compression should be associated with a pulse. If no pulse is palpable, change technique (or operator).

Small dogs: Wrap a single hand around the sternum at the level of the heart and compress the thorax between your thumb and fingers; or use the technique for deep and narrow-chested dogs.
Medium and large dogs: Place the palm of one hand over the back of the other hand with your fingers interdigitated. Apply the palms of the hands to the dog's thorax. Keep your elbows locked in extension and push downwards through the palms of your hands. For most dogs, place your hands centrally over the thorax, such that compressive force acts on the widest part of the chest.
Deep and narrow-chested dogs: Place your hands directly over the area of the dog's heart.

Ventilation

1 Intubate the dog *in lateral recumbency* using a laryngoscope.

2 Secure the ET tube to the animal's muzzle or mandible.

3 Inflate the cuff of the ET tube.

4 Attach an Ambu bag to the ET tube.

5 Ventilate at 10 breaths/min. The aim is to expand the chest gently; breaths should not be excessively large.

Advanced life support (ALS)

Monitoring

- Attach an ECG monitor, capnograph and pulse oximeter
- Electrolytes and arterial blood gas analysis: not mandatory but useful where electrolyte disturbance may be involved in causing CPA

1 Supplement inspired oxygen.

- If arterial blood gas data are available, titrate to P_aO_2 of 80–105 mmHg or S_pO_2 >95%.
- If arterial blood gas data are unavailable, giving 100% of F_iO_2 is reasonable.

2 Establish vascular access via an intravenous catheter (preferable) or intraosseous cannula.

PRACTICAL TIPS

- Intratracheal drug dosing can be considered for adrenaline (0.02–0.1 mg/kg) and atropine (0.15–0.2 mg/kg), though it may be ineffective:
  - Insert a dog urinary catheter via the ET tube to the level of the carina
  - Dilute the drug with saline or sterile water prior to administration and follow up with a breath
- Intracardiac administration of drugs is NOT recommended

3 Give low-dose adrenaline (0.01 mg/kg i.v.) during every other cycle of BLS. If CPA persists for >10 minutes, consider single high-dose adrenaline injection (0.1 mg/kg i.v.).

4 If there is pulseless electrical activity or vagally induced cardiopulmonary arrest, give atropine (0.04 mg/kg iv).

5 If there is ventricular fibrillation (VF) or pulseless ventricular tachycardia (VT), perform electrical defibrillation:

- If VF or pulseless VT is detected within 4 minutes of CPA, perform defibrillation immediately
- If VF or pulseless VT is detected after 4 minutes of CPA, perform 1 cycle of BLS before defibrillation.

For information on defibrillation protocols, see the *BSAVA Guide to Procedures in Small Animal Practice*.

PRACTICAL TIP

If electrical defibrillation is unavailable, perform a precordial thump with the heel of your hand

6 Administer reversal agents for opioids (naloxone), alpha-2 agonists (atipamezole) or benzodiazepines (flumazenil) if these drugs are implicated in CPA (see table above for doses).

7 Consider intravenous fluid therapy.

- **In euvolaemic or hypervolaemic patients, do not give fluids.**
- In hypovolaemic patients, give intravenous fluids to restore blood volume.   ▶

QRG 8.1 *continued*

8 Open-chest CPR. *Only consider this if a specialist veterinary team and a dedicated intensive care unit are available.*

Post-CPR care

- Referral to a specialist centre should be considered.
- Continue monitoring: ECG; $ETCO_2$; S_pO_2; arterial blood gases; blood pressure; blood electrolyte, lactate and glucose concentrations; and body temperature.

Basic life support (BLS)

Perform in uninterrupted cycles of 2 minutes each:
- Chest compressions: 100–120/min; compress thorax width by one-third to one-half
- Intubate and ventilate: 10 breaths/min; tidal volume 10 ml/kg; inspiratory time 1 second

↓

Monitoring
- ECG to check for arrhythmias
- $ETCO_2$: >15 mmHg
- Palpate pulse between and during BLS cycles

↓

Supplement oxygen
- Give F_iO_2 of 100%, or titrate to P_aO_2 of 80–105 mmHg

↓

Obtain vascular access

↓

Treat arrhythmias
- Asystole or pulseless electrical activity:
  - Give low-dose adrenaline every other BLS cycle
  - Give atropine every other BLS cycle
  - *If no response after 10 minutes*, give high-dose adrenaline

↓

Administer reversal agents
- For opioids: naloxone
- For alpha-2 agonists: atipamezole
- For benzodiazepines: flumazenil

Reproduced from the *BSAVA Guide to Procedures in Small Animal Practice, 2nd edn*

Acute collapse

Mark Maltman

Acute collapse is a common presenting complaint in first-opinion practice and can be a source of enormous stress for inexperienced clinicians. There is a vast list of differential diagnoses (Figure 9.1), ranging in severity from conditions requiring only simple treatment (e.g. osteoarthritis in an old dog) to those where there is immediate life-threatening compromise (e.g. haemoperitoneum).

It is easy to be drawn into the panic of the owner and start clutching at diagnoses, but a logical approach which builds on history and thorough physical examination with a simple minimum database of

---

Cardiac disease

- Dilated cardiomyopathy
- Endocardiosis
- Endocarditis
- Angiostrongylosis
- Pericardial effusion and other forms of pericardial disease
- Outflow tract obstruction: aortic stenosis, pulmonic stenosis, hypertrophic obstructive cardiomyopathy

- Tachyarrhythmia: atrial fibrillation, ventricular tachycardia
- Bradyarrhythmia: profound sinus bradycardia/arrhythmia, sinus arrest/block, atrioventricular block
- Mixed tachy/bradyarrhythmia: sick sinus syndrome
- Vasovagal syncope secondary to gastrointestinal disease or abdominal pain
- Postural hypotension

Respiratory disease (including pleural space and chest wall)

- Laryngeal obstruction: laryngeal paralysis, eversion of laryngeal saccules, neoplasia
- Brachycephalic obstructive airway syndrome (BOAS)
- Tracheal collapse
- Pulmonary oedema
- Pulmonary thrombosis

- Pneumothorax
- Pleural effusion: haemothorax, pyothorax, non-septic exudate, modified transudate, transudate, chylothorax
- Chest wall disease: tumour, trauma
- Ruptured diaphragm

Endocrine/metabolic disease

- Hypoadrenocorticism
- Hyperadrenocorticism (via muscle weakness)
- Hypoglycaemia: insulinoma, hunting dog hypoglycaemia, liver dysfunction, sepsis, non-pancreatic neoplasia, xylitol toxicity
- Diabetic ketoacidosis
- Phaeochromocytoma
- Hepatic encephalopathy
- Hypercalcaemia: malignancy, renal dysfunction, hypoadrenocorticism, hypervitaminosis D, primary hyperparathyroidism

- Hypocalcaemia: primary hypoparathyroidism, pancreatitis, renal dysfunction
- Hyperkalaemia: hypoadrenocorticism, acute kidney injury, urinary obstruction, urinary tract rupture
- Hypokalaemia: chronic renal dysfunction, anorexia, vomiting and diarrhoea, hyperaldosteronism
- Hyponatraemia: hypoadrenocorticism
- Acidaemia
- Shock: hypovolaemic, cardiogenic, endotoxic

Gastrointestinal disease

- Gastric dilatation–volvulus (GDV)
- Gastroenteritis: vomiting and diarrhoea: fluid loss, pain
- Ulceration: idiopathic; secondary to inflammation, neoplasia or non-steroidal anti-inflammatory drugs (NSAIDs)

- Intestinal obstruction: foreign body, intussusception, neoplasia, torsion
- Severe constipation/obstipation
- Severe colitis
- Dysautonomia

Genitourinary disease

- Pyometra
- Prostatitis
- Pyelonephritis
- Acute kidney injury
- Chronic renal failure

- Urolithiasis
- Ruptured urinary tract: ureter, bladder or urethra
- Urinary obstruction: calculus, prostatic enlargement, bladder neck or urethral tumour, urethral dyssynergia

9.1 Differential diagnoses for acute collapse. Common examples are given in each category. (continues) ▶

Abdominal disease

- Hepatic dysfunction, including xylitol toxicity
- Cholangiohepatitis
- Biliary mucocele of the gall bladder
- Biliary rupture

- Pancreatitis
- Peritonitis
- Haemoperitoneum (e.g. splenic rupture)
- Uroperitoneum

Musculoskeletal disease

- Osteoarthritis
- Immune-mediated polyarthritis: primary; secondary to gastrointestinal disease, neoplasia, inflammation or tick-borne disease

- Myositis
- Fractures
- Bilateral disease: cruciate disease, bilateral elbow dysplasia

Neurological disease

- Sterile (steroid-responsive) meningitis ± arteritis
- Cerebrovascular accident
- Neoplasia
- Prolapsed intervertebral disc
- Status epilepticus
- Idiopathic peripheral vestibular syndrome
- Granulomatous meningioencephalitis

- Fibrocartilaginous embolism
- Myasthenia gravis
- Peripheral polyneuropathy
- Metaldehyde toxicity
- Avermectin toxicity (inadvertent ingestion of parasiticides containing avermectins)
- Dysautonomia

Haematological disease

- Anaemia: haemorrhage, haemolysis, bone marrow disease
- Myeloproliferative disorders: lymphoma, leukaemia, multiple myeloma

- Polycythaemia: polycythaemia vera, kidney disease, chronic hypoxia
- Secondary clotting dysfunction (e.g. rodenticide toxicity) leading to anaemia through accumulation of blood in body cavities

Miscellaneous

- Non-specific pain
- Pyrexia of unknown origin

- Behavioural: response to fear
- Slippery flooring

9.1 (continued) Differential diagnoses for acute collapse. Common examples are given in each category.

blood tests, urinalysis and survey imaging should be practised in a calm and consistent manner. If this is done, the diagnosis is often surprisingly obvious without too much stress. Even when this is not the case, large parts of the differential list can be ruled out and thus leave one much nearer the answer.

PRACTICAL TIPS

- There may or may not be forewarning that such an animal is about to arrive at the clinic. Having the requisite equipment to hand at all times eliminates the problem of an owner arriving in an unannounced panic
- Inexperienced clinicians would be well advised to learn and practise a consistent approach and to role play the stages of this in their mind, with or without a collapsed patient, such that it becomes second nature

Immediate considerations

First Aid

The basics of first aid must be immediately considered in ensuring that there is:

- A patent airway
- Good respiratory function
- Adequate circulation

External bleeding requires pressure to be applied whilst measures are taken to re-establish the circulation with a blood transfusion or crystalloid fluid therapy

In general, it is always good practice to take a thorough history and perform a diligent clinical examination. However, there may be situations where immediate action is required in order to save the patient's life. For example, a cyanosed dog with severe respiratory compromise due to a pharyngeal foreign body, such as a ball or rawhide chew, will receive far greater benefit from examination of this area and foreign body removal than it will from further delay. If one focuses on the primary considerations of **A**irway, **B**reathing, **C**irculation and haemorrhage control, then cases requiring immediate intervention should be easily recognized. General supportive nursing with warmth and oxygen is helpful; analgesia should be considered in the early stages.

Such attention to basic first aid may be life-saving and at the very least will turn an emergency situation into a stable patient, giving the clinician time to obtain a thorough history and plan the line of investigation.

In less urgent cases, once the history and clinical examination have been completed, the following minimum database should be acquired in all acute collapse patients:

- Haematology: if not complete, then a centrifuged in-house haematocrit (packed cell volume, PCV) is vital and also allows for measurement of total solids (TS) in the serum using a refractometer
- Chemistry: the minimum would be considered to be urea, creatinine, alanine aminotransferase (ALT), alkaline phosphatase (ALP) and blood glucose ± bile acids
- Electrolytes: sodium, potassium, chloride, calcium
- Urinalysis: specific gravity measured on a refractometer; dipstick chemistry
- Survey radiography of the chest and abdomen
- Survey abdominal ultrasonography to rule out free peritoneal fluid.

An animal collapsed with seizures or status epilepticus will need anticonvulsant therapy concurrently with the establishment of this database (see Chapters 8 and 11).

History

Taking a careful history can reveal subtle signs that may have been present prior to collapse, and will allow the list of differentials to be reduced. For example:

- An untreated cough will allow one to focus on differential diagnoses associated with cardiothoracic disease
- Weight loss may suggest neoplasia
- The presence of polyuria/polydipsia (PU/PD) highlights its own differentials from the list of those associated with collapse.

General questions should be asked, in particular regarding:

- Levels of food and water intake
- The presence or absence of vomiting and diarrhoea
- Observation of any other signs such as coughing, sneezing, bleeding, vaginal discharge, seizures and other neurological signs.

Other pertinent history includes the possibility of trauma or access to obvious toxins (e.g. rodenticide, ethylene glycol, metaldehyde, pesticides) and to substances that owners may not recognize as toxic (e.g. grapes, sultanas, raisins, currants, dark chocolate and, in certain chewing gums, xylitol). Parasiticides containing avermectins may lead to coma and seizures when inadvertently administered orally or chewed by a dog, especially in certain breeds such as collies.

Signalment is important, as younger dogs are likely to experience a different set of conditions from older dogs (e.g. neoplasia is more common with advancing age). Certain breed dispositions can help but one must not jump to conclusions. For example: a collapsed Dobermann with pale mucous membranes and increased respiratory rate probably has dilated cardiomyopathy; but it could also have immune-mediated haemolytic anaemia or splenic rupture causing the same clinical signs.

The point in the oestrous cycle is helpful in cases of pyometra and type II diabetes mellitus.

In some cases, there may be no relevant history prior to the onset of clinical signs.

Observation

Observation will allow assessment as to whether collapse is complete, partial or intermittent.

Is there any ability to walk?

- Dogs with immune-mediated polyarthritis may be able to shuffle along with multiple sore joints but collapse regularly due to pain.
- Dogs with severe metabolic, circulatory or cardiorespiratory disease may not be able to rise at all.
- Dogs with hypoglycaemia or myasthenia gravis may have collapse interspersed with periods of normality.

Assessment of respiration may be made simply by watching the patient before examination; signs such as tachypnoea, hyperpnoea, orthopnoea and dyspnoea point towards a cardiorespiratory origin, but can also be present with increased respiratory drive associated with anaemia, acidaemia, pain or pyrexia, or less commonly with respiratory muscle failure in cases with peripheral neuromuscular disorders.

Physical examination

Head and neck

Mucous membrane colour should be examined, but capillary refill time is a less reliable indicator. Pale membranes (Figure 9.2a) are associated with poor peripheral perfusion (shock – hypovolaemic, cardiogenic, endotoxic) or anaemia (haemorrhage, haemolysis or bone marrow dysfunction) (see also Chapter 20).

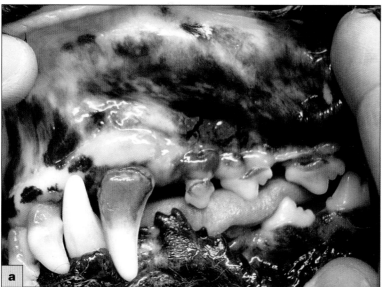

9.2 A 13-year-old Labrador Retriever that presented acutely collapsed. **(a)** The mucous membranes were pale and the dog had a PCV of 19%. (continues) ▶

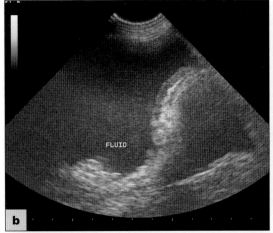

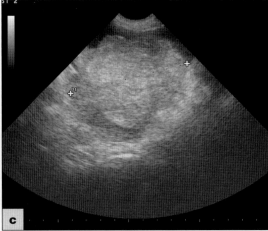

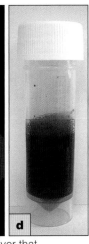

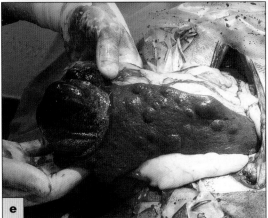

9.2 (continued) A 13-year-old Labrador Retriever that presented acutely collapsed. Free peritoneal fluid was found on abdominal palpation and confirmed with ultrasonography **(b)**, which also showed a large splenic mass **(c)** and facilitated guided abdominocentesis to yield frank blood **(d)**. Surgery removed a large spleen with multiple nodules and one large ruptured mass **(e)** which was found to be non-malignant on histopathology. It should be noted that ruptured splenic masses should not be assumed to be malignant haemangiosarcomas, as haematomas, splenic hyperplasia and haemangiomas are also possible. The dog made a good recovery.

Significant enlargement of peripheral lymph nodes may be associated with lymphoma, but can also be a non-specific response to inflammatory diseases.

Thoracic auscultation

Auscultation of the thorax will provide information that can be tied in with that gleaned from the initial observation. Abnormal cardiac sounds such as murmurs (see Chapter 24), or pulmonary noise such as crackles or wheezes may be present. Alternatively, these sounds may be muffled in cases with pleural or pericardial effusion, and lung sounds may be lost altogether when lungs are collapsed in the presence of pneumothorax. The heart rate and rhythm should be noted; many cases with heart disease of sufficient severity to cause collapse will have concurrent cardiac arrhythmias, but ventricular arrhythmias are also commonly present with non-cardiac disease such as gastric dilatation–volvulus (GDV), splenic disease, pancreatitis and severe sepsis.

Combining auscultation with assessment of the **peripheral pulse** allows one to assess the state of the circulation, as well as to identify pulse deficits associated with arrhythmias. A strong pulse is an appropriate response to sympathetic stimulation associated with physical disease of sufficient severity to induce collapse, unless that disease is characterized by low blood pressure in cases of shock, classified as:

- Hypovolaemic: acute, internal or external haemorrhage or severe fluid loss
- Cardiac (cardiogenic or obstructive): low cardiac output associated with any cardiac disease

- Endotoxic (also known as distributive or septic shock): classically seen with pyometra.

In contrast to acute anaemia, patients with chronic anaemia of mild to moderate severity, where there has been time for the body to compensate, are likely to have good pulse quality.

Abdominal palpation

Palpation of the abdomen may reveal (see Chapter 25):

- Gaseous distension associated with GDV
- Ascites associated with:
  - Right-sided cardiac failure (including cases caused by pulmonary hypertension, possibly induced by *Angiostrongylus vasorum*)
  - Pericardial effusion
  - Portal hypertension
  - Hypoproteinaemia (protein-losing enteropathy or nephropathy, or end-stage liver disease)
  - Abdominal neoplasia
  - Pancreatitis
  - Torsion of a liver lobe, the spleen or mesenteric root
  - Peritonitis.

More specific fluid can accumulate with haemoperitoneum (traumatic or neoplastic organ rupture, coagulopathy) and urinary or biliary tract rupture.

In the absence of fluid, enlargement of the liver and/or spleen, and the presence of solid neoplastic masses may be detected. Generalized enlargement of the liver and spleen can be seen with cardiac disease, lymphoma, leukaemia and multifocal abdominal neoplasia. Abdominocentesis will assist in narrowing the list of differentials for free peritoneal fluid.

Body temperature

Pyrexia (see Chapter 18) may be associated with any inflammatory or infectious process in the body and, even where this can be easily addressed with antibiosis, may lead in the short term to collapse purely through malaise. If there is ongoing pyrexia of unknown origin, one should consider the possibility of intractable infectious or septic disease, immune-mediated disease or neoplasia.

Orthopaedic examination

A common cause of collapse in older dogs, especially in first-opinion practice and involving large breeds, is an acute flare-up of osteoarthritic pain (see Chapter 15). Care should be taken not to confuse symmetrical orthopaedic disease, such as immune-mediated polyarthritis or bilateral cruciate rupture, with spinal lesions. Polyarthritis is usually associated with pyrexia. The stress caused by pain in these dogs may present as changes in cardiac rhythm, which may settle when the pain is controlled.

Neurological examination

A neurological examination is vital in cases of collapse. Specific points to consider are as follows:

- Have there been any seizures? If so, are these ongoing such that anticonvulsant treatment is required (see Chapter 11); or is the collapsed patient post-ictal, with the owners having found it after the seizure had finished?
- One should assess the animal for its general demeanour. Obtundation is non-specific for intracranial disease (e.g. space-occupying lesion, raised intracranial pressure, cerebrovascular accident) or extracranial disease (e.g. hepatic encephalopathy, hypoglycaemia)
- Proprioception should be assessed (see Chapter 16):
  - Unilateral proprioceptive deficits of both the forelimb and hindlimb are indicative of contralateral cerebral disease
  - Bilateral proprioceptive deficits in only the hindlimbs points toward spinal disease caudal to T3 (upper motor neuron signs: T3–L3; lower motor neuron signs: L4–S3)
  - Proprioceptive deficits in all four limbs suggests generalized brain disease, spinal lesions C1–T2 (Figure 9.3) or peripheral neuropathies. The latter may be distinguished by the absence of withdrawal reflexes

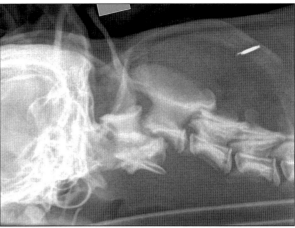

9.3 Radiograph of the cervical spine of an 8-month-old Norfolk Terrier that was presented with quadriparesis after trauma. Severe neck pain was noted, and radiography showed a fracture/luxation of C1–C2.

- Vestibular disease, presenting with ataxia, nystagmus, head tilt and/or vomiting is very common in general practice and is most often caused by idiopathic peripheral vestibular syndrome, which can be identified as such by the presence of normal proprioception; abnormal proprioception suggests that vestibular dysfunction is central in origin.

Diagnostic tests

The minimum database outlined above leads to a diagnosis in many cases.

Blood tests

Haematology

The most commonly identified haematological cause of collapse is anaemia. A slide agglutination test is an easy patient-side test to perform and is used to identify immune-mediated haemolytic anaemia.

Slide agglutination test

1. One drop of blood from an EDTA tube is applied to a warm slide and one drop of 0.9% saline added, before gently rolling the fluid round on the slide
   - Failure to add a drop of saline does not allow for the possibility of rouleaux formation; this is not abnormal but has a granular gross appearance that can produce a false-positive result. Saline will disperse any rouleaux.
2. A negative result is seen when the blood continues to show a homogeneous watery appearance
3. A positive result is seen when granular autoagglutination is present, confirming immune-mediated haemolytic anaemia

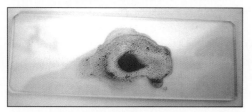

4. Agglutination may also be confirmed on the slide microscopically where the red cells are seen adhered together like 'bunches of grapes', whereas the microscopic appearance of rouleaux is that of 'stacks of coins'

Internal blood loss as a cause of anaemia may be identified as free pleural and/or peritoneal fluid using radiography or ultrasonography, but internal haemorrhage may still occur insidiously through the gastrointestinal system or urinary tract, so tests to identify blood in faeces or urine may be required.

Hypercoagulable conditions may be identified where there is: marked polycythaemia (primary polycythaemia vera or secondary to kidney disease, or as an appropriate response to chronic hypoxia) on haematology; or monoclonal hyperproteinaemia (multiple myeloma, lymphoma) on serum protein electrophoresis.

Biochemistry

Biochemistry may identify: liver or kidney dysfunction; hypoalbuminaemia as a cause of effusions; hyper/hypoglycaemia; and electrolyte derangements. Pancreatic-specific lipase is assayed when pancreatitis is suspected from vomiting and/or abdominal pain.

Reductions in either plasma potassium or sodium may lead to weakness, whilst the combination of azotaemia, hyperkalaemia and hyponatraemia is indicative of hypoadrenocorticism or acute kidney injury. An adrenocorticotrophic hormone (ACTH) stimulation test is used to confirm hypoadrenocorticism in such situations, but may also be required for those cases where sodium and potassium are normal (so-called 'atypical hypoadrenocorticism'), although this latter subset is more likely to present with gastrointestinal signs than with acute collapse.

Azotaemia may be prerenal or primary renal in origin (or postrenal in cases of urinary rupture or blockage) and urine specific gravity (USG) must also be assessed:

- Prerenal azotaemia (e.g. in hypovolaemia, severe dehydration, cardiac failure) will be notably hypersthenuric (USG >1.030, usually >1.050) owing to the kidneys producing an appropriate response in an attempt to conserve fluid
- In primary renal failure there is an inability to concentrate urine (USG <1.030, usually <1.020)
- The exception to this rule is in hypoadrenocorticism, which leads to azotaemia due to hypovolaemia but is characterized by isosthenuria because hyponatraemia means there is insufficient sodium in the renal interstitium for concentration to occur.

Occasionally, myopathy (including that secondary to severe exertion in trialling dogs or racing Greyhounds) may be seen, shown by a marked increase in creatine kinase (CK) and aspartate aminotransferase (AST). These cases may also present with acute kidney injury. Myoglobin in the urine causes red discoloration of the supernatant after urine centrifugation; this is distinguished from haemoglobinuria by inspecting the colour of the patient's plasma: this is not discoloured in myoglobinaemia, but in haemoglobinaemia the plasma will also be red.

Diagnostic imaging

Radiography of the chest may reveal cardiorespiratory causes of collapse, such as: cardiac failure (cardiomegaly and pulmonary oedema); lung disease; pleural space disease (pneumothorax or effusion); neoplasia; or trauma to the chest wall. Echocardiography can be used to evaluate the function of the heart in cases where murmur, cardiac failure or cardiomegaly have been identified and will allow easy visualization of pericardial fluid in cases of pericardial effusion. Electrocardiography must be undertaken to assess the rate and rhythm of the heart, with severe bradyarrhythmias (most commonly, 3rd degree atrioventricular block) and tachyarrhythmias (e.g. ventricular tachycardia or atrial fibrillation) both potentially causing collapse. Intermittent arrhythmias in dogs with episodic weakness or collapse may be investigated using a Holter monitor. Electrolytes (sodium, potassium, chloride, calcium) and thyroid function (hypothyroidism for bradyarrhythmia and, rarely in dogs, hyperthyroidism for tachyarrhythmia) should be considered as systemic causes of disturbance to cardiac function. Further discussion on cardiorespiratory disease may be found in Chapter 24 and its associated suggested reading.

Imaging of the abdomen allows assessment for: gastric dilatation ± volvulus (Figure 9.4); free peritoneal fluid; neoplasia (intact or ruptured) of the major organs; intestinal obstruction; abdominal lymphadenopathy; pancreatitis; biliary obstruction; and adrenal gland hyperplasia/neoplasia.

Radiography of the skeleton is needed to assess for generalized osteoarthritic pain or multiple myeloma (multiple lucencies seen in the long bones, pelvis and/or vertebrae).

Further tests

More specific diagnostic tests include arthrocentesis and cerebrospinal fluid (CSF) analysis, most commonly used to assess immune-mediated polyarthritis and sterile steroid-responsive meningitis, respectively. The latter condition is most commonly seen in young Beagles in conjunction with arteritis an marked neck

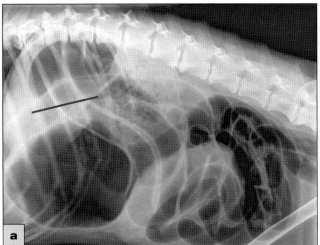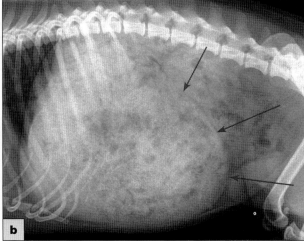

9.4 Gastric dilatation, with or without volvulus, is a common presentation as a cause of acute collapse in first-opinion practice, often as an out-of-hours emergency. **(a)** Abdominal radiograph from a 10-year-old Flatcoated Retriever with GDV and mesenteric torsion. The GDV is seen as the stomach distended in the cranial abdomen with radiolucent gas, divided into two sections by a central radiopaque line; this line is somewhat obscured here by the gaseous distension of the small intestinal loops, but has been marked in red to highlight it. The entire small intestine is markedly dilated with gas, owing to a concurrent mesenteric torsion. The patient was euthanased at surgery because of necrosis of the torsed small intestine, which was a far more insurmountable problem than the GDV. **(b)** Abdominal radiograph from a 6-year-old small cross-breed terrier who had broken into the feed cupboard and gorged on dry food. The caudal borders of the stomach (red arrows) are seen projecting almost to the pelvic inlet. Surgical decompression of huge quantities of swollen dry dog food was required.

pain. Aspiration of synovial fluid from multiple joints in a collapsed patient, especially if pyrexic, should be undertaken early on if the minimum database does not yield a result, as immune-mediated polyarthritis is not that uncommon and, in such cases, one must consider whether the arthropathy is primary or secondary to distant inflammation or neoplasia, gastrointestinal disease or tick-borne infections.

Suspicion of central nervous system disease may dictate the need for magnetic resonance imaging (MRI) of the brain and/or spine in order to arrive at a definitive diagnosis. Serology for *Toxoplasma* and *Neospora* may be indicated in neurological cases; alternatively, PCR may be carried out on CSF when available.

Angiostrongylosis is diagnosed by detection of parasite antigen on patient-side blood testing, or identification of the parasite in faeces or bronchoalveolar lavage fluid, as well as assessment of clotting function (platelet numbers, prothrombin time (PT) and activated partial thromboplastin time (APTT)). Secondary coagulation function tests (PT, APTT) are also required to confirm other forms of coagulopathy such as rodenticide toxicity and disseminated intravascular coagulation.

References and further reading

King L and Boag A (2007) *BSAVA Manual of Canine and Feline Emergency and Critical Care.* BSAVA Publications, Gloucester

The trauma patient: assessment, emergency management and wound care

10

Julian Hoad

Wounds may be caused by a number of different insults to the body, and may involve just the skin, or many body systems. Correct management of trauma relies on being able to make a fairly rapid assessment of the patient as a whole, identifying injuries, coming up with a plan for treatment, estimating the prognosis, and conveying all that to the client, together with an estimation of costs involved. Clearly, doing all this from first principles would be difficult and time-consuming. Thus it is important to develop or follow various action plans for initial triage, wound assessment, wound management and on-going patient care. Only in this way can one be sure of covering all eventualities and not missing a serious complicating factor. This chapter attempts to provide a basic understanding of the principles involved in developing a standard procedure for trauma patients.

Triage and emergency stabilization

Triage involves an initial assessment to determine whether the patient should be dealt with immediately or whether it is stable enough to wait while more urgent cases are seen. For notes on triage over the telephone and subsequent preparation, see Chapter 8.

When a trauma patient is presented at the surgery, it is very important to establish some idea of:

- The severity of the injuries
- The signalment of the patient
- The time elapsed since the injury
- Any pertinent facts relating to the patient's medical history (e.g. presence of a chronic illness such as diabetes, heart disease, hypoadrenocorticism).

The process of asking the owner questions can often do much to reduce stress or panic, and may allow a really anxious owner some time to calm down. Watching the patient while questioning the client allows an appreciation of the dog's respiratory function so that assessment can begin.

PRACTICAL TIPS

- It is useful to have a checklist of questions, although it is better to have a mental checklist than to present the client with a long and tedious form, which will do nothing to allay their anxiety
- Talking reassuringly *to the patient* will allow an assessment of consciousness (whether or not a response is obtained) and will help calm the dog

---

Visual examination

Whilst asking the owner questions, a full visual examination of the animal can be performed. However, if the dog is obviously collapsed, haemorrhaging or seizuring, or the owner is distressed or showing signs of panic, it is best to separate the dog and owner at this stage.

Initially, a superficial 'hands-off' examination should be done, checking for:

- Breathing
- Consciousness (and whether the dog is alert)
- The presence of bleeding (with a rough visual estimate of amount: this need be no more involved than 'a lot' or 'a little' at this stage).

WARNING

Before touching or palpating the patient, it should be established whether or not the dog is usually aggressive, or whether it has bitten anyone. Regardless of this, precautions should be taken to avoid anyone being bitten, as even the friendliest dog may exhibit aggression when in pain; but forewarned is forearmed

---

D–ABC

D: Danger (to yourself or others from an aggressive dog)
A: Airway
B: Breathing
C: Circulation

This initial check should take no more than 2 or 3 minutes. If any immediate life-threatening problem is identified during this process, the dog should be removed to the treatment room and emergency procedures instigated (e.g. cardiopulmonary resuscitation (CPR; see Chapter 8), assisted ventilation, tourniquet for arterial bleeding).

Main body systems

Provided there is no immediately life-threatening problem, at this stage a more in-depth assessment can be made. This should include (see Chapter 8 for more detail):

- Respiratory rate and effort
- Heart rate and evaluation of the mucous membranes
- A brief evaluation of the nervous system (to include presence of anisocoria, pupillary light reflex (PLR), limb movement (ability to walk))
- Presence or absence of a palpable bladder.

The above checks cover the four main body systems: dysfunction of any of these can rapidly become life-threatening. This does not mean that any other injuries or problems can be forgotten, but assessing and attending to the above buys time for further examination and further investigation. It may be helpful for a veterinary nurse or another suitably trained member of staff to take notes.

Additional checks

- Wounds should be assessed for ongoing blood loss. Haemorrhage from an extremity may be addressed at this time by swift application of a sterile non-adhesive dressing, held in place by a conforming bandage; definitive wound care can be carried out later.
- Limbs should be palpated for fractures and the whole patient should be examined for the presence of bulges or asymmetry, which may indicate body wall rupture.
- The anus and vulva should be examined for prolapse.

By this stage it should be fairly well established whether the patient needs to be admitted immediately for intensive emergency stabilization (see Chapter 8), or whether the injuries can be dealt with over a longer time. These latter cases will clearly require attention, but immediate care may simply include:

- Application of a wound dressing
- Administration of analgesia and/or antibiotics (see later)
- Regular (every 5–10 minutes) checks to ensure there is no deterioration in the dog's condition and vital signs: temperature, pulse, respiration (TPR); mucous membrane colour; assessment of mentation; palpation of the bladder.

Figure 10.1 demonstrates a simplified triage algorithm.

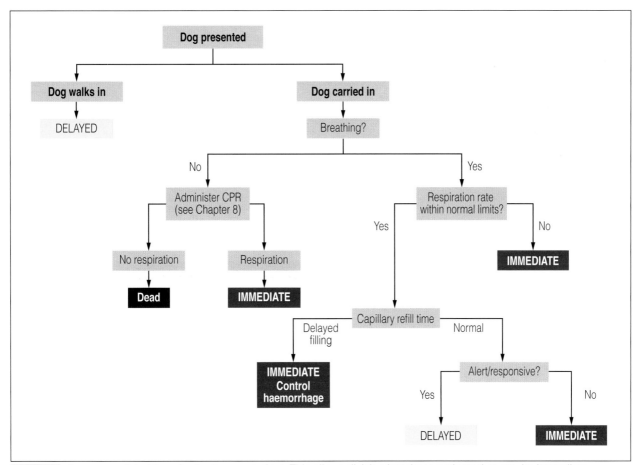

10.1 An approach to triage for the trauma patient. This allows division into those patients that require immediate treatment or else death may ensue, and those for whom treatment can be delayed. Note that 'delayed' treatment does not mean that the patient may be sent home and seen later: any trauma patient should be admitted and assessed every 5–10 minutes. The acceptable delay will depend on the nature of the injury and treatment required.

Informed consent

- It is vital to obtain informed consent from the owner (see also Chapter 6) and to give some estimate of costs
- Informed consent should be as detailed as possible and should cover all eventualities: it is not acceptable to fail to mention the possibility of death occurring in order to spare an owner's feelings. An agreement to contact the owner with updates must be adhered to: it is both frustrating and worrying not knowing what is happening to one's pet

- It may not be possible to state exactly what the costs will be, as the full extent of injury may not be apparent until further investigations have been performed; however, a 'ball park' figure should be given that can be revised later in the light of further information. It is important to phrase discussions about money carefully, to avoid giving the client the impression that money is the overriding concern, rather than the wellbeing of their pet. It may be useful to ask a more experienced colleague for advice on delivery

---

Emergency stabilization and treatment

Once the patient's status has been determined, treatment can commence.

Fluid therapy

In all cases an intravenous catheter should be placed: this is not only helpful for correction of fluid loss or circulatory function, but also ensures that there is intravenous access if required for the administration of emergency drugs. Fluid therapy (including blood transfusion if appropriate) should be given unless there are specific contraindications (see Chapter 8). For details of fluid therapy see Chapter 8 and the *BSAVA Manual of Canine and Feline Emergency and Critical Care*. For details of blood transfusion protocols see the *BSAVA Manual of Canine and Feline Haematology and Transfusion Medicine*.

Any patient with blood loss should have its packed cell volume (PCV) assessed, although initially this may remain within normal limits as whole blood is lost and it is only as circulating volume recovers that the haematocrit drops. Blood biochemistry may be useful to rule out the presence of contemporaneous disease (see Chapters 8 and 9).

Analgesia

Analgesia should be a high priority: patients in pain may rapidly deteriorate and are at greater risk of cardiorespiratory decompensation. In any trauma case, a pure opioid (e.g. morphine) is the first-line drug of choice (Figure 10.2). Local analgesia is extremely effective and should be considered wherever possible, following initial stabilization of the patient. Wound infiltration, local nerve blocks, intravenous regional analgesia (IVRA) and epidural administration are all possible, though care must be given not to exceed the toxic dose.

Figures 10.3 and 10.4 suggest ongoing analgesics for stabilized and discharged patients.

Analgesic class	Example	Dose and route	Duration of action	Contraindications and cautions
Opioids	Buprenorphine	0.02 mg/kg i.v., i.m., s.c.	6–8 hours	All full-opioid agonists cause dose-dependent respiratory depression and should be used with caution in respiratory-compromised cases. Advise client that the use of morphine is 'off label'; client must sign an 'off-label' drug consent form
	Methadone	0.1–0.5 mg/kg i.m.	3–4 hours	
	Morphine	0.5 mg/kg i.v., i.m., s.c.	2–4 hours	
		Epidural: 0.1 mg/kg, diluted with 0.26 ml/kg sterile saline (max. total volume 6 ml)	18–24 hours	
	Pethidine	2–10 mg/kg i.m., s.c.	1–2 hours	

10.2 Commonly used analgesics for trauma cases: first-line drugs. Morphine is the first-line analgesic drug of choice.

Analgesic class	Example	Dose and route	Duration of activity	Contraindications, cautions and comments
NSAIDs	Carprofen	4 mg/kg i.v., s.c.	24 hours	Do not use in dehydrated, hypovolaemic patients, or those with coagulopathies. Do not use if there has been damage to the gastrointestinal tract
	Meloxicam	0.2 mg/kg s.c.		
	Tolfenamic acid	4 mg/kg i.m., s.c.		
Opioids	See Figure 10.2			
	Fentanyl patch	4 µg/kg/h	72 hours	May take up to 24 hours to begin providing appreciable analgesia
Local anaesthetics	Bupivacaine	Local: no more than 1–2 mg/kg (usually a dose of 1–2 ml of a 0.5% solution will suffice)	6–8 hours	Avoid overdosage and inadvertent intravenous administration. Much smaller amounts than the suggested doses are usually effective. There are many useful specific nerve blocks which can be used. Spraying a little directly on to a wound is also effective ('splash block')
		Epidural: 1.6 mg/kg		
	Lidocaine	Local: no more than 4 mg/kg	1–2 hours	

10.3 Commonly used analgesics for trauma cases: in-house treatment of the stabilized patient. (continues) ▶

Analgesic class	Example	Dose and route	Duration of activity	Contraindications, cautions and comments
Alpha-2 agonists	Dexmedetomidine	3–5 µg/kg i.v., i.m., s.c.	1 hour	Doses are based on combination with an opioid to provide neuroleptanalgesia. Do not use medetomidine in dogs with cardiac disease. Remember that reversal with atipamezole also reverses analgesia
	Medetomidine	10–20 µg/kg i.v., i.m., s.c.		
Adjunct	Ketamine	250 µg/kg i.v. loading dose and 10 µg/kg/min CRI intraoperatively; 5–7 mg/kg i.m. combined with dexmedetomidine or medetomidine	1–2 hours (variable)	Ketamine has been shown to be effective at reducing 'wind up' pain. Ketamine may cause hyperexcitability on recovery

10.3 (continued) Commonly used analgesics for trauma cases: in-house treatment of the stabilized patient.

Analgesic class	Example	Dose and route	Duration of activity	Contraindications, cautions and comments
NSAIDs	See Figure 10.3			
	Firocoxib	5 mg/kg orally	24 hours	Stop administering if signs of gastrointestinal upset are seen
Opioids	Fentanyl patch	4 µg/kg/h	72 hours	Owners should be cautioned as to the dangers of pets and children ingesting fentanyl patches. Advise clients that the use of these drugs is 'off label'; client must sign an 'off-label' drug consent form
	Tramadol	2–5 mg/kg orally	?8 hours (pharmacodynamics uncertain)	
Adjunct	Gabapentin	10–60 mg/kg orally (total daily dose, divided q8–12h)	Not known	Gabapentin takes 1–2 days to reach a steady state, and may not provide adequate analgesia within 2 hours of administration. Gabapentin has been shown to be effective at reducing 'wind up' pain. Use with caution in renal and hepatic disease. Advise clients that the use of gabapentin is 'off label'; client must sign an 'off-label' drug consent form

10.4 Commonly used analgesics for trauma cases: ongoing analgesia (or for the discharged patient).

'Soft' analgesia

Other forms of analgesia – such as cold compress, bandage/dressing, petting/stroking – are often neglected, but do play an important role in patient recovery. There are few contraindications to stroking, but the patient's demeanour should be appraised beforehand

Antibiosis

Antibiotics should always be used in cases with:

- Diaphragmatic hernia with liver entrapment
- Compound (or 'open') fractures
- Severe tissue damage.

Broad-spectrum, intravenous antibiotics (Figure 10.5) should be used in trauma patients. Antibiotics should be administered following current guidelines and indications (see *BSAVA Small Animal Formulary*).

Drug	Intravenous dose (mg/kg)	Dosing frequency	Authorized for use in dogs in the UK?
Amoxicillin	16–33	q8h	No
Ampicillin	10–20	q6–8h	No
Cefotaxime	20–40 (some authors suggest 10–20 q12h)	q6–8h	No
Ceftazidime	20–50	q8–12h	No
Cefuroxime	10–15	q8–12	No
Clarithromycin	4–12	q12h	No
Co-amoxiclav	8.75 (combined dose of both drugs)	q8h	No
Enrofloxacin	5	q24h	Yes (NB: Intravenous route not authorized)
Flucloxacillin	15	q6h	No
Lincomycin	11–22 (slow infusion)	q12–24h	Yes
Marbofloxacin	2	q24h	Yes
Metronidazole	10 (slow infusion)	q12h	No
Penicillin G	15–25	q4–6h	No
Ticarcillin	40–100	q4–6h	No (NB: Reserve for life-threatening *Pseudomonas* infection)
Tobramycin	2–4 (slow infusion)	q8–24h	No

10.5 Antibiotics appropriate for intravenous use in trauma patients.

An approach to the road traffic accident case

A common presentation of trauma, potentially involving many body systems, is the road traffic accident (RTA) case. When presented with a dog involved in an RTA, the triage procedure above should be followed. *The driver of the car should be aware that the RTA should be reported to the police as soon as possible and certainly within 24 hours under the provision of the Road Traffic Act 1988.*

Once the triage assessment has been performed, and any immediate life-threatening injuries have been dealt with, a problem list should be drawn up of all injuries to the body systems.

Physical examination

This should begin with the head, and progress along the body in the usual way.

1. Examine the head.
   - Check jaw alignment: if possible, gently open the mouth to check for damage to the temporomandibular joint. Sedation may be necessary for this; if so, it is best to wait until other checks have been completed, to ensure the patient is as stable as possible prior to sedation.
   - Re-examine the pupils for pupillary light reflex (PLR) and anisocoria.
   - Re-assess mentation.
   - Perform an otoscopic examination: the presence of blood near the tympanum can indicate severe skull fracture.
   - The skull should be examined for symmetry and any swelling or fluctuant masses which could suggest skull fracture.
   - If it has been possible to open the mouth, then the tongue and as much of the oral cavity as possible should be examined for any bleeding, which could affect airway patency.
   - Examine the nostrils for any bleeding.
   - A microscope slide held up to the nostrils will help indicate any blockage of the nasal cavity.
2. Palpate the neck and spine for any injury.
   - Take care if the patient is paralysed: such patients should have a full neurological assessment performed (see Chapters 11 and 16 and the *BSAVA Manual of Canine and Feline Neurology*).
   - Since nerve damage can often improve once neuropraxia has resolved, or worsen with ongoing inflammation, it is wise to be cautious in giving any prognosis at the time of injury.
   - Intense pain and shock can affect deep pain assessment: it is important to allow time for stabilization and analgesia before repeating neurological tests.
3. Palpate the trunk for any sign of rib or body wall damage.
   - Rib fractures may be felt as lumps or painful areas. If several ribs are fractured in two or more places, this can lead to 'flail chest', in which there is an incongruous dipping of a region of the chest wall on inspiration, and bulging on expiration. Although several

methods of complex splinting procedures have been reported for this condition, in practice no treatment is required in most cases. The dyspnoea tends to improve after analgesia and the ribs usually 'knit' without surgical intervention.
   - Any crepitus under the skin should alert one to the possibility of subcutaneous emphysema, which may be caused by puncture to the lungs, or by a 'sucking' skin wound. Radiography will help distinguish these conditions.
   - Any bulges in the abdominal wall may be due to subcutaneous bleeding, or may indicate ruptures and herniation.
   - It may be possible to palpate a tear in the abdominal musculature; this can be confirmed by radiography and/or ultrasonography.
4. Palpate the abdomen. This should initially be done with the dog conscious. Sedation may be required to assess the viscera adequately: if so, it is best to wait until the rest of the checks have been completed and the animal is as stable as possible prior to sedation.
   - Free fluid palpated may be blood, urine, or the result of over-vigorous fluid replacement. Haemoabdomen is usually associated with marked abdominal pain, and so increasing tenseness on abdominal palpation should be a warning sign.
   - Care should be taken to try to identify the bladder, although its presence does not rule out bladder rupture or leakage. If bladder rupture is suspected, measurement of raised urea and creatinine within aspirated abdominal fluid compared with systemic blood proves the presence of urine. This test may be performed on most in-house biochemistry machines.
5. Examine the external genitalia for any injury that might interfere with voiding urine.
   - If necessary, insert a urinary catheter (Figure 10.6).
6. Examine the anus and tail, including checking for traumatic rectal prolapse, bleeding from the anus and neurological assessment of the tail.

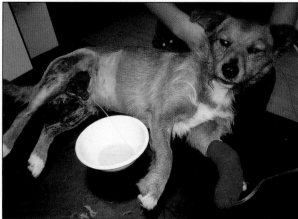

10.6 Placement of a urinary catheter is a priority when there is damage to the urethra and external genitalia. This 3-year-old male cross-breed dog suffered extensive trauma to the hindlimbs and penis. Treatment involved amputation of one hindlimb and a perineal urethrostomy. The dog went on to make a good recovery.

- A flaccid tail with no deep pain response should prompt radiography of the pelvic spine and close monitoring for urination.
7. Finally, carefully examine the limbs for any skin wounds, luxations, fractures or neurological dysfunction.

Diagnostic imaging

Once the problem list has been drawn up, imaging should be the next step (provided no new life-threatening injury has been discovered).

In any RTA victim, chest radiography should be performed to rule out diaphragmatic hernia, rib fracture, pneumothorax, thoracic haemorrhage and pulmonary contusion, although the latter may not be apparent for 12–24 hours following injury. Radiographs of the rest of the body and limbs should be performed on the basis of clinical findings.

Ultrasonography is useful for detecting and monitoring fluid accumulation in the abdomen, and for examination of the urinary system. In cases of diaphragmatic hernia, ultrasound examination is invaluable for identifying the organs involved in the hernia.

WARNING

Fractures are rarely life-threatening; emergency stabilization should *not* be compromised in order to obtain a perfect radiographic view

---

Diaphragmatic hernia

- Diaphragmatic hernia is much less common in dogs following an RTA than in cats
- It results from increased intra-abdominal pressure against a closed glottis. This causes rupture of the diaphragm and herniation of some of the abdominal contents into the thorax, or occasionally into the pericardial sac (traumatic peritoneopericardial diaphragmatic hernia)
- The increased intra-abdominal pressure is likely to have caused additional damage, and so careful radiographic examination of the pelvis and urinary bladder is strongly advised
- In most cases the liver is involved in the hernia; however, it is not unusual for other abdominal organs to herniate, particularly the stomach and intestines
- The reduction of thoracic space causes dyspnoea, which may worsen dramatically if incarcerated viscera become bloated. Respiratory function can be assisted in the short term by maintaining the patient in a confined and calm environment to utilize its respiratory reserve
- Strangulation of the herniated contents may sometimes occur and lead to compromise of the vasculature, resulting in tissue necrosis and further inflammation
- Timing of repair is a balance between the need to restore pulmonary function and prevent ischaemic injury of incarcerated viscera on the one hand, and the risk of general anaesthesia in an animal with potential pulmonary and cardiac contusions on the other
- For further discussion see the *BSAVA Manual of Canine and Feline Abdominal Surgery*

Wound management

Basic wound management should include immediate bandaging of bleeding wounds to reduce ongoing blood loss and also to reduce the risk of infection. More precise wound care will depend on the type of wound (Figure 10.7) and the degree of contamination (Figure 10.8). For detailed treatment of degloving injuries and for wound care in general, the reader is recommended to consult the *BSAVA Manual of Canine and Feline Wound Management and Reconstruction*.

For the first 6 hours after trauma, the proliferation of microorganisms within a wound is insufficient to cause infection: the wound is considered to be *contaminated*. This is known as the 'golden period' and wounds treated appropriately within this period are amenable to primary wound closure. Contaminated wounds should be flushed with copious amounts of sterile lactated Ringer's solution; attaching a fluid bag to a 19 G needle using a giving set, syringe and three-way tap is an excellent way to facilitate this (Figure 10.9).

Wound type	Characteristics
Abrasion (graze)	Shearing or friction injury. Usually superficial, but can expose bone. There is minimal bleeding, but the wounds tend to be very painful when touched
Avulsion (tear)	Includes degloving injuries, and involves creation of skin flaps by tearing the skin away from its attachment. Depending on the direction of tear, the flap may dehisce if the blood supply is lost
Burn (chemical or thermal)	Necrosis of skin and subcutaneous layers by contact with heat or certain chemicals. Thermal burns tend to be extremely painful. Chemical burns should be lavaged copiously to remove any residual chemical. The true extent of any burn may take several days to become apparent
Contusion (bruise)	Haematoma caused by blunt trauma. Haematomas within muscle bellies can reduce blood flow and constrict nerves, causing compartment syndrome
Incision	A cut or breach in the skin and deeper tissues caused by a sharp object or instrument
Laceration	Tearing of the skin and deeper tissues with a blunt object. Often confused with incision. No skin flap is produced (compare with Avulsion)
Puncture (with or without foreign body)	Caused by a pointed implement penetrating the skin (e.g. tooth, stick, thorn). There is usually only a small entry wound, but there may be much damage to underlying tissues and organs. These wounds often require multimodal imaging and extensive surgical exploration
Firearm	These wounds may range from 'puncture wounds' caused by airgun pellets, to devastatingly damaging wounds caused by bullets. Fortunately, the incidence of the latter in the UK is very low; shotgun wounds may be seen, especially in rural areas
Crush	Crush wounds show aspects of several types of wound. They are caused by squeezing between two hard objects. Crush injuries may result in fractures, lacerations, contusions or nerve injury (directly and as a result of compartment syndrome) and are prone to infection due to the low redox potential of the devitalized tissue

10.7 Classification of wounds by type.

Classification	Characteristics
Clean	A surgically incised wound that does not enter a visceral cavity (e.g. gut, oral, respiratory, genitourinary). Can be assumed to have little or no bacterial presence. Primary repair is possible. Antibiotics are generally not required unless infection would be catastrophic (e.g. spinal surgery, orthopaedic surgery when implants are placed)
Clean–contaminated	A surgically incised wound in which there has been entry to a visceral cavity but no leakage has occurred. Primary repair is possible. Prophylactic antibiotics are generally indicated
Contaminated	A surgically incised wound that has experienced leakage of gut contents or infected urine, or where a major disruption to aseptic technique has occurred. Also traumatic wounds within the 'golden period'. Prompt attention to debridement and lavage can alter these to clean wounds, and primary repair is often possible. Prophylactic antibiotics are required
Dirty	Traumatic wounds with infection. There may be necrotic tissue, purulent exudate or foreign bodies present. Also surgical wounds with faecal contamination. Primary repair is not possible in these cases and they must be managed by antibiotic therapy, lavage, and often several cycles of dressings and debridement

10.8 Classification of wounds by degree of contamination.

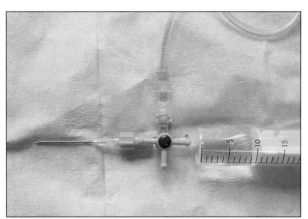

10.9 A flushing catheter can be easily constructed from a sterile saline bag, giving set, three-way tap, 20 ml syringe and large-bore needle.

After this initial period, the burden of pathogens should be assumed to have risen above the critical infectious level (around 10^5 colony-forming units (CFU) per gram of tissue) and the wound is considered to be *infected*. Such wounds may require debridement and several days of wound management and antibiosis prior to closure.

A summary of dressing types and their uses is given in Figure 10.10.

PRACTICAL TIP

The requirement for repeated ongoing dressing changes can often be very expensive (especially if sedation or anaesthesia is required) and should be included in any estimate given to owners

---

Type of dressing	Examples	Comments and indications for use
Adherent dressings		
Dry-to-dry	Dry sterile gauze swabs	Very painful to remove and have been almost completely superseded by hydrogel dressings
Wet-to-dry	Sterile swabs soaked in Hartmann's (lactated Ringer's) solution. Adding 0.05% chlorhexidine solution may reduce bacterial growth	Initial stages of treatment of contaminated wounds. Aid debridement of necrotic wounds, especially when there is viscous exudate. Must be changed at least every 24 hours
Hydrogels	Intrasite gel (Smith and Nephew); Granugel (ConvaTec)	Use is as for wet-to-dry dressings, but are more absorptive and less painful to remove. May be left in place for 48 hours in most wounds
Semi-permeable adhesive film	Opsite (Smith and Nephew); Tegaderm (3M)	For use primarily on clean or minimally contaminated wounds, closed surgical incisions, or to hold a non-adherent primary layer dressing in place
Non-adherent dressings		
Foam	Allevyn (Smith and Nephew); Tielle (Johnson and Johnson)	For use in contaminated necrotic wounds; suitable for most stages of wound closure
Perforated film, absorbent	Melolin (Smith and Nephew); Skintact (Robinson Healthcare)	Although termed non-adherent, these dressings do tend to adhere to exuding wounds. Their use is mainly limited to covering closed surgical wounds
Hydrocolloid	Duoderm (ConvaTec); Tegasorb (3M)	Useful for primary treatment of wounds with extensive necrotic tissue and large amounts of exudate
Alginate	Sorbsan (Animalcare Ltd); Kaltogel (ConvaTec)	Use is as for hydrocolloid dressings, but have advantages in that they may promote fibroblast activity, are non-painful to remove, and act rapidly to aid autolysis of necrotic tissue. May be left in place for 2–3 days
Silicon	Silflex (Advancis Medical); Mepiform (Mölnlycke)	Main use is in the reduction of scar tissue which may otherwise form cicatrix

10.10 Types of wound dressing and their use. Only a few examples are given, for clarity. For more details see the *BSAVA Manual of Canine and Feline Wound Management and Reconstruction*.

Burns

Burns are less common in veterinary practice than in human trauma units. Unfortunately, a common cause remains iatrogenic burn from incorrect use of patient heating devices, especially microwaveable heating pads (Figure 10.11) or discs.

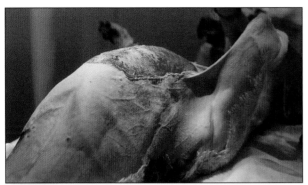

10.11 This 5-year-old female neutered Greyhound suffered a full-thickness burn over the ventral chest while lying on a heat pad at the owner's kennel. The wound has been treated with wet-to-dry dressings for 48 hours and is now being prepared for delayed primary closure.

Thermal burns cause tissue breakdown secondary to cell death. The cell death may be immediate or it may be ongoing, due to infection or the release of vasoactive compounds. Initially, there may be little evidence of tissue damage unless the burn has been caused by a naked flame. Hair loss and tissue sloughing may only occur several days after a low-intensity contact burn. A burn wound is characterized by a necrotic, exudative central area, demarcated by a line of hyperaemia, sometimes referred to as the 'tide mark'. Until this line has appeared, it is difficult to assess the true extent of a burn, and this must be borne in mind when attempting to debride the wound margins. It may be more appropriate to dress the wound for another 24 hours or so to allow the margins to 'declare'.

Assessment

A full triage assessment should be carried out on a burn victim: it may be that other injuries are present. Additionally, burn wounds often result in the loss of considerable amounts of protein and fluid: blood biochemistry should be assessed to evaluate total protein (TP) and albumin. An estimate should be made of the size of the burn with respect to the affected body surface area (ABSA).

Affected body surface area

The ABSA can be estimated using the 'rule of nines':

- Each forelimb = 9% TBSA
- Each hindlimb = 18% TBSA
- Ventrum = 18% TBSA
- Dorsum = 18% TBSA
- Head and genitalia account for the rest
- **Dogs with >15% of their total body surface area (TBSA) affected will require intensive emergency stabilization**
- **Patients with >50% TBSA burns rarely survive, and so consideration should be given to euthanasia**

Treatment

Emergency treatment is aimed at replacing fluid loss and providing analgesia. In acute presentations it may be appropriate to use shock doses of intravenous fluids (see Chapter 8); caution is warranted with chronic burns, however, as these patients may be hypoproteinaemic and thus less tolerant of fluid overload. It is worth advising an owner to run cool tap water over a burn for 20 minutes before driving to the practice. This reduces the heat transfer to deeper tissues, improves analgesia and reduces healing time. There may be some benefit to trying to cool a burn in the practice, if it has happened within 3 hours of presentation.

Attention to analgesia is important, as burn wounds are not only painful at the time of presentation and treatment, but can also lead to wind up and chronic pain. Neuroleptanalgesia (e.g. combination of an opioid with an alpha-2 agonist), non-steroidal anti-inflammatory drugs (NSAIDs) and topical or infiltrative local analgesics should be used together and 'topped up' at appropriate intervals.

WARNING

Care should be taken to ensure that fluid loss has been corrected before administering NSAIDs

---

The burn wound should be covered with a sterile, non-adherent dressing as soon as possible, reducing the risk of infection and providing analgesia. Once the patient has been stabilized, debridement of a large burn should be carried out without delay. The hard leathery covering of a burn wound, the eschar, should be removed by sharp dissection. It has been shown that early removal of this necrotic tissue improves healing and reduces infection rates. At this stage, silver sulfadiazine-containing dressings may be used, as these reduce the incidence of sepsis in burn wounds.

Definitive closure of burn wounds will depend on the size, depth and position of the wound. More detailed treatment protocols are given in the *BSAVA Manual of Canine and Feline Emergency and Critical Care* and there is an excellent review of burn pathophysiology and treatment by Bohling (2012).

Dog fight injuries

The most common presentation of dog fight injuries is biting to the head and neck (see also Chapter 23), but a surprise attack can result in an injury anywhere on the body. It is likely also to be quite a traumatic experience for the owner, as they may be shocked to see true aggression from or toward their pet. It is very important to question the owner as to exactly how the fight occurred. The incidence of dogs attacking other dogs is closely linked to dogs attacking people.

Triage assessment for a dog fight injury is carried out as above, with damage to the airways and blood vessels being of overriding importance. Although puncture wounds may be the only superficially obvious injury, the bitten dog will tend to pull away from the aggressor in any fight, causing a tooth that has penetrated the skin to gouge through underlying tissues. Even if there is only damage to the subcutaneous fat, there can still be ongoing tissue necrosis and discharge. Such wounds should always be left open to drain and heal by secondary intention.

PRACTICAL TIP

Meticulous examination of the patient is required, as puncture wounds may be easily missed in haired areas

Where skin damage requires excision and primary closure, temporary drainage is strongly recommended (Figure 10.12). Broad-spectrum antibiotic cover should be commenced and continued for at least 5 days; bacteria commonly isolated from dog bites include *Pasteurella canis*, *Staphylococcus* and *Fusobacterium* spp.

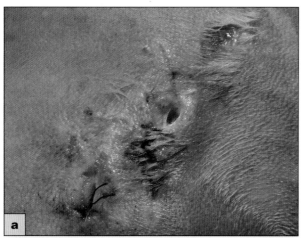

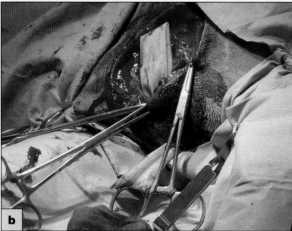

10.12 **(a)** This dog bite wound on the flank of a 7-year-old male Golden Retriever had been sutured 5 days previously using inadequate wound care. Infection is present and the wound is reopening. **(b)** The wound has been extensively debrided and flushed and a Penrose drain is being placed prior to closure. The drain was removed after 3 days and the wound healed uneventfully.

Dogs' jaws can inflict a massive biting pressure, and it is quite common for a seemingly insignificant small wound to overlie a severe injury. Bite wounds over the thorax should be carefully palpated for any sign of subcutaneous emphysema, which could be a sign of tearing of the intercostal muscles or rib fracture. Wounds over the abdominal cavity should be checked for bulges that could indicate body wall rupture and herniation. If these are suspected, radiography or ultrasonography may be useful to demonstrate ruptures, although it may be necessary to investigate the bite tract of each wound surgically to ensure that no tears in the muscle have been missed. If an abdominal tear is discovered, exploration of the entire abdominal cavity may be justified to rule out the presence of damage to the viscera.

Fractures

Specific fracture treatment is described in the *BSAVA Manual of Small Animal Fracture Repair and Management*. The following points should be borne in mind.

- As fractures are rarely life-threatening, they should take second place to emergency treatment and stabilization.
  - However, a judiciously applied support dressing can dramatically improve analgesia for distal limb fractures. *The dressing must immobilize the joint above the fracture site or the extra weight of the bandage will actually increase movement at the fracture site and lead to increased discomfort and the potential for further damage of adjacent soft tissues.*
  - With proximal limb fractures it may be more appropriate to rely on analgesia and padded bedding than to concoct complex splints.
- Luxations should similarly await patient stabilization, although if the patient is already sedated or anaesthetized for investigation, then it would make sense to attempt a non-surgical reduction and placement of a support bandage.

References and further reading

Boag A and Hughes D (2007) Fluid therapy. In: *BSAVA Manual of Canine and Feline Emergency and Critical Care, 2nd edn*, ed. LK King and A Boag, pp.30–45. BSAVA Publications, Gloucester.

Bohling MW (2012) Burns. In: *Veterinary Surgery: Small Animal*, ed. KM Tobias and SA Johnston, pp.1291–1302. Elsevier Saunders, St. Louis

Brown AJ and Drobatz KJ (2007) Triage of the emergency patient. In: *BSAVA Manual of Canine and Feline Emergency and Critical Care, 2nd edn*, ed. LG King and A Boag, pp.1–7. BSAVA Publications, Gloucester

Carroll GL (2003) Anesthesia and analgesia for the trauma or shock patient. In: *Textbook of Small Animal Surgery, 3rd edn*, ed. D Slatter, pp.2538–2544. Saunders, Philadelphia

Coughlan AR and Miller A (2006) *BSAVA Manual of Small Animal Fracture Repair and Management* (revised reprint). BSAVA Publications, Gloucester

Hellyer PW *et al.* (2007) Pain and its management. In: *Lumb and Jones' Veterinary Anaesthesia and Analgesia, 4th edn*, ed. WJ Tranquilli *et al.*, pp.31–60. Blackwell, Iowa

Platt S and Olby N (2013) *BSAVA Manual of Canine and Feline Neurology, 4th edn*. BSAVA Publications, Gloucester

Ramsey I (2014) *BSAVA Small Animal Formulary, 8th edn*. BSAVA Publications, Gloucester

Seim III HB and Willard MD (2002) Surgical infections and antibiotic selection. In: *Small Animal Surgery, 2nd edn*, ed. TW Fossum, pp.60–68. Mosby, St. Louis

Seymour C and Duke-Novakovski T (2007) *BSAVA Manual of Canine and Feline Anaesthesia and Analgesia, 2nd edn*. BSAVA Publications, Gloucester

Williams JM and Moores A (2009) *BSAVA Manual of Canine and Feline Wound Management and Reconstruction, 2nd edn*. BSAVA Publications, Gloucester

Williams JM and Niles J (in production) *BSAVA Manual of Canine and Feline Abdominal Surgery, 2nd edn*. BSAVA Publications, Gloucester

Seizures, ataxia and other neurological presentations

Alex Gough

Dogs presented with neurological problems are often viewed as particularly challenging to diagnose and manage.

Animals with neurological diseases may present with a variety of clinical signs, including seizures, ataxia, pain, paresis/paralysis and behavioural changes.

Neurological emergencies may present as:

- Status epilepticus
- Severe cluster seizures
- Stupor/coma
- Ataxia
- Paresis or paralysis (see also Chapter 16)
- Pain.

History

As with all medical investigations, the neurological work-up should begin with a detailed medical history. Certain questions become more pertinent for the neurological patient. Some clinicians prefer to take a full history before becoming more focused. However, the owner will often want to discuss the chief complaint straight away, and it can be useful to clarify their concerns at the start of the consultation, both to make the owner feel they are being listened to, and to direct further enquiries. For example: an animal presenting with a history of seizures should prompt more in-depth questioning regarding other forebrain signs such as behavioural changes and pacing; for an animal presenting with a head tilt, details of any history of ear disease could be important. **NB: An animal presenting in status epilepticus requires immediate emergency treatment.**

It is also important at this stage to clarify the owner's description. Seizures, faints and collapses can all mean different things to different people, so the owner should be asked to describe exactly what they have observed, including:

- Time/date of onset
- Association with pain
- Speed of progression
- Associations with the animal's activity (e.g. rest or exercise)

- Whether the complaint is of an episodic nature
- What happens immediately before, during or after an episodic event
- Frequency of episodic events.

PRACTICAL TIPS

- It can be extremely useful to view episodic events on video; if the owners do not have any video footage at the time of consultation they should be encouraged to obtain some, for example on a mobile phone
- There are many examples on the Internet of animals showing neurological signs and for the clinician unfamiliar with different types of movement disorders and seizures, viewing these can be useful, as can showing a typical video to the owner and asking if their pet is behaving the same way. Be wary, as the diagnosis accompanying these videos is not always correct!

Specific historical information that should be obtained includes:

- Signalment
- How long the animal has been in the owner's possession
- Vaccination status
- Parasite treatment
- Travel history
- Current medication and recent changes in medication
- Diet
- Similar problems in animals in the same household or in related animals
- Exposure to toxins.

Questions relating to the animal's general health should include details about:

- Appetite
- Thirst
- Urinary and faecal continence
- Exercise tolerance

- Vision
- Vomiting/regurgitation
- Diarrhoea
- Respiratory problems such as coughing, sneezing or dyspnoea.

> **PRACTICAL TIP**
>
> While the history is being taken, allowing the animal to wander freely in the consulting room allows observation of gait and behaviour

Physical examination

Once the history has been taken, a full physical examination should be undertaken, including:

- Temperature
- Pulse rate
- Respiratory rate
- Thoracic auscultation (see Chapter 24)
- Mucous membrane assessment (see Chapter 20)
- Abdominal palpation (see Chapter 25).

If the problem is still deemed to be neurological at this stage, a full neurological examination should be performed; an example of a results form is given at the end of the chapter. This can take half an hour to perform in detail, and so time needs to be allowed in the consulting schedule for this. Alternatively, the animal can be admitted for examination at a later stage.

> **PRACTICAL TIPS**
>
> A quick 'screening' neurological examination may be of use in a short consultation to help confirm the presence or absence of common neurological deficits. QRG 11.1 shows the author's suggestion for a 'screening' neurological examination, which should take around 5 minutes
>
> - A full neurological examination and further investigations should be undertaken in cases where neurological deficits are found or the history is suggestive of neurological disease
> - The short neurological examination may be of more use in animals with vague signs or history to give some clues as to whether resources should be concentrated on the neurological system or elsewhere

After the history has been taken and the neurological examination performed, it should be possible to classify the disease using the *aide mémoire* of five categories corresponding to the five fingers of a hand (Holger Volk, personal communication):

- Onset
- Clinical course
- Lateralization
- Pain
- Neurolocalization.

For example: a thoracolumbar disc extrusion may present as an acute-onset, static, left-sided, painful myelopathy; whereas seizuring due to a brain tumour may be characterized as a chronic, progressive, right-sided, non-painful forebrain disease.

Common conditions

Seizures and other forebrain disease

An epileptic seizure is the physical manifestation of abnormal electrical activity in the cerebral cortex. Seizures always originate in the forebrain (cerebrum and thalamus), although the underlying cause may be intracranial or extracranial. Seizures may or may not be accompanied by other signs of forebrain disease, including:

- Behavioural changes (e.g. aggression, loss of house training, disorientation, hemi-inattention)
- Depression
- Stupor (response only to aversive stimuli; more commonly associated with brainstem disease)
- Head pressing
- Paresis (mild).

Figure 11.1 lists some common causes of forebrain disease.

> - Degenerative (e.g. cognitive dysfunction syndrome)
> - Anomalous (e.g. hydrocephalus)
> - Metabolic (e.g. hepatic encephalopathy, hypoglycaemic encephalopathy)
> - Neoplastic, including primary tumours (e.g. glioma, meningioma) and secondary tumours (metastatic and locally invasive)
> - Nutritional (e.g. thiamine deficiency)
> - Inflammatory (e.g. meningoencephalitis of unknown origin)
> - Infectious (e.g. canine distemper virus, Protozoa, bacteria)
> - Toxic (e.g. lead, organophosphate)
> - Vascular (e.g. thromboembolic disease, haemorrhage)

11.1   Common causes of forebrain disease.

Clinical signs and history

Seizures can be recognized by certain characteristics that help differentiate them from other intermittent events such as syncope and movement disorders.

- There is occasionally a prodromal phase, a change in mood or behaviour that can last for 1 to 24 hours before the seizure occurs.
- A little more frequently, there is a pre-ictal phase or aura, which lasts for a few seconds to minutes before a seizure starts. The aura may involve behaviour such as agitation, seeking the owner or vomiting.
- After the seizure, there is often a post-ictal phase in which the animal may be lethargic and sleepy, wander aimlessly, appear blind, exhibit depression and urinate/defecate involuntarily. This phase can last for minutes to days.

The seizure event itself can present in several ways:

- **Generalized seizures:**
  - Characterized by loss of consciousness, involuntary motor activity of the whole body and autonomic signs such as salivation, defecation and urination

- May be clonic (rhythmic muscle contractions), tonic (increased muscle tone) or have tonic and clonic phases
- Rarely, may be atonic (lack of muscle tone; can be hard to differentiate from syncope) or myoclonic (spasmodic jerky contractions of groups of muscles; myoclonus can occur because of non-seizure causes).

■ **Partial seizures:**
- Involve only part of the forebrain and may or may not be associated with altered consciousness
- Simple partial seizures are characterized by brief, recurring, stereotypical movements or autonomic signs, such as flexion of a paw or hypersalivation
- Complex partial seizures usually involve altered consciousness and abnormal behaviour such as fly catching, star gazing, chewing, barking at nothing or unprovoked aggression.

Seizures should be differentiated from other causes of collapse or abnormal movement and behaviour such as syncope, vestibular disease, episodic weakness, behavioural disorders, movement disorders and pain and/or pruritus. This is best achieved by obtaining a detailed history and ideally observation of the event.

PRACTICAL TIP

Ask the owner to video an event. This gives a much clearer assessment than a simple description

---

Diagnosis

The diagnostic approach to forebrain disease is similar, whether the manifestation is seizure, disorientation or head pressing. Once the history has been obtained, and physical and neurological examinations carried out, a full blood count, urinalysis and routine serum biochemistry panel help rule out the common metabolic causes. A bile acid stimulation test is also important at this stage, as seizures can occur due to hepatic encephalopathy at any age and in some cases without any other clinical signs.

If no cause of the seizures has been identified, advanced imaging and cerebrospinal fluid (CSF) analysis should be considered. The utility of this should be weighed against the financial costs and risks to the animal of anaesthesia and CSF collection. Details of the technique for CSF collection are given in the *BSAVA Guide to Procedures in Small Animal Practice*.

The most common cause of seizures in dogs that have their first seizure at an age between 1 and 6 years, that have generalized seizures and that are normal inter-ictally, is idiopathic epilepsy. These patients usually have normal magnetic resonance imaging (MRI) and CSF findings. It is therefore acceptable in these cases to treat on this presumptive diagnosis if the owner is unwilling or constrained from pursuing advanced imaging. Owners may still want to proceed with these investigations to rule out more unusual conditions such as early-onset neoplasia (Figure 11.2), or late onset of signs related to congenital disease, but they should be warned of the low diagnostic yield. Duration of signs may also assist in diagnosis: if seizures have been occurring

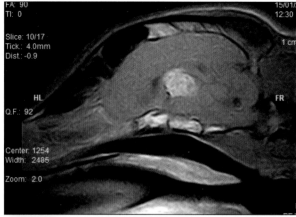

11.2 T1-weighted sagittal MRI scan of a 3-year- old Beagle with depression, head pressing and neck pain. The gadolinium contrast material is enhancing an intracranial mass, suspected to be a choroid plexus tumour.

for weeks to months without progressing, then inflammatory brain disease is less likely; whereas, if seizures have been present for over 6 months without progressing, then intracranial neoplasia is less likely.

Advanced imaging should be encouraged in dogs under 1 or over 6 years of age, to look for congenital (Figure 11.3) or neoplastic disease. Dogs with abnormal findings on inter-ictal neurological examinations will often have abnormalities on brain MRI. If there is neck pain or pyrexia, CSF analysis becomes more important for investigating inflammatory and infectious brain disease. MRI is preferred to computed tomography (CT) for the investigation of brain disease, due to its superior resolution of soft tissue and the difficulty of viewing the caudal brain with CT due to artefacts.

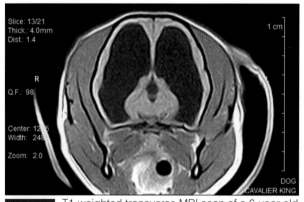

11.3 T1-weighted transverse MRI scan of a 6-year-old Cavalier King Charles Spaniel with seizures. The image shows hydrocephalus.

Treatment

Emergency treatment: Emergency treatment is re-quired if an animal is in status epilepticus, i.e. a seizure that is not self-limiting, or is having clusters of seizures (several close together). Since the onset of status epilepticus cannot be predicted, it can be useful to supply the owner with rectal diazepam, to be administered in the event of a seizure lasting more than 5 minutes, with advice that the vet should be called if it is necessary to use this. For a dog presenting to a surgery in status epilepticus, the first priority is to stop the seizure; a protocol is given in QRG 11.2. Although some dogs may be heavily sedated for

24–48 hours, many cases of status epilepticus can be controlled with this protocol and, although they may have post-ictal signs that can last 1–2 weeks, many dogs will return to a good quality of life, depending on the underlying cause.

PRACTICAL TIPS

- Do not confuse the gentle paddling associated with recovery from sedation or anaesthesia with the more jerky violent movements associated with seizure activity
- Familiarize yourself with animals in your surgery recovering from general anaesthesia
- If you have seen few seizuring animals before, examples can be found on the Internet

---

Long-term management: Treatment of underlying causes of epilepsy is beyond the scope of this chapter, but even serious brain diseases may respond for variable lengths of time to treatment. For example, dogs with brain tumours can have extended survival times following various combinations of radiotherapy, surgery and chemotherapy, and even prednisolone can have a palliative effect for weeks to months in some cases. Meningoencephalitis of unknown origin is associated with a guarded prognosis, but extended survival times or remission can be seen in animals treated with combinations of immunosuppressive drugs.

Owner education

Owner education is important in the management of seizures

- Owners need to be aware that it is rarely possible to prevent seizures completely, the aim being to reduce them to a frequency compatible with a good quality of life
- If seizures are occurring more frequently than every 2–3 months, seizure control should be considered suboptimal and treatment should be commenced, or ongoing treatment reviewed. However, it is not always possible to achieve a level of control in which seizures only occur every 3 months, and the dog's quality of life regarding seizure frequency and severity should be balanced against drug side effects when reviewing treatment
- The owners should be aware that side effects from treatment are common, although many of these are self-limiting within the first couple of weeks after starting treatment
- Beneficial effects of drugs may also take some time to be established
- Owners need to be aware of the importance of regular blood testing for therapeutic levels of the drug, and blood testing for adverse effects such as liver disease
- The owners should know that missing doses of drugs, or stopping them abruptly, may cause rebound seizures
- The owners should keep accurate records of seizure frequency, character and timing, and seek advice if the frequency increases, occurs in clusters, or the dog has a seizure lasting more than 5 minutes

---

There are three drugs authorized in the UK for the long-term treatment of epilepsy in dogs.

Phenobarbital is the first-line treatment, as it is generally better tolerated and more effective than potassium bromide (Boothe *et al.*, 2012).

- The initial dose is around 2–3 mg/kg twice daily. Data sheet recommendations for initial dose are either 2.5 mg/kg twice daily or 2–5 mg/kg twice daily, depending on brand. However, the dosage is best adjusted by monitoring serum concentration.
- As the drug has a long half-life, blood testing should be performed 2 weeks after starting therapy or 2 weeks after a dose change to ensure that drug concentration is steady. The blood test is generally performed 1–2 hours before a dose is due, to obtain a trough level, although in most cases the timing of blood sampling is not significant.
- Hepatic enzyme induction can mean the amount of drug required increases over time, so 6-monthly monitoring of serum concentration is recommended.
- Common side effects include sedation and ataxia after initiating treatment or increasing the dose. This is usually self-limiting over a period of 2 weeks. Increased thirst and appetite may be seen.
- Rarely, hepatotoxicity occurs, and this is more common at higher serum concentrations. As hepatic enzymes are induced by the drug, monitoring of these is not helpful, but liver function should be monitored regularly by checking dynamic bile acids, albumin and urea.

Imepitoin is a new anti-epileptic drug that was authorized in the UK in 2013 for 'the reduction of the frequency of generalized seizures due to idiopathic epilepsy in dogs... after careful evaluation of alternative treatment options'.

- The dose is 10–30 mg/kg twice daily, with the dose being varied depending on the severity of the disorder. It is recommended to start with an initial dose of 10 mg/kg twice daily, and if the drug is well tolerated but seizure control is not adequate after a minimum treatment duration of 1 week, the dose can be increased in 50 to 100% increments up to the maximum dose.
- As bioavailability is greater in fasted dogs, the timing of tablet administration in relation to feeding should be kept constant.
- Adverse effects, including polyphagia, polydipsia, polyuria and hyperactivity, have been reported to be generally mild and transient.
- Imepitoin should not be used as the primary treatment for cluster seizures or status epilepticus.
- The efficacy as an add-on drug has not been evaluated, but the author has used imepitoin in combination with phenobarbital, potassium bromide and/or levetiracetam in a small number of cases without adverse effect.
- Transition to or from other types of anti-epileptic therapy should be done gradually and with close supervision.

Potassium bromide is authorized in the UK as an anti-epileptic agent for use as an adjunct to pheno-barbital in the control of refractory cases of epilepsy in dogs. A patient may be considered refractory to phenobarbital when its quality of life is affected by frequent and/or severe seizures, despite an adequate serum concentration of the drug. Approximately 50% of dogs that are resistant to phenobarbital achieve good control of seizures with the addition of potassium bromide. Potassium bromide can be considered as a sole agent if there is a reason not to use phenobarbital, e.g. pre-existing hepatic disease.

- The recommended dose in the data sheet is 15 mg/kg twice daily with food.
- The half-life of potassium bromide is 24 days, so it can take weeks to months to achieve an adequate steady concentration.
- If more rapid control is required (such as in a dog with cluster seizures), a loading dose of potassium bromide can be given (e.g. 600–1000 mg/kg orally) but this has an increased risk of adverse reactions, such as sedation and ataxia, and the author's preference is to add one of the quicker acting anti-epileptic drugs such as levetiracetam, either long term or temporarily while adequate serum concentrations are achieved.
  - Alternatively, giving a loading dose of potassium bromide of 200 mg/kg orally q24h for 5 days may reduce the incidence of side effects, after which the dose can be decreased to the maintenance dose.
- Serum concentrations should be assessed at 2 and 4 months after initiation or a dose change.
- Side effects include sedation, ataxia, vomiting, polyuria, polydipsia, polyphagia, an erythematous rash, and possibly pancreatitis.

Diazepam has too short a half-life in dogs to be of use in maintenance therapy. However, tactical use of the oral or rectal form may be of benefit in controlling cluster seizures. It is also prudent to give the owner of an epileptic dog a small supply of rectal diazepam to be used in the event of a prolonged seizure (the author recommends that this is used in the event of a seizure lasting 5 minutes or more).

Levetiracetam has a short half-life and appears to be very well tolerated. It appears to be effective as a third anti-epileptic drug in cases refractory to phenobarbital and potassium bromide, and may be superior to those drugs in the treatment of partial seizures. It can also be used tactically for a few days in the event of cluster seizures, as it has a rapid onset of activity. It can be very expensive for bigger dogs and tolerance may develop to it in the long term, which can limit its usefulness.

Other anti-epileptic drugs that may be used include gabapentin and zonisamide. **Gabapentin** appears to decrease seizure frequency. It is also effective as an analgesic in cases of neuropathic pain. It can be difficult in some cases to distinguish between unusual behaviour due to intermittent pain and complex partial epilepsy; gabapentin can some-times be of use in these cases, though it will not be possible to know whether a response to treatment is due to analgesic or anticonvulsant effects.

Refractory cases

If a dog fails to respond to anti-epileptic treatment, or becomes refractory at a later stage, consider or investigate:

- Owner compliance: it is important that doses are not missed as this can lead to rebound seizures
- Incorrect dosage: check therapeutic levels
- Malabsorption, e.g. due to gastroenteritis
- Drug interactions affecting metabolism
- Incorrect diagnosis: are these really seizures? Is there an underlying cause that has not been diagnosed, or has newly occurred?

Epilepsy is a treatable condition in dogs, but the owners should be aware that not all dogs can have their seizures controlled adequately and that there is a significant emotional and financial commitment to owning an epileptic dog. Euthanasia may be considered in cases where the owner is not prepared to make that commitment, or in cases where the dog is refractory to treatment and its quality of life is adversely affected

---

Ataxia and gait abnormalities

Ataxia is a failure of muscle coordination, excluding weakness, musculoskeletal problems and abnormal movements such as tremor. It can be classified as:

- **Cerebellar ataxia:**
  - Loss of ability of fine control of movement
  - Characterized by high stepping or over-reaching gait (hypermetria)
  - May be accompanied by intention tremor and loss of menace response
- **Vestibular ataxia:**
  - Characterized by leaning, falling or tight circling to one side with unilateral disease
  - Usually accompanied by head tilt and nystagmus
  - In bilateral disease the patient is reluctant to move, and will often stay crouched and show side-to-side movements of the head
- **Sensory ataxia:**
  - Loss of sensation of limb position (conscious proprioception)
  - Characterized by clumsiness and incoordination, leading to a wide-based stance, swaying gait, scuffing of toes and a longer than normal stride length
  - May be accompanied by a variety of signs, depending on neurolocalization.

Observation of gait and head position, along with conscious proprioception testing in the neurological examination will usually allow neurolocalization of ataxia.

- Cerebellar ataxia is usually caused by cerebellar disease.
- Vestibular ataxia may be due to peripheral (i.e. middle/inner ear disease) or central vestibular disease (i.e. brainstem and parts of the cerebellum).

- Sensory ataxia may be due to a lesion involving the forebrain, brainstem, spinal cord (see Chapter 16) or peripheral nerves.

Figure 11.4 indicates ways of differentiating peripheral from central vestibular disease.

Characteristic	Central vestibular disease	Peripheral vestibular disease
History of otitis externa	+	+
History of ototoxins	–	++
Conscious proprioceptive deficits	++	–
Head tilt	++	++
Spontaneous nystagmus	+	++
Positional nystagmus	++	–
Vertical nystagmus	++	–
Rotatory nystagmus	+	+

11.4 Differentiating central from peripheral vestibular disease. – = rarely associated; + = sometimes associated; ++ = frequently associated.

Localizing the lesion in ataxic animals is important in directing further investigation, treatment and prognosis. For example:

- A dog with acute-onset head tilt, horizontal spontaneous nystagmus, ataxia with no conscious proprioceptive deficits and no history of otitis externa would be strongly suspected to have idiopathic vestibular syndrome, and a limited investigation with monitoring might be appropriate
- A dog with gradual-onset vestibular signs accompanied by lateralized conscious proprioceptive deficits would prompt an investigation of central disease, such as MRI of the brain
- A dog with hindlimb proprioceptive deficits only, and brisk segmental spinal reflexes, would benefit from a spinal investigation such as myelography or MRI/CT of the spine.

Figure 11.5 lists the most common causes of ataxia.

Weakness

Weakness may be episodic, exercise-induced (more properly termed fatigue) or persistent. It can be difficult to differentiate from other causes of reluctance to move, such as pain and paresis. A physical examination can help identify areas of pain, and assessing reflexes such as the withdrawal reflex can help identify reduced strength. Consideration should be given as to whether the weakness is persistent, or worsens with exercise as in the case of myasthenia gravis (see below). The approach to weakness (see Chapter 17) involves careful history-taking and physical examination; blood testing (e.g. haematology, biochemistry, electrolytes) is usually appropriate. Common differential diagnoses for weakness are listed in Figure 11.6.

Intracranial disease

- Trauma
- Meningoencephalitis
- Neoplasia
- Cerebrovascular accident
- Toxicity
- Extension of otitis media into brain

Peripheral vestibular disease

- Idiopathic
- Otitis interna
- Iatrogenic (ear cleaning)
- Trauma
- Neoplasia
- Hypothyroidism
- Toxicity

Spinal disease

- See Chapter 16 for further details

Peripheral neuropathy

- Toxicity
- Trauma
- Idiopathic/inherited (e.g. sensory neuropathy)
- Metabolic (e.g. diabetes mellitus, hypothyroidism)
- Neoplastic/paraneoplastic
- Inflammatory/infectious (e.g. protozoal)

11.5 Common causes of ataxia. See Chapter 17 for details of endocrine causes.

Metabolic disorders

- Hypoglycaemia
- Hypocalcaemia

Endocrine disorders

- Hypoadrenocorticism
- Hypothyroidism

Haematological disease

- Anaemia

Immune-mediated disorders

- Myasthenia gravis
- Immune-mediated polyarthritis

Cardiovascular disease

- Arrhythmia
- Heart failure
- Pericardial effusion
- Aortic thromboembolism

Respiratory disease

- Obstructive (e.g. asthma, foreign body)
- Intrathoracic neoplasia
- Severe pulmonary parenchymal disease

Neuromuscular disorders

- Myasthenia gravis
- Tick paralysis
- Myopathies

Nutritional disorders

- Malabsorption
- Anorexia
- Cachexia

11.6 Common causes of weakness. See Chapter 17 for details of endocrine causes.

Neuromuscular diseases and myopathies

Weakness and fatigue are common signs of neuromuscular diseases and myopathies. Common myopathies include polymyositis and masticatory myositis.

Polymyositis can be suspected when generalized weakness is present, together with muscle pain on palpation (although some dogs will be more sensitive than others) and pyrexia. Muscle biopsy is required for definitive diagnosis, and electromyography can be supportive. Testing for infections that can affect the muscles, e.g. *Neospora*, is important, as treatment of idiopathic polymyositis involves immunosuppression.

Myasthenia gravis and other neuromuscular junction diseases often present with generalized weakness. Acute flaccid tetraparesis is more likely to be seen with tick paralysis and botulism, whereas generalized myasthenia gravis is more likely to be characterized by weakness occurring after a short period of exercise. Diagnosis is by detection of anti-acetylcholine receptor antibodies on serology, although an edrophonium response test (see *BSAVA Guide to Procedures in Small Animal Practice*) is supportive. Myasthenia gravis may also present in a focal form, characterized by regurgitation due to megaoesophagus, although this sign is also often present in the generalized form. Megaoesophagus worsens the prognosis due to the common sequel of aspiration pneumonia. A chest radiograph of the conscious dog will aid in the diagnosis of megaoesophagus.

Masticatory myopathy is a type of myositis confined to the masticatory muscles of the head and is usually an idiopathic immune-mediated disease. It can present either with muscle weakness and inability to close the jaw, or with trismus (locked jaw) due to fibrosis of atrophied muscles. In the acute stages the masticatory muscles may be swollen, but more commonly the condition is noticed in the chronic form when they become atrophied. Diagnosis is by muscle biopsy and serology for anti-2M antibodies, and ruling out infectious diseases such as toxoplasmosis and neosporosis using serology. Treatment is with immunosuppression: steroids are useful in this condition for their antifibrotic effects as well as their immunosuppressive effects. Other causes of masticatory muscle atrophy include hyperadrenocorticism/glucocorticoid administration, cancer cachexia and other systemic diseases.

Cranial nerve disorders

Certain cranial neuropathies present in characteristic ways. Treatment and prognosis will depend on the underlying cause.

A dropped jaw can be a sign of bilateral trigeminal nerve lesions. Diseases that might cause a dropped jaw include: idiopathic trigeminal neuropathy, which is often self-limiting; infections; inflammatory diseases; and lymphoma.

WARNING

Be aware of animals that have been in countries where rabies is endemic, as a dropped jaw can also be a sign of rabies

Lesions affecting a single trigeminal nerve can lead to severe unilateral masticatory muscle atrophy (Figure 11.7). These lesions are often neoplastic. As a rule of thumb, unilateral masticatory muscle atrophy is likely to be neurogenic, whereas bilateral is likely to be due to masticatory myopathy (see earlier). Further testing is required to clarify this.

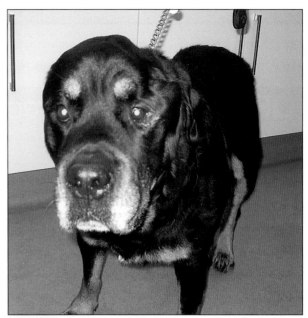

11.7 This 8-year-old Rottweiler shows marked left-sided masticatory muscle atrophy, due to a trigeminal nerve sheath tumour.

Facial paralysis can be idiopathic and self-limiting. It may also be related to brainstem or middle ear disease, or to trauma. Flaccid paralysis of the facial muscles is noted, together with a loss of the palpebral reflex.

Horner's syndrome is characterized by miosis, narrowing of the palpebral fissure and protrusion of the third eyelid (Figure 11.8). It is caused by a lesion affecting the autonomic nerve supply to the eye. This is a complicated pathway, and so the lesion can be anywhere from the midbrain, through the spinal cord to T1–T3, up the vasovagal sympathetic trunk in the neck, to near the middle ear. The condition can be idiopathic, and Golden Retrievers are over-represented (Boydell, 1995).

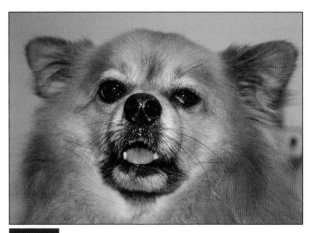

11.8 Horner's syndrome in a Pomeranian.

References and further reading

Bagley RS (2005) *Fundamentals of Veterinary Clinical Neurology.* Blackwell, Iowa

Bexfield N and Lee K (2014) *BSAVA Guide to Procedures in Small Animal Practice, 2nd edn.* BSAVA Publications, Gloucester

Boothe DM, Dewey C and Carpenter DM (2012) Comparison of phenobarbital with bromide as a first-choice antiepileptic drug for treatment of epilepsy in dogs. *Journal of the American Veterinary Medical Association* **240**, 1073–1083

Boydell P (1995) Idiopathic Horner's syndrome in the golden retriever. *Journal of Small Animal Practice* **36**, 382–384

Hardy B, Patterson EE, Cloyd J, Hardy R and Leppik I (2012) Double-masked, placebo-controlled study of intravenous levetiracetam for the treatment of status epilepticus and acute repetitive seizures in dogs. *Journal of Veterinary Internal Medicine* **26**, 334–340

Jaggy A (2010) *Small Animal Neurology.* Schlütersche, Hannover

Platt SR and Garosi L (2012) *Small Animal Neurological Emergencies.* Manson Publishing, London

Platt SR and Olby NJ (2013) *BSAVA Manual of Canine and Feline Neurology, 4th edn.* BSAVA Publications, Gloucester

---

QRG 11.1 Short 'screening' neurological examination

1 Visual assessment of the head: look from the front for signs of asymmetry, e.g. masticatory muscles, head tilt, anisocoria, drooping lip.

2 With a bright light, look for evidence of strabismus and nystagmus, and check pupillary light reflexes (see Chapter 21).

3 Palpate the head and neck for pain.

4 Open the mouth wide to assess for pain, jaw strength and the presence of trismus. Test gag reflex at this time *if it is safe to do so.*

5 Tilt the head upwards, to assess for both neck pain and positional nystagmus.

- Move the head from side to side to assess for neck pain and for normal physiological nystagmus. A normal young dog should be able to have its neck gently flexed: laterally in both directions so that its nose is flat along its flank; upwards so it is looking at the ceiling; and downwards so its mandible is flat along its chest.

WARNING

Downward flexion of the neck should be avoided in dogs at risk of atlantoaxial subluxation, such as young small-breed dogs

- If possible, turn the dog on its back to assess for positional nystagmus.

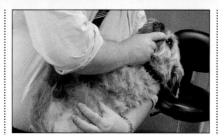

6 Check palpebral and menace reflexes.

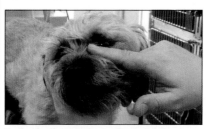

Testing for the palpebral reflex by lightly tapping the medial canthus of the eye. A normal response is a brisk blink.

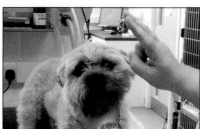

Testing for the menace response by making a threatening gesture towards the eye. A normal response is a blink. *Be careful not to make a draft of air, which will trigger the palpebral or corneal reflexes.*

7 Palpate the spine for pain, and the limbs for pain, muscle tone and atrophy.

8 Check the paw placing response on all four feet.

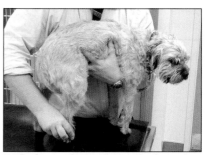

Testing for conscious proprioception by turning the paw on to its dorsal aspect. A normal response is briskly returning the foot to its normal position.

9 Check withdrawal response in all four feet by pinching between the toes.

QRG 11.2 Emergency treatment of status epilepticus

For a dog presenting to a surgery in status epilepticus, the first priority is to stop the seizure. The following protocol can be followed in these cases.

1 Administer diazepam: 0.5–1.0 mg/kg i.v. or rectally, for up to three doses, 5 minutes apart.

2

■ If this stops the seizure, administer a loading dose of phenobarbital slowly intravenously:
  • If the dog has not previously been on phenobarbital treatment, the dose is 12 mg/kg
  • If the dog is already on phenobarbital treatment, 4–6 mg/kg of phenobarbital can be given slowly intravenously to increase the blood levels slightly
■ If the diazepam does *not* stop the seizure, administer phenobarbital 2–4 mg/kg i.v. every 20–30 minutes to effect, *not exceeding 24 mg/kg over 24 hours*. The dose will be lower if the animal is already being treated with oral phenobarbital.

3 If diazepam and phenobarbital fail to halt seizure activity, other options include:

■ A continuous diazepam infusion of 0.1–0.5 mg/kg/h
  • Note that diazepam can become adsorbed on to the plastics of syringes and giving sets, but once the initial dose has passed through them, the plastic should become saturated, allowing further diazepam to pass through normally
  • *Diazepam should not be diluted or mixed with other agents*
■ Propofol, initially in boluses of 1–2 mg/kg i.v., followed by 0.1–0.6 mg/kg/min constant rate infusion
■ Intravenous levetiracetam (20 mg/kg q8h) has recently been shown to have some effect and to be well tolerated in status epilepticus (Hardy *et al.*, 2012). It also has the advantage or causing minimal sedation, which is useful in assessing response, although it is very expensive
■ Inhalant anaesthesia with isoflurane is a last resort.

4 Supportive care should be instituted, including: airway support; oxygenation or ventilation if required; fluid therapy to maintain hydration; and treatment of hyperthermia.

5 Blood tests for electrolytes, glucose, calcium, packed cell volume (PCV) and total protein should be performed and deviations corrected where possible.

6 Monitor blood pressure, body temperature and hydration status.

7 Turn the patient every 4 hours, express the bladder as required and keep the patient warm, clean and dry.

8 Give a loading dose of an anticonvulsant drug if not already given. Start maintenance treatment (see main text).

9 Continue to monitor for 24–48 hours.

Although some dogs may be heavily sedated for 24–48 hours, many cases of status epilepticus can be controlled with the above protocol, and although they may have post-ictal signs that can last 1–2 weeks, many cases will return to a good quality of life, depending on the underlying cause.

OBSERVATION

Mental state: Alert ❑   Obtunded ❑   Stuporous ❑   Comatose ❑

Posture: Standing ❑   Sitting ❑   Lying ❑

Stance...

Head tilt ❑   Lameness ❑   Involuntary movement ❑

Gait: Normal ❑   Circling ❑   Ataxic ❑   Knuckling ❑

Stride length...

PALPATION/MANIPULATION

Muscle tone...

Muscle atrophy...

Skeletal abnormalities...

Neck pain...

Joint pain...

Spinal pain..

POSTURAL REACTIONS

Score 0 for absent, 1 for reduced, 2 for normal and 3 for exaggerated

Reaction	L thoracic limb	R thoracic limb	L pelvic limb	R pelvic limb
Hopping				
Knuckling				
Wheelbarrow				
Hemiwalking				
Tactile placing				
Visual placing				
Extensor postural thrust				

CRANIAL NERVE TESTS

Smelling non-irritant substance (I) ❑
Pupil size/anisocoria (retina, II, III) ❑
Pupillary light reflex (II, III, sympathetic, retina) ❑
Menace (II, VII, forebrain, cerebellum, brainstem) ❑
Corneal reflex (V, VI, VII) ❑
Throw cotton wool (II) ❑
Auditory response (VIII) ❑
Strabismus:
    Permanent: III, IV, VI ❑
    Positional: VIII ❑
Spontaneous nystagmus:
    Horizontal ❑
    Vertical ❑
    Rotatory ❑
Positional nystagmus (III, VIII, brainstem) ❑
Facial sensation, nasal stimulation (V, forebrain) ❑
Facial symmetry (VII) ❑
Palpebral reflex (V, VII) ❑
Swallowing/gag reflex (IX, X) ❑
Tongue (XII) ❑
Oculocardiac (V, X) ❑
Jaw tone (V) ❑

SPINAL REFLEXES

Thoracic withdrawal (C6–T2) ❑
Pelvic withdrawal (L6–T2) ❑
Patellar (L4–L6) ❑
Gastrocnemius (L6–S1) ❑
Perineal (S1–S3) ❑
Extensor carpi radialis (C7–T2) ❑
Tail movement ❑

URINARY FUNCTION

Voluntary urination?   Yes ❑   No ❑
Full bladder?   Yes ❑   No ❑
Easily expressed?   Yes ❑   No ❑

PAIN SENSATION

Sensation	L thoracic limb	R thoracic limb	L pelvic limb	R pelvic limb
Deep pain				
Hyperaesthesia				
Superficial pain				

PANNICULUS REFLEX
CUT-OFF POINT ....

An example of a form that can be used for a neurological examination.

Behaviour problems: a brief guide

Tiny De Keuster, Joke Monteny and Christel P.H. Moons

Behavioural problems may be a reason for presentation by the owner or may be noted during a consultation for another reason. In either event it is important to investigate them. As well as affecting the dog itself, behavioural problems can threaten the human–animal bond, and society itself: a behaviour problem in an otherwise healthy animal may result in re-homing or euthanasia of the dog, social stress for owners, or even injury to third parties. It is important for the practitioner to realize that giving advice about behavioural problems has broad consequences beyond the patient itself.

Behavioural complaints may appear simple ("My dog is just pulling on the lead") and are coloured by the owner's interpretation ("It is just a disobedient dog"). Owners may ask for a quick fix, such as a drug to calm the dog down or a few tips and tricks. However, as for signs of any disease, behavioural signs deserve a full clinical and behavioural examination; a symptomatic approach should be avoided at all times. If no in-house expertise is available, referral to a specialist in behavioural medicine should be considered.

A detailed discussion of multiple behavioural conditions is beyond the scope of this chapter. Brief guidelines are given concerning a range of topics that are frequently presented as problems in general practice (see *BSAVA Manual of Canine and Feline Behavioural Medicine* for more details).

Canine body language

Humans and dogs are both social species, which means that not only do they enjoy the presence of a companion, but they also exhibit decreased functioning in isolation and may experience reduced welfare. Optimal functioning is dependent upon social relationships with other members of society, and this requires effective communication and a mutual understanding of species-specific signalling, social gestures and interactions.

Important concepts in canine communication

Perception
Perception is the process by which individuals register and evaluate information detected from the internal and external environment, consciously or unconsciously (Burn, 2009). The quality and quantity of stimuli that can be perceived depends on the sensory apparatus of the animal, whilst the complexity of perception depends on the cognitive abilities and previous experiences of the individual. When dealing with dogs, it is important to understand that some actions, which are perceived as benign by humans, can be perceived as threatening by dogs (Figure 12.1).

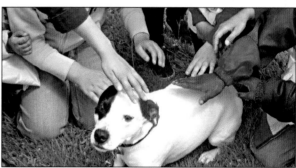

12.1 Human *versus* dog perception of the interaction. The children were allowed to pet the dog in a friendly manner. However, the dog is signalling that it is not comfortable with this interaction. Unfortunately, people often miss such subtle canine communication or interpret it incorrectly. (© K Buysse)

Cognition
Cognition refers to the mechanism by which animals acquire, process, store and act on information from the environment (Shettleworth, 2001). For veterinary surgeons, it is important to be aware that health or age-related factors influencing information retrieval (sensory function), information processing (central nervous system, CNS) or executive functioning (cardiovascular, musculoskeletal or neurological systems) may affect the cognitive and communicative functioning of the dog (Figure 12.2).

Arousal
Arousal is a state of psycho-physiological activation that determines the responsiveness of an individual to environmental stimuli. From a behavioural point of view, arousal is characterized by increased alertness, sensory sensitivity and readiness to respond to

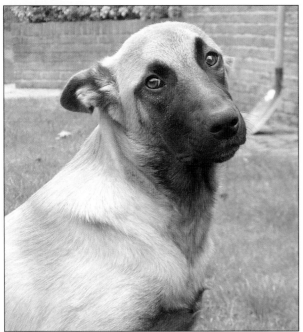

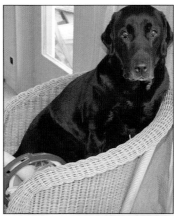

12.3 Children tend to approach and pet a dog that is lying down or sitting in a chair. This dog is feeling cornered in the chair and is emitting conflict avoiding signals, including averting its gaze and turning its head away. As the petting continues and the level of stress increases, the sclera becomes visible. (© M Vermeulen)

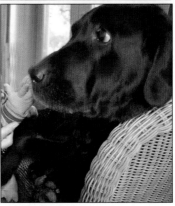

12.2 Disease or pain may impair communication and body language. This Malinois puppy has been hit by a car and is in pain. (© J Monteny)

stimulation through faster cognitive processing and more response (Ligout, 2009). However, when arousal is too high it interferes with the acquisition and assimilation of information and consequently with proper cognitive processing (Overall, 2013).

Stress

Stress is the the biological response elicited when an individual perceives a threat to its homeostasis (Moberg, 2000). Previous research has indicated that an individual's *perception* of the stressor (through predictability and control) plays an important role in the effects of stress (Weiss, 1972; Yang *et al.*, 2011), even more so than the physical characteristics of the stressor (such as intensity or duration).

How dogs react in social stress situations: The way a dog copes with a perceived social threat in a specific context (e.g. veterinary examination) depends on dog-related factors (physical health, emotional state) influenced by actual context (owner present or absent, previous experience of the car ride, waiting room or clinic). When a perceived threat cannot be resolved by emitting conflict avoiding signalling, the dog will try strategies higher up the 'ladder of aggression' (see Figures 12.3, 12.4 and 12.14).

How dogs communicate

Communication is the transfer of information between a sender and a receiver, where both the sender and the receiver map a signal to a particular meaning. When signal-to-meaning mapping involves a syntax (a formal structuring of the signals in relation to each other), the type of communication is called *language* (van der Zee, 2009). As dogs have no spoken language, their communication mainly relies on body language combined with odour signalling and vocalization (Figures 12.5 and 12.6).

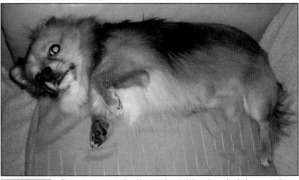

12.4 Owners may believe that this dog is lying on its back to have its stomach rubbed, but this is not always the case. This dog is showing indications of tension and stress, including open eyes, dilated pupils, gazing at the perceived threat (i.e. the approaching person) and growling when being touched (see also Figure 12.14). Hence the importance of the correct interpretation of the message ('please go away'). (© G Van Grembergen)

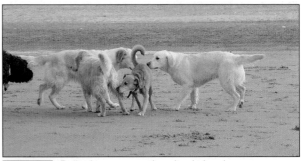

12.5 Polite human greeting rituals involve eye contact, static encounters and often a handshake. Polite dog greetings involve dynamic encounters that are commonly characterized by curved approaches, avoidance of eye contact and reciprocally sniffing genital regions whilst moving around. (© H Blancke)

Communication	Emotion/motivation	Message(s)	Sensory organs picking up the message
Body language: Face Body Skin Posture Action	Positive or negative emotion Positive or negative arousal Perceived threat Perceived conflict	Social approach Social distancing Play	Visual system – note that a dog's eyes are very sensitive to movement, even when far away Tactile system
Vocalizations: Bark Growl Howl Yelp Scream			Auditory system – harsh low frequency, unmodulated barks are more commonly the response to a perceived threat. The more tonal, higher pitched, modulated barks are more commonly seen during play and isolation
Odour signalling: Urine Anal glands	Positive sexual arousal Negative stress arousal	Oestrus Perceived competition Perceived threat	A dog's sense of smell exceeds that of humans. This is important to consider for veterinary clinic hygiene management (e.g. remaining scent from a fearful dog in a previous consultation may 'worry' the next dog entering the room)

12.6 It is important to realize that most signals used in canine body language have more than one meaning, depending upon the situation. Hence, the importance of observing the behaviour of the dog in the relevant context.

How well are dogs able to understand human language?

It is thought that ten thousand years of cohabitation between humans and dogs may have enabled dogs to understand quite a lot of human communication. However, it is important to understand what dogs are actually responding to.

The meaning of words

According to a recent study, attempts to teach dogs words outside an associative context (e.g. by human referential actions only) were not successful. However, dogs can learn words by association (through classical conditioning) (Tempelmann *et al.*, 2014; see also Puppy development and behaviour, below).

Feelings of guilt

In contrast to belief, studies have found no relationship between the 'guilty look' on a dog's face and the fact that it had engaged in disobedient behaviour. However, researchers did find that the dog's 'guilt admitting' behaviour occurred in response to owner cues (e.g. scolding) (Horowitz, 2009).

Human non-verbal cues

Research has shown that 'what' we say is highly influenced by 'how' we say it, i.e. the role of non-verbal communication is unmistakable and it is likely that this influences our communication with dogs. Dogs are able to comprehend a variety of human non-verbal cues, such as pointing and gazing, which makes them more able than primates to read human non-verbal gestures (Kaminski *et al.*, 2012; Kirchhofer *et al.*, 2012).

Understanding human intentions

Dogs are able to treat human communication in a flexible way and can discriminate between communication that is intended towards them and that intended towards third parties. Dogs do not need eye contact to know if a human gesture is intended for them. These characteristics of understanding human communication have been demonstrated in puppies as young as 6–10 weeks old (Kaminski *et al.*, 2012).

Potential pitfalls

As humans are largely unaware of their own body language, and unaware that dogs pick up the non-verbal cues they emit, this could lead to misunderstanding.

For veterinary professionals, it is important to look at these human gestures from the dog's perspective: do dogs meet and greet in the same way, how are 'human gestures' like extending a hand or hugging perceived, how could problems arise and how should they be dealt with?

How well are humans able to understand dog language?

Importance of dispelling myths

Dogs that cohabit with humans are capable of bonding with other dogs and species within the family and forming stable, lifelong attachments. Unfortunately, for more than half a century, human vision of dog behaviour has been influenced by our own social constructs. For example, dominance has been (incorrectly) perceived as an individual dog trait and the interpretation of certain types of canine signalling has been (incorrectly) linked to status (i.e. dogs with their tail up and ears forward have been thought to be 'dominant' and dogs with their tail tucked under and ears back have been thought to be 'submissive') (Bradshaw *et al.*, 2009). Such associations have not been helpful in promoting safe and animal-friendly interactions between humans and dogs. For veterinary professionals working with dogs, it is therefore crucial to dispel myths and adopt a scientific approach.

Breed differences

In addition to the differences between individual dogs in terms of reaction to stimuli, the selection and breeding of dogs for certain characteristics has resulted in a range of phenotypes for head and body size, hair coat, skin folds, ear and tail position and tail length, which influence the way emotions and motivations are expressed by dogs and are observed by humans (Rimbault and Ostrander, 2012). For example, some breeds (e.g. Beagles) spontaneously hold the tail in an elevated position, whilst others (e.g. Chow Chow) hold the tail in an upright curved position. However, some breeds may only raise the tail in response to a (pleasant or unpleasant) stimulus. In addition, some breeds may have no discernible facial expressions because of the presence of skin folds or overlapping hairs surrounding the eyes and face (e.g. Bull Terriers, Cavalier King Charles Spaniels). Thus, veterinary professionals should remember that just looking at a few body parts is not an accurate way to assess a dog's emotion or motivation; it is important to interpret dog language by looking at the entire dog (face, eyes, ears, skin, hairs, posture, sounds, smells and movement) within a given context.

Dog barking

Barking in dogs appears to be characterized by acoustic parameters specific for the context and animal's emotional state (tonality, peak frequency and inter-bark intervals). Consequently, barking has more than one meaning. For example, when dogs bark they can be aroused or excited in a positive (i.e. during play) or a negative (i.e. when isolated or feeling threatened during exposure to visual or auditory stimuli) way. Research indicates that humans, in general, are quite skilled at recognizing different types of bark and underlying emotional state (Pongrácz *et al.*, 2005, 2011). Unfortunately, human society in general does not take kindly to barking by dogs and this kind of canine vocalization may lead to serious conflicts between neighbours, the filing of official complaints and could potentially result in relinquishment or euthanasia of the dog. For further information on barking, see the *BSAVA Manual of Canine and Feline Behavioural Medicine*.

Prevention is key

Be aware of human pitfalls

- Human social gestures, such as sitting close to show affiliation, putting one's arm around someone's shoulders and restraining someone in a friendly hug, are positive signals from a human perspective. Young children, especially, like to pet dogs as a sign of their friendship, not realizing that their (benign) actions might intimidate a dog and induce fear. The fact that the dog freezes and does not move, may lead parents and/or teachers to think that the dog feels happy with the well-intended attention.
- Humans might interpret subtle signs such as yawning as the dog being 'bored' or 'tired'. However, it should be explained to owners that this may, in fact, be a subtle sign relating to conflict avoidance.
- It is important to be aware of why an unfamiliar dog might approach you in the veterinary practice. When an unknown dog approaches you and sniffs (e.g. your hand), this is most likely not a request to be petted; it only means that the dog is exploring you.

Be aware of dog language pitfalls

- When dogs meet humans or other dogs, they are not trying to sort out who is the boss; they just want to investigate and pick up information. Problems may arise when dogs are restricted in their movement (e.g. when they are on a lead) or when owners with a dog on a lead approach the other dog from the front and stand still. Dogs may interpret this encounter as a potential threat (Figure 12.7).
- When a dog raises its tail and bristles, this does not signal status. Instead, it relates to arousal and, perhaps, threat perception.
- When a dog wags its tail, this does not necessarily mean it is friendly and wants to be petted. Tail wagging represents a state of arousal that might be pleasant (play, greeting) or unpleasant (threat, incentive for attack). Translating dog language based on tail movements is not helpful.

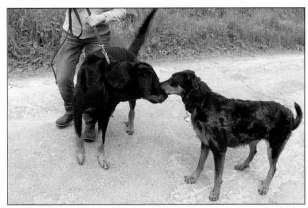

12.7 Meeting an unknown dog when on a lead and standing still may change the dynamics of communication between the dogs. (© J Monteny)

- Always interpret behaviour within a context (Figure 12.8). The way a dog reacts to environmental and social stimuli depends on its perception, cognition, threshold for arousal and the type of emotional response that is triggered in the brain. The individual behavioural strategy (i.e. signalling of the response) depends on several factors such as genetic predisposition, behavioural development, health status, past learning experiences and context.
- Important note: aggression is not a trait or characteristic inherent to an individual. Aggression is a strategy that dogs use when conflict avoiding signalling does not have the desired outcome from the dog's point of view (Figure 12.9).

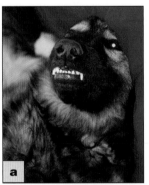

a

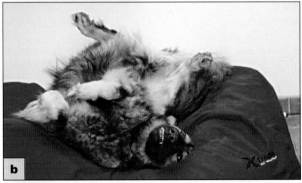

b

12.8 Behaviour should always be interpreted within a context. **(a)** What signs (if any) may indicate stress or feeling threatened? What do you think the dog is communicating? **(b)** The sclera are visible and the corners of the lips appear to be retracted backwards, revealing the teeth. This could have led to the assumption that the dog is bearing its teeth as an act of aggression. However, when considering the entire dog, it becomes clear that the puppy is completely relaxed and having an upside down nap. (© E Larmuseau)

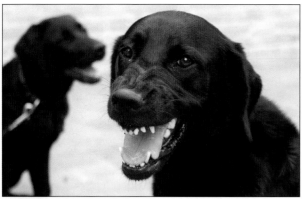

12.9 This type of signalling could lead humans to concluded that this is an aggressive dog. However, aggression is a strategy that dogs use when conflict avoiding signalling does not have a successful outcome. Thus, aggression should be considered a strategy and not a personality trait. (© J Monteny)

Puppy development and behaviour

A puppy's development is influenced by its genetic makeup, its environment and learning experiences. Lack of exposure to social and environmental stimuli, or exposure to stimuli that overtaxes the puppy's ability to cope, may induce chronic stress and lead to developmental disorders (Weiss, 1972). The socialization period (between 3 and 14 weeks of age) is a particularly sensitive time during which puppies develop strategies to cohabit with conspecifics or other species (socialization) and learn how to respond to environment stimuli (environmental learning). Both socialization and environmental learning should be continued throughout a dog's life and owners should be informed correctly by trained professionals (McBride, 2009).

Owners should speak to experts before and after buying a puppy to avoid unrealistic expectations and maximize the chances of a successful adoption (Hetts *et al.*, 2004; Gazzano *et al.*, 2008; Marder and Duxbury, 2008). The role of the veterinary practice is to provide animal health care and to support the owner in ensuring good pet welfare. For the latter, the role of the veterinary practice is to *educate owners* about everyday life of a puppy within a household, the importance of puppy socialization classes and the need for using training methods conducive to good welfare. Attending puppy classes has been found to be associated with less behavioural problems later in life (Sterry *et al.*, 2005; Blackwell *et al.*, 2008) and a lower chance of relinquishment (Duxbury *et al.*, 2003).

Organizing puppy classes entails a responsibility towards dogs and their owners, and strongly influences the functionality of the human–dog relationship within society. Puppy classes, therefore, should be run by professionals with a number of theoretical and practical skills related to learning theory, dog training, observation and awareness of dog language, as well as sufficient interpersonal skills to provide smooth and friendly owner guidance (ABTC, 2012).

When setting up puppy classes in veterinary practice, or when referring clients to puppy classes, it is important for the veterinary team to be aware of what a 'good' puppy class is and how to screen for it.

Puppy welfare

According to the Animal Welfare Act 2006 (which applies in England and Wales), the Animal Health and Welfare (Scotland) Act 2006 and the Welfare of Animals (Northern Ireland) Act 2011, the person responsible for the animal has a duty to meet its welfare needs, which are for a suitable environment, a suitable diet, to exhibit normal behaviour patterns, to be housed with or apart from other animals (if applicable) and to be protected from pain, suffering, injury and disease. Whilst veterinary surgeons are trained to monitor the physically-related needs, there is a lack of information about what constitutes appropriate canine (social) behaviour and how to offer preventive care related to puppy fear and anxiety.

When thinking about raising puppies to balanced adults, veterinary surgeons must not only promote techniques conducive to welfare, but also inform owners about their individual puppy's developmental needs and limitations due to genetic background (e.g. dogs will react differently when bred as companion animals *versus* when bred selectively from a working line or a 'show' line). The expectations of the owner and the needs of the puppy should both be taken into account.

What types of tools can my practice recommend to help owners achieve a minimum set of expectations in their puppy?

1. Prevention

Although the exact minimum set of expectations may depend on the specific household, in general, owners will expect a puppy to be housetrained, to be able to be left home alone, to allow human contact, to discriminate human objects from toys, and to be friendly to people without jumping and biting. As neurological and physical development is ongoing, most of these behaviours will take time for a puppy to learn. The owner needs to be aware that the puppy cannot be perfectly educated and well behaved from day one.

For example, puppies explore the world by taking random objects in their mouth, chewing on them and sometimes even ingesting them. A puppy will not initially discriminate between objects and toys. This chewing behaviour is nonetheless part of normal behavioural development, but problems can arise, including:

- Health problems when the puppy ingests harmful items (sharp objects, toxic plants or substances, irritating liquids)
- Dissatisfaction in the owner when the puppy chews a valuable object (mobile phone, tablet, clothes/shoes).

Action points:

- Avoid situations where puppies can perform unwanted behaviour.
- Plan ahead, prepare the environment and make it puppy-proof.
- Use appropriate tools (puppy safety gates, puppy kennels).
- Teach owners the correct way to introduce these tools (associate with something rewarding).

2. Positive reinforcement

Reinforcing desirable behaviours is a puppy-friendly way to learn, and will increase the odds that they happen. In addition to the minimum set of skills, there are others that may be useful and many of these can be taught during puppy classes: coming when called (recall), going to a dog bed or crate when requested, performing behaviours such as sitting or lying down on cue, loose lead walking, greeting humans and dogs on walks, getting along with other dogs, going on car journeys, going to the vet, and anything else that is physically possible for the puppy and that the owner requires. The rationale for using positive reinforcement should be clarified to the owner along with an explanation about how it should be applied (see Figure 12.10). In addition, a reinforcing stimulus can be primary (inherently rewarding, such as food or play) or secondary (associated with a primary stimulus such as a clicker).

Action points:

- List desirable behaviours according to the owner's viewpoint. Some behaviours owners will readily list, such as "we want him to be housetrained" and "we want him to greet people in a friendly way". Other behaviours are taken for granted by the owner and may not be mentioned, such as "lying quietly on his bed" or "playing with his own toys".
- Avoid the pitfall of wording such as "we want him to stop jumping", as reinforcement is not about stopping, but encouraging behaviour.
- Explain the importance of timing. Reinforcing the action needs to be done immediately and before the puppy engages in a new action (or shows the intention to).
- Explain the importance of being consistent. A puppy will learn faster if the desired behaviour is initially followed by a reward every time.
- A reward is not necessarily what humans find rewarding – it is something that the puppy finds worthwhile at that moment. The value of the reward can change: the perception of a treat may be different in terms of quantity (being hungry or not), quality (bread *versus* chicken) and variation (always the same treat may reduce motivation).
- Some behaviours may be self-rewarding for the puppy, such as chewing, destructive behaviour, digging or barking. Preventing eliciting situations is important (see above). In addition, when observing such behaviours, consider that they may be coping mechanisms due to the lack of environmental stimulation.

3. Why, how and what to ignore
Ignoring unwanted puppy behaviour may be tough for owners. Good preventive behavioural practice requires that the veterinary team explains why ignoring certain behaviours is important, *how* to do it, and *what* situations can or cannot be ignored.

Action points:

- *Why.* Puppies learn by trial and error. The puppy may feel rewarded for actions that trigger a response. When an owner tells a puppy off (e.g. "stop doing that"), the puppy does not

understand the content of what is being said (Horowitz, 2009). Instead it may experience the 'talking to' as rewarding attention and not as a punishment.
- *How.* To ignore a puppy's undesirable behaviour means continuing to do what you were doing and not performing any action related to the puppy's behaviour. Interaction with the puppy (talking to, looking at, touching, moving towards) must be avoided. Leaving the room to give the puppy a 'time-out' is not the same as ignoring the puppy's behaviour.
- *What can be ignored.* Ignoring a puppy's behaviour should be limited to those behaviours that are harmless for the puppy and the environment. For example, stealing a towel or a newspaper are actions that might be better ignored to avoid the risk of inadvertently rewarding the stealing behaviour. Preventing eliciting situations (see above) is also important.
- *What cannot be ignored.* Other actions cannot be ignored and require immediate intervention (interrupt the puppy and remove it from the situation), including:
  - Actions that may be harmful to the puppy's health (e.g. swallowing a handkerchief or chewing sharp, toxic or hazardous objects)
  - Painful or potentially harmful actions towards humans or other animals (e.g. biting a person or clothes).

4. Anticipate and redirect unwanted behaviour
Teach owners to observe their puppy's behaviour and recognize signs of imminent undesirable behaviour. For example, an owner anticipates a puppy taking a towel from a rack because it approaches the towel. It is important to intervene before the puppy actually takes the towel by redirecting the puppy's interest to another target. When owner intervention occurs after the towel has been removed, a puppy can learn that stealing towels (and other objects) is a good way to elicit (rewarding) attention from the owner.

Action points:

- Observe early signs of imminent undesirable behaviour and redirect the puppy's interest.
- Ensure redirecting occurs in a positive and encouraging way.
- Be aware of the fact that dogs are able to differentiate between positive and negative emotional messages. The latter may lead to stress and conflict between the owner and the puppy.

5. Encourage and guide alternative behaviour
Puppy owners often want to stop a particular behaviour. However, *teaching a puppy what not to do is not very useful*, since the dog still does not know what it can do. It is better to focus on teaching the dog desirable behaviours, preferably those that are incompatible with undesirable ones.

Action points:

- *Be patient.* Wait for the puppy to spontaneously perform behaviour that is on the list of desirable

behaviours. For a puppy that jumps up against people while greeting them, the desired behaviour could be standing with all four feet on the floor.
- *Be aware of timing* (see above).
- *Prepare a reward.* Choose a type of reward in advance (primary and/or secondary) and make sure the puppy understands it (the secondary reward has been associated with the primary). When using a secondary reward, always present it before the primary one, not after. For the primary reward, choose something you know will be rewarding and that you can reach quickly.

6. Understand the puppy's perspective
In order for a puppy to function as part of a family, it is not only important that it understands the owner, but also that the owner understands the puppy. Understanding the puppy's perspective means learning how the puppy experiences the world around it and to be aware of dog language (see above). This will help an owner to interpret whether a puppy has understood what is required of it, what a puppy is signalling and how the puppy responds emotionally to certain events (getting upset/stressed, becoming over enthusiastic).

7. Clarify the role of punishment
While punishment is perceived as an acceptable regulator in human society (e.g. not stopping at a red traffic light may result in a fine), in dog training it is rather a loaded term. Dog owners and dog professionals often engage in emotional disputes about the usefulness, or abusiveness, of punishment. When teaching puppy classes it is important to clarify the meaning (see Figure 12.10).

Action points:
- Clarify that punishment is only about *suppressing* behaviour or reducing the chance that the behaviour may be performed in the future. If something does not suppress the behaviour, it is not a true punishment. Instead, it will only be something annoying for the puppy.
- Merely trying to suppress an undesirable behaviour without indicating to the dog what is expected instead does not provide a long-term solution.
- Be aware of *different types of punishment.*
- The use of *physical punishment* needs to be restricted to emergency situations. There are too many welfare risks involved when applying it.
- *Negative punishment techniques can be very useful* (be aware of pitfalls), whereas positive punishment has many risks (see Figure 12.10).
- Try to avoid being judgemental when owners speak of punishment. Instead, try to listen critically – analyse and reflect what they are telling you in terms of learning principles.

Frequently asked questions

Q: Are puppies sensitive to stress?
A: Recent research indicates that the Stress Hypo Responsive Period (SHRP) ends at 4 weeks of age, and that from the age of 5 weeks the impact of behavioural and emotional responses to external stressors needs to be taken into account in puppies (Nagasawa *et al.*, 2013).

Q: At what age should puppies attend socialization classes?
A: Healthy puppies can start socialization classes 1 week after their primary vaccination as the benefits of early socialization on reducing behavioural problems outweighs the risk of infection in most cases.

Q: When should socialization start?
A: Socialization in the broad sense of social contact with conspecifics (littermates and the dam) or humans, starts at the breeder's facility right after birth. Even when the puppy still has closed eyes and ear canals, the olfactory and tactile perception is functional and will influence brain development. When referring to real social interaction, this starts between week 2 and week 3 after birth when the eyes and ear canals open, so the early experiences at the breeder's premises are very important. According to Howell and Bennett (2011), breeders would benefit from starting to exercise puppies as young as 3 weeks of age. Breeders can also help with environmental learning by habituating puppies to different environmental stimuli (smells, surfaces, materials, human social contact).

Q: What skills and knowledge should a puppy class instructor possess?
A: The UK Animal Behaviour Training Council (ABTC) published a set of standards in 2012 listing the knowledge and skills required for different types of animal behaviour and training professionals (www.abtcouncil.org.uk), including for people who teach animal (puppy) training classes.

Q: What are the key learning principles a puppy class instructor should know?
A: An overview is provided in Figure 12.10. (For more detailed information, the reader is referred to the *BSAVA Manual of Canine and Feline Behavioural Medicine.*)

Q: What clinical signs should be screened for in a puppy socialization class and what action(s) should be taken?
A: An overview is provided in Figure 12.11.

Q: What is the problem with the use of aversive training methods to stop problem behaviour?
A: When looking at problem behaviours frequently encountered in puppies, such as chewing household objects or stealing objects/food, 78% and 83%, respectively, of dog owners in a UK-based study mentioned using techniques based on physical or verbal punishment to stop the behaviour (Hiby *et al.*, 2004). In addition, results showed that the use of training methods based on physical punishment were correlated with a higher incidence of problem behaviours. Problem behaviours need to be considered as a welfare issue for the animal, as they may result in relinquishment or euthanasia of the dog at some point in life.

Non-associative learning

Habituation

Repeated or prolonged exposure to a non-harmful stimulus (or set of stimuli) that results in cessation or decrease in the response to the stimulus (Meunier, 2006)

Benefits of the technique:

- Very important in puppy training and education
- Recommended for normal attenuation of a response to something novel in the environment
- Easy technique (does not require timing and consistency)
- Requires frequent exposure to mild stimuli in multiple contexts (below the threshold of arousal)

Examples:

- Surfaces – a puppy is exploring a novel surface (e.g. grass in the garden). After a short while, the brain will habituate and the surface becomes a stimulus without meaning
- Household noises – a puppy habituates to everyday mild household sounds (washing machine, refrigerator, radio) and they soon become background noises
- Objects – an item introduced to the house (e.g. large plant) will be novel in the beginning, but after a short while the object in this context will be ignored
- Social cues – a puppy habituates to the movement of the owner and this becomes background information

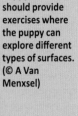

Puppy classes should provide exercises where the puppy can explore different types of surfaces. (© A Van Menxsel)

Risks of the technique:

- Habituation is context-specific
  - A change in the stimulus or environment in which it is presented may undo the process. Example: moving a large plant from the living room to the kitchen may require another period of habituation
- Habituation requires frequent exposure to mild stimuli
  - When stimuli are presented above the threshold for arousal/stress, the brain may not be able to attenuate the importance of the stimulus. Example: an owner is walking the puppy down the street, when a passing truck makes a sudden and loud noise. The puppy is startled and reacts with a fear response. This experience will not be helpful to habituate the puppy to the sound of trucks as the noise was above the puppy's threshold for stress
- When stimuli are presented above the threshold for stress, sensitization may occur
  - Example: a puppy that reacts with a fear response to the loud noise of a truck may respond more fearfully with repeated exposure to truck noise, and may even start responding fearfully to milder noises such as cars
- Associative learning may still occur
  - In the long-term, habituation may induce a conditioning process whereby a puppy comes to expect certain stimuli in specific contexts. Example: a puppy is habituated to the owner moving around the kitchen. In the long-term, the puppy may learn that at a specific time of day, the movement of the owner (e.g. towards the refrigerator) has a pleasant outcome (e.g. opening the refrigerator and preparing the puppy's meal). In this instance, habituating to the owner's movement may be replaced by associative learning (expecting food)

Flooding

Flooding involves prolonged exposure to a worrisome stimulus that provokes a response. The aim of flooding is that, with exposure, the puppy will stop reacting to the stimulus.

- Flooding techniques represent a welfare issue and should **never** be used in puppy training. The inability to escape (whether from a cage or a stimulus that the puppy views as fearful) can cripple the animal behaviourally for life because they experience a condition called learned helplessness (Overall, 2013)
- Example: a puppy that has been living in a kennel environment for 5 months behaves extremely fearfully towards all outside stimuli. Once adopted, the owners try to help the puppy by taking it for a walk in a busy street and sitting down on a bench for a few hours. Although the owner's intention is for the puppy to get used (habituate) to the noise and movement, it is unavoidable that the overload of stimuli at high intensity (vehicles and people) terrifies the puppy and the flooding will lead to a state of learned helplessness

Associative learning

Classical conditioning

Pairing of two stimuli. Usually it is a neutral stimulus that is timely and consistently followed by a meaningful stimulus. As a result, the neutral stimulus acquires the same meaning and becomes a 'conditioned' stimulus (Pavlov, 2003)

Benefits of the technique:

- Very important in puppy education and training
- Acquisition of associations is a passive process for the puppy (no action is required)
  - Example: a leash originally has no meaning for a puppy. In this case attaching the leash is followed each time by 'going out for a walk'. The original neutral stimulus (the leash) becomes the predictor of 'expecting a walk'
- Strong and lasting associations are made. Once classical conditioning is installed, extinction is difficult and eradication of the association is impossible
- Emotions can be conditioned along with the stimuli
  - On its first visit to the veterinary practice, the puppy is placed on the examination table and given treats. Consequently, the examination table will become associated with a pleasant emotion (i.e. the anticipation of food). Note: The effect of the examination table being conditioned to something pleasant will also have a protective effect towards a third (potentially unpleasant) stimulus. When the vet gives the puppy on the examination table an injection (unpleasant), the chance that the puppy now associates the table with something unpleasant is much less likely

Risks of the technique:

- Long lasting and strong associations. Humans may accidentally create associations or chains of associations that are undesirable
  - Example: the owner uses a can opener to open the puppy's canned food. Every time the puppy hears the owner enter the kitchen, open the cupboard and take out the can opener, the puppy expects the owner to prepare its food; the puppy gets aroused and starts salivating
- Unpleasant emotions can be conditioned along with the stimuli
  - When specific stimuli are followed by a significant unpleasant event and/or stress, they can become associated with an unpleasant emotional reaction. Therefore, it is crucial to look at the puppy's threshold for arousal and/or stress and evaluate learning from the puppy's perspective. Example: the sound of the doorbell predicts the entering of visitors. A puppy that feels stressed when visitors enter the home will soon become stressed at the sound of the doorbell (as this predicts the sight of visitors)

12.10 Review of non-associative and associative learning techniques. (continues) ▶

Associative learning continued

Operant conditioning
The puppy learns that there is a certain consequence to its behaviour (Skinner, 1951). When the puppy experiences the outcome as pleasant ('reward' or 'reinforcement'), the behaviour is more likely to occur in the future. When the puppy experiences the outcome as unpleasant ('punishment'), the behaviour is less likely to occur (Thorndike, 1927). There are different forms of reinforcement and punishment:

- Positive reinforcement (or R+)
- Negative reinforcement (or R−)
- Positive punishment (or P+)
- Negative punishment (or P−)

Positive reinforcement (R+ = adding something pleasant)
The behaviour results in something pleasant being added from the puppy's perspective (pleasant outcome)

Benefits of the technique:

- **Very important tool** in puppy training and education
- Proven positive effect on welfare when applied correctly. Enhances the relationship between the puppy and the owner (focuses on desired behaviour)
- Focuses on desired behaviour. Teaching the puppy 'what to do' instead of 'what not to do'
- Owners learn to observe behaviour and assess the motivation of the puppy (i.e. the likelihood of the desired behaviour occurring)
- No risk of the owner doing anything unpleasant that the puppy might associate with the owner rather than its own behaviour

Examples:

- Learning to sit and wait at the door – a puppy is outside and only when it is sitting quietly and relaxed at the door does the owner open it. The puppy has now learned that the behaviour (sitting at the door) has a positive outcome (the door opens)
- Playing with dog toys – when the puppy takes its toy and starts chewing it, the owner pays attention to the puppy and praises it. The puppy learns that chewing its toys has a positive outcome. In combination with prevention (see text), puppies can be easily taught to increasingly chew on their own toys instead of the owner's objects or furniture

Risks of the technique:

- Owners need to think about and focus on desired (rather than undesired) behaviours
- Implementation of positive reinforcement requires skill and practice in order for the owner to perform this correctly (timing and being consistent). Lack of timing and consistency may induce frustration in puppies
- Unwanted behaviour may be unintentionally reinforced (by the owner or in the owner's absence)
  - Example: chewing on inappropriate objects – a puppy plays with its toys but nobody is paying attention. However, as soon as the puppy starts chewing on the owner's shoe, the owner reacts, talks to the puppy and tries to recover the shoe. From the puppy's point of view, stealing and chewing a shoe has a favourable outcome and such behaviour is likely to occur more often
  - Learning to scratch at the door – a puppy is outside and wants to come indoors. It paws at the kitchen door. Because the owner is worried about damage to the door, it is opened for the puppy to enter. From the puppy's point of view, scratching at the door had a favourable outcome and it is likely the puppy will repeat this behaviour when wanting to come inside
- If the puppy's threshold for arousal is exceeded, then it may not be able to perform the desired behaviour (and using positive reinforcement may not be possible)
  - Example: a puppy reacts with arousal when watching a cat and starts a pursuit. As watching the cat induces a state of arousal in the puppy, the chances that the puppy will perform a calm behaviour that can be reinforced are low. In these cases, the owners often fall into the trap of performing positive punishment (shouting, reprimanding the puppy). The key is to prevent the situation from happening in the first place (see text)

Negative reinforcement (R− = removing something unpleasant)
The behaviour results in something unpleasant being taken away (pleasant consequence)

Benefits of the technique:

- Easy technique to perform, at least from a human perspective
- Can be useful in rare cases during puppy upbringing, providing the unpleasant stimulus is mild and not perceived by the puppy as painful/harmful or fear-/anxiety-inducing
  - Example: learning to walk on a loose lead – an owner is walking a puppy and the puppy has reached the end of the leash. The moment the puppy wants to walk further away, the owner stops (resulting in more tension on the leash). As soon as the puppy stops pulling, the owner starts walking again. Note: This type of exercise can only be performed with puppies that have a normal threshold of arousal/frustration and have already learned a range of strategies to 'solve' these situations

Risks of the technique:

- **Not a good instrument** in puppy training and education
- Difficult to carry out without stressing the puppy
- Negative reinforcement has to be used with caution, as taking away something unpleasant means that something pleasant was administered previously. Examples that should be considered harmful include:
  - Learning to sit – an owner wants to make a standing puppy sit and pushes on the hindquarters. When the puppy sits, the pressure on the hindquarters is removed
  - Learning to lie down – an owner wants a puppy to lie down and therefore places their foot on the leash (putting tension on the puppy's neck). Once the puppy lies down, the foot is removed from the leash

Positive punishment (P+ = adding something unpleasant)
The behaviour results in something unpleasant for the puppy (unpleasant outcome)

Benefits of the technique:

- Can be effective in an emergency situation or for self-preservation
  - Emergency situation – a puppy is walking on the pavement and jumps towards the street where a motorbike is approaching. The owner pulls the lead with a firm jerk, preventing the animal from being hit by the vehicle. Similar situations are conceivable where an owner provides an unpleasant action (shouting, grabbing, pulling, pushing) in situations associated with danger around stairs, windows or swimming pools, or in situations with children. It is important to note that none of these represents a training situation, all are emergency situations
  - Self-preservation – a puppy spots a hedgehog and tries to bite it, but biting the hedgehog results in painful contact with the spikes and the puppy no longer bites the hedgehog. In future encounters, the puppy may have learned to avoid hedgehogs

12.10 (continued) Review of non-associative and associative learning techniques. (continues) ▶

Associative learning continued

Risks of the technique:

- **Not a good instrument** in puppy training and education
- It is difficult to apply correctly and without causing harm to the puppy. There is evidence of inducing fear, anxiety and an elevated risk of aggression towards the owners (Herron *et al.*, 2008). Teaching a puppy what it cannot do also does not help it understand what it should do
- Applying positive punishment (particularly with aversive stimuli) in training is likely to induce reduced interactivity during play and lower levels of interaction with new people (Rooney and Cowen, 2011)
- The puppy may associate the unpleasant stimulus with the person applying it (owner) or the context in which it is administered.
  - Example: making wrong associations – each time the owner sits on the sofa, the puppy approaches, jumps on their knees and bites their clothing, all with the intention to play. The owner reacts by pushing the puppy away, while telling them off ("no, stop doing it"). For this puppy, the situation (approaching the owner on the sofa) will become associated with an unpleasant outcome (negative message and being pushed away). Because a puppy cannot understand the reason when humans respond unpleasantly to playful interaction, it may not know how to solve the situation, and instead become frustrated and bark
  - Example: learning the wrong skills – an owner is walking the puppy on a leash. When they meet another dog, the puppy starts pulling towards the dog (out of curiosity and desire to play). The owner responds by giving a firm jerk on the leash. The puppy has now learned that the sight of a dog approaching is associated with something unpleasant happening. In the future, the puppy might anticipate and start barking when it sees a dog while on the leash
- There is a risk that the puppy links the aversive stimulus with a different behaviour than the owner had in mind
  - Example: avoidance conditioning – a 5-month-old puppy while in the garden was barking incessantly at passers-by, and the owners were advised to use an electric shock collar whenever it barked. Instead of associating the shocks with its own barking, the puppy quickly learned that the sight of people passing by was linked to an unpleasant outcome (the shock). Consequently, the sight of people will induce a strong emotional response in the puppy's brain, enhancing strategies to cope with fear, such as flight (trying to get away) or fight (aggressive response aimed at chasing away the threat). In both scenarios, the puppy's welfare will be compromised
- Positive punishment is no long-term solution for situations in which undesirable behaviour occurs. Prevention is the key (see text)

Negative punishment (P- = removing something pleasant)
The behaviour is followed by something pleasant being taken away (unpleasant consequence)

Benefits of the technique:

- **Very important tool** in puppy training and education
- In contrast to positive punishment, there are less risks for harmful consequences for the puppy. Less risk for damage to the relationship between the owner and the puppy
- Constructive method to use in puppies with normal thresholds of arousal. Can be combined with positive reinforcement once the puppy shows a desired behaviour
  - Example: puppy education – a puppy is playing with its owner and gets a bit excited: it jumps and starts nipping clothes. Because the owner does not want the puppy to become overexcited, they end the play session by stopping all movements and releasing the play objects. By depriving the puppy of pleasant things (i.e. interaction with the owner), the excited behaviour is 'punished' and the puppy stops jumping, barking and nipping

Risks of the technique:

- It takes skill for owners to see whether they are taking away something pleasant or accidentally applying something unpleasant (e.g. putting the puppy in another room, away from people)
- There is a risk of frustration when the puppy cannot obtain success or when the objectives of the owner are too difficult for the puppy
  - Example: frustration – particularly in puppies with a very low threshold for frustration, in a play setting (as described above), the moment the owner stops the interaction and lets go of the toys, the puppy tends to get frustrated and more aroused. Such puppies will increasingly growl, bite and snap at the owner. (Frustration is a status that may arise when the puppy's expectation and what is really happening are perceived to be too far away from one another)
  - Example: stress and conflict – an owner wants to teach a puppy to only start eating on cue, after the bowl has been placed on the floor. To train this, each time the owner puts down the food bowl and the puppy approaches, the owner withdraws the food bowl. However, as the puppy is not aware of the owner's intentions, it just learns that the outcome of being presented with a food bowl results in a stressful situation. If the owner expresses negative emotion when the puppy does it 'wrong', feeding will now also equal conflict. At this point the puppy may start presenting conflict avoidance behaviours (see text)
- Relies on extinction of behaviour and can, in some cases, initially lead to an increase in the undesired behaviour due to frustration. Owners may not be able to persist with negative reinforcement and instead begin to intermittently reward the behaviour or even use positive punishment

12.10   (continued) Review of non-associative and associative learning techniques.

Social/non-social environmental stimuli above the puppy's threshold for arousal (can be pleasant)	Clinical signs that may be observed
Physiological signs of arousal	Dilated pupils, panting, increased motor actions
Behavioural signs of arousal	Excitement, jumping, pulling, chewing, scratching, biting
Social/non-social environmental stimuli above the puppy's threshold for stress	**Clinical signs that may be observed**
Physiological signs of an acute stress response	Dilated pupils, panting, salivating, trembling, urinating, defecating, stopping eating
Behavioural signs of an acute stress response	Loud noises and new/moving objects – freezing, sitting, laying down, trying to get away, panic Social conflict – lip licking, pawing, turning body away, lying down, trying to leave, restlessness Escalation of social conflict – barking, biting, growling, lunging, staring, bearing teeth

Immediate actions

- Stop the exercise and examine what is happening
- Depending on the intensity, duration and frequency of the behaviour, ignore the behaviour or stop lesson and give the puppy a break
- Adapt solution according to the core problem (was the exercise above the threshold? Or is it a fearful puppy with a lowered threshold?)
- In the case of a noise context, instantly remove the puppy from the situation and provide a quiet environment where the puppy is able to calm down
- In all cases where the puppy is not immediately recovering and presenting functional behaviour, it should be seen by a veterinary surgeon for a clinical and behavioural health check

12.11   Clinical signs that may be observed with social/non-social environmental stimuli above a puppy's physiological threshold for arousal and stress.

A clinical approach to behaviour problems

Dealing with behaviour cases is comparable to dealing with veterinary internal medicine, in that the dogs are presented with signs observed by the owner that do not necessarily present during the clinical examination: a coughing dog might cough, but a vomiting dog will not necessarily vomit in the surgery. As with other conditions, to interpret behavioural signs in context, owners should be questioned and asked to describe their observations.

Behavioural examination

The consultation for a behavioural problem will take the following course. Often, considerable time is required for a behavioural consultation and it may be necessary to schedule an additional appointment to allow a full investigation.

1. The complaint

This is essentially the signs displayed – as perceived by the owner. Owners should be encouraged to describe the behavioural signs but it is important to distinguish these from an owner's interpretation of them (e.g. "We think he is jealous"). Open questions (see Chapter 2) should be used to guide the conversation: What happened? With whom? What happened next? How did you solve it?

At this stage of the consultation it may be appropriate to screen the information for the degree of emergency or for potential harm to people or pets, e.g. a dog bite might happen again and harm people or other pets. Behaviour problems might be so extreme (e.g. destruction, aggression, house soiling) that they could be a reason for relinquishment or even euthanasia at this stage.

It is important to respond in a client-centred way (e.g. "I understand that you feel upset about Bono destroying the new sofa, and our team is happy to help you solve Bono's problem"). Communication techniques such as rephrasing, emphatic listening and summarizing might be helpful (Cornell and Kopcha, 2007; see also Chapter 2).

2. History-taking

Open-ended questions should be used with the client. It is important to investigate the incidence, frequency, extent and evolution of the problem signs over time, together with details of how the owners have reacted and what therapeutic steps have already been tried. An example of a canine behaviour questionnaire can be found at the end of the chapter.

It can be helpful to draw a timeline (letting the owner participate), using colours when necessary to indicate problem-free periods (green) and problem situations (red) (Figure 12.12).

3. Observation

It is of critical importance to spend time observing the dog, both for the signs it displays and also to see its interaction with its owner.

- What behaviour triggers a response from the owner?
  - Dog being relaxed and calm (owner is reinforcing relaxed behaviour).
  - Dog showing signs of arousal (e.g. jumping up, pacing; owner is reinforcing arousal/excitement).
- How does the owner respond?
  - Does the owner respond verbally or with physical restraint?
  - Is the owner's response calm or angry?
  - Is the response consistent with what the owner described during the history-taking process?

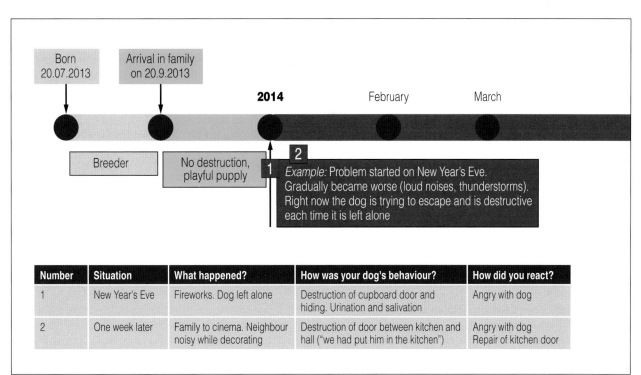

12.12 A timeline can be helpful. In this example, green periods are problem-free and red indicates when problems occurred. The problem contexts are explored.

The context is important, as behaviour is context-dependent: a dog behaving calmly in the clinic might behave differently at home or on walks. **Never rely on behaviour observed in only one context.** It can be useful to observe the dog–owner interaction in the home setting. If a home visit is not possible (or safe), the owner should be asked to provide video footage a few days before an appointment, so that the veterinary team can review it prior to the consultation. Both relaxed and problem situations should be observed, noting the response of the owner (and other family members) in each case and the outcome. Careful note should be taken of how the dog behaves in the owner's absence.

4. Differential diagnosis

It is essential to investigate any potential underlying disease, pain or physical impairment, and to consider the potential side effects of any medication that might produce behavioural signs (e.g. metoclopramide, phenylpropanolamine). It is also helpful to define any underlying motivation (e.g. play, solving conflict, avoiding threat, competition, frustration) and any underlying emotion (positive or pleasant – negative or unpleasant). Factors (pertaining to the dog or its environment) that elicit the behaviour should be differentiated from those that maintain it.

5. Diagnosis

Whereas diagnosing the cause of a physical disease is commonly based on laboratory and clinical evidence, a diagnosis of the cause of a behavioural problem should be considered more as a working hypothesis, to be checked and rechecked. It may be helpful to consider this in terms of functional and contextual diagnosis.

- **Functional diagnosis** relates to the motivation for the behaviour and any underlying emotion.
- **Contextual diagnosis** relates to the factors that elicit and/or maintain the behaviour. These can be:
  - Dog-related (e.g. the dog lacks self-control and reacts to low-level stimuli)
  - Owner-related (e.g. age group, socioeconomic situation)
  - Environmental (e.g. home location, neighbours).

6. Risk assessment

A risk assessment should be performed in every situation where the dog's behaviour may result in harm to people or other animals. The risk assessment investigates the risk a dog may represent within a given context (De Messter *et al.*, 2011).

i.   **Identify the hazards.** Investigate how often, when and where a dog might be exposed to the threatening triggers (sounds, social stimuli, situations). This should include not only an assessment of the animal's physical and behavioural characteristics but also its physical and social environment.

ii. **Decide who might be harmed or at risk and how.** Identify people or other pets that might potentially interact with the dog and, for each of them, identify: contexts (action, time, place, frequency, who will be present); the most likely strategy the dog will adopt; and the likely consequence in terms of injury or trauma.

iii. **Evaluate the risks and decide on precautions.**
   - What are the safety measures necessary to make sure the dog can find safety and comfort and will NOT be exposed to EACH of the risk situations?
   - What is necessary to prevent injury or trauma?
   - What are the options/limitations for implementation of each of the safety measures in the dog's living environment in the short term (human-, dog- and context-related factors).

iv. **Record your findings and implement them.**
   - Write down the findings and proposed safety measures.
   - Check that the clients have fully understood, and determine what further help they may need for implementation.
   - In most cases a safety protocol is part of a behaviour modification therapy (BMT) plan (see later); talk to the client and check how they see the plan (practically, financially and in terms of follow-up).

7. Prognosis

Owners will hope to hear a prediction on future developments. However, this will not be possible at the outset, as the prognosis depends on assessment of all the diagnostic factors (dog, human and environmental) and is influenced by the owner's willingness, compliance and the response to therapy.

8. Treatment options

- **Treat underlying or concomitant physical disease.** Be aware that some conditions (e.g. chronic pain conditions, sensory impairment, cognitive decline) might need a continuous follow-up and communication with colleagues treating that part of the dog's condition.
- **Management.** Provide comfort and safety zones for the dog; suggest immediate measures such that the dog is no longer exposed to threatening stimuli. Make sure management tips are applicable and understood by the owners (explain to owners what to do and how to do it) and refer to a behavioural counsellor when necessary.
- **Cognitive approach.** Owner misconceptions and beliefs must be identified and addressed. This must not be judgemental, as owners may be distressed and react defensively to the ongoing behavioural problem of their dog. It is important to use appropriate communication techniques to put the dog's behavioural condition into the correct context. These techniques can be learned (see Cornell and Kopcha (2007) and Chapter 2).
- **Behaviour modification therapy (BMT).**
  - *Communication* – whilst clients may focus on stopping the dog's unwanted behaviours, it is advisable to investigate thoroughly how far the BMT plan that you have in mind for the dog fits in with the owners expectations in terms of:
    - Type of behavioural improvement (e.g. "we want our dog to be sociable with children of all ages" or "we want our dog to stay home alone for 5 hours a day")

- Owner engagement (e.g. "we would like to solve the noise problem by Christmas, but our working schedule will not allow us to put a lot of effort into rehabilitation training")
- The extent of professional help the owners are willing to accept (e.g. "we are happy to have a rehabilitation trainer helping us" or "we would prefer you to write it down and we will do it ourselves")
- The cost of the therapy
- The duration of the BMT plan (e.g. weeks, months, years).

- **Plan:**
  - Identify comfort zones (increases the dog's perception of predictability and control)
  - Explore the type and number of functional behaviours (e.g. relaxed behaviour)
  - List new behavioural strategies for the dog to achieve in terms of progress
  - Plan how these strategies can be implemented (protocols should be based on learning theory)
  - Check feasibility of the rehabilitation training in terms of the dog's threshold to arousal/stress
  - Check the owner's understanding and skills in relation to the plan
  - Determine whether psychotropic drugs are required (which drug(s), for what purpose, at what dosage and for how long)
  - Recheck and follow up how implementation of the plan can be maximized (owner agreement in terms of training goals and the use of drugs, as well as the role of the owner, the skills they need for implementation of the plan and the engagement required in the short and long term).

- **Psychotropic drugs** – Psychotropic drugs can be used to achieve different goals:
  - Strategic administration – for the treatment of profound anxiety or panic associated with sporadic events
  - Long-term administration – with the aim of influencing reactivity, self-control, emotional responses and cognitive function in order to raise the threshold for arousal and stress, and allow the dog to respond in a more functional manner to adverse stimuli
  - The psychotropic drugs most commonly used include benzodiazepines (diazepam, midazolam, lorazepam and temazepam) for short-term use and antidepressants (tricyclic antidepressants, e.g. clomipramine; selective serotonin reuptake inhibitors, e.g. fluoxetine, fluvoxamine, sertraline; monoamine oxidase inhibitors, e.g. selegiline) for long-term use. For specific indications, administration, side effects and potential risks, see the *BSAVA Small Animal Formulary*
  - Before prescribing a psychoactive substance for a behaviour problem, it is important to consider the following:
    - The medical history and health status of the dog

    - The functional and contextual behaviour diagnosis
    - Is the psychotropic agent authorized for use in dogs? If not, then written informed consent for off-label drug use should be obtained from the owner
    - Evidence-based medicine – what is known about the indications, effects and side effects of the drug from the veterinary literature?
    - How experienced is the veterinary team with using the drug?
    - What are the expected side effects in this patient and how could they affect the dog's welfare?
    - Is the veterinary team aware of any medical contraindications for use of the drug?
    - What psychotropic drugs have been used in this dog previously (relating to the actual problem), when were they used and what were the results?
    - What is the cost of the drug and how does it relate to owner compliance to complete the entire treatment course?
    - How will the owner administer the drug to the dog and who should they contact in the event of problems
    - What is the risk to family members (including children) from accidental/abusive ingestion of this drug.

- **Nutraceuticals:**
  - The use of diets, nutraceuticals and supplements may appeal to clients and be preferred to the use of medicines, as they are felt to affect behaviour in a more 'natural' way
  - Although nutraceuticals offer tremendous promise for favourably influencing behaviours at the molecular level in the brain in a way that may have fewer side effects than traditional psychotropic drugs (Overall, 2013), more research is needed regarding the underlying mechanisms of action (Galan *et al.*, 2014; Dodd *et al.*, 2015)
  - Supplements such as alpha-casozepine and L-theanine have been studied for use in animals with anxiety disorders (Beata *et al.*, 2007; Arauyo *et al.*, 2010)
  - The strongest evidence for the use of nutraceuticals has been shown in age-related brain neurodegenerative changes. Diets enriched with neuroprotectives/antioxidants (Cotman, 2002) or nutraceuticals containing a combination of phosphatidylserine, a standardized extract of Ginkgo biloba, D-alpha-tocopherol and pyridoxine have been shown to be effective in canine cognitive dysfunction syndrome (Osella *et al.*, 2007).

- **Tranquillizers** (e.g. butyrophenones and phenothiazines) are not useful for BMT because they decrease spontaneous activity, resulting in a decreased response to external and social stimuli and thus interfere profoundly with any behaviour modification.

- **Referral to a behaviour specialist.** Modifying dog behaviour requires different skills such as insight (what needs to be changed and why) and theoretical understanding (what is the problem and how can it be changed), as well as practical and professional skills (what methods to apply in order to maximize the animal's comfort and progress). For veterinary practices that offer behavioural services in-house, it may be constructive to collaborate with professional rehabilitation trainers in order to maximize therapy implementation. Whenever the veterinary team feels that the professional skills to achieve these goals are not present in-house, referral to a veterinary behaviour specialist is advised.

The authors are opposed to the use of therapies based on physical punishment (e.g. kicking, hitting, scruff grabbing and shaking) or tools that function as such (e.g. choke chains, citronella collars, electric shock collars and electric fences) as these tools are aimed only at suppressing behavioural signs and fail to address the underlying motivational, emotional and welfare aspects of the problem

The British Small Animal Veterinary Association (BSAVA) recommends against the use of electronic shock collars and other aversive methods for the training and containment of animals. Shocks and other aversive stimuli received during training may not only be acutely stressful, painful and frightening for the animals, but may also produce long-term adverse effects on behavioural and emotional responses

The Association recognizes that all electronic devices that employ shock as a form of punishing or controlling behaviours and other means that rely on aversive stimuli are open to potential abuse and that incorrect use of such training aids has the potential to cause welfare problems

Apart from the potentially detrimental effect on the animal receiving shocks, there is also anecdotal evidence that there is a risk to public safety from the use of shock systems, as they evoke aggression in dogs under certain circumstances

The BSAVA strongly recommends the use of positive reinforcement training methods that could replace those using aversive stimuli

Euthanasia is a valid outcome in cases where treatment options are incompatible with basic welfare issues: i.e. the dog's quality of life cannot be restored, or the safety of people, pets or the environment cannot be ensured (due to risk factors relating to the dog, owners and/or the environment itself)

Clinical approach to some common presentations

The following discussion of presenting signs is arranged in alphabetical order, which does not reflect commonness or severity. The reader is referred to the *BSAVA Manual of Canine and Feline Behavioural Medicine* for further details of the conditions and their management. A range of client handouts is available on a CD that accompanies that Manual and also at www.bsava.com for members of BSAVA.

It is important first to exclude medical problems that might contribute to the problem. For the purposes of this chapter, it is assumed that any underlying medical problems have been addressed

Aggression

Aggression against familiar people or pets

- **Triggers:** There is often a perceived conflict over 'resources' (food, bones (Figure 12.13), toys, objects, resting places, human attention). This perceived threat may be triggered by various interactions:
  - Benign – approaching, walking by, petting, talking, gazing
  - Aversive – pulling, pushing, picking up
  - Aversive painful – inflicting pain.

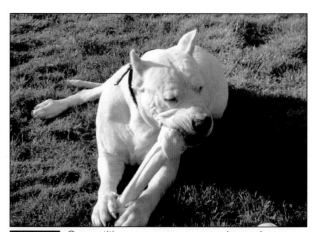

12.13 Competition over resources, such as a bone, can be perceived as a threat and may lead to aggression. (© B Boerner)

- **Features:** Dogs use a number of strategies to avert threat or to solve a conflict; these may be viewed as a ladder of intensity (Figure 12.14). The actual strategy (behaviour) employed will depend on the individual dog, the behaviour of the victim, and the context.
- **Comments:** There is a negative emotion, associated with an unpleasant event and the dog is aroused. Aggression towards familiar people or pets is mostly initiated by an action from the victim (human or pet).
- **Clinical approach and management:**
  - Explore contexts, eliciting trigger(s), outcomes and owner responses. Differentiate contributing factors (Figure 12.15)

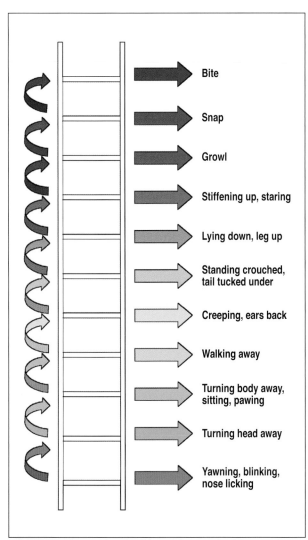

	Bite
	Snap
	Growl
	Stiffening up, staring
	Lying down, leg up
	Standing crouched, tail tucked under
	Creeping, ears back
	Walking away
	Turning body away, sitting, pawing
	Turning head away
	Yawning, blinking, nose licking

12.14 The canine 'Ladder of Aggression': how a dog reacts to stress or threat. It is important to note that dogs may not follow all steps on the ladder in a consecutive manner. The strategies employed depend on the individual animal and the context. (Reproduced from the *BSAVA Manual of Canine and Feline Behavioural Medicine, 2nd edn*)

Types of factors	Examples
Physical problems	Disease Pain Sensory impairment Drugs
Behavioural disturbances	Emotional disorders Reduced threshold of self-control Reduced control of bite response
Genetic predisposition	Cocker Spaniel Bernese Mountain Dog
Early life experience	Sensory deprivation Social deprivation
Training	Use of physical punishment
Human factors	Children (unpredictable behaviour) Owner beliefs Miscommunication
Sociocultural environment	Poor housing conditions Overcrowded housing (people) Other pets

12.15 Factors contributing to aggression in dogs.

- Perform risk assessment. Decide on safety precautions, risk of injury and risk of recurrence
- The primary aim of veterinary intervention should be to prevent aggression occurring.

Aggression against unfamiliar people or pets

- **Triggers:** A perceived threat following mostly benign actions, such as movement (walking, cycling, jogging, approaching; see Figure 12.3) of a social stimulus (people, pets). Dogs may be triggered to react aggressively by subtle cues predicting a potential action from the social stimulus (e.g. gazing, reaching out) before it moves.
- **Features:** The behavioural features depend on the context.
  - In public places this is commonly directed at chasing people or pets, or attacking whilst the person or pet is moving or just passing by.
  - Dogs behind a fence will usually bark or perform threatening postures and attack.
  - Dogs that feel threatened if approached while walking on a lead may use the strategies on the 'ladder of aggression' (see Figure 12.14) and/or immediately bark, launch and attack, as the behavioural response is modified over time (operant learning).
- **Comments:** The negative emotion associated with an unpleasant event is triggered by the appearance of a person or pet. The fact that the dog feels threatened by benign actions, such as people walking, cycling or running, is difficult to understand from the human perspective. This is the typical setting for attacks in public places and may be compounded by predation (Figure 12.16).

Element	Aggression	Play	Predation
Goal	Threat aversion Conflict resolution	Development of social skills No threat; no conflict	Killing prey; feeding No threat; no conflict
Emotion	Negative Unpleasant	Positive Pleasant	Positive Pleasant
Vocalization			
Growling	+++	+++	–
Barking	+/–	+/–	–
Visual signalling			
Play bow	–	+	–
Threatening body postures	+++	–	–
Baring teeth	+++	+++	–
Snapping	+++	+++	–
Staring	+++	+++	+++
Stalking	+/–	+/–	+++
Chasing	+/–	+	+++
Biting	+++	+++	+++

12.16 A comparison of motivation and behaviour associated with aggression, play and predation.

■ **Clinical approach and management:**
  • Explore contexts, eliciting trigger(s) and outcomes
  • Perform a risk assessment. Public safety is paramount
  • It is important that the owner develops the correct attitudes, being able to exert control over the dog without physical force and can understand and implement appropriate safety measures, such as confinement of the dog (garden, lead).

Biting

Bites resulting from aggression

■ **Triggers:** A perceived threat or social conflict.
■ **Features:** Dogs use a range of strategies (see Figure 12.14) to avert threats and solve conflicts. The goal of these behavioural sequences is to deflect the threat and to restore harmony. A bite represents the last resort for a dog that is trying to solve a conflict or avert a threat.
■ **Comments:** When bites are directed toward familiar people after no apparent trigger, or after a benign trigger, it is always important to look for signs of *physical disease* (e.g. abnormalities or reduction in general activity, exploratory behaviour, food and water intake, wakefulness, play or social interaction) as well as signs of *behavioural* problems (e.g. anxiety, social fear, hyperactivity/hyper-reactivity).
■ **Clinical approach and management:**
  • See Aggression, above. Behavioural investigation should include a full behavioural consultation and risk assessment
  • Perform a standard medical investigation. Consider rabies in a dog that has recently travelled abroad
  • When considering biting in puppies, it is essential to differentiate aggression from play biting (see below). Aggression in puppies should always be considered an emergency and necessitates investigation of underlying physical or emotional disorders.

Bites resulting from frustration
Preventing access to motivating stimuli results in a negative emotion and can lead to a bite. Frustration can also arise when using 'negative' punishments, such as the removal of something pleasant.

Bites resulting from play

■ **Triggers:** Arousal and movement.
■ **Features:**
  • Excitement, jumping and snapping
  • No threatening postures.
■ **Comments:** Play biting in puppies is a normal behaviour within the development of social and predatory skills.
■ **Clinical approach and management:**
  • Avoid triggering contexts (movement) and reinforce more controlled play
  • Avoid the pitfall of physical punishment as it will eventually lead to conflicts
  • Play biters that persist and/or cause injury to the owners should be given a behavioural consultation.

Biting linked to predation

■ **Triggers:** Moving potential prey or non-socialized species.
■ **Features:**
  • Chasing, stalking, launching, biting and killing
  • No threatening body postures, growling or baring of teeth
  • The goal of the dog's behaviour is catching and killing prey.
■ **Comments:**
  • Predation stimulates a positive emotion in the dog and there is no threat or conflict involved
  • Selective breeding for specific aspects of predation (e.g. hunting behaviour) may intensify different elements of these responses (e.g. chasing, stalking, rounding up)
  • Be aware of the differences between dogs that chase potential prey (predation) and dogs that chase people or animals in the context of a perceived threat (aggression).
■ **Clinical approach and management:**
  • Lifelong safety measures – there is no curative BMT
  • Prevention is the key (i.e. socializing dogs with different species; Figure 12.17).

Redirected biting

■ **Triggers:** Physical restraint or control in a highly aroused or excited dog.

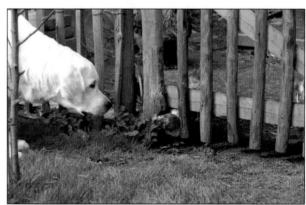
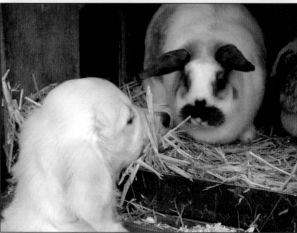

12.17 Early exposure to prey species helps to prevent predatory behaviour later in life and may even encourage social behaviour toward these individuals. (Courtesy of H Blancke and reproduced from the *BSAVA Manual of Canine and Feline Behavioural Medicine, 2nd edn*)

- **Features:**
  - Impulsive bite
  - No warning signals
  - The target is usually the hand or leg that performs the restraining action.
- **Comments:** Always obtain a full behavioural history to differentiate between dogs with problems of self-control, dogs with lowered thresholds for arousal and bite control problems, and dogs suffering from hyperactivity/compulsive disorders.
- **Clinical approach and management:**
  - Clarify the risks of inappropriate physical restraint when the dog is aroused
  - Address the underlying behavioural problem and determine risk contexts
  - Implement management and owner education.

Compulsive behaviours

Compulsive behaviours include:

- Locomotion – spinning, tail chasing, pacing, jumping in place, digging and scratching
- Oral – self-licking, self-chewing and flank sucking
- Vocalization – repetitive barking, whining and howling
- Hallucinatory – shadow chasing and fly snapping
- Aggressive – self-directed growling, biting and attacking.

The following breed predispositions have been noted:

- Dobermann – flank sucking
- English Bull Terrier – spinning in circles, sticking head between objects and freezing
- Staffordshire Bull Terrier – spinning in circles
- German Shepherd Dog – tail chasing
- Australian Cattle Dog – tail chasing
- Miniature Schnauzer – checking hind end
- Border Collie – shadow chasing
- Large-breed dogs – persistent licking.

Causes may be behavioural or medical:

- Normal behaviour in acute conflict/frustration – the behaviour is shown in situations with motivational conflict or resulting from frustration, or another situation in which a dog does not have an appropriate response for reducing arousal
- Attention-seeking – owner attention may condition normal conflict behaviours or reinforce existing compulsive behaviours
- Medical disorder – central nervous system (CNS) disease, skin disease, degenerative disease, toxin exposure or trauma.

Coprophagia

Puppy behaviour

- **Triggers:** Often simply a puppy picking up faeces amongst other objects and chewing on it or ingesting it.
- **Features:**
  - Puppy exploring its environment and picking up objects (faeces)
  - Owner may be present or absent.

- **Comments:**
  - Normal exploratory behaviour in puppies, but generally considered repulsive to owners
  - Some dogs may develop a dietary preference for faeces and may find ingestion of animal faeces rewarding due to smell, flavour and texture (frozen in winter).
- **Clinical approach and management:**
  - Exclude underlying disease or anomaly (e.g. hydrocephalus)
  - Control defecation setting (supervise puppy when toileting)
  - Reinforce acceptable behaviours (retrieving treats instead of faeces)
  - Clean up in the absence of the puppy using appropriate cleaning products.

Attention-seeking or learned behaviour

- **Triggers:**
  - Owner presence or intervention
  - Anticipation of owner intervention.
- **Features:**
  - With the owner present, the dog defecates and ingests its faeces; this is followed by a negative response from the owner
  - Or, to avoid a negative reaction, the dog defecates and ingests the faeces immediately, before the owner can respond.
- **Comments:** Dogs may use several behaviours at random while seeking attention from the owner. Dogs will learn from the outcome (operant learning), so faeces-eating can be involuntarily reinforced by owner attention (whether positive or negative) and the dog usually eats faeces in the owner's presence.
- **Clinical approach and management:** Owner education:
  - Clarify the difference between anthropomorphism and the dog's perspective
  - Explain operant learning (how the dog learns from the outcome of the situation)
  - Explain why owner attention reinforces the behaviour (initiating factor) and why it is maintained (positive and negative attention will both reinforce the coprophagia).

As part of a behavioural disorder

- **Triggers:** May have unapparent triggers or can be secondary to anxiety or part of a compulsive disorder.
- **Features:**
  - Dog spends time scavening for faeces instead of exhibiting adaptive behaviour (sniffing, exploring, playing)
  - Owner may be present or absent.
- **Comments:** Absence of normal sniffing, with coprophagia or pica instead, can be a coping strategy to divert stress in hyperactivity, compulsive disorders and emotional disorders.
- **Clinical approach and management:**
  - Inform the owner that coprophagia is a coping mechanism for an underlying behavioural disorder
  - It is important to stress the detrimental effects of physical punishment on the problem
  - Treat the underlying behavioural disorder and use psychotropic drugs when indicated.

Secondary to a medical condition

- **Triggers:**
  - Hunger (polyphagia, malabsorption, exocrine pancreatic insufficiency, inadequate diet)
  - CNS disease.
- **Features:**
  - Dog scavenges for faeces (and/or other abnormal food items – pica)
  - Owner may be present or absent.
- **Comments:**
  - Polyphagia can be iatrogenic (e.g. corticosteroid therapy, over-supplementation of thyroxine)
  - In senior pets always consider canine cognitive function.
- **Clinical approach and management:** Treat the underlying medical condition.

Destructive behaviour

Puppy behaviour

- **Triggers:** Normal puppy behaviour (puppies have a high propensity to chew on anything they find).
- **Features:** Exploring, chewing on objects (sometimes ingesting).
- **Comments:** An active under-stimulated puppy is more likely to destroy objects and furniture.
- **Clinical approach and management:** Prevention is key! Provide environmental diversity, mental and physical stimulation and a safe environment with appropriate objects to chew on. Pay special attention to puppies from working breeds.

Attention-seeking or learned behaviour
See Coprophagia: attention-seeking behaviour, above.

As part of a behavioural disorder

- **Triggers:**
  - There is often a specific external trigger, such as a sound or visual or social stimulus
  - The stimulus may occur in the presence or absence of the owner.
- **Features:**
  - Chaotic destruction, selection of objects, only destroying doors and windows blocking the way out
  - May occur with owner present or absent
  - Video monitoring is crucial for differentiating types of activity and stimuli.
- **Comments:** The type of destruction will reflect the underlying motivation/emotion. For example:
  - Points of egress, small items: sound sensitivity
  - Objects in reach, random, chaotic: self-control problems (Figure 12.18a)
  - Selective to chaotic destruction when owner absent: separation-related behaviour (Figure 12.18b)
  - Near point of exposure to moving social stimuli: perception of unsolvable stress/threat (territorial behaviour).
- **Clinical approach and management:**
  - Avoid eliciting triggers
  - Treat any underlying behavioural disorder and provide comfort zones
  - Consider BMT
  - Use psychotropic drugs when indicated.

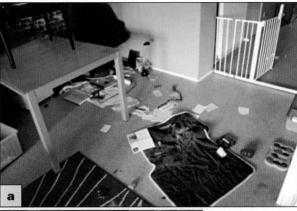

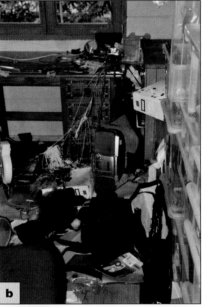

12.18 Separation-related destruction related to **(a)** self-control problems and **(b)** separation anxiety. With self-control problems, destruction may start with object-related play or with gathering of objects and then destroying them. In these cases destruction can be seen as the result of high arousal and motoric activity. With separation anxiety, the destruction is chaotic and random, and is often accompanied by physiological signs of stress (salivation, urination and defecation). (a, © G Pyka; b, © A Vergauwen)

Digging

Normal behaviour

- **Triggers:**
  - Lack of appropriate outlet for exercise
  - Opportunity to dig (soft ground) and the presence of potential prey (such as rats or mice)
  - Some working breeds might dig as part of hunting behaviour (terriers, Dachshunds)
  - Dogs may bury items and dig them up again
  - Inside the home digging may be targeted; for example, at carpets and floors (see Destructive behaviour, above).
- **Features:** Digging in the garden, furniture (e.g. sofa, bed), floors and carpets.
- **Comments:** Normal canine behaviour (Figure 12.19), but may be unacceptable to owners. Normal digging is inherently rewarding! Search for the motivation.
- **Clinical approach and management:** Owner education.

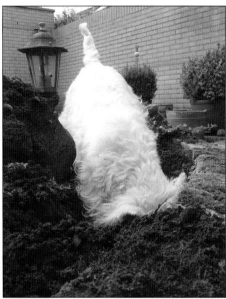

12.19 Digging is normal canine behaviour, but may be unacceptable to the owner. (© J Monsieur)

Attention-seeking or learned behaviour

- **Triggers:** Owner presence at first, but then owner absence in the long term.
- **Features:** Dog is digging and behaviour is reinforced by the owner's response, whether positive or negative.
- **Comments:**
  - Owner intervention will result in increased digging and, eventually, in digging in the owner's absence only
  - Differentiate from dogs that perform digging because they wish to escape or roam.
- **Clinical approach and management:**
  - Address the underlying problem
  - Provide suitable environmental enrichment
  - Educate the owner
  - Physical punishment must be avoided as it may lead to conflict, human-directed aggression and jeopardy of the human–animal bond.

As part of a behavioural disorder

- **Triggers:** May be unapparent or specific (e.g. sound, visual, social stimulus, presence or absence of the owner).
- **Features:** Digging may be an attempt to hide or seek comfort zones, or performed selectively at barriers blocking the exit. Video monitoring is crucial for differentiation.
- **Comments:** The context/place of digging will reflect the underlying motivation/emotion:
  - Aim to escape or to access comfort zone: sound sensitivity
  - Random, chaotic: hyperactivity, self-control problems
  - Search for comfort zone: separation-anxiety.
- **Clinical approach and management:**
  - Avoid eliciting triggers
  - Treat underlying behavioural disorder and provide comfort zones
  - BMT
  - Use of psychotropic drugs when indicated.

Fear of objects, places or people
Fear due to limited experience

- **Triggers:** Unapparent, usually casual benign triggers.
- **Features:** The dog displays acute stress signalling, including withdrawal, avoidance, turning the body away and trying to escape (Figure 12.20). When escape is not possible, other strategies may be used (e.g. aggression, self-directed behaviours and compulsive behaviours).

- Urination and defecation/diarrhoea
- Increased motor activity
- Vocalizations
- Salivation
- Piloerection
- Trembling
- Polypnoea/panting
- Looking away
- Protrusion of the tongue
- Muzzle licking
- Yawning
- Paw lifting (front paw held at 45 degrees)
- Frequent shifting of body position
- Low postures

12.20 Behavioural and somatic signs of acute stress in dogs.

- **Comments:**
  - There may be a genetic predisposition (selective breeding for certain characteristics/abilities)
  - There has often been regular exposure to stimuli during the key developmental period
  - Fearful responses towards people are usually misinterpreted by owners and thought to be linked to a 'traumatic event' (dog has been abused by someone); owner education is the key.
- **Clinical approach and management:**
  - Provide a safe environment for the dog (Figure 12.21)
  - Make use of BMT. Introduce environmental stimuli gradually whilst monitoring, to allow the dog to stay in its comfort zone (a comfort zone is a place where the dog perceives predictability and control over its environment, i.e. a place without threatening stimuli).

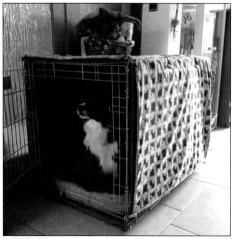

12.21 Comfort zone for a dog presenting with aggression towards unknown people entering the home. Visual protection prevents the dog from seeing visitors entering the home. (© T De Keuster)

Fear due to trauma

- **Triggers:** Often physical trauma and/or loud noises.
- **Features:** Behavioural responses within the normal range that have abruptly changed following the traumatic event.
- **Comments:** Genetic predisposition will determine the emotional response and related emotional reactions (dogs without a genetic predisposition may have no negative consequences following the same trauma).
- **Clinical approach and management:**
  - Provide a safe environment for the dog
  - Make use of BMT
  - Use of psychotropic drugs when indicated.

As part of a behavioural disorder

- **Triggers:** May be unapparent or specific (sound, visual, social stimulus, presence or absence of owner).
- **Features:** Video monitoring is crucial for differentiation.
- **Comments:** Explore the underlying motivation/emotion:
  - Social fear (withdrawal or aggressive response)
  - Sound sensitivity (trying to escape or move into comfort zone)
  - Separation-related (search for comfort zone).
- **Clinical approach and management:**
  - Treatment goals are to make the dog's behaviour functional and will not necessarily lead to normal behaviour
  - Avoid eliciting triggers
  - Treat any underlying behavioural disorder
  - Always provide comfort zones (Figure 12.22)
  - Consider BMT and the use of psychotropic drugs when indicated.

Secondary to a medical condition

- **Triggers:** Any disorder that alters sensory function, stimulus interpretation or behavioural response.
- **Features:** Head down, trembling, backing away, acute stress signalling or active escape behaviours.
- **Comments:**
  - Think of cognitive dysfunction in senior dogs
  - Consider possible drug effects.
- **Clinical approach and management:** Treat the underlying medical condition.

House soiling

Secondary to a medical condition

- **Triggers:**
  - Increased volume
  - Increased frequency
  - Problems influencing control.
- **Features:** Inappropriate urination or defecation.
- **Comments:** Investigate for the underlying medical disorder.
- **Clinical approach and management:** Treat the underlying medical condition.

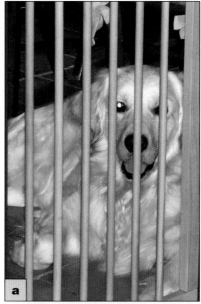

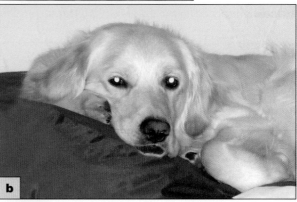

12.22 Treatment options for fear-related behaviour may include: **(a)** providing mechanically protected safe zones, so that the dog has a predictable environment; and **(b)** providing the dog with an area in which to relax. (© A Demunck)

Incomplete housetraining

- **Triggers:**
  - Urge to eliminate
  - Inadequate cleaning after a previous episode
  - There may be a substrate or location preference.
- **Features:** Inappropriate urination or defecation.
- **Comments:**
  - There are often owner misconceptions and physical punishment may exacerbate the problem so that the dog will urinate or defecate only in the owner's absence
  - Some dogs have 'learned' to soil indoors for various reasons (e.g. poor supervision, lack of access to outdoors). Dogs with learned preferences may not eliminate outdoors and show preferential elimination on arrival in the home environment.
- **Clinical approach and management:** Owner education and application of learning principles.

As part of a behavioural disorder

- **Triggers:** There may be unapparent or specific triggers (sound, visual, social stimulus, presence or absence of the owner).

- **Features:** Inappropriate urination/defecation due to various scenarios:
  - Separation-related problems (urination/defecation occurs in the absence of the owner)
  - Hyperactivity (elimination following arousal or a greeting)
  - Sound sensitivity (in the absence of the owner the dog will eliminate following fear-inducing noise stimuli; outdoors the dog may refuse to eliminate in the presence of a fear-inducing noise stimuli)
  - Fear of places (fearful animals may wait rather than eliminate outdoors, and may eliminate in an appeasing environment, often at home – indoors).
- **Comments:** Differential diagnosis is key.
- **Clinical approach and management:**
  - Owner education
  - Treat any underlying behavioural disorder and use psychotropic drugs when indicated.

Urine marking

- **Triggers:**
  - A normal behaviour in canine communication, triggered by odours (urine) or context (vertical objects)
  - May also be stress-related or conflict-related (social stress, either visual or olfactory) and a sign of an underlying behavioural problem.
- **Features:**
  - A small amount of urine on vertical surfaces, novel items or prominent surfaces
  - The classical posture is the cocked leg (male and female dogs after sexual maturity).
- **Comments:** Marking indoors may be considered to be 'naughty' behaviour by owners and may lead to physical punishment.
- **Clinical approach and management:**
  - Owner education
  - Appropriate cleaning of urine indoors
  - Treat any underlying behavioural disorder and use psychotropic drugs when indicated.

Hyperactivity
As learned behaviour

- **Triggers:** Owner's presence.
- **Features:** Dog behaves in a hyperactive way (jumping, panting, vocalizing, destructive behaviour, stealing, inability to be trained or walked) in different contexts but always in the presence of the owner.
- **Comments:**
  - Owners may not be aware of learning principles and may involuntarily reinforce unwanted behaviours in a normally active dog
  - Inexperienced owners may be more prone to bad timing, involuntarily reinforcing wrong behaviours
  - Dogs from selective working breeding lines may be more at risk
  - Over time this may result in conflicts or physical punishment and risk escalation towards aggression.
- **Clinical approach and management:** Owner education.

As part of a behavioural disorder

- **Triggers:**
  - Often unapparent
  - Lack of habituation to normal environmental (social or non-social) stimuli.
- **Features:**
  - Dog appears agitated and unable to settle, displaying signs including jumping, panting, vocalizing, destructive behaviour, coprophagia, stealing and an inability to be trained
  - This may be in the presence or absence of the owner.
- **Comments:**
  - Dogs present with a lack of focus and are easily distracted
  - It is difficult to reinforce desired behaviours.
- **Clinical approach and management:**
  - Differentiate from a normal dog with a lack of physical activity and stimulation, or inexperienced owners reinforcing unacceptable behaviours
  - Be aware of risk of escalation if physical punishment is used. Implement safety management (BMT)
  - The support of psychotropic drugs is indicated.

Redirected behaviour
See Biting, above.

Resource guarding
See Aggression, Biting, above.

Sound sensitivity

> Sensitive breeds may include shepherds, collies and other herding dogs. Certain lines may be considered 'noise-sensitive' or 'noise-stable'

Resulting from a lack of exposure early in life

- **Triggers:** Noise not previously experienced.
- **Features:** Salivation, urination, defecation, destruction, trembling, vocalization, freezing, escape attempts (Figure 12.23), restlessness, scanning and hiding.

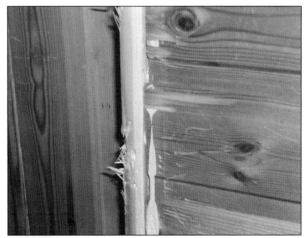

12.23 Destruction of potential escape locations by a dog with separation-related destruction noise sensitivity. (© R Van Hyfte)

- **Comments:** A high variability of signs can occur between individuals.
- **Clinical approach and management:**
  - BMT, taking into account reserved prognosis
  - Aim is for functional behaviour, not necessarily 'perfect' behaviour.

Resulting from sensitization

- **Triggers:** Repeated exposure to noise (e.g. fireworks) (Figure 12.24).
- **Features:** Increasing signs of inability to cope with stimulus.
- **Comments:** May be induced following the misconception that the dog should eventually habituate to the sound when exposed on a regular basis. In reality, the opposite will happen in a noise-sensitive dog – the animal will become sensitized to minimal intensity of the presented noise.

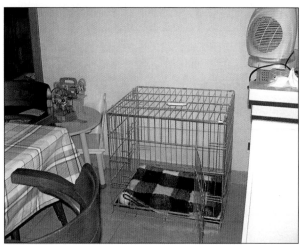

12.24 This location is subject to noise from kitchen appliances, family dining and children playing. Enclosing the noise-sensitive dog in a kennel here triggers vocalization and soiling and represents a welfare problem for the animal. (© R Van Hyfte)

- **Clinical approach and management:**
  - Address the underlying emotional disturbance
  - BMT
  - May need the support of psychotropic drugs.

As a result of a traumatic experience

- **Triggers:** Physical trauma associated with loud noises (e.g. shotgun, heavy thunderstorms).
- **Features:** Behavioural responses were within the normal range, but abruptly changed following the traumatic event.
- **Comments:** Genetic predisposition will determine the emotional response and related emotional reaction. Dogs without a genetic predisposition may have no negative consequences following the same traumatic events.
- **Clinical approach and management:**
  - Provide a safe environment for the dog
  - Use BMT (desensitization and counter-conditioning should be used with care)
  - Provide support of psychotropic drugs when indicated.

Separation-related problems

As part of a medical problem

- **Triggers:** Painful process or CNS disease (i.e. cognitive decline).
- **Features:** Vocalizing, salivating, panting, house soiling, destruction and escape attempts. As these features are signs of emotional arousal and distress (and not necessarily linked to the physical disease itself), the dog may initially present them only in the owner's absence and behave 'normally' when the owner is present. With progressing CNS decline, arousal and distress may become chronic and signs may be present with or without the owner.
- **Comments:** Use of video footage is recommended to investigate behaviour.
- **Clinical approach and management:**
  - Treat the underlying medical condition
  - Provide comfort zones
  - A BMT plan may be indicated in order to create predictable routines and comfort zones for the dog, which reduce stress and improve wellbeing.

As part of a behavioural disorder

- **Triggers:** Varied and may be linked to anxiety of being separated from attachment figure (human/dog). Can also occur in dogs that suffer from different anxiety problems, such as sound (e.g. fireworks, thunderstorms) or visual cues (e.g. humans, other animals or vehicles passing by). These animals might behave in a functional way when the owners are present (due to no exposure or the comfort of owner presence) and in a dysfunctional way when the owner is absent (a dog in a garden or behind a window exposed to visual and auditory cues). Dogs with low arousal thresholds and lack of self-control (hyperactivity) may be presented for 'separation-related problems'. As these dogs might be physically managed and/or reprimanded in the owner's presence, absence of owner control may lead to destruction and vocalization.
- **Features:** Destruction, vocalization, house soiling, self-trauma and licking behaviours when separated from the owner.
- **Comments:** Destructive behaviour, soiling and vocalization reflect the underlying motivation/emotion:
  - Destruction of points of egress and small items – sound sensitivity
  - Destruction of objects at reach, at random and chaotic – hyperactivity
  - Problems only in the absence of an attachment figure (human/animal) – separation anxiety
  - Target is near point of exposure to social stimuli – territorial
  - Video monitoring is crucial to differentiate the type of destruction and behaviour.
- **Clinical approach and management:**
  - Avoid eliciting triggers and/or contexts
  - Treat any underlying behavioural disorder and provide comfort zones
  - BMT
  - Use psychotropic drugs when indicated
  - Barking.

Normal behaviour linked to arousal

- **Triggers:** Visual or auditory external stimulus.
- **Features:** Barking can be seen as a normal response in a context of arousal, excitement, distress or threat.
- **Comments:**
  - Positive or negative emotion possible. The emotional state is not always easy to distinguish from the owner's description and use of video is recommended
  - Dogs will learn from the outcome of a situation and the owner's reaction (whether verbal or physical) to the dog's barking will intensify the problem (operant learning).
- **Clinical approach and management:** Owner education.

As attention-seeking behaviour

- **Triggers:** Dog wants to be with the owner.
- **Features:** Repetitive high-pitched barking.
- **Comments:** Dogs may use several behaviours at random while seeking attention from the owner.
- **Clinical approach and management:** Owner education.

As sign of hyperactivity

- **Triggers:** Occurs with minimal environmental or social stimuli.
- **Features:** There is high arousal and an excessive vocal and motor/social response to minimal stimuli.
- **Comments:**
  - Dog appears agitated and unable to settle
  - Must be differentiated from learned/conditioned hyperactivity (see above).
- **Clinical approach and management:**
  - Treat the underlying behavioural disorder
  - Be aware of the consequences of physical punishment (evolution towards an aggressive response).

While hunting or chasing prey

- **Triggers:** Moving prey.
- **Features:**
  - Positive emotion
  - Chasing and stalking.
- **Comments:**
  - High state of arousal
  - Positive emotion
  - Desired behaviour in hunting breeds – bark when they locate prey but do not proceed to eating it.
- **Clinical approach and management:** No curative treatment. Avoidance is the best strategy (e.g. keep away from prey species and provide alternative exercise).

As a sign of frustration

- **Triggers:** Discordance between the expected outcome of a situation versus reality.
- **Features:**
  - High arousal
  - Repetitive high-pitched bark.

- **Comments:**
  - High arousal, negative emotion
  - Frustration may lead to conflict and aggressive strategies from the animal.
- **Clinical approach and management:**
  - Owner education
  - Avoiding frustrating situations
  - BMT.

As learned behaviour

- **Triggers:** External triggers, visual or auditory.
- **Features:** Barking occurs following external trigger and is involuntarily reinforced by owners, by reacting each time the dog barks.
- **Comments:** Very popular miscommunication, and perhaps the most difficult to treat, as owner intervention often stops the barking in the short term.
- **Clinical approach and management:**
  - Trigger identification (e.g. social, noise, doorbell) and counter-conditioning
  - Provide safe environment from the dog's perspective
  - Owner education.

During play

- **Triggers:** Arousal and movement.
- **Features:**
  - Play bow, play face
  - Other behavioural elements may include growling, biting and jumping.
- **Comments:** Barking may be more common in certain breeds (e.g. herding dogs).
- **Clinical approach and management:**
  - Advise owners to focus on playing games with a lower degree of arousal (e.g. search games or intelligence games)
  - Note that punishment of the aroused dog might induce redirected behaviours of conflict.

As territorial or fear-based behaviour

- **Triggers:**
  - External trigger (exposure to moving stimuli – social (people, pets) or non-social (vehicles))
  - Dogs bred for guarding and territorial behaviours might be presented more often for barking in this context.
- **Features:**
  - Barking is used as a distance-increasing signal (rising frequency and ferocity of bark)
  - Other body signalling may be present (tense body posture).
- **Comments:**
  - The visual or auditory stimulus is perceived as a threat or conflict, resulting in high arousal, negative emotion and distress
  - Owners may not be aware of the dog's emotion and/or motivation for the response. This is especially so in relation to barking in social situations
  - There is no such thing as the standard, and different dogs will react in different ways
  - Social conflicts can arise in the context of resources (competition) or interactions (benign, aversive, painful)

- Other aggressive signalling may be present (see Figure 12.14).
- **Clinical approach and management:**
  - Owner education (conflict solving, threat-averting signalling)
  - Provide a safe environment for the dog (e.g. fencing)
  - Address any underlying behavioural disorder.

As separation-related behaviour

- **Triggers:** Absence of owner or attachment figure.
- **Features:**
  - Negative emotion
  - Vocalization indicating distress (howling, distress barking).
- **Comments:** Differentiate from vocalizing related to sound sensitivity and hyperactivity (video footage may be helpful).
- **Clinical approach and management:**
  - Avoid eliciting triggers and contexts
  - Treat any underlying behavioural disorder
  - Provide comfort zones
  - Use BMT
  - Use psychotropic drugs when indicated.

Reflecting a medical problem

- **Triggers:** Medical condition and an inability to respond appropriately (e.g. pain or cognitive decline).
- **Features:**
  - Besides vocalizing, other signs may be present (e.g. salivating, panting, house soiling, destruction or escape attempts)
  - Older dogs suffering from cognitive decline often display monotonous barking at night, in the owner's absence or in the owner's presence.
- **Comments:** Use of video footage is recommended to investigate further.
- **Clinical approach and management:**
  - Treat the underlying medical condition
  - Provide comfort zones
  - A BMT plan may be indicated.

References and further reading

Araujo J, de Rivera C, Ethier J, Landsberg G, Denenberg S et al. (2010) Anxitane tablets reduce fear of human beings in a laboratory model of anxiety-related behaviour. Journal of Veterinary Behavior 5, 268–275

Beata C, Beaumont-Graff E, Diaz C et al. (2007) Effects of alpha-casozepine (Zylkene) versus selegiline hydrochloride (Selgion, Anipryl) on anxiety disorders in dogs. Journal of Veterinary Behavior 2(5), 175–183

Blackwell EJ, Twells C, Seawright A and Casey RA (2008) The relationship between training methods and the occurrence of behavior problems, as reported by owners, in a population of domestic dogs. Journal of Veterinary Behavior 3, 207–217

Bowen J and Heath S (2005) Behaviour Problems in Small Animals: Practical Advice for the Veterinary Team. Elsevier Saunders, Philadelphia

Bradshaw J, Blackwell E and Casey R (2009) Dominance in domestic dogs: useful construct or bad habit? Journal of Veterinary Behavior 4, 135–144

Burn C (2009) Cognition. In: The Encyclopaedia of Applied Animal Behaviour and Welfare, ed. D Mills et al., pp. 459–462. CABI Publishing International, Oxon

Cornell K and Kopcha M (2007) Client–veterinarian communication: skills for client centered dialogue and shared decision making. Veterinary Clinics of North America: Small Animal Practice 37(1), 37–47

Cotman CW, Head E, Muggenburg BA, Zicker S and Milgram NW (2002) Brain aging in the canine: a diet enriched in antioxidants reduces cognitive dysfunction. Neurobiology of Aging 23, 809–818

De Meester RH, Mills DS, De Keuster T et al. (2011) ESVCE position statement on risk assessment. Journal of Veterinary Behavior 6, 248–249

Dodd FL, Kennedy DO, Riby LM and Haskell-Ramsay CF (2015) A double-blind, placebo-controlled study evaluating the effects of caffeine and L-theanine both alone and in combination on cerebral blood flow, cognition and mood. Psychopharmacology DOI 10.1007/500213-015-3895-0

Dreschel N (2010) The effects of fear and anxiety on health and lifespan in pet dogs. Applied Animal Behaviour Science 125, 157–162

Duxbury MM, Jackson JA, Line SW and Anderson RK (2003) Evaluation of association between retention in the home and attendance at puppy socialization classes. Journal of the American Veterinary Medical Association 223, 61–66

Galan A, Carletti BE, Morgaz J, Granados MM, Mesa I et al. (2014) Comparative study of select biochemical markers in cerebrospinal fluid of healthy dogs before and after treatment with nutraceuticals. Veterinary Clinical Pathology 43(1), 72–77

Gazzano A, Mariti C, Alvares S, Cozzi A, Tognetti R and Sighieri C (2008) The prevention of undesirable behaviors in dogs: effectiveness of veterinary behaviorists' advice given to puppy owners. Journal of Veterinary Behavior 3, 125–133

Herron ME, Shofer FS and Reisner IR (2009) Survey of the use and outcome of confrontational and non-confrontational training methods in client-owned dogs showing undesired behaviors. Applied Animal Behaviour Science 117, 47–54

Hetts S, Heinke ML and Estep DQ (2004) Behavior wellness concepts for general veterinary practice. Journal of the American Veterinary Medicine Association 225, 506–513

Hiby EF, Rooney NJ and Bradshaw JWS (2004) Dog training methods: their use, effectiveness and interaction with behaviour and welfare. Animal Welfare 13, 63–69

Horowitz A (2009) Disambiguating the 'guilty look': salient prompts to a familiar dog behaviour. Behavioural Processes 81, 447–452

Horwitz DF and Mills DS (2009) BSAVA Manual of Canine and Feline Behavioural Medicine, 2nd edn. BSAVA Publications, Gloucester [contains CD of client handouts; these handouts are also available to members of BSAVA at www.bsava.com]

Howell T and Bennett P (2011) Puppy power! Using social cognition research tasks to improve socialization practices for domestic dogs (Canis familiaris). Journal of Veterinary Behavior 6, 195–204

Kaminski J, Schulz L and Tomasello M (2012) How dogs know when communication is intended for them. Developmental Science 15(2), 222–223

Kirchhofer KC, Zimmermann F, Kaminski J and Tomasello M (2012) Dogs (Canis familiaris) but not chimpanzees (Pan troglodytes) understand imperative pointing. PLoS ONE 7(2), doi: 10.1371/journal.pone.0030913

Landsberg G (2005) Therapeutic agents for the treatment of cognitive dysfunction syndrome in senior dogs. Progress in Neuro-Psychopharmacology and Biological Psychiatry 29, 471–479

Levine C and Ambady N (2013) The role of non-verbal behaviour in racial disparities in health care: implications and solutions. Medical Education 47, 867–876

Ligout S (2009) Arousal. In: The Encyclopaedia of Applied Animal Behaviour and Welfare, ed. D Mills et al., p. 36. CABI Publishing International, Oxon

Luescher A, Flannigan G, Frank D and Mertens P (2007) The role and limitations of trainers in behavior treatment and therapy. Journal of Veterinary Behavior 2, 26–27

Marder A and Duxbury MM (2008) Obtaining a pet: realistic expectations. Veterinary Clinics of North America: Small Animal Practice 38, 1145–1162

McBride EA (2009) It's a dog's life – the what and who of training and behavior. In: Proceedings of the CABTSG Study Day

Merola I, Prato-Previde E, Lazzaroni M and Marshall-Pescini S (2014) Dogs' comprehension of referential emotional expressions: familiar people and emotions are easier. Animal Cognition 17, 373–385

Meunier LD (2006) Selection, acclimation, training and preparation of dogs for the research setting. ILAR Journal 47, 326–347

Moberg GP (2000) Biological response to stress: implications for animal welfare. In: The Biology of Animal Stress – Basic Principles and Implications for Animal Welfare, ed. GP Moberg and JA Mench, pp. 1–21. CABI Publishing International, Oxon

Nagasawa M, Shibata N, Yonezawa A, Morita T, Kanai M, Mogi K and Kikusui T (2014) The behavioral and endocrinological development of stress response in dogs. Developmental Psychobiology 56(4), 726–733

Osella MC, Re G, Odore R, Girardi C, Badino P, Barbero R and Bergamasco L (2007) Canine cognitive dysfunction syndrome: prevalence, clinical signs and treatment with a neuroprotective nutraceutical. Applied Animal Behaviour Science 105, 297–310

Overall KL (2013) Manual of Clinical Behavioral Medicine for Dogs and Cats. Elsevier Mosby, Missouri

Pavlov IP (2003) Conditioned Reflexes. Dover Publications Inc., Mineola, NY

Pongrácz P, Molnár C, Dóka A and Miklósi A (2011) Do children understand man's best friend? Classification of dog barks by pre-adolescents and adults. Applied Animal Behaviour Science 135, 95–102

Pongrácz P, Molnár C, Miklósi A and Csanyi V (2005) Human listeners are able to classify dog (*Canis familiaris*) barks recorded in different situations. *Journal of Comparative Psychology* **119(2)**, 136–144

Ramsey IK (2014) *BSAVA Small Animal Formulary, 8th edn.* BSAVA Publications, Gloucester

Rimbault M and Ostrander E (2012) So many doggone traits: mapping genetics of multiple phenotypes in the domestic dog. *Human Molecular Genetics* **21**, 52–57

Rooney N and Cowan S (2011) Training methods and owner–dog interactions: links with dog behaviour and learning ability. *Applied Animal Behaviour Science* **132**, 169–177

Shaw JR and Lagoni L (2007) End-of-life communication in veterinary medicine: delivering bad news and euthanasia decision making. *Veterinary Clinics of North America: Small Animal Practice* **37**(1), 95–108

Shettleworth S (2001) Animal cognition and animal behaviour. *Animal Behaviour* **61**, 277–286

Skinner BF (1951) How to teach animals. *Scientific American* **185**, 26–29

Sterry J, Appleby D and Bizo L (2005) The relationship between measures of problematical behaviour in adult dogs and age of first exposure outside the first owner's home and attendance at puppy classes. In: *Proceedings of the CABTSG Study Day*

Tempelmann S, Kaminski J and Tomasello M (2014) Do domestic dogs learn words based on humans' referential behaviour? *PLoS ONE* **9(3)**, doi: 10.1371/journal.pone.0091014

Thorndike EL (1927) The law of effect. *American Journal of Psychology* **39**, 212–222

Van der Zee E (2009) Communication. In: *The Encyclopaedia of Applied Animal Behaviour and Welfare*, ed. D Mills *et al.*, pp. 116–118. CABI Publishing International, Oxon

Wei C (2009) Cognition. In: *The Encyclopaedia of Applied Animal Behaviour and Welfare*, ed. D Mills *et al.*, pp. 110–113. CABI Publishing International, Oxon

Weiss JM (1972) Psychological factors in stress and disease. *Scientific American* **226**, 104–113

Yang L, Wellman LL, Ambrozewicz MA and Sanford LD (2011) Effects of stressor predictability and controllability on sleep, temperature and fear behavior in mice. *Sleep* **34(6)**, 759–771

Yin S and McCowan B (2004) Barking in domestic dogs: context specificity and individual identification. *Animal Behaviour* **68**, 343–355

Useful websites

American Veterinary Society of Animal Behavior (AVSAB) – Position Statement on Puppy Socialization (2008) www.AVSABonline.org

Animal Behaviour Training Council (ABTC) – Standards for Practitioners (2012) www.abtcouncil.org.uk/standards-for-practitioners.html#2

Association of Pet Behaviour Counsellors (APBC) www.apbc.org.uk/apbc

Association of Pet Dog Trainers (APDT) www.apdt.co.uk/dog-trainers

British Small Animal Veterinary Association (BSAVA) – Aversive training methods https://www.bsava.com/Resources/Positionstatements/Aversivetrainingmethods.aspx

British Veterinary Behaviour Association (BVBA) www.bvba.org.uk

European College of Animal Welfare and Behavioural Medicine (ECAWBM) www.ecawbm.com

BSAVA CLIENT QUESTIONNAIRES: BEHAVIOUR SERIES

Canine behaviour questionnaire

Date _____

Owner details

(Mr/Mrs/Miss/Ms) Surname/Family name _____ First name or Initials _____

Address _____
_____ Postcode _____

Phone (day) _____ (evening) _____
(mobile) _____ Fax _____
Email _____

Please include as much information as possible. The more detail available, the more accurate our assessment of the case can be. Please use additional sheets where necessary.

Have you owned a dog before?   [   ] Yes   [   ] No
Have you owned this breed of dog before?   [   ] Yes   [   ] No
Have you owned other pets previously?   [   ] Yes   [   ] No

Please list other current household pets

Type and breed	Name	Age	Spayed/neutered?	Relationship with dog (e.g. avoids, plays, fights)

Please list the names, ages and occupations of other family members who live at home

Name	Age	Occupation

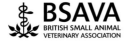
BSAVA
BRITISH SMALL ANIMAL
VETERINARY ASSOCIATION

Canine behaviour questionnaire
© BSAVA 2009
BSAVA Manual of Canine and Feline Behavioural Medicine, 2nd edition

BSAVA CLIENT QUESTIONNAIRES: BEHAVIOUR SERIES

Patient details

Name _____ Breed _____

Sex   [   ] Male   [   ] Female   [   ] Male neutered   [   ] Female spayed

Date of birth _____ Age when obtained (if known) _____

Date first acquired _____ Source _____

Reason(s) for obtaining this dog
_____
_____
_____

Has the dog ever been used for breeding?   [   ] Yes   [   ] No
If yes, at what age?   _____

How would you describe your dog's personality?
_____

Do you consider your dog to be:

[   ] Aggressive? (growling, snarling, snapping, nipping or biting in any circumstances)
[   ] Destructive?   [   ] Hyperactive/restless?   [   ] Disobedient?   [   ] Housetrained?
[   ] Nervous?   [   ] Excitable?   [   ] Noisy/excessive vocalization?
[   ] Depressed?   [   ] Demanding attention?   [   ] Playful?

A   Medical history

1.   Please give a brief medical history, especially recurrent problems and treatment.
      Use an extra sheet if necessary
      _____
      _____
      _____

2.   Vaccination status   _____

3.   Date last wormed   _____

4.   Is your dog currently on any regular medications (such as allergy medication, heartworm
      treatment, herbal or homeopathic remedies)?

Drug/remedy	Dose

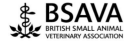

BSAVA CLIENT QUESTIONNAIRES: BEHAVIOUR SERIES

5.   Has your dog been on medication for his/her behaviour in the past?
      If yes, please list name and dosage (include herbals and homeopathics)

Drug/remedy	Dose

6.   Is your dog on any medication for his/her behaviour now?
      If yes, please list name and dosage (include herbals and homeopathics)

Drug/remedy	Dose

B   Early history

1.   Please give details of the dog's early life, if known, including litter size, age of weaning, age when obtained, whether raised outside or indoors, if orphan or stray, whether hand-reared, etc.
      _____
      _____
      _____

2.   How much interaction did the puppy have with people in the first year of his/her life?_____
      _____

3.   What method of housetraining was used?_____

4.   How did you react to any mistakes during housetraining?_____

5.   Did your puppy attend puppy 'parties' or classes? If so, please give details_____
      _____

C   Training and obedience

1.   Has your dog ever attended training classes?   [   ] Yes   [   ] No

2.   If Yes, please give details (when, where, age of dog, who took it to the class) _____
      _____

3.   What types of training techniques were used in the class? _____
      _____

4.   What training methods have you used?_____
      _____

5.   How well did your dog do in the class?   [   ] Very well   [   ] Average
                                                    [   ] Poor   [   ] Was asked to leave
      If asked to leave, please say why _____

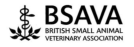
BSAVA
BRITISH SMALL ANIMAL
VETERINARY ASSOCIATION

Canine behaviour questionnaire
© BSAVA 2009
BSAVA Manual of Canine and Feline Behavioural Medicine, 2nd edition

BSAVA CLIENT QUESTIONNAIRES: BEHAVIOUR SERIES

6.   Do you think your dog is Good, Average or Poor at learning?   [   ] Good   [   ] Average   [   ] Poor

7.   What tasks will the dog reliably perform for you on command?
      [   ] Sit   [   ] Stay   [   ] Down   [   ] Fetch   [   ] Other _____

8.   Does your dog do 'tricks' (such as shake, rollover)? _____

9.   Does your dog pull when on the lead?   [   ] Yes   [   ] No

10.   Is your dog more obedient in some places than in others?   [   ] Yes   [   ] No
      If Yes, please give details: _____
      _____

11.   Is your dog more obedient with some people than with others?   [   ] Yes   [   ] No
      If Yes, please give details: _____
      _____

12.   How do you correct your dog when he/she misbehaves? _____
      _____

D   Diet and feeding

1.   What types of food (and brands) do you give your dog? _____
      _____

2.   How much does he/she eat a day? _____

3.   When and where is the dog fed? (how often and at what time) _____

4.   If there is more than one dog in the home, how many food bowls are provided? _____
      Where are the food bowls situated? _____

5.   Who feeds the dog? _____

6.   Is the dog protective (stiffening, growling, snapping or biting) around the food?   [   ] Yes   [   ] No
      Details _____

7.   Is his/her appetite Good or Poor?   [   ] Good   [   ] Poor

8.   Does your dog eat Quickly or Slowly?   [   ] Quickly   [   ] Slowly

9.   What are his/her favourite foods? _____

10.   Do you have to be present for him/her to eat?   [   ] Yes   [   ] No

11.   How much does your dog drink each day (in pints or litres)? _____

12.   Do you add supplements or titbits to the diet?   [   ] Yes   [   ] No
      If yes, what and why? _____

13.   Is he/she given bones or chews? _____
      Is he/she possessive with these? _____

14.   Do you consider your dog to be at the correct weight?   [   ] Yes   [   ] No
      Please fill in your dog's weight _____

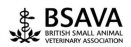
BSAVA
BRITISH SMALL ANIMAL
VETERINARY ASSOCIATION

Canine behaviour questionnaire
© BSAVA 2009
BSAVA Manual of Canine and Feline Behavioural Medicine, 2nd edition

BSAVA CLIENT QUESTIONNAIRES: BEHAVIOUR SERIES

E   Daily activities

Sleeping and waking
1.   Where does your dog sleep? _____

2.   If your dog sleeps on the bed, who invites him/her up? _____

3.   When does the dog get up in the morning? _____

4.   Does your dog ever wake you at night?   [   ] Yes   [   ] No
     If yes, how often and why? _____

Going outside
5.   When does your dog go outside and for how long? _____

6.   How does your dog ask to go outside? _____

7.   Does he/she roam free in a garden or yard? _____

8.   What type of fencing is used to restrain the dog? _____

9.   Is your dog keen to explore when on its own? _____

Toileting
10.   Where does your dog tend to go to the toilet? _____

11.   Does your dog spot mark with small amounts of urine?   [   ] Yes   [   ] No
     If so, where? _____

12.   How often does he/she empty his/her bladder in a day? _____

13.   How frequently does he/she empty his/her bowels? _____

Exercise
14.   What sort of exercise (e.g. walking on/off lead, running off lead, agility training) does your dog receive and how much?

Type	Purpose	Amount	Frequency

15.   Who takes the dog for exercise?

Play/training
16.   Is there any specific time devoted to play and/or training on a daily basis?   [   ] Yes   [   ] No

17.   Does your dog play games with you or other family members?   [   ] Yes   [   ] No
     Details _____

18   Who initiates play: people or the pet? _____

19   What types of toys does your dog play with? _____

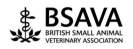
BSAVA
BRITISH SMALL ANIMAL
VETERINARY ASSOCIATION

Canine behaviour questionnaire
© BSAVA 2009
BSAVA Manual of Canine and Feline Behavioural Medicine, 2nd edition

BSAVA CLIENT QUESTIONNAIRES: BEHAVIOUR SERIES

'Home alone'

20. Is your dog left home alone in the house? _____

21. Where does the dog stay during the day when no one is home? _____

22. What does he/she do as you prepare to depart? _____

23. Does your dog ever bark or whine when you leave?   [ ] Yes   [ ] No

24. Does your dog ever [   ] vocalize, [   ] toilet, or [   ] engage in destructive behaviour while you are gone?

25. Typically, how long is your dog alone without people on any given day? _____

26. What arrangements are made for your dog when you go on holiday? _____

Family routine

27. What does he/she do during family meals? _____

28. Has there been a change in your household routine (e.g. new work hours, new baby, moving, new roommate or visitors, boarding, diet change)?   [   ] Yes   [   ] No
    Details _____

Favourite things

Please list 5 things your dog enjoys most; these may be foods, toys or activities

_____ _____ _____ _____ _____

F   Interaction with family members

The home environment

1. What type of home do you have (e.g. flat/apartment, house) _____

2. What areas of the house does your dog have access to? _____

3. Where does your dog sleep at night? _____

4. Does he/she have their own bed? _____

Reaction to handling by family members

5. Is there aggression in the following circumstances? This can include growling, snarling (showing teeth), lunging, nipping, snapping or biting. Please fill in the chart: (Y=Yes, N=No, N/A=doesn't apply). If biting has occurred in any of these circumstances, please describe the wound (tear, puncture, bruising)

	Adult owner (female)	Adult owner (male)	Children	Any specific individual
Handling/grooming				
Petting or hugging				
Disturbed when resting				
Disciplining				
Walking on the lead				
Taking food away				
Taking other objects				

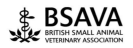

BSAVA
BRITISH SMALL ANIMAL
VETERINARY ASSOCIATION

Canine behaviour questionnaire
© BSAVA 2009
BSAVA Manual of Canine and Feline Behavioural Medicine, 2nd edition

BSAVA CLIENT QUESTIONNAIRES: BEHAVIOUR SERIES

G   Interaction with others

Reaction to visitors

1.   How does your dog behave when visitors come to the house (e.g. barking, door charging)?
_____

2.   Is the behaviour different toward familiar and unfamiliar people?   [   ] Yes   [   ] No
If yes, describe_____

3.   Is the behaviour different toward people outside the house and people inside the house?
[   ] Yes   [   ] No
If yes, describe_____

4.   Does your dog display aggression (growling, snarling, snapping or biting) to visitors to your home?
[   ] Yes   [   ] No
If yes, describe_____

5.   Has your dog ever bitten or attacked anyone?   [   ] Yes   [   ] No

6.   Please fill in details of any regular visitors to the home

Name (if known)	Purpose	Time & Days	Dog's reaction

7.   What is the dog's response to other visitors?

Frequent visitors	Occasional visitors	Rare visitors

Reactions to other people

8.   Please describe your dog's reaction to each of the following:

	In the home	Out of the home
Familiar men		
Familiar women		
Familiar children		
Unknown men		
Unknown women		
Unknown children		
Familiar dogs		
Unknown dogs		
Other animals		
Crowds/busy areas		

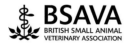
BSAVA
BRITISH SMALL ANIMAL
VETERINARY ASSOCIATION

Canine behaviour questionnaire
© BSAVA 2009
BSAVA Manual of Canine and Feline Behavioural Medicine, 2nd edition

BSAVA CLIENT QUESTIONNAIRES: BEHAVIOUR SERIES

Reactions to other animals

9. What is the reaction to other dogs when out at exercise?
    On a lead _____
    Free exercise _____

10. What is the reaction to other animals, e.g. squirrels, unfamiliar cats? _____
    _____

H Other behaviours

1. Does your dog ever show inappropriate mounting or other sexual activity?   [   ] Yes   [   ] No
    If so, to whom or what? _____

2. Is your dog ever protective over parts of his/her body (especially ears and feet)?   [   ] Yes   [   ] No
    If yes, which regions? _____

3. Does your dog lick or chew on themselves more than you would expect?   [   ] Yes   [   ] No

I The current problem

1. What is the current problem(s) you are having with your dog? Please describe it briefly _____
    _____
    _____

2. When did it begin? _____

3. How long has it been present? _____

4. How old was the dog when it began? _____

5. Where does the problem occur? _____

6. With whom? _____

7. How often? _____

8. Other details _____
    _____
    _____

J Aggression

Please answer the questions below if the problem is aggression:

1. Describe the most recent incident and the setting it occurred in (try to be very precise, as if you were drawing a picture):

    a) Where was the dog? _____
    b) Where was everyone in relation to the dog? _____
    c) What was everyone doing before the incident? _____
    d) What did the dog do? _____
    e) What was the dog's body posture? Describe the position of ears, tail, face, hair on back, or draw a picture if necessary _____
        _____
        _____

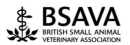
BSAVA
BRITISH SMALL ANIMAL
VETERINARY ASSOCIATION

Canine behaviour questionnaire
© BSAVA 2009
BSAVA Manual of Canine and Feline Behavioural Medicine, 2nd edition

BSAVA CLIENT QUESTIONNAIRES: BEHAVIOUR SERIES

2.   What was your reaction to the behaviour?_____

3.   How did the dog react to your reaction? _____

4.   Was there any punishment? _____

5.   If there was a bite wound was it a puncture wound or a tear?_____

6.   Going back in time, describe the 3 most recent incidents of the behaviour. Please use additional
      pages for this _____

7.   How frequently does the problem occur?   [   ] Times per day   [   ] Times per week
                                                  [   ] Times per month   [   ] Times per year

8.   When does the problem occur?
      When left alone?   [   ] Always   [   ] Usually
                                                   [   ] Rarely   [   ] Never
      When family members are present?   [   ] Always   [   ] Usually
                                                   [   ] Rarely   [   ] Never

9.   What has been done to correct the problem?_____

10.   Is the problem getting: [   ] Better   [   ] Worse   [   ] No change?

11.   Do you suspect any cause?_____

K   House soiling

      If the problem is house soiling, does it take place:
      When you are not present?   [   ] Yes   [   ] No
      When someone is home?   [   ] Yes   [   ] No

L   Destruction

      If the problem is destruction, does it take place:
      When you are not present?   [   ] Yes   [   ] No
      When you are home?   [   ] Yes   [   ] No

M   Other problems
      What other behaviours does your dog engage in that are objectionable to you? _____
      _____
      _____

      Does his/her behaviour cause arguments at home? _____
      _____
      _____

N   You and your dog

1.   How would you describe your relationship with this dog?
      Adult owners (female) _____
      Adult owners (male)_____
      Children _____

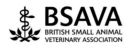

Canine behaviour questionnaire
© BSAVA 2009
BSAVA Manual of Canine and Feline Behavioural Medicine, 2nd edition

BSAVA CLIENT QUESTIONNAIRES: BEHAVIOUR SERIES

2.   What are your feelings about the dog's present behaviour?
     Adult owners (female) _____
     Adult owners (male)_____
     Children _____

3.   How would you ideally like your dog to be? _____

4.   Under what circumstances would you consider euthanasia? _____
     _____

5.   What is your expectation for change? _____

6.   Is there anything else you would like to add about your dog and its behaviour?
     Please give any other information you think is relevant to the case _____
     _____
     _____
     _____
     _____
     _____
     _____
     _____
     _____
     _____
     _____
     _____
     _____
     _____

Questionnaire completed by (print) _____

Signature _____ Date_____

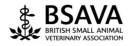

BSAVA BRITISH SMALL ANIMAL VETERINARY ASSOCIATION

Canine behaviour questionnaire
© BSAVA 2009
BSAVA Manual of Canine and Feline Behavioural Medicine, 2nd edition

Regurgitation, vomiting and diarrhoea

Sara Gould

Vomiting and diarrhoea are extremely common reasons for owners to present their dogs at veterinary clinics. A logical systematic approach, beginning with a full history and thorough physical examination, is necessary to ensure that appropriate further investigations and treatments are instigated.

The majority of acute vomiting/diarrhoea cases are self-limiting. However, a small but significant minority have potentially life-threatening problems. Severe vomiting itself can result in fluid and electrolyte depletion and occasionally aspiration pneumonia. Care of emergency patients is discussed in Chapter 8.

Presenting signs and causes

Regurgitation

Regurgitation is the passive expulsion of undigested saliva-covered food from the oesophagus, and is the most important clinical sign of oesophageal disease. It is essential to differentiate clearly between vomiting and regurgitation (Figure 13.1), as a failure to make this distinction will invariably lead to a misdiagnosis.

Regurgitation	Vomiting
Usually immediately after eating or soon after	May be immediate but often delayed
Passive, no abdominal effort	Abdominal effort, retching
Unchanged food and saliva present	Digested or partially digested food present
Food may be re-eaten	Food is not re-eaten in most cases
No bile present	Bile may be present

13.1   Differentiation of regurgitation and vomiting.

The severity of the clinical signs depends on the underlying cause. Retching and dysphagia suggest oropharyngeal disease (see Chapters 20 and 23). Severe regurgitation can result in aspiration pneumonia; these patients will present with a cough, fever and harsh lung sounds (see Chapter 24). Common causes of regurgitation are listed in Figure 13.2.

- **Megaoesophagus** (Figure 13.3) is probably the most common cause of regurgitation in the dog,

although in the majority of adult-onset cases no cause is identified (idiopathic). Megaoesophagus may be secondary to myasthenia gravis, hypoadrenocorticism, polymyositis or thymoma.

Cause of regurgitation	Presentation
Oesophageal foreign body	Often in small terrier breeds. Radiodense foreign body (FB) visible on thoracic radiography
Oesophagitis	Secondary to physical damage (FB), chemical injury or gastro-oesophageal reflux
Megaoesophagus	Dilated air-filled oesophagus often visible on plain thoracic radiographs. Congenital or acquired disease
Oesophageal stricture	Secondary to FB or following gastro-oesophageal reflux under general anaesthesia
Hiatal hernia	Congenital hiatal hernia seen in Shar Pei, Chow Chow, French Bulldog, Bulldog
Congenital vascular ring anomalies	Young puppies often regurgitate from the time of weaning

13.2   Common causes of regurgitation.

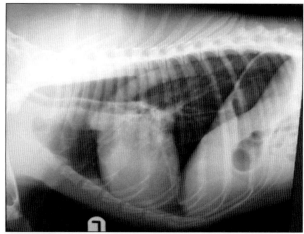

13.3   A lateral thoracic radiograph of a 7-year-old Whippet with regurgitation, pyrexia and a soft cough. A large gas-filled megaoesophagus is visible, and there is patchy increased opacity in the cranioventral lung lobes consistent with aspiration pneumonia.

- **Oesophageal foreign bodies** (FBs) occur frequently in small terriers, although any breed can be affected. The commonest oesophageal FBs are bones. Dogs with complete oesophageal obstruction present with *acute* signs, whereas those with partial obstruction may have a *chronic* history of regurgitation. FBs lodged in the cervical oesophagus may be palpable. Survey radiography will identify a radiodense FB. Radiolucent FB identification may require contrast studies or direct visualization using endoscopy.
- **Oesophagitis** may be a result of ingestion of irritants, or secondary to an oesophageal FB (Figure 13.4), or may follow gastro-oesophageal reflux. Chronic vomiting, hiatal hernia, gastric motility disorders and anaesthesia are all potential causes of gastro-oesophageal reflux. If damage to the oesophagus is severe, scarring and fibrosis can result in an oesophageal stricture.

Vomiting

Vomiting is defined as the forceful ejection of stomach contents, and involves three stages:

1. Nausea.
2. Retching.
3. Vomition.

It is essential to differentiate clearly between vomiting and regurgitation (see Figure 13.1), as a failure to make this distinction will invariably lead to a misdiagnosis. The onus is on the clinician to obtain sufficient historical information to make the distinction. Occasionally it may not be clear from the history obtained and it may be necessary to observe the patient. Occasionally patients may regurgitate and vomit concurrently.

Vomiting is initiated by the vomiting centre in the medulla oblongata that can be triggered either directly or indirectly (via the chemoreceptor trigger zone, CRTZ) (Figure 13.5).

> **PRACTICAL TIP**
>
> Whilst the majority of cases of vomiting are linked to gastrointestinal disorders, it is important not to forget non-gastrointestinal causes (e.g. pyometra, prostatitis) when compiling lists of differential diagnoses (see Figure 13.6)

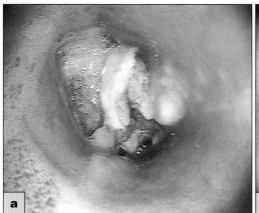
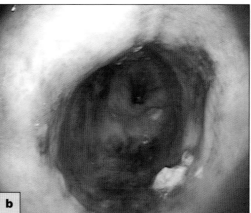

13.4
(a) An oesophageal foreign body (bone) viewed endoscopically in a West Highland White Terrier with acute regurgitation.
(b) Oesophagitis is evident following removal of the foreign body. The dog was treated with gastroprotectants for 7 days.

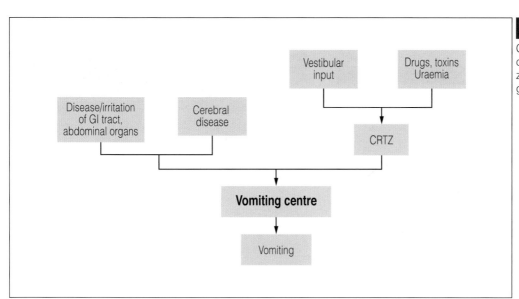

13.5 Initiation of vomiting. CRTZ = chemoreceptor trigger zone; GI = gastrointestinal.

Diarrhoea

If the predominant sign is diarrhoea attempts should be made to distinguish between small intestinal (SI) and large intestinal (LI) diarrhoea. This distinction is most relevant in chronic diarrhoea.

- Small intestinal diarrhoea results in increased faecal volume, usually without urgency. Melaena may be evident.
- Large intestinal diarrhoea usually results in urgency, mucus, tenesmus and, occasionally, fresh blood and increased faecal frequency. Tenesmus is often associated with diseases of the rectum and the anus (see Chapter 30).

It is beyond the scope of this chapter to list every known cause of vomiting/diarrhoea; the common differential diagnoses seen in practice will be considered. With the aid of historical and clinical information, an appropriate differential list can be formulated (Figure 13.6).

Gastric disorders
- Dietary indiscretion/intolerance/allergy
- Gastritis
- Haemorrhagic gastroenteritis (HGE)
- Foreign body
- Gastric ulceration (e.g. non-steroidal anti-inflammatory drugs (NSAIDs), steroids)
- Neoplasia

Intestinal disorders
- Foreign body
- Inflammatory bowel disease
- Antibiotic-responsive enteropathy
- Intussusception
- Ulceration
- Neoplasia
- Exocrine pancreatic insufficiency

Extra-gastrointestinal abdominal disorders
- Pancreatitis
- Liver disease
- Pyometra
- Prostatitis
- Peritonitis
- Nephritis

Metabolic/endocrine disorders
- Renal failure
- Diabetic ketoacidosis
- Hypercalcaemia
- Hypoadrenocorticism

Infections
- Parvovirus
- *Leptospira*
- *Campylobacter*
- *Salmonella*
- *Clostridium*
- *Giardia*

Drug/toxin-induced
- Examples: ethylene glycol; morphine; chemotherapy drugs; erythromycin

Neurological disorders
- Vestibular disease
- Neoplasia

13.6 Common differential diagnoses of vomiting and/or diarrhoea.

Diagnostic approach

History

Signalment may allow the clinician to consider specific conditions or breed predispositions to certain gastrointestinal (GI) diseases: young dogs are more likely to have infectious, congenital or hereditary causes; older dogs are more likely to have acquired disease or neoplasia. The dog's previous medical history should be obtained, with particular reference to previous GI problems, vaccination status, worming history, medications, diet and environment.

Key information to obtain is:

- Signalment and medical history
- Vaccination status, worming history and current medications
- Duration, nature and severity of signs
- Time in relation to eating (ensure clear differentiation from regurgitation)
- Environment and diet: is the dog a scavenger?, have there been changes in diet or appetite?
- Content of vomitus: food, bile, blood, foreign material
- Appearance of diarrhoea: melaena, mucus, blood, steatorrhoea; small intestinal *versus* large intestinal
- Other systemic signs: e.g. polyuria/polydipsia (PU/PD), fever.

> **PRACTICAL TIP**
>
> It is important to consider all body systems, as many systemic diseases have gastrointestinal signs. For example, if PU/PD is identified prior to the onset of vomiting, then metabolic/endocrine disorders are likely differentials

Physical examination

A careful and thorough clinical examination may help identify the underlying cause (Figure 13.7), as well as assessing the severity of the vomiting and/or diarrhoea.

- Careful attention should be paid to the hydration status of the patient (pulse rate, quality, skin tenting, mucous membrane colour) and abdominal palpation.

Physical examination finding	Possible causes
Tympanic abdomen and unproductive retching	Gastric dilatation–volvulus
Abdominal pain	Pancreatitis, hepatitis, peritonitis, prostatitis, nephritis
Abdominal mass	Foreign body, neoplasia, intussusception, lymph nodes
Jaundice	Pancreatitis, liver disease
Vaginal discharge	Pyometra
Uraemia/stomatitis	Chronic renal failure
Enlarged peripheral lymph nodes	Lymphoma (and hypercalcaemia)

13.7 Physical examination findings and possible causes of vomiting and/or diarrhoea.

- Abdominal palpation should be performed in a methodical way, considering the abdomen in four quadrants and carefully assessing the abdominal organs. Pain, if present, should be reproducible. Excessive force applied suddenly to the abdomen can result in abdominal guarding.
- In some individuals abdominal palpation may be made difficult due to temperament, physical size and/or abdominal guarding. In these cases the possibility of abdominal pain/masses should not be excluded.
- Rectal examination should be performed to assess the prostate gland in male dogs, and may assist in the identification of melaena and rectal abnormalities. Further discussion of rectal disorders can be found in Chapter 30.

Further investigation

The further investigations that are most appropriate are usually dictated by the historical and clinical findings. If self-limiting disease is suspected, further investigations may not be necessary (Figure 13.8). Dogs with severe vomiting/diarrhoea that are systemically unwell, or those with chronic relapsing gastrointestinal signs, warrant further investigation (Figure 13.9).

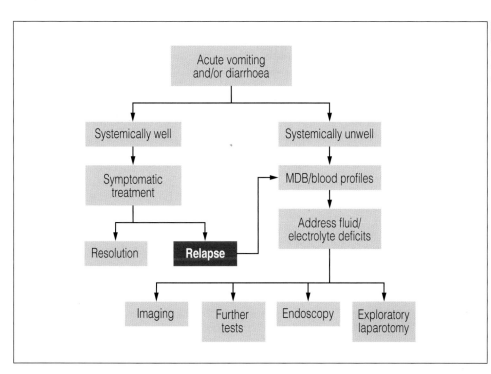

13.8 A suggested approach to acute vomiting and/or diarrhoea. MDB = minimum database.

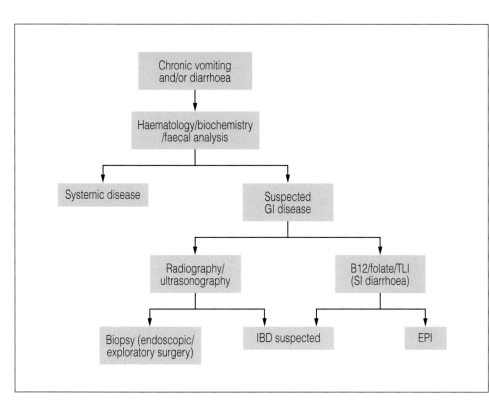

13.9 A suggested approach to chronic vomiting and/or diarrhoea. EPI = exocrine pancreatic insufficiency; GI = gastrointestinal; IBD = inflammatory bowel disease; SI = small intestinal; TLI = trypsin-like immunoreactivity.

> **WARNING**
>
> It is important to remember that animals that are significantly dehydrated or are suspected of having significant life-threatening GI or systemic disease, need to have their fluid and electrolyte deficits corrected whilst further investigations are undertaken. Failure to correct fluid and electrolyte abnormalities before general anaesthesia, for example, is likely to lead to increased patient morbidity and mortality

Laboratory tests

Minimum database: Basic information can be obtained rapidly and for relatively little expense. Packed cell volume (PCV) and plasma protein can easily be determined from a microhaematocrit. Additionally, a crude assessment of white cell numbers can be obtained by examining the buffy coat, and the appearance of the plasma may give clues as to the cause of the vomiting (i.e. icteric plasma). A blood glucose measurement can also be obtained easily. Urine dipstick tests and urine specific gravity (USG) can give additional information about renal function and help establish whether any azotaemia is caused by renal (increased urea and creatinine; USG <1.030) or prerenal (increased urea and creatinine; USG >1.030) disease.

Biochemistry and complete blood count: Serum biochemistry (Figure 13.10) and complete blood count (CBC) (Figure 13.11) are useful to identify non-GI causes of vomiting/diarrhoea and to assess the effects

Abnormality	Possible causes
Hypoglycaemia	Sepsis. Severe liver disease. Hypoadrenocorticism
Hyperglycaemia	Diabetes mellitus/diabetic ketoacidosis
Elevated urea and creatinine	Prerenal (dehydration). Renal failure. Postrenal obstruction
Hyperkalaemia ± hyponatraemia	Hypoadrenocorticism
Hypokalaemia ± hyponatraemia	GI fluid and electrolyte losses
Hypoalbuminaemia	GI loss (chronic). Liver disease (chronic). GI blood loss
Hypercalcaemia ± azotaemia	Hypercalcaemia of malignancy. Hypoadrenocorticism
Elevated bilirubin	Liver disease. Pancreatitis
Hypocholesterolaemia	GI loss. Chronic liver disease
Hypercholesterolaemia	Acute obstructive liver disease. Pancreatitis
Increased liver enzymes	Acute liver disease (massive increases expected). Mild to moderate increases in chronic liver disease, secondary to other inflammatory/infectious diseases
Elevations in amylase/lipase	Mild elevations suggest decreased renal clearance or are a non-specific finding. Massive elevations may suggest pancreatitis, so testing for specific canine pancreatic lipase is recommended (see text)

13.10 Some differential diagnoses for commonly identified abnormalities seen on biochemistry in dogs with vomiting and/or diarrhoea.

Abnormality	Possible causes
Increased PCV and increased plasma protein	Dehydration. Marked increase in PCV often seen in haemorrhagic gastroenteritis
Leucocytosis	Pancreatitis. Pyometra. Prostatitis
Leucopenia	Parvovirus. Sepsis
Eosinophilia	Parasitism. Eosinophilic enteritis. Hypoadrenocorticism
Neutrophilia, lymphopenia ± eosinopenia	Stress leucogram
Thrombocytosis	Chronic GI blood loss
Anaemia	GI blood loss. Hypoadrenocorticism
Microcytic hypochromic anaemia	Chronic GI blood loss

13.11 Some differential diagnoses of commonly identified abnormalities seen on CBC in dogs with vomiting and/or diarrhoea.

of profuse vomiting/diarrhoea. Even if the signalment, history and clinical examination are suggestive of an underlying cause, further testing can confirm suspicion and also check for concurrent disease.

Blood gas analysis: If facilities exist to determine acid–base status, then this can assist the management of acutely unwell patients. Metabolic acidosis is generally more common than metabolic alkalosis in dogs with GI disease. However, abnormalities in acid–base status rarely require addressing in their own right, and the focus should remain on treating the underlying cause and correcting fluid deficits and electrolyte abnormalities.

Faecal analysis: Full faecal analysis including culture is one of the first tests that should be performed, especially in young animals with vomiting/diarrhoea. Faecal PCR tests are now available for *Giardia*, *Salmonella*, *Clostridium perfringens* and parvovirus. A parvovirus ELISA is also available.

> **WARNING**
>
> *Campylobacter*, *Salmonella* and *Giardia* are zoonotic infections

Tests for pancreatitis: Pancreatitis is probably an underdiagnosed disease in general practice. Whilst it may be relatively easy to diagnose severe acute pancreatitis, many more dogs suffer from chronic pancreatitis that may be harder to diagnose. Any dog can get pancreatitis, but certain breeds including Cocker Spaniels, Miniature Schnauzers, Boxers and Cavalier King Charles Spaniels appear to be over-represented (Watson *et al.*, 2007). A presumptive diagnosis of pancreatitis should be made on the basis of a combination of historical, clinical and laboratory testing (see Figures 13.10 and 13.11). The lack of sensitivity of amylase and lipase is well known, but even newer tests including canine pancreatic lipase immunoreactivity (cPLI) and SNAP cPL are not 100% sensitive or specific. SNAP cPL and Spec cPL have the advantage of improved sensitivity and specificity compared with amylase or lipase, but results should always be interpreted in light of clinical, biochemical and imaging results (McCord *et al.*, 2012). The gold standard diagnostic test is pancreatic biopsy, though this is rarely performed.

Tests of exocrine pancreatic function: Inadequate production of digestive enzymes by the pancreatic acinar cells, due to atrophy, leads to maldigestion and malabsorption of nutrients. The persistence of undigested food within the small intestine often results in bacterial overgrowth. Voluminous, pale, often malodorous, small intestinal diarrhoea is present and many dogs are clinically malnourished. Exocrine pancreatic insufficiency (EPI) can affect any breed, but German Shepherd Dogs are over-represented. EPI can also develop as a consequence of chronic pancreatitis. Dogs with EPI have low trypsin-like immunoreactivity (TLI) and will often have cobalamin and folate abnormalities (see Tests of intestinal absorption, below).

Tests of liver function: Many dogs with severe GI disease have abnormalities of liver enzymes, but it may not be easy to decide whether the changes are due to a primary liver disease or reflect a secondary hepatopathy. For example, dogs with severe inflammatory bowel disease will have changes in liver enzymes as a consequence of increased metabolic demand and increased toxins/bacteria in the portal blood. Successful treatment of the primary disease should resolve the changes in liver enzymes. Dogs with both acute and chronic liver disease can present with vomiting and diarrhoea, and recognizing patterns that are suggestive of acute liver disease, chronic liver disease and secondary hepatopathies requires evaluation of liver enzymes and liver function tests (Figure 13.12), together with historical and clinical information. Dogs with significant inflammatory diseases such as pancreatitis, inflammatory bowel disease, pyometra or prostatitis could all have biochemical changes consistent with a secondary hepatopathy.

Parameter	Acute liver disease	Chronic liver disease	Secondary hepatopathy
ALT/ALP/GGT	Marked increase	Mild/moderate increase	Mild to moderate increase
Albumin	Usually normal/low normal	Reduced	Depends on primary disease
Cholesterol	Increased/normal	Often low/normal	Depends on primary disease
Bile acids	Moderate/marked increase	Marked increase	Mild/moderate increase
Bilirubin	Normal/increased	Normal/increased	Usually normal

13.12 Biochemical changes in acute, chronic and secondary hepatopathies. ALP = alkaline phosphatase; ALT = alanine aminotransferase; GGT = gamma-glutamyl transferase.

Bile acids

- A serum bile acids concentration of <40 μmol/l is typical in secondary hepatopathies
- Dogs with primary liver disease, either acute or chronic, would be expected to have bile acids >60 μmol/l, and levels can be >100 μmol/l

---

Testing for hypoadrenocorticism: Hypoadrenocorticism is an uncommon cause of vomiting and/or diarrhoea. Many cases are presented in acute crisis; others can have a more chronic, waxing and waning disease, making diagnosis a challenge. Hypoadrenocorticism is most common in young to middle-aged dogs and certain breeds are over-represented (e.g. poodles, West Highland White Terrier, Bearded Collie, Nova Scotia Duck Tolling Retriever). Most dogs with hypoadrenocorticism have classical electrolyte abnormalities (hyperkalaemia, hyponatraemia, with sodium:potassium ratios <27:1, and hypochloraemia) but these electrolyte abnormalities are not pathognomonic for hypoadrenocorticism and many dogs with acute vomiting/diarrhoea have electrolyte disturbances. Other abnormalities can include azotaemia and a relatively dilute USG. Hypercalcaemia and hypoglycaemia may also be seen.

Diagnosis of hypoadrenocorticism is made using the adrenocorticotrophic hormone (ACTH) stimulation test, confirming suboptimal cortisol before and after stimulation:

- In hypoadrenocorticism cortisol levels are typically <20 nmol/l both pre- and post-stimulation
- It is important to remember that pretreatment with steroids can blunt the adrenocortical response
- Measuring resting cortisol levels may be useful to exclude hypoadrenocorticism: if cortisol is >55 nmol/l hypoadrenocorticism is unlikely (Lennon *et al.*, 2007).

Tests of intestinal absorption: Folate/B12 (cobalamin) tests are most often utilized in cases of chronic vomiting and/or diarrhoea, to assess intestinal absorptive function. They can be helpful in confirming a suspicion of inflammatory bowel disease or bacterial overgrowth. The tests should be interpreted in the context of known exocrine pancreatic function. Deficiencies in cobalamin can be supplemented parenterally.

Coagulation profiles: Testing coagulation by activated partial thromboplastin time (APTT) and prothrombin time (PT) is indicated in patients with haematemesis or melaena, or in systemically unwell dogs with an acute abdomen, in order to detect disseminated intravascular coagulation (DIC). Platelet counts should be verified by checking a blood film prior to undertaking coagulation profile testing. Animals with severe thrombocytopenia (<50 x 10^9/l) can bleed spontaneously.

Diagnostic imaging

A structured examination of all abdominal contents is essential to avoid missing abnormalities that were not anticipated.

Survey abdominal radiography: Abdominal radiography can assist in the diagnosis of many GI diseases, such as gastric dilatation–volvulus (GDV), and is a priority in suspected cases of intestinal obstruction. Classic signs of GDV are: dilatation of the stomach with gas ± food/fluid; and malposition of the fundus and pylorus. The pylorus rotates to the left and becomes more cranial and dorsal relative to the fundus (Figure 13.13).

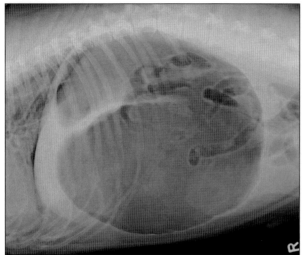

13.13 Right lateral radiograph of a large-breed dog with gastric dilatation–volvulus. The pylorus can be seen in the dorsocranial abdomen and is gas-filled, giving a 'boxing glove' or reverse c-shape appearance.

Small intestinal obstruction may be evident on plain abdominal radiographs. Dilated loops of small intestine may be seen in association with obstruction caused by a foreign body (Figure 13.14), neoplasia or intussusception. The exact criteria upon which dilatation is diagnosed is variable, though most authors agree that a small intestinal width greater than the height of the vertebral endplate of L2 is significant.

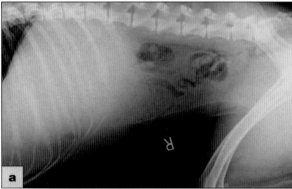

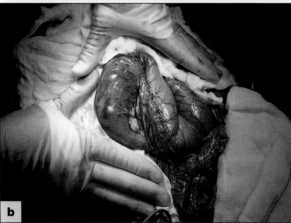

13.14 **(a)** Lateral abdominal radiograph showing a small region of gaseous distension of the small intestine, and a more obvious increased soft tissue opacity in the cranial abdomen consistent with a fluid-filled distended stomach, in a Labrador Retriever bitch with acute vomiting. **(b)** During surgery, a proximal duodenal foreign body was identified. An enterotomy was performed and the dog recovered uneventfully.

(The measurement of intestinal wall thickness cannot be reliably assessed on plain abdominal radiographs, and can only be measured during contrast studies or ultrasonographically.) Linear foreign bodies may be suspected on the basis of clumping of intestines, tight bends or C-shaped loops and ovoid gas pockets. Not all foreign bodies are radiodense.

A loss of serosal detail may suggest free abdominal fluid and direct further investigations such as ultrasonography to establish a diagnosis and obtain fluid samples (see Chapter 25). The best determination of liver size is based on the appearance of the gastric axis and the extent beyond the costal arch on plain abdominal radiographs. Abnormalities in organ size and shape can be further investigated by ultrasonography.

> **PRACTICAL TIP**
>
> It is important to remember that not all foreign bodies are visible on plain radiographs and that a normal abdominal radiograph does not exclude the possibility of gastrointestinal or systemic disease

Abdominal ultrasonography: Image quality is dependent on machine-related factors and also on the skill and experience of the operator. Large amounts of gas, food and faeces can also make abdominal imaging difficult. A methodical assessment of the GI tract and other intra-abdominal organs is essential. Readers are directed to specific imaging texts (e.g. *BSAVA Manual of Canine and Feline Ultrasonography*) for detailed information; a guide to some of the more common abnormalities that might be seen in cases of acute vomiting and diarrhoea, that may not have significant abnormalities on clinical examination, is given in Figure 13.15.

Ultrasonographic finding	Possible causes
GI wall thickening with no loss of layering	Inflammatory disease
GI wall thickening with loss of layering	Neoplasia more likely
Enlarged abdominal lymph nodes	Mild increases: reactive lymph node. Moderate/marked increases: diffuse or metastatic neoplasia
Free abdominal fluid	Peritonitis. Liver disease
Microhepatica	Chronic end-stage liver disease. Portosystemic shunts
Hepatomegaly	Acute hepatitis or cholangiohepatitis. Neoplasia
Enlarged hyperechoic /hypoechoic pancreas (often painful)	Acute pancreatitis. Pancreatic tumour

13.15 Possible causes of some ultrasonographic abnormalities in patients with vomiting and/or diarrhoea.

> **PRACTICAL TIPS**
>
> - Not all causes of vomiting and/or diarrhoea will result in obvious ultrasonographic changes
> - Gastric foreign bodies can easily be missed if there is a lot of gas present in the stomach

Ultrasonography can also be used to confirm the nature of abnormalities identified on clinical examination, in assessing the nature of abdominal masses (e.g. foreign body, neoplasia, intussusception; Figure 13.16), or in screening to exclude potential differential diagnoses. If neoplasia is suspected it is important to evaluate the abdomen thoroughly for evidence of metastatic spread, but to remember that ultrasonography cannot be used to diagnose a particular tumour type and that not all 'nodules' or 'masses' are neoplastic. Thoracic radiographs (ideally two inflated views) should be obtained to assess for pulmonary metastases if neoplasia is suspected.

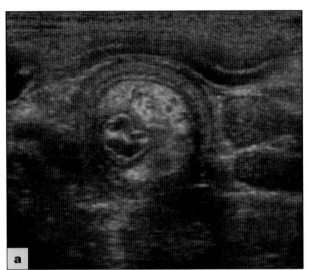

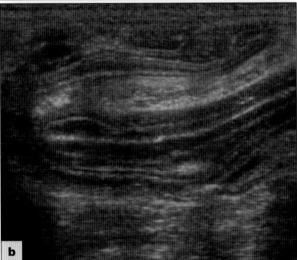

13.16 Ultrasound images from a 1-year-old dog with diarrhoea and a palpable abdominal mass. The images show an intussusception in **(a)** cross-section and **(b)** longitudinal section. (Courtesy of M Costello)

Endoscopy

In the *acute* setting endoscopy may be used to investigate haematemesis, to look for gastroduodenal ulceration or neoplasia, or occasionally to retrieve gastric foreign bodies. *It is essential to ensure that patients are haemodynamically stable before being anaesthetized for endoscopic procedures.*

Endoscopy is mainly used for biopsy in chronic inflammatory GI conditions, after many other potential differential diagnoses have been excluded. Multiple biopsy samples should be taken from both the stomach and small intestine when investigating vomiting or small intestinal diarrhoea. Large amounts of food or fluid in the stomach, despite adequate starving, can hamper gastroduodenoscopy, and is suggestive of a gastric motility disorder.

WARNING
Care should be taken if gastroduodenal ulcers are seen. Biopsy samples should not be taken from the centre of ulcers, to avoid the risk of perforation

Colonoscopy is indicated for dogs with large bowel diarrhoea, tenesmus and haematochezia. Patients need to be adequately prepared with 24 hours' starvation, oral cleansing solutions and warm water enemas.

Pros and cons of endoscopy

■ Benefits:
  • Potentially reduced morbidity and mortality compared with surgery
■ Limitations:
  • Operator skills
  • Biopsy samples often small
  • Can only identify mucosal disease
  • Not all portions of the GI tract can be visualized/sampled

Exploratory laparotomy

Laparotomy to obtain full-thickness biopsy samples as part of a thorough examination of the abdominal cavity still has a useful role in general practice, though surgeons should be adequately prepared for such procedures (see *BSAVA Manual of Canine and Feline Abdominal Surgery*). Exploratory surgery is part of the treatment process for GDV (Figure 13.17), intestinal foreign bodies (Figure 13.18), intussusceptions, most discrete intestinal tumours and perforated ulcers (Figure 13.19).

It is important to remember that chronic inflammatory GI disease may not be visible to the surgeon.

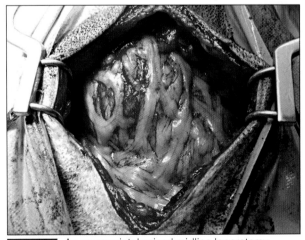

13.17 An appropriately sized midline laparotomy incision in a large-breed dog with a GDV. A gaseous distended stomach can be seen covered in greater omentum.

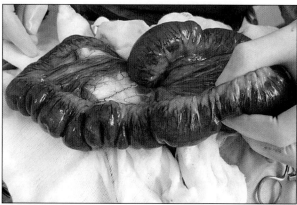

13.18   The appearance of a linear intestinal foreign body on exploratory laparotomy. Note the bunching of the intestines.

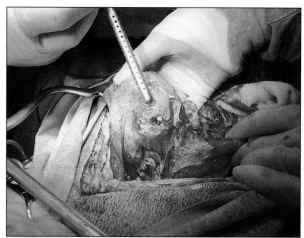

13.19   A perforated gastric ulcer at laparotomy in a dog presenting with haematemesis and signs of an acute abdomen. The ulcer was thought to have been caused by long-term NSAID medication.

Only histopathology can confirm that disease is present, so gut biopsy samples should be taken even if the bowel looks 'normal'. A thorough assessment of the entire GI tract should be performed in a logical manner, ensuring that all loops of intestine have been palpated, as foreign bodies and small intraluminal lesions can be missed. Any enlarged lymph nodes can be sampled, as can other abdominal organs.

Full-thickness gut biopsy carries a slightly increased risk of complications, and owners should be made aware of the risks. The likelihood of wound breakdown is increased in patients with significant hypoalbuminaemia, in those that are profoundly anorexic, and with poor surgical technique. Most dehiscence occurs within 72 hours of surgery.

Principles of treatment

Dogs that are systemically well and suspected to have self-limiting disease can be treated symptomatically.

Systemically well patients
The dog should be starved for 12–24 hours, followed by the introduction of small quantities of a low-fat highly digestible diet. Veterinary prescription diets can be used, but home-cooked diets (chicken/cottage cheese/egg and rice) are also suitable. If the clinical

signs resolve, the dog can then be gradually reintroduced to its normal diet over several days. Water should be offered little and often, and oral electrolyte solutions can be offered in addition to water.

In addition:

- Anti-emetics can be used, provided GI obstruction has been excluded
- Antibiotics are not indicated in acute vomiting or diarrhoea, unless a specific infection has been identified (e.g. *Campylobacter*)
- Anthelmintics should be considered in puppies
- If haematemesis is a clinical feature, gastroprotectants such as sucralfate, omeprazole or H2 blockers (e.g. cimetidine, ranitidine) can be used
- Products such as prebiotics, probiotics and clay based medications are often used to treat diarrhoea but there is limited published evidence of efficacy.

WARNING

Owners must be made aware that if the patient does not respond as expected and clinical signs continue, further investigations and treatment will be necessary. For example, a dog with a gastric foreign body may be systemically well and only vomit occasionally, but if the foreign body moves into the duodenum and causes obstruction the patient will quickly deteriorate

Systemically unwell patients
Patients that are significantly dehydrated, or have suspected systemic or severe GI disease will benefit from correction of fluid deficits and electrolyte abnormalities. Assessing hydration status should be part of the clinical assessment.

PRACTICAL TIP

It is important to remember that dogs that are nauseous or vomiting will often not have dry mucus membranes, and hence their level of dehydration may be underestimated

The choice of fluid depends on the underlying disease and the type of fluids available. The priority is always to correct dehydration and electrolyte imbalances and the commonest error in practice is failure to give sufficient fluids, rather than giving the 'wrong' fluids.

- For dogs with hypercalcaemia, hyperkalaemia (suspected hypoadrenocorticism) and pyloric/jejunal obstruction, the crystalloid of choice would be 0.9% NaCl.
- In the majority of other causes of acute vomiting/diarrhoea, Hartmann's solution would be appropriate.
- Colloids (10–20 ml/kg) or plasma may be useful in markedly hypoproteinaemic patients.
- Blood transfusion is indicated in cases of severe GI blood loss.

Potassium supplementation

Many animals with vomiting and diarrhoea are hypokalaemic, and additional potassium supplementation should be given. Clinicians are often concerned about the risks of potassium supplementation in practice, but it can be undertaken safely if the following guidelines are followed:

- Wherever possible, adjust potassium supplementation based on plasma potassium levels
- Always ensure potassium is well mixed in the fluid bag
- Ensure the bag is labelled appropriately with the amount of potassium added
- Use a fluid pump/syringe driver
- Do not exceed infusion rates of 0.5 mmol K⁺ per kg per hour

Fluid rates are calculated based on the level of dehydration and the underlying disease. Crystalloid fluid rates can be calculated based on deficits, sensible and insensible losses. Many clinicians use multiples of maintenance requirements to guide fluid rates (Figure 13.20). These guide rates are then modified based on clinical response. Wherever possible, fluids – especially those with added potassium – should be given using fluid pumps/syringe drivers to ensure accurate delivery of fluids.

Whatever the fluid type or rate of administration, frequent monitoring of the patient should be undertaken, with particular reference to urine output, heart rate, pulse quality and hydration status.

In addition to fluid therapy:

- Anti-emetics can be used to reduce fluid and electrolyte losses, but should not be used in cases of GI obstruction, or for prolonged periods without a diagnosis
- Gastroprotectants can also be given
- Antibiotics should be reserved for cases with identified infections, or those at risk of sepsis.

Details of specific treatments for specific conditions can be found in appropriate BSAVA manuals.

Condition	Suggested initial fluid therapy rate
Mild vomiting ± diarrhoea with no obvious evidence of dehydration	1–1.5 x maintenance
Moderate vomiting ± diarrhoea with clinical evidence of dehydration	2–2.5 x maintenance
Severe vomiting ± diarrhoea with marked dehydration	2–3 x maintenance ± bolus fluids (20–30 ml/kg over 15–20 minutes)
Gastric dilatation–volvulus	Bolus fluids; shock rate 90 ml/kg/h

13.20 Suggested crystalloid fluid therapy rates in dogs with vomiting ± diarrhoea. Maintenance rate = 2–4 ml/kg/h.

References and further reading

Barr F and Gaschen L (2011) *BSAVA Manual of Canine and Feline Ultrasonography*. BSAVA Publications, Gloucester

Hall EJ, Simpson JW and Williams DA (2005) *BSAVA Manual of Canine and Feline Gastroenterology, 2nd edn.* BSAVA Publications, Gloucester

Lennon EM, Boyle TE, Hutchins RG *et al.* (2007) Use of basal serum or plasma cortisol concentrations to rule out a diagnosis of hypoadrenocorticism in dogs: 123 cases (2000–2005). *Journal of the American Veterinary Medical Association* **231**, 413–416

Lhermette P and Sobel D (2008) *BSAVA Manual of Canine and Feline Endoscopy and Endosurgery*. BSAVA Publications, Gloucester

McCord K, Morley PS, Armstrong J *et al.* (2012) A multi-institutional study evaluating the diagnostic utility of the spec cPLTM and SNAP CPLTM in clinical acute pancreatitis in 84 dogs. *Journal of Veterinary Internal Medicine* **26**, 888–896

O'Brien R and Barr F (2009) *BSAVA Manual of Canine and Feline Abdominal Imaging*. BSAVA Publications, Gloucester

Villiers E and Blackwood L (2005) *BSAVA Manual of Canine and Feline Clinical Pathology, 2nd edn.* BSAVA Publications, Gloucester

Watson PJ, Roulois AJ, Scase T, Thompson H and Herrtage ME (2007) Prevalence and breed distribution of chronic pancreatitis at post-mortem examination in first opinion dogs. *Journal of Small Animal Practice* **48**, 609–618

Abnormalities of eating and drinking

Nick Bexfield

Dogs presenting with polydipsia, polyuria, polyphagia or weight loss are seen relatively commonly in clinical practice. There are multiple causes for each of these problems, and it is important that the clinician formulates a complete list of differential diagnoses prior to undertaking diagnostic investigations. It is very unusual for patients with these clinical signs to present as an emergency, so there is time for a methodological work-up. However, the investigation can be challenging, and it is vital that a logical approach to each case is employed. This chapter will provide an overview of the causes of each of these clinical signs and cover the diagnostic approach, including how the signalment, history and results of the physical examination can be helpful, and how to interpret results of routine and more specific laboratory tests and diagnostic imaging. Helpful practical tips and warnings related to case investigation are also included.

Polydipsia and polyuria

Drinking and the renal control of salt and water excretion are the main mechanisms for balancing water intake with water loss.

Definitions

- A healthy dog drinks approximately 20–90 ml/kg/day, depending on the moisture content of its diet
- Normal urine output varies between 20 and 45 ml/kg/day
- **Polydipsia** (PD) in dogs is defined as a fluid intake of >100 ml/kg/day
- **Polyuria** (PU) in dogs is defined as a urine output of >50 ml/kg/day

---

The causes of PU/PD (Figure 14.1) can be divided into:

- Those that cause primary polydipsia (with secondary polyuria)
- Those that cause primary polyuria (with a compensatory polydipsia).

Primary polydipsia is very uncommon and is usually psychogenic. Psychogenic polydipsia, or compulsive water drinking, is usually a manifestation of a behavioural problem triggered by an environmental or emotional stimulus (see Chapter 12).

In contrast, the causes of primary polyuria are much more numerous. The more common causes of PU/PD in dogs (including chronic renal failure, hyperadrenocorticism, hypercalcaemia, hyperthyroidism, liver failure and pyometra) are those that induce *secondary* nephrogenic diabetes insipidus (NDI), in which the renal tubules are insensitive to antidiuretic hormone (ADH). It should be noted that central diabetes insipidus (CDI) and primary NDI are uncommon but should always be considered as differential diagnoses in cases of PU/PD.

- Diabetes mellitus
- Chronic renal failure
- Hyperadrenocorticism
- Pyometra
- Drug administration (e.g. diuretics)
- Liver failure
- Hypercalcaemia
- Protein-losing nephropathy
- Hypoadrenocorticism
- Pyelonephritis
- Post-obstructive diuresis
- Psychogenic polydipsia
- Central diabetes insipidus (idiopathic, trauma-induced, neoplastic)
- Primary renal glycosuria
- Acromegaly
- Primary nephrogenic diabetes insipidus

14.1 Causes of polyuria and polydipsia in dogs, listed in approximate order from most to least common.

Osmotic diuresis

Osmotic diuresis occurs when the concentration of an osmotic solute, such as glucose present in the glomerular filtrate, exceeds the proximal tubular capacity for reabsorption. This impairs the passive reabsorption of water and results in increased obligatory water loss. By far the most common cause of osmotic diuresis leading to PU/PD is diabetes mellitus. Other causes include primary renal glycosuria, seen in the Norwegian Elkhound and Basenji, and the diuresis that follows relief of a postrenal obstruction (e.g. following urethral catheterization in an animal with urethral obstruction).

Diagnostic approach

The first step for any dog suspected of having PU/PD is to establish that the problem truly exists, preferably by home measurement of daily water consumption over 2–3 days and random urine specific gravity (USG) measurements on submitted samples.

Confirming PU/PD

- If daily water intake is normal, or if a random USG determination is >1.030, additional history should be obtained to rule out other urinary tract disorders (e.g. urinary incontinence or dysuria; see Chapter 26) that are commonly confused with polyuria
- If random USG measurements are consistently <1.030 and daily water consumption is >100 ml/kg, PU/PD is deemed to be present, and a diagnostic work-up to determine the cause is warranted

---

Sometimes the signalment, history and physical examination findings are very suggestive of a cause for the PU/PD, but it is often necessary to perform additional diagnostic tests. Figure 14.2 shows the general diagnostic approach to the patient with PU/PD.

History

Signalment: Some disorders that cause PU/PD develop more commonly in certain breeds or age groups of dog. For example:

- Hyperadrenocorticism (see Chapter 17) typically develops in middle-aged to older small breeds, such as the Miniature Poodle, Dachshund, West Highland White Terrier and Yorkshire Terrier
- The Standard Poodle, Bearded Collie, Rottweiler and Great Dane appear to be predisposed to developing hypoadrenocorticism (see Chapter 17); whilst this is a much less common condition, it should be considered in such a breed presenting with vague but consistent clinical signs

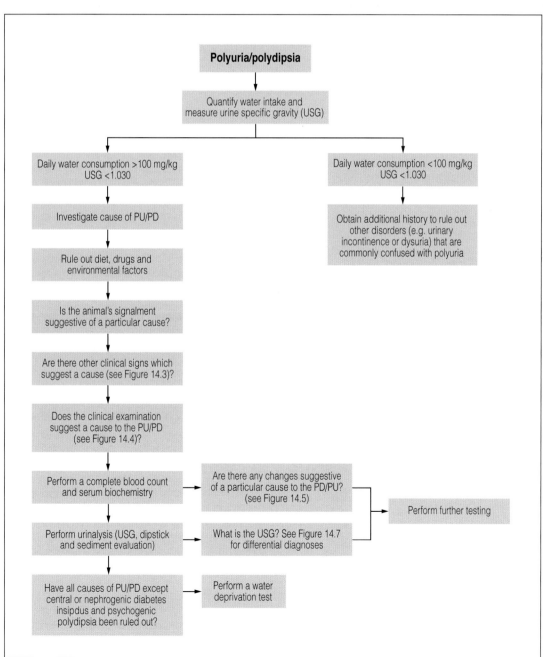

14.2

A general diagnostic approach to a dog with polyuria (PU) and polydipsia (PD).

■ Many of the other common causes of PU/PD (e.g. diabetes mellitus, chronic renal failure, liver failure and pyometra) are often found in older animals
■ Psychogenic polydipsia occurs more frequently in young, hyperexcitable, large-breed dogs
■ Pyometra should be high on the list of differential diagnoses in an intact bitch developing PU/PD during or immediately after the dioestrus phase of the oestrous cycle.

Diet: When evaluating an animal with PU/PD, the nature and composition of the diet should be taken into account, especially if clinical signs develop around the time of a dietary change. Food is an important source of water, and dogs fed on dry food invariably drink more water than those fed on moist food.

Drugs: Current or recent drug administration should also be ruled out as a cause of PU/PD. Medications that are frequently associated with PU/PD include glucocorticoids, phenobarbital and diuretics. Chronic administration of progestogens to intact bitches for oestrous suppression can lead to acromegaly (growth hormone excess), which can cause secondary diabetes mellitus.

Environmental factors: Environmental factors can trigger PU/PD in some animals. In dogs with psychogenic polydipsia it may be possible to identify a stressful environmental change that preceded the onset of clinical signs; examples include the arrival of a new baby or pet, or moving house. PU/PD that develops after head trauma could suggest damage to the ADH-secreting neurons or disruption to the pituitary stalk, resulting in CDI.

Clinical history: The presence of other clinical signs in the history may be helpful in determining the cause of PU/PD. Clinical signs more commonly associated with the different causes of PU/PD are listed in Figure 14.3.

Additional clinical signs	Possible causes of PU/PD
Progressive weight loss	Chronic renal failure, diabetes mellitus, hypercalcaemia, liver failure, protein-losing nephropathy
Weight gain	Hyperadrenocorticism
Anorexia or inappetence	Chronic renal failure, hypercalcaemia, pyometra, liver failure, hypoadrenocorticism, pyelonephritis
Polyphagia	Hyperadrenocorticism, diabetes mellitus
Gastrointestinal signs, e.g. vomiting, diarrhoea	Chronic renal failure, hypercalcaemia, liver failure, hypoadrenocorticism
Behavioural or neurological signs	Liver failure, psychogenic polydipsia, central diabetes insipidus
Very marked polydipsia in which patients almost continuously seek and consume water	Psychogenic polydipsia, central diabetes insipidus, primary nephrogenic diabetes insipidus
Recent oestrus (previous 2 months) in a middle-aged bitch	Pyometra

14.3 Additional clinical signs commonly associated with diseases causing PU/PD.

Physical examination
A careful clinical examination can help to identify many of the more common causes of PU/PD (Figure 14.4).

> **PRACTICAL TIP**
>
> Dogs with psychogenic polydipsia, CDI or primary NDI are typically alert and active, and seldom show any abnormalities on physical examination

Physical examination findings	Possible causes of PU/PD
Small or irregular kidneys	Chronic renal failure, protein-losing nephropathy
Large kidneys	Pyelonephritis, lymphoma (with hypercalcaemia)
Painful kidneys/sublumbar pain	Pyelonephritis
Hepatomegaly	Hyperadrenocorticism, diabetes mellitus
Alopecia, pot belly	Hyperadrenocorticism
Cataracts	Diabetes mellitus
Abdominal distension	Liver failure, hyperadrenocorticism, pyometra
Peripheral lymphadenopathy	Lymphoma (with hypercalcaemia)
Perianal mass	Anal sac adenocarcinoma (with hypercalcaemia)
Vaginal discharge	Pyometra
Fever, peri-renal pain	Pyelonephritis
Uraemic breath or stomatitis	Chronic renal failure

14.4 Physical examination findings associated with diseases causing PU/PD.

Laboratory tests
Even if the signalment, history and physical examination findings are suggestive of an underlying cause, it is usually prudent to perform further testing to confirm the suspicion or evaluate for concurrent disease. This is most important in older animals, as these patients may have more than one disease process present (e.g. the elderly dog with chronic renal failure and liver failure).

Complete blood count and serum biochemistry: A complete blood count (CBC) and serum biochemistry are the most useful initial screening tests when investigating dogs with PU/PD. These baseline tests often allow a diagnosis immediately; or they may offer clues as to the underlying cause of the PU/PD. Figure 14.5 shows differential diagnoses for some of the more commonly identified abnormalities on CBC and serum biochemistry, and suggests further tests. For example, dogs with hyperadrenocorticism commonly have elevated alkaline phosphatase (>90% cases), hypercholesterolaemia (>50% cases) and a stress leucogram (neutrophilia, lymphopenia ± eosinopenia).

Urinalysis: Urinalysis is a vital test when investigating the patient with PU/PD. The most important features are: USG; presence or absence of glucose, protein or bacteria; and the cellularity of the sample. Urine collection techniques are described in Chapter 26.

Parameter	Possible causes of PU/PD	Suggested further tests
Elevated urea and creatinine	Chronic renal failure, pyelonephritis, (protein-losing nephropathy)	Urinalysis, ultrasound evaluation of the kidneys
Decreased BUN	Liver failure (can be non-specific sign)	Measure bile acids
Hypercalcaemia (total and ionized)	Hypercalcaemia of malignancy, hypervitaminosis D, primary hyperparathyroidism, granulomatous disease, idiopathic, chronic renal failure, skeletal lesions	Identify source of hypercalcaemia with: thorough clinical examination; thoracic and abdominal imaging; ± measurement of PTH; ± measurement of PTHrP
Elevated liver enzymes	Liver failure	Measure bile acids
	Hyperadrenocorticism (especially if ALP>ALT)	ACTH stimulation tests ± LDDS test, abdominal imaging
	Diabetes mellitus	Measure blood and urine glucose
	Pyometra	Abdominal imaging
Hyperglycaemia	Diabetes mellitus	Measure urine glucose
	Hyperadrenocorticism (very mild increase)	ACTH stimulation tests ± LDDS test, abdominal imaging
Hyperkalaemia ± hyponatraemia	Hypoadrenocorticism	ACTH stimulation test
Hypercholesterolaemia	Hyperadrenocorticism	ACTH stimulation tests ± LDDS test, abdominal imaging
	Diabetes mellitus	Measure blood and urine glucose
	Protein-losing nephropathy	Quantify urine protein loss
	Liver failure	Measure bile acids
Hypoalbuminaemia	Liver disease	Measure bile acids
	Protein-losing nephropathy	Quantify urine protein loss
Stress leucogram (neutrophilia, lymphopenia ± eosinopenia)	Hyperadrenocorticism	ACTH stimulation tests ± LDDS test, abdominal imaging
	Any 'stressful' disease	Tests specific to the disease suspected

14.5 Abnormalities that may be identified on CBC and serum biochemistry, the diseases they are associated with, and suggested further tests. ACTH = adrenocorticotrophic hormone; ALP = alkaline phosphatase; ALT = alanine aminotransferase; BUN = blood urea nitrogen; LDDS = low-dose dexamethasone suppression; PTH = parathyroid hormone; PTHrP = PTH-related protein.

PRACTICAL TIP

Analysis of a urine sample should ideally be performed within 30 minutes of collection. Delayed analysis will allow any bacteria within the sample to proliferate, and the urine pH then becomes alkaline. Casts and cells may degrade as the urine 'ages', and crystals may either sediment out of solution or dissolve

---

Urinalysis should include:

- **Specific gravity:** must be done using a refractometer, as dipstick measurement of USG is unreliable
- **Dipstick evaluation:** for pH, protein, glucose, ketones, urobilinogen, bilirubin, blood, etc. (Figure 14.6)
- **Sediment examination:** for casts, erythrocytes, leucocytes, bacteria, yeast, crystals, abnormal cells, etc.
  - The sediment should be prepared by centrifuging a standardized volume of urine (1–5 ml) at 2000 rpm for 5 minutes. The supernatant is decanted and the remaining sediment resuspended in about 0.5 ml of supernatant or water

- A drop of urine is placed on a slide and can be examined stained or unstained
- **± Culture:** for bacteriology and sensitivity testing (samples should be obtained by cystocentesis)
- **± Urine protein:creatinine (UPC) ratio:** for diagnosis of protein-losing nephropathies.

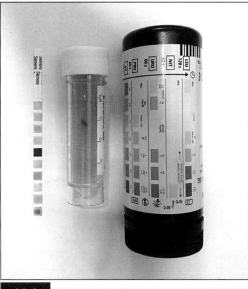

14.6 An example of a commercial dipstick testing kit.

Protein-losing nephropathies

Protein-losing nephropathies (e.g. glomerulonephritis, amyloidosis) are an important cause of PU/PD in dogs. They are addressed separately from 'chronic renal failure', as these animals **are often not azotaemic on presentation**. In a patient with PU/PD and a reduced USG (1.008–1.029), it is very important to measure urinary protein excretion by way of a UPC ratio, as part of the diagnostic work-up. Urine dipstick evaluation for protein can be unreliable, especially in the patient with very dilute urine

- A UPC of >0.5 with inactive urine sediment supports a diagnosis of a protein-losing nephropathy
- Significant proteinuria (UPC >0.5) in the presence of an inactive urine sediment *and dilute urine* can be associated with hyperadrenocorticism, pyelonephritis and pyometra

Additional diagnostic tests (see Figure 14.5) will help differentiate these various causes

Urine specific gravity:

- A USG of <1.030 suggests a concentrating defect and is consistent with PU/PD. The direction of further work-up can often be based on the USG (Figure 14.7). Note that glucosuria increases the measured USG; therefore the value will not be entirely representative of renal tubular concentrating function.
- A USG consistently 1.001–1.007 in a middle-aged to older dog is usually associated with hyperadrenocorticism, or less commonly with CDI (complete or partial), primary NDI or psychogenic polydipsia. It is important to remember that not all dogs with hyperadrenocorticism show 'classic' signs of disease, and PU/PD may be the only abnormality present. Moreover, these animals may lack the serum biochemistry abnormalities commonly associated with hyperadrenocorticism (see Figure 14.5). In a dog with a USG 1.001–1.007, hyperadrenocorticism should be ruled out before testing for CDI, primary NDI and psychogenic polydipsia. This should be done by performing tests including an adrenocorticotrophic

hormone (ACTH) stimulation test and low-dose dexamethasone suppression (LDDS) test, in combination with other investigations such as abdominal ultrasonography (see QRG 14.1).

- A USG of 1.008–1.029 can be associated with hyperadrenocorticism, chronic renal failure, hypercalcaemia, protein-losing nephropathies or pyelonephritis, as well as psychogenic polydipsia. Hyperadrenocorticism, chronic renal failure, hypercalcaemia and protein-losing nephropathies should be ruled out first (see Figure 14.5), followed by pyelonephritis, before evaluating the patient for psychogenic polydipsia.

PRACTICAL TIP

Pyelonephritis can sometimes be difficult to diagnose, but a positive bacterial culture, active urine sediment (red and white blood cells, casts, protein) and a dilated renal pelvis on ultrasonography are supportive of this diagnosis. If these changes are not present, a therapeutic trial with an appropriate antibiotic (e.g. potentiated amoxicillin, fluoroquinolone) could be instigated

Water deprivation test

The water deprivation test is used for the final evaluation of the patient with PU/PD. **Its only indication is to distinguish between CDI, primary NDI and psychogenic polydipsia.** In theory, urine will become concentrated in animals with psychogenic polydipsia but will remain dilute in animals with CDI and primary NDI.

WARNING

- The water deprivation test should be performed only after all other causes of PU/PD have been ruled out, limiting the differential diagnoses to CDI, primary NDI and psychogenic polydipsia
- Dogs with many of the more common causes of PU/PD may respond to a water deprivation test in a similar manner to a dog with CDI, primary NDI or psychogenic polydipsia. Even more importantly, use of the water deprivation test in such patients may be dangerous
- The test should be performed with great care, as it can result in rapid alterations of water and electrolyte balance that can be life-threatening
- It is **contraindicated** in azotaemic and/or dehydrated patients and in patients with known renal disease. Patients that are dehydrated have, by definition, already failed the test

Urine specific gravity	Differential diagnoses (in approximate order from most to least common)
1.001–1.007	Hyperadrenocorticism Psychogenic polydipsia CDI (complete or partial) Primary NDI
1.008–1.029	Hyperadrenocorticism Chronic renal failure Protein-losing nephropathies Hypercalcaemia Pyelonephritis Psychogenic polydipsia
>1.030 without glycosuria	Unlikely to be polyuric or polydipsic: no further work-up required

14.7 Differential diagnoses for causes of PU/PD based on urine specific gravity.

Because use of the water deprivation test is limited to differentiating between some of the less common causes of PU/PD it is beyond the scope of this chapter and readers are referred to the *BSAVA Manual of Canine and Feline Nephrology and Urology* and the *BSAVA Guide to Procedures in Small Animal Practice*.

Notes on treatment

The treatment of every disorder causing PU/PD is beyond the scope of this chapter (the reader is referred to the relevant BSAVA Manuals), but some general points should be noted.

- Until the mechanism of PU/PD is understood, water intake should **not** be restricted.
- Dogs with PU/PD should be provided with free access to water unless they are vomiting. In the vomiting patient, parenteral fluids should be administered along with other supportive therapies.
- Parenteral fluids should also be provided when other conditions limit oral intake or the dog appears to be dehydrated despite oral intake.
- The hypercalcaemic animal may require additional parenteral fluid therapy and other measures (e.g. furosemide) to reduce serum calcium. Prolonged hypercalcaemia can lead to irreversible renal damage and other detrimental effects.
- In most cases, directly treating the underlying cause will improve or resolve the PU/PD.
- PU/PD will likely continue in a dog with chronic renal failure, and some animals benefit from additional fluid therapy via subcutaneous administration.
- Treat psychogenic polydipsia by gradually limiting water intake to a normal daily volume (20–90 ml/kg/day). Animals should probably have their water intake reduced over days to weeks to avoid undesirable behavioural side effects that could occur.

Diabetes mellitus: treatment overview

For more details see the *BSAVA Manual of Canine and Feline Endocrinology* and the *BSAVA Manual of Canine and Feline Rehabilitation, Supportive and Palliative Care*. See also Chapter 17

- Once the diagnosis is established, all dogs require insulin. Most dogs respond well to subcutaneous lente insulin administered at a dose of 0.5–1.0 IU/kg q12h. Owners should be instructed on the handling, storage and administration of insulin
- Commercial diets are available for diabetic dogs; if these are not used, the diet should contain digestible carbohydrates and increased fibre. Feed half the calorific requirement at the time of insulin administration
- Consider weight reduction in obese dogs
- Dogs should be exercised at approximately the same time each day and the amount of exercise should be roughly the same each day
- Assess the control of glycaemia primarily by monitoring clinical signs. Additional testing such as the measurement of fructosamine or serial blood glucose measurements are also required in some dogs
- Monitor for complications including: blindness and anterior uveitis resulting from cataract formation; hypoglycaemia; recurring infections, especially those of the lower urinary tract; and ketoacidosis

---

Chronic renal failure: treatment overview

For more details see the *BSAVA Manual of Canine and Feline Nephrology and Urology* and the *BSAVA Manual of Canine and Feline Rehabilitation, Supportive and Palliative Care*

- Once the diagnosis is established, management is supportive
- Nutrition plays a central role in the management of chronic renal failure, and diet should be tailored to the individual patient
- It is vital that dogs are encouraged to eat
- If blood phosphate is elevated, consider a phosphate-restricted diet
- If blood phosphate is still elevated after starting a phosphate-restricted diet, consider phosphate binders
- Encourage water intake
- Monitor for proteinuria and treat if present (e.g. an angiotensin-converting enzyme (ACE) inhibitor, protein-restricted diet, omega-3 fatty acid supplementation)
- Monitor for hypertension and treat if present (e.g. ACE inhibitor, calcium channel blocker)

Polyphagia

Polyphagia is an increased food intake, which can be manifested by the dog eating either more frequently and/or consuming a greater quantity than normal. Some animals that are polyphagic may also show signs of excessive food-seeking and food-stealing behaviour.

Polyphagia may be prompted by:

- Failure to assimilate nutrients or an increased loss of nutrients (e.g. exocrine pancreatic insufficiency)
- Inability to use nutrients (e.g. diabetes mellitus, gastrointestinal parasites, poor-quality diet)
- Hypoglycaemia (e.g. insulinoma, insulin overdose)
- Increased metabolic rate or demand (e.g. cold environment, pregnancy, lactation)
- Psychological or learned behaviour (e.g. palatable diets, competition with others for food)
- Endogenous or exogenous glucocorticoids or other drugs (e.g. anticonvulsants).

The causes of polyphagia are listed in Figure 14.8.

Diagnostic approach

History

A complete history should be obtained for the polyphagic patient, with particular attention to the type and quantity of food fed.

Signalment: Some disorders causing polyphagia develop more commonly in certain breeds or age groups. For example:

- Hyperadrenocorticism typically occurs in middle-aged to older small breeds
- In an entire bitch, pregnancy or lactation should be considered as possible causes of polyphagia

Pathological
■ **Diabetes mellitus** ■ **Hyperadrenocorticism** ■ **Gastrointestinal parasites** ■ **Exocrine pancreatic insufficiency** ■ Inflammatory bowel disease ■ Lymphangiectasia ■ Insulinoma

Physiological
■ **Pregnancy** ■ **Lactation** ■ Growth ■ Cold environment ■ Increased exercise

Pharmacological and dietary
■ **Poor diet** ■ **Overfeeding** ■ **Corticosteroids** ■ **Anticonvulsants** ■ Benzodiazepines ■ Progestins ■ Insulin overdosing ■ Competition for food

14.8 Causes of polyphagia in dogs. Those more commonly identified in small animal practice are shown in **bold**.

- The young German Shepherd Dog or Rough-Coated Collie with polyphagia should raise the suspicion of exocrine pancreatic insufficiency (EPI)
- Diabetes mellitus is often found in older dogs
- Gastrointestinal parasites are more common in young animals
- Inflammatory bowel disease and lymphangiectasia can occur in animals of any age.

Diet: It is advisable to ask owners to bring in the dog's normal food and for them to show the quantity fed per day. To determine whether sufficient food is being given, the caloric value of the diet should be noted from the container, and the dog's resting energy requirement (RER) calculated (see Chapter 4). The amount of exercise the dog receives should be considered in light of the amount of food fed. Questions should also be asked about the dog's environment, with particular reference to competition for food in a multi-animal household.

Other considerations:

- Current or recent drugs should be ruled out as a cause of polyphagia, especially corticosteroids, anticonvulsants, benzodiazepines and progestins.
- A history of weight loss suggests the presence of a concurrent disease, whereas weight gain, or a change in body shape, may suggest hyperadrenocorticism.
- A concurrent history of PU/PD (see above) suggests diabetes mellitus or hyperadrenocorticism.
- Chronic vomiting, diarrhoea and weight loss raise the suspicion of gastrointestinal parasites (in puppies and adolescent dogs), lymphangiectasia or inflammatory bowel disease.
- The presence of voluminous faeces and steatorrhoea supports the diagnosis of EPI, although it should be noted that this is not a consistent finding in all cases.

Physical examination

Findings on physical examination may be helpful when investigating the patient with polyphagia (Figure 14.9). Particular attention should be paid to the dog's body condition, quality of the hair coat, presence of organomegaly or abdominal enlargement.

Physical examination findings	Possible causes of polyphagia
Poor body condition (<2 on a 5-point scale)	Gastrointestinal parasites, diabetes mellitus, exocrine pancreatic insufficiency, lymphangiectasia, inflammatory bowel disease, pregnancy, lactation
Excessive body fat	Does not suggest a particular underlying medical condition. Consider: overfeeding, drug administration, hyperadrenocorticism, insulinoma
Hepatomegaly	Hyperadrenocorticism, diabetes mellitus
Alopecia, pot belly	Hyperadrenocorticism
Poor-quality hair coat	Hyperadrenocorticism, exocrine pancreatic insufficiency
Abdominal enlargement	Pregnancy, hyperadrenocorticism
Cataracts	Diabetes mellitus

14.9 Physical examination findings in patients with polyphagia, and possible underlying causes.

Laboratory tests

When the cause of polyphagia is not apparent from the signalment, history or physical examination findings, a CBC and serum biochemistry can offer clues as to the underlying cause (Figure 14.10).

Additional tests may include:

- Faecal analysis to rule out gastrointestinal parasites. Alternatively, a therapeutic trial with a suitable anthelmintic could be performed
- Measurement of trypsin-like immunoreactivity (TLI) for the diagnosis of EPI. As noted earlier, the young German Shepherd Dog or Rough-Coated Collie with voluminous faeces, diarrhoea, weight loss and polyphagia should prompt the suspicion of EPI. However, not all dogs with EPI develop voluminous faeces or diarrhoea. Older dogs of any breed can sometimes also develop EPI, usually a result of end-stage chronic pancreatitis.

Notes on treatment

The treatment of every disorder causing polyphagia is beyond the scope of this chapter (see relevant BSAVA Manuals), but some general points should be noted.

- Animals without weight gain, or with weight loss, should **not** have food restricted, as an underlying disorder is likely.
- In dogs with a pathological cause of polyphagia, treatment of the underlying disease usually resolves or significantly reduces the polyphagia.
- In dogs with a physiological cause of polyphagia, increasing their energy intake is usually all that is required. Consideration should also be given to using a diet with a higher energy density, especially if the volume of food becomes excessive.

Parameter	Possible cause of polyphagia	Suggested further tests
Elevated liver enzymes	Hyperadrenocorticism (especially if ALP>ALT)	ACTH stimulation tests ± LDDS test, abdominal imaging
	Diabetes mellitus	Measure blood and urine glucose
	Corticosteroid administration (ALP>ALT)	
	Anticonvulsants (phenobarbital) (ALP>ALT)	
Hyperglycaemia	Diabetes mellitus	Measure urine glucose
	Hyperadrenocorticism (very mild increase)	ACTH stimulation tests ± LDDS test, abdominal imaging
Hypoglycaemia	Insulinoma	Measure serum insulin, abdominal ultrasonography, exploratory laparotomy
	Insulin overdose	
Hypercholesterolaemia	Hyperadrenocorticism	ACTH stimulation tests ± LDDS test, abdominal imaging
	Diabetes mellitus	Measure blood and urine glucose
Hypoalbuminaemia ± hypoglobulinaemia	Lymphangiectasia, inflammatory bowel disease	Ultrasonography and biopsy of the gastrointestinal tract
Stress leucogram (neutrophilia, lymphopenia ± eosinopenia)	Hyperadrenocorticism	ACTH stimulation tests ± LDDS test, abdominal imaging
	Any 'stressful' disease	Tests specific to the disease suspected

14.10 Abnormalities that may be identified on CBC and serum biochemistry, the diseases they are associated with, and suggested further testing. ACTH = adrenocorticotrophic hormone; ALP = alkaline phosphatase; ALT = alanine aminotransferase; LDDS = low-dose dexamethasone suppression.

- Owners should measure food given, to assess intake accurately.
- Some dogs may benefit from the addition of low-calorie bulking foods to the diet.
- Feeding smaller meals several times per day may be beneficial in some animals.
- Polyphagia as a result of drug administration may decrease if a dose alteration is made. Alternatively, different therapy protocols can be considered.

Inappetence

Inappetence refers to a loss or lack of appetite and the term is often used interchangeably with anorexia.

Inappetence is a common but usually non-specific complaint in small animal practice and is often associated with a systemic disease process (Figure 14.11). The pathophysiology is complex. For example: in part, inflammatory, immune-mediated and neoplastic diseases cause inappetence due to the release of pro-inflammatory cytokines such as interleukin-1 and tumour necrosis factor; endogenous toxins contribute to the decreased appetite seen in renal, liver and other diseases; altered gastrointestinal tract motility associated with metabolic disorders, gastrointestinal tract disease and neoplasia contribute to inappetence; fear, pain and stress may also decrease appetite in some patients; decreased appetite has also been associated with aging, and is thought to be mediated in part by cholecystokinin released from the gastrointestinal tract and an enhanced satiating effect of intestinal carbohydrates.

Inappetence can also occur in dogs that have any disease causing painful or dysfunctional prehension, mastication and swallowing (Figure 14.12); these animals may display an interest in food but be unwilling to eat.

- Gastrointestinal disease
- Renal disease
- Liver disease
- Neoplasia
- Cardiac disease
- Respiratory disease
- Endocrine disease
- Metabolic disease
- Infectious disease
- Neurological disease
- Toxicities and drugs
- Motion sickness
- Pain, fear, stress
- Anorexia of aging

14.11 Major causes of inappetence in dogs.

- Stomatitis/gingivitis/glossitis/pharyngitis
- Retropharyngeal abscess/haematoma/lymphadenopathy
- Dental or periodontal disease
- Retrobulbar disease
- Salivary gland inflammation or neoplasia
- Masticatory myositis
- Fractures of the jaw
- Diseases of the temporomandibular joint
- Oesophagitis
- Cranial nerve V, VII, IX and X neuropathies
- Central nervous system diseases

14.12 Examples of conditions that cause problems with prehension, mastication and swallowing.

Diagnostic approach

History

It is important first to determine whether the dog has an interest in food and the ability to prehend, masticate and swallow. Patients with disorders causing dysfunction or pain of the oral cavity, oropharynx, other regions of the head or the oesophagus, may show interest in food but cannot eat. These patients commonly display weight loss with halitosis and excessive salivation. Conversely, animals with systemic disease usually have little interest in food.

A thorough general history should be obtained to evaluate for clinical signs that may be associated with diseases leading to inappetence. In order to identify any psychological causes, details about the dog's environment, diet, other pets and people should be obtained. Current or recent drug administration should also be ruled out as a cause.

Physical examination

A multitude of physical examination findings may be present in the inappetent patient and these vary with the underlying cause. A complete physical examination is therefore required to determine the presence of systemic disease leading to inappetence. Findings may include fever, icterus, pain, changes in organ size, abdominal distension, masses and abnormal heart or lung sounds.

A thorough ophthalmic, dental, oropharyngeal, facial and cervical examination is required to identify diseases causing painful or dysfunctional prehension, mastication and swallowing (see Chapter 20). Sedation or general anaesthesia may be necessary. The patient can also be observed while feeding, noting signs of pain or dysfunction.

Laboratory tests

Complete blood count, biochemistry, urinalysis: If the dog has a lack of interest in food and therefore a systemic disease is suspected, a CBC, serum biochemistry and urinalysis are the most useful initial screening tests. Abnormalities will vary with the different underlying diseases.

PRACTICAL TIP

Test results can sometimes be normal, especially in patients with conditions causing painful or dysfunctional prehension, mastication and swallowing

---

Other more specific laboratory tests may be required to rule out diseases suggested by the history, physical examination and initial diagnostic tests. For instance, investigating for the presence of liver disease as a cause of inappetence may require the measurement of pre- and post-feeding bile acids.

Diagnostic imaging: Radiography and ultrasonography are often required to detect thoracic and abdominal pathology. More advanced imaging modalities such as computed tomography (CT) or magnetic resonance imaging (MRI) may be performed if there is a suspicion of central nervous system (CNS) disease. Fluoroscopy is useful when evaluating the ability of a patient to prehend, masticate and swallow food. Additional diagnostic procedures such as endoscopy to investigate gastrointestinal disease or biopsy of abdominal organs may also be required.

Notes on treatment

The mainstay of treatment is aimed at identifying and correcting the underlying disease causing the inappetence. Some general rules in the management of the inappetent dog can be noted. More detail can be found in the *BSAVA Manual of Canine and Feline Rehabilitation, Palliative and Supportive Care: Case Studies in Patient Management.*

- Modification of the diet may improve palatability. Consider warming food to body temperature, adding flavoured toppings and increasing the fat content.
- As a general rule, animals should not remain inappetent or anorexic for longer than 3–5 days

before alternative feeding methods (e.g. a naso-oesophageal tube, Figure 14.13) should be instigated.
- Animals with severe weight loss, hypoproteinaemia or a chronic disease likely to cause continued inappetence should ideally receive supplemental nutrition.
- An appetite stimulant for use in dogs is mirtazapine (0.6 mg/kg orally q24h).
- Analgesics may improve appetite in painful conditions.
- Anti-emetics such as metoclopramide and maropitant are useful to decrease nausea-associated inappetence.

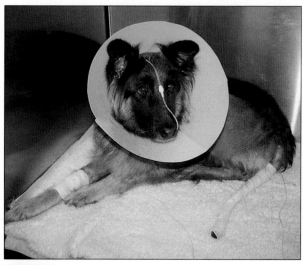

14.13 A German Shepherd Dog with a naso-oesophageal feeding tube in place. The tube is secured by glue and sutures. An Elizabethan collar prevents the dog interfering with the tube.

Weight loss

Definitions

- Weight loss here refers to an unintended loss of bodyweight
- Cachexia, often considered a state of severe weight loss, is usually secondary to a severe underlying disease

---

Weight loss is a non-specific clinical sign in dogs and is caused by a multitude of conditions. Weight loss may occur due to decreased nutrient intake, increased loss of nutrients, increased nutrient use, maldigestion, malabsorption or malassimilation (Figure 14.14). Weight loss of >10% of bodyweight is particularly significant.

PRACTICAL TIP

If other problems with a more defined list of differential diagnoses (e.g. PU/PD, polyphagia, jaundice) are also present, they should be investigated first

---

Decreased nutrient intake

- Anorexia
- Poor-quality diet
- Underfeeding
- Competition for food
- Dysphagia, regurgitation, vomiting

Increased nutrient loss

- Protein-losing enteropathy
- Protein-losing nephropathy
- Intestinal parasites
- Neoplasia
- Chronic blood loss (epistaxis, haematemesis, haematuria, melaena)
- Diabetes mellitus
- Effusions

Increased nutrient use

- Neoplasia
- Physiological (e.g. cold environment, exercise, fever, pregnancy, lactation)

Maldigestion and malabsorption

- Inflammatory and infiltrative small intestinal disease
- Lymphangiectasia
- Severe intestinal parasitism
- Exocrine pancreatic insufficiency

Malassimilation

- Hepatic failure
- Cardiac failure
- Renal disease
- Hypoadrenocorticism
- Neoplasia

14.14 Causes of weight loss in dogs.

Diagnostic approach

History

Figure 14.15 provides an overview of the diagnostic approach to the dog with unintended weight loss. It is vital to determine whether the dog has a history of a normal, increased or decreased appetite. Weight loss despite a good appetite usually indicates maldigestion, malabsorption, increased utilization or physiological factors.

A complete dietary history is required in order to determine nutrient intake, the type and quantity of food consumed and any changes to the diet. The caloric value of the diet should be noted and the dog's resting energy requirement (RER) calculated (see Chapter 4) to determine whether sufficient food is being fed.

- Questions should also be asked about the dog's environment, with particular reference to competition for food in a multi-animal household.
- Information on the patient's activity and environment can help to determine calorie expenditure.
- The dog's history should be reviewed for evidence of dysphagia, regurgitation, vomiting, or increased use of calories (e.g. pregnancy, lactation, a cold environment, exercise).
- Questions should be asked about the consistency of the faeces to indicate whether malabsorption may be present.

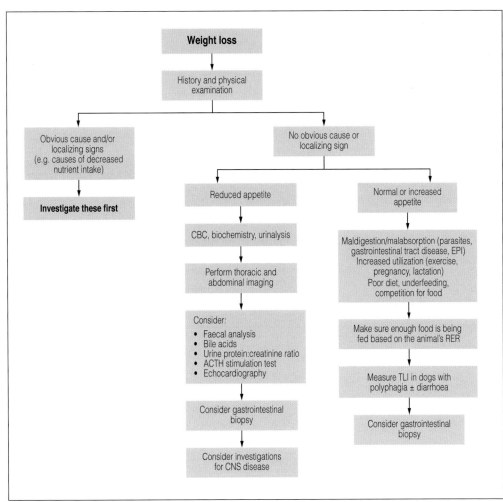

14.15 A diagnostic approach to the dog with unintended weight loss. ACTH = adrenocorticotrophic hormone; CBC = complete blood count; CNS = central nervous system; EPI = exocrine pancreatic insufficiency; RER = resting energy requirement; TLI = trypsin-like immunoreactivity.

- Other historical findings such as PU/PD, lethargy, vomiting, exercise tolerance, coughing, changes in body size and neurological signs may help to identify an underlying disease.

Physical examination

Physical examination should include measurement of bodyweight, body condition score (see Chapter 4) and an assessment of muscle wasting. Bodyweight can be compared against historical data for the dog to determine the exact amount of weight lost. Muscle wasting is assessed by palpating over the skull and scapulae, as well as palpation of the longissimus and gluteal muscles.

A complete physical examination should be performed to identify abnormalities that might help localize the problem to a particular organ or body system. Fever suggests an underlying infectious, inflammatory or immune-mediated disease. Lack of fever is more consistent with metabolic causes of weight loss such as renal, hepatic, cardiac or gastrointestinal disease.

Diagnostic tests

A CBC, serum biochemistry and urinalysis are the most useful initial screening tests to identify the presence of an underlying disease such as organ failure or inflammation. Abnormalities will vary with the different underlying diseases causing weight loss.

PRACTICAL TIP

Test results can sometimes be normal, especially in patients with decreased nutrient intake leading to weight loss

---

Other more specific laboratory tests may be required, determined by the most likely differential diagnoses, on the basis of findings on the history, physical examination and initial diagnostic tests. The following is a suggested list of further investigations when considering the dog with weight loss:

- Thoracic and abdominal imaging to detect neoplasia or the presence of systemic disease
- Examination of serial (ideally three) faecal samples, for intestinal parasites
- Measurement of pre- and post-feeding bile acids, to rule out liver dysfunction
- Determination of UPC ratio, to detect protein-losing nephropathy
- ACTH stimulation test in dogs with intermittent lethargy, gastrointestinal signs and/or PU/PD

- Measurement of serum TLI for dogs with polyphagia and/or diarrhoea
- Gastrointestinal endoscopy and biopsy to identify inflammatory and infiltrative small intestinal disease and lymphangiectasia. The majority, but not all, patients with these disorders will have diarrhoea and/or vomiting
- Echocardiography in animals with suspected cardiac disease, even if thoracic radiographs are normal
- Evaluation of the CNS for causes of anorexia or infectious, inflammatory or neoplastic diseases leading to weight loss.

PRACTICAL TIPS

- If the cause of weight loss remains undetermined, daily physical examination should be carried out to localize any disease
- For example, pyrexia may be intermittent in some animals with immune-mediated or inflammatory disease. In the older animal with unexplained and significant weight loss, neoplasia is the major differential diagnosis. In such cases, one may have to wait until the tumour progresses enough to be detectable

---

Treatment

The most important consideration is to treat the underlying cause of the weight loss.

Additionally, appropriate nutritional support should be provided, based on the dog's RER. If the dog is able to ingest, digest and absorb nutrients, oral nutrition is the preferred route. If the dog is unable or unwilling to ingest food, but can digest and absorb nutrients, enteral nutrition should be provided. Methods for providing enteral nutrition include the use of a naso-oesophageal, oesophageal or gastrostomy feeding tube (see *BSAVA Guide to Procedures in Small Animal Practice* for details).

References and further reading

Barr F and Gaschen L (2011) *BSAVA Manual of Canine and Feline Ultrasonography*. BSAVA Publications, Gloucester

Bexfield N and Lee K (2014) *BSAVA Guide to Procedures in Small Animal Practice, 2nd edn*. BSAVA Publications, Gloucester

Elliott J and Grauer GF (2007) *BSAVA Manual of Canine and Feline Nephology and Urology, 2nd edn*. BSAVA Publications, Gloucester

Lindley S and Watson P (2010) *BSAVA Manual of Canine and Feline Rehabilitation, Supportive and Palliative Care: Case Studies in Patient Management*. BSAVA Publications, Gloucester

Mooney CT and Peterson ME (2012) *BSAVA Manual of Canine and Feline Endocrinology, 4th edn*. BSAVA Publications, Gloucester

QRG 14.1 Testing for hyperadrenocorticism: some important considerations

ACTH stimulation test

Details of how to perform this test can be found in the *BSAVA Guide to Procedures in Small Animal Practice*.

The ACTH stimulation test only reliably identifies ~50% of dogs with adrenal-dependent disease and ~85% of dogs with pituitary-dependent disease. This means that significant numbers of cases will be missed if only an ACTH stimulation test is performed. Moreover, this test incurs false-positive results relatively frequently. For example, dogs with 'chronic stress' due to the presence of another disease may have adrenal gland hyperplasia and thus an abnormal ACTH test response.

Low-dose dexamethasone suppression test

Details of how to perform this test can be found in the *BSAVA Guide to Procedures in Small Animal Practice*.

The LDDS test is more reliable than the ACTH test in confirming hyperadrenocorticism, as the results are diagnostic in the majority of adrenal-dependent cases and in ~90–95% of pituitary-dependent disease. However, the LDDS test is also prone to false-positive results, generally due to stress during the 8-hour period over which the test is performed.

PRACTICAL TIP

In a patient that becomes stressed during hospitalization, consideration should be given to sending the animal home during the period between blood sampling

Adrenal gland ultrasonography

Adrenal gland ultrasonography is an important technique to aid the diagnosis of hyperadrenocorticism. The adrenal glands of a dog with pituitary-dependent hyperadrenocorticism (PDHAC) are symmetrically enlarged; a thickness of >7.5 mm for the left adrenal gland is considered to provide the best sensitivity and specificity as a diagnostic test for PDHAC. However, increases in adrenal gland thickness are not specific enough to warrant the use of adrenal ultrasonography as a screening test for hyperadrenocorticism, as there is considerable overlap between normal and hyperplastic adrenal glands.

Adrenal gland hyperplasia can occur in animals with chronic stress, such as in a variety of diseases including diabetes mellitus and pyometra.

If one adrenal gland is enlarged, and the other is hypoplastic, especially if the larger gland is asymmetrical or invasive, this supports a diagnosis of adrenal-dependent hyperadrenocorticism.

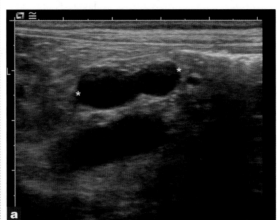

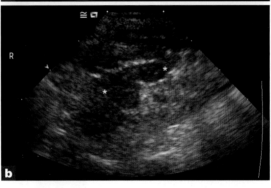

Ultrasonograms of the bilaterally enlarged (a) left and (b) right adrenal glands in a dog with PDHAC. Note that the shape of the glands is bilaterally preserved; however, both glands appear 'plump'. Asterisks indicate the long axis of the gland. Reproduced from the *BSAVA Manual of Canine and Feline Ultrasonography*.

Lameness

15

Tim Hutchinson

The lame dog is one of the more common presentations to first-opinion vets and any vet working in a busy general practice will be faced with such a case on a daily basis. Rather than a systematic review of all causes of lameness (which is covered elsewhere – especially the *BSAVA Manual of Canine and Feline Musculoskeletal Disorders*), this chapter will focus on the initial approach to the lame dog, to help the clinician develop a list of the common differential diagnoses for further investigation and treatment. Neurological causes and generalized weaknesses that may present with a gait abnormality are dealt with in Chapters 11 and 17. Lameness associated with acute trauma (such as a road traffic accident) is of secondary concern to the assessment and stabilization of the traumatized patient, which is considered in Chapter 10. Essentially, this chapter will consider the approach to the orthopaedic patient.

The aim of the first-opinion 10-minute consultation should be to work through the following plan:

1. Is the dog lame?
2. Which limb is affected?
3. Gathering baseline data.
4. The seat of pain – which part of the limb is affected?
5. What are the most common differentials?
6. What further investigations or treatment are appropriate?

Observation

> **Definition of lameness**
>
> For the purposes of this chapter, lameness will be considered to be: reduced or absent use of one or more limbs, associated with discomfort

With moderate to severe unilateral lameness the affected limb will be readily apparent as the animal hobbles into the consulting room. However, observation should begin as early as possible: preferably with the posture of the dog as it sits in the waiting room and how it rises as the client is called. For example, dogs with stifle discomfort will often sit on one haunch with both hindlegs to one side of the body (Figure 15.1) because the full flexion of the stifle required to sit normally will be painful.

Watching how the dog moves (from behind, in front and from the side) in straight lines and turning can be very useful, but should always be *on a flat surface*. For subtle lameness this may be the best way to identify which leg is affected (this may differ from the owner's opinion).

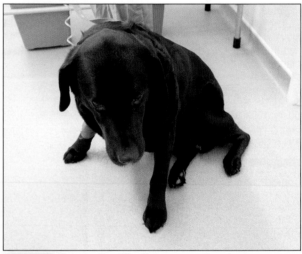

15.1 Dogs with stifle disease usually adopt a characteristic sitting posture, with both hindlegs to one side of the body.

With any lameness the dog will be willing to place more weight on the unaffected leg(s):

- For the forelimb, this will mean that as the sound leg contacts the ground the dog's head will sink, but as the painful leg bears weight the dog's head will rise
- For hindlimbs, the gluteal region will lift as the painful leg strikes the ground
- With bilateral hindlimb lameness, there may be 'bunny hopping', which is particularly noticeable with increased speed of movement
- Young dogs with bilateral forelimb disorders (e.g. medial compartment elbow disease) may have a shuffling gait or seem alternately lame on each limb.

Observation of the moving dog should also note the passage of the *affected* leg through the swing phase:

- Is it flicked out?
- Is it swung laterally, to avoid flexion of the joints required to maintain normal sagittal movement?

There may also be hints (such as ataxia, weakness or spasticity) that the problem may be something other than orthopaedic (see relevant chapters).

History: baseline data

Clinical training in the university environment usually involves extremely thorough history-taking, relating not just to the presenting condition but to all aspects of the animal and its environment. Whilst the importance and value of such a thorough approach should not be underestimated, it is time-consuming beyond the scope of most first-opinion consultations and will often merely duplicate data already in the clinical records. Instead, it is important to establish the key facts relating to the presenting complaint, expanding as required, and reserve a full history for those cases that require significant further investigation. With experience these data may be obtained in tandem with the clinical examination for greater efficiency.

The most important points to be addressed for a lame dog include:

- **Age:** Is the patient:
  - A skeletally immature dog: Raises the suspicion of a developmental disorder:
    - Most developmental disorders will become apparent at 5–8 months
    - Skeletal maturity can be considered to be present at 12 months (up to 15 months in giant breeds)
  - A young adult (typically 1–6 years): Trauma is more likely
  - An older dog: Osteoarthritis is likely
- **Breed:** Certain conditions are more common in specific breeds, which can affect how much weight should be given to a specific differential.
  - For example, hip dysplasia is rife amongst German Shepherd Dogs, but rarely, if ever, seen in Greyhounds
- **Duration:** When did the owner first notice the problem and has it been constant since then?
  - This should be viewed in light of the physical examination, and the degree of muscle atrophy present, which might conflict with the reported onset. For example, a dog with cruciate disease may have been lame for several months, with a marked degree of muscle atrophy, but may only be presented by the owner when that lameness worsens suddenly, as the ligament finally snaps completely or the meniscus tears
- **Was there an obvious inciting cause?**
  - There may be a history of obvious trauma or acute lameness after vigorous exercise
  - An owner may relate the lameness to a less specific insult that resulted in worsening of a previously unnoticed condition

- **Is there any history of previous orthopaedic problems (in the affected limb or another limb) or past trauma?**
- Can the owner describe the lameness? For example:
  - Is the lameness worse after rest, but eases with gentle exercise (might be consistent with osteoarthritis)
  - Is the lameness constant and restrictive to exercise (might suggest a muscle problem).

Physical examination: identifying the seat of pain

Although time may be limited, and there is a desire to get to the cause of the problem as quickly as possible, rushing straight to the affected limb is never indicated. A lame dog is likely to be in pain and anxious; taking time to ensure that it is relaxed and comfortable in the consulting environment will greatly enhance the results of the physical examination. This time can be used for assessing the general physical state of the dog (see Chapter 3) and gathering data from the owner; it may also give an indication as to whether further restraint (or protection) is required before manipulating a painful area.

The approach taken to the examination of a limb may differ from one clinician to another, but it is vital that whatever approach is adopted, it is systematic, thorough and involves examination of the contralateral limb for comparison. The author's preference is to work from the distal extremity of the limb proximally, and to split the examination into palpation and manipulation.

Palpation
Without moving the limb, all aspects are palpated – from the toes to the dorsal midline. This allows the identification of any particularly sensitive areas, which may then modify how the joints are examined and manipulated. For example, if long bone palpation produces a pain response, then to examine the joints at either end of the bone will necessitate manipulation without holding the painful long bone area. Also, if joint pain is identified through palpation alone then it can be predicted that manipulation of the joint will be even more painful, and flexion and extension examinations should be carried out with care.

Pain from palpation of the long bones is unusual in dogs, but is seen relatively commonly in four conditions:

- Panosteitis (Figure 15.2): usually affects juvenile dogs; German Shepherd Dogs are over-represented
- Neoplasia (Figure 15.3): middle-aged and older larger breeds usually affected; key sites of predilection are the metaphyseal regions close to the stifle and away from the elbow
- Metaphyseal osteopathy: metaphyses will be markedly misshapen, hot and painful
- Physeal injuries: e.g. Salter–Harris type II fracture (Figure 15.4).

Particular attention should be paid to the feet, as conditions of the feet and digits can be acutely

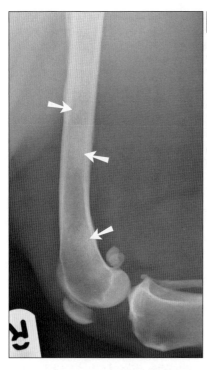

15.2

Panosteitis is one of the few common causes of bone pain. Radiographically it presents as radiodense 'thumbprint' lesions on the long bones (arrowed).

15.3

Primary bone neoplasia, most commonly osteosarcoma, usually affects the extremities of the long bones away from the elbow and towards the stifle. Unusually, the distal tibia was involved in this case.

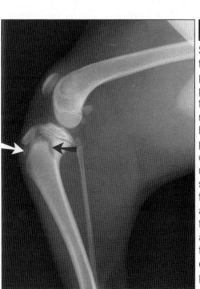

15.4

Salter–Harris type II fracture of the proximal tibia. On presentation, such fractures are often remarkably stable, but there is marked pain and swelling of the metaphyseal region. Note the small bone fragment below the avulsed tibial tuberosity (white arrow) and the fracture line extending from the physis (red arrow).

painful, with dramatic and severe lameness resulting from small focal areas such as sepsis around a nail. Conditions of the feet are discussed in detail in Chapter 29.

Note should be made of the shape of the long bones and the angles of the joints with the dog standing, to assess for valgus or varus deformity. Some breeds with naturally bowed legs can be difficult to assess and it may be useful to gauge valgus together with palpation of the metaphyseal region to feel for any obvious thickenings. Any areas of thickening or swelling (especially compared with the contralateral limb) should be noted, as well as heat consistent with acute inflammation.

Joints should be palpated for effusions. These are readily identified in the carpus, elbow, hock and stifle, but are very hard to discern in the hip and shoulder:

- Carpus: pouching of the joint is easily identified on the dorsal aspect
- Elbow: effusions can be voluminous and are most prominent on the lateral aspect caudal to the lateral humeral epicondyle (Figure 15.5)
- Tarsus: there will be distension of the joint around the collateral ligaments, both medially and laterally, at the tarsocrural joint
- Stifle: joint effusion is easily palpated to either side of the straight patellar ligament (Figure 15.6).

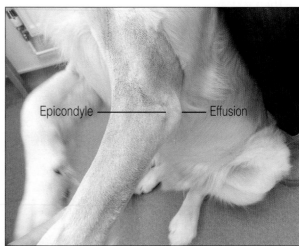

15.5 Elbow effusions can be particularly voluminous, as in this 6-month-old Golden Retriever with osteochondrosis dissecans (OCD). There is a large distension caudal to the lateral epicondyle.

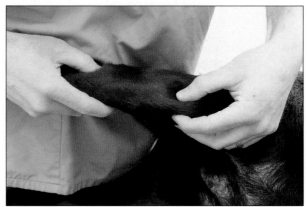

15.6 Stifle effusion is easily palpated as a bulging of the joint capsule to either side of the straight patellar ligament.

Manipulation

Following palpation, examination should proceed to manipulation of the joints. This should be done in such a way as to be able to flex and extend one joint at a time, avoiding direct pressure on any previously identified sensitive regions. Joints should be carefully flexed and extended, noting: the range of motion (again, using the contralateral limb as reference); any evidence of crepitus; and any pain response.

Examining specific joints

Interphalangeal and metacarpo/tarsophalangeal joints

Injuries to the digital joints are common at any age, but especially in very energetic dogs.

- With ligament disruption or fractures there is usually obvious swelling and deformity and a history of acute onset.
- For subtle injuries it is helpful to apply pressure from all angles to each digit separately. for signs of excessive movement.
- Osteoarthritis of the interphalangeal and metacarpo/tarsophalangeal joints is often seen in older animals. The foot tends to collapse, taking on a flatter appearance with splayed digits and joint thickenings. It should not be underestimated as a cause of lameness.

Carpus

Acute trauma to the carpus is usually associated with profound and obvious swelling. Common injuries to the carpus involve hyperextension or damage to the collateral ligaments.

- Hyperextension can be assessed by extending the joint from the elbow (pushing distally on the olecranon) whilst exerting an opposing force on the palmar aspect of the foot with the other hand (Figure 15.7). Note: If there is obvious joint swelling, this is likely to be extremely painful and such examination should be carried out under sedation.
- Laxity in the collateral ligaments can be assessed by holding the foot firmly and moving from side to side; however, the carpus is a very lax joint generally, and any movement must be referenced against the normal limb.
- Carpal bone fractures are commonly seen (and will be accompanied by diffuse joint swelling and acute onset). Fractures to the proximal portions of metacarpals II and V can cause significant joint instability due to the effective avulsion of the collateral ligament.

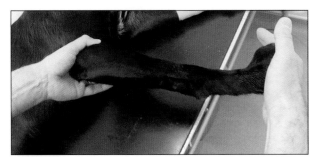

15.7 Examining the carpus for hyperextension injury is best achieved by simultaneously compressing from the olecranon and the palmar aspect of the foot.

Elbow

The elbow is a very rewarding joint to examine.

- Effusions are readily palpated, especially caudal to the lateral epicondyle.
- Deposition of new bone associated with chronic disease is easily identified as firm thickenings medially and laterally around the insertions of the joint capsule. This can be so pronounced that it is not possible to feel the fossa between the lateral epicondyle and the olecranon.
- In young dogs with medial compartment disease, the medial aspect of the joint, just distal to the medial epicondyle, can be exquisitely painful as pressure is applied directly over the region of the medial coronoid process. As the elbow is a hinge joint, it is easy to assess objectively the range of motion and the degree of flexion or extension that produces a pain response. In advanced osteoarthritis, where periarticular new bone can produce massive thickening of the joint (Figure 15.8), flexion can be severely restricted. This in turn will lead to a very clumsy gait as the leg is swung away from the body. In early elbow disease where changes may be subtle, it can be useful to flex and extend the joint in varying degrees of pronation and supination, which will affect the pressure through the medial compartment.

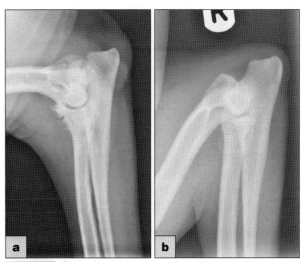

15.8 Periarticular new bone formation can be **(a)** dramatic compared with **(b)** the normal joint causing marked thickening which is readily palpable.

Shoulder

The shoulder is an unusual joint, in that movement is often minimal during walking, with the whole limb swinging in a sagittal plane through the actions of the extrinsic shoulder muscles and the majority of limb shortening to permit the swing occurring at the carpus and elbow. Shoulder lameness may therefore be much less obvious than lameness associated with the more distal joints.

- Palpation of both shoulders simultaneously (from the dorsal aspect, standing astride the dog) can be useful to detect muscle atrophy – especially in the supra- and infraspinatus muscle groups.
- Three important manipulations can be used for the shoulder to assess for a pain response:

- Cranial traction of the limb, pulling the leg forward with one hand and pushing back on the shoulder with the opposite hand. Note: This can also produce a pain response in dogs with cervical disc disease due to traction on the nerve roots
- Caudal traction of the limb, to flex the shoulder and simultaneously palpate around the biceps tendon. In a normal joint there must be reciprocal flexion of the elbow to facilitate shoulder flexion, due to the limiting action of the biceps. With the shoulder flexed, pressure can be exerted to extend the elbow to assess the pain response through the biceps. In cases of biceps tendon rupture or avulsion of the supraglenoid tubercle, extension of the elbow with the shoulder in flexion will be possible
- Abduction of the shoulder joint, i.e. abduction of the humerus and distal limb with the scapula held flat. This puts strain through the medial glenohumeral ligament, which is a common site of shoulder ligament injury.

Tarsus

- Tarsal lameness is invariably accompanied by swelling (acute) or thickening (chronic) of the joint, which may significantly reduce the range of movement.
- Injuries or degeneration of the intertarsal or tarsometatarsal joints will be accompanied by inappropriate movement of these tight joints, dorsoplantar deviation, or thickening around the supporting ligaments. Particular attention should be paid to the Achilles tendon, feeling for areas of thickening. Fractures of the proximal portion of metatarsals II and V will have a destabilizing effect similar to the carpus.

PRACTICAL TIP

The talocrural joint is remarkably mobile, and this mobility can easily be confused with ligament damage

---

Stifle

The stifle is the single most common joint implicated in orthopaedic lameness in the dog. A thorough examination should include:

- Palpation for evidence of joint effusion
- Palpation for thickening of the fibrous soft tissues around the medial collateral ligament (medial buttressing)
- Assessment of muscle atrophy in the thigh: quadriceps atrophy is a particular feature of stifle disease
- Assessment of the mobility of the patella. The patella should be pushed medially and laterally, with the joint in varying degrees of flexion, to assess whether it will luxate and, if so, in which direction and at which stifle position. Patellar luxation is a very common orthopaedic disorder
- Assessment for anterior cruciate ligament instability, using cranial drawer and tibial thrust (see QRG 15.1)

- The joint should be flexed and extended fully, to feel for crepitus or any clicks or even clunks, the latter often associated with a tear in the medial meniscal cartilage
- In cases of acute lameness, especially in small terrier puppies, palpation around the tibial tuberosity should be performed to detect signs of avulsion (Figure 15.9).

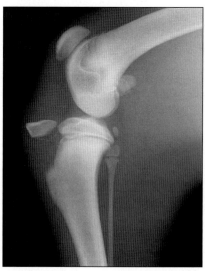

15.9

Avulsion of the tibial tuberosity is a common injury in juvenile dogs, requiring prompt surgical attention.

Hip

As a true ball and socket joint, the hip should be free to move through a global range without evidence of pain. Palpation for effusion is invariably unrewarding.

Pain from hip disease is most frequently encountered with the limb fully extended caudally, or abducted. It is helpful to rest one hand over the hip joint whilst the other manipulates the limb to feel for crepitus and laxity. Young dogs with markedly dysplastic hips may exhibit palpable (and sometimes audible) subluxation as the femoral head slips over the dorsal acetabular rim. In extreme cases this can be apparent by resting the hands over the hips with the dog standing and rocking the hindquarters from side to side. In less severe cases, and especially if painful, hip laxity is best assessed with the dog sedated (see QRG 15.2).

It is worth noting that many young dogs with extremely lax hips may not display overt discomfort, but may present with a 'bunny hopping' gait.

PRACTICAL TIPS

When recording findings in the clinical records it is helpful to be as descriptive as possible. Lameness scales (e.g. 7/10 lame) are subjective and may vary from one observer to another, so describing the lameness may be more useful

- Be precise about any anatomical landmarks that are associated with pain on palpation and try to quantify the degree of manipulation of a joint that produces a reaction
- Always double check that the correct limb has been recorded, as some conditions may be bilateral and it is important for future examination to know for certain on which limb the dog was previously lame

---

Differential diagnosis

Common conditions associated with specific joints are listed in Figure 15.10. The suspicion of a particular condition may be raised when a susceptible joint in an over-represented breed is identified as the source of lameness (Figure 15.11).

Because of the frequency of occurrence of developmental orthopaedic disorders, it is helpful to refine the list of the more common differentials with the consideration of juvenile (<1 year old) *versus* adult dogs.

Juvenile dogs

Many young dogs presenting with lameness concurrent with acute inflammation will have an underlying developmental disorder. It is important to detect these at as early an age as possible, as this may significantly affect the outcome. Common conditions include:

Condition	Breeds commonly affected
Medial compartment elbow disease (fragmented coronoid process; osteochondrosis dissecans, OCD)	Retrievers, Bernese Mountain Dog, Rottweiler
Ununited anconeal process	German Shepherd Dog, giant breeds (especially Great Dane, Mastiff)
Incomplete ossification of the humeral condyle	Spaniels
Shoulder OCD	Gundogs (e.g. Vizsla, retrievers)
Tarsal OCD	Labrador Retriever, Bull Terrier
Achilles tendinopathies	Can occur in any breed if traumatic; idiopathic in Dobermann
Plantar ligament disorders	Collies
Anterior cruciate ligament disease	Can occur in any breed, but very common in retrievers, Rottweiler, Mastiff, Boxer, and in small breeds with overly steep tibial plateau angles
Luxating patella	Medial luxation: terrier breeds, spaniels, Labrador Retriever. Lateral luxation: giant breeds, Labrador Retriever
Tibial tuberosity avulsion	Very common in small terriers, especially West Highland White Terrier
Hip dysplasia	Found in most breeds except for racing breeds. Over-represented in retrievers, German Shepherd Dogs, spaniels
Avascular necrosis of the femoral head (Legg–Calvé–Perthes disease)	Small terrier breeds

15.11 Breeds commonly affected by specific orthopaedic disorders. This list is far from exhaustive, but picks out some of the more commonly presented breeds and conditions.

Digital joints
- Fractures
- Luxations
- Ligament damage

Carpus
- Hyperextension injuries
- Collateral ligament tears/avulsion
- Metacarpal fractures (proximal fractures of metacarpals II or V may lead to carpal instability)
- Carpal bone fractures

Elbow
- Fragmented coronoid process
- Osteochondrosis dissecans (OCD) of medial aspect of humeral condyle
- Ununited anconeal process
- Incongruency
- Luxation
- Incomplete ossification of the humeral condyle

Shoulder
- OCD
- Medial glenohumeral ligament tears
- Bicipital tendonitis
- Luxation

Tarsus
- OCD
- Achilles tendinopathies
- Plantar ligament disorders
- Metatarsal fractures (proximal fractures of metatarsals II and V may lead to tarsometatarsal instability)
- Tarsal bone fractures

Stifle
- Anterior cruciate ligament disease
- Luxating patella
- Tibial tuberosity avulsion

Hip
- Hip dysplasia
- Avascular necrosis of femoral head
- Luxations
- Fractures of femoral head/neck

15.10 Some of the more commonly presented problems of specific joints. This list is far from exhaustive, but includes those conditions that should be excluded first in any investigation.

- Osteochondrosis dissecans (OCD)
- Joint incongruency
- Subluxations (especially the hip)
- Physeal injuries.

It is important to remember that skeletal growth is rapid and precedes the development of supporting muscle mass. Also, the supporting capsule and ligaments are considerably more elastic in juvenile dogs than in their adult counterparts. The implication of this is that a joint may feel adequately reduced and congruent on a basic examination, but may actually be quite lax when subjected to the rigours of boisterous puppy exercise. Careful questioning regarding lifestyle and diet is necessary, as owners may have been given inappropriate advice by breeders (e.g. to restrict exercise in a young growing dog of a breed susceptible to joint disease). Bone is a very plastic tissue and develops around the forces applied through it. Consequently, it is the type of exercise that is more damaging than the amount. Five minutes of bounding around the garden and jumping up and down at the fence to get to the cat next door can be far more damaging than several miles of controlled lead walking; there will be good bone-to-bone contact in the latter, with movement within an appropriate and controlled range, which will encourage good joint development.

Adult dogs

The increased muscle bulk associated with physical maturity and the decreased elasticity of supporting fibrous structures reduces the injury that can occur to joints through subluxation associated with joint laxity. Consequently, strain injuries are more common.

Occasionally, acute inflammation may still be the result of a previously quiescent developmental abnormality, for example late fragmentation of the coronoid process, but usually lameness associated with such conditions in adults will be due to the secondary osteoarthritis (see below).

Geriatric dogs

With advancing age the incidence of osteoarthritis increases. Any breed that is over-represented for a developmental disorder as a puppy should be considered to be over-represented for arthritis in that same joint when older.

Further investigations

Radiography

Radiography is the primary tool of choice for first-opinion investigation of orthopaedic disease. However, radiography of an entire limb in the absence of a thorough physical examination may be unrewarding or dangerously misleading. Rather, it should be used for further investigation of a specific painful or deformed anatomical region.

Radiographic abnormalities may be detected that do not correlate with clinical lameness. For example, moderate to advanced remodelling of the hip may be present in dogs with little or no hip pain, and may cause the clinician to overlook the subtle changes associated with a more clinically relevant condition, such as early cruciate disease (Figure 15.12).

Occasionally clients may present a young dog with acute-onset lameness following an apparent inciting cause. Examination may reveal a painful swollen joint and the decision to move straight to radiography may be hard to justify before empirical treatment (rest and anti-inflammatory medication) has ruled out a sprain injury. More frequently, however, a young dog is presented with a history of several days (or even weeks) of intermittent or persistent lameness, with pain localized to a specific joint on examination. In these cases it is almost always justified to admit the dog for examination and radiography under sedation. Such cases may be very early in the course of a developmental disorder and radiographic changes may be subtle. It is important to obtain good quality images that are well positioned (Figure 15.13) and appropriately collimated and exposed, in order to increase the likelihood of a diagnosis (see *BSAVA Manual of Canine and Feline Radiography and Radiology*). Further opinions from more experienced colleagues should be sought, if in doubt; they will also be able to advise on the limitations for further investigation and treatment within the individual practice and when referral may be necessary.

In younger adult dogs with lameness associated with a specific anatomical region and minimal gross thickening, the presumptive diagnosis of a sprain or strain injury may be top of the list of differentials, and empirical treatment is frequently justified. However,

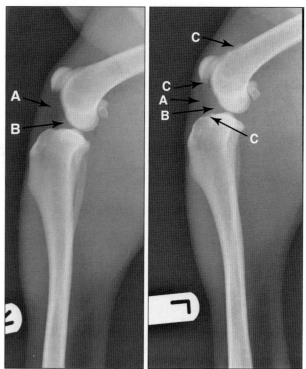

15.12 It is important not to overlook early changes in a joint that, although subtle, may be more significant than advanced changes elsewhere that may be quiescent. Comparison with the contralateral limb can be useful, as in this case of early cruciate disease: early changes are shown by joint effusion and subtle new bone deposition. A = fat pad; B = synovial fluid; C = osteophytes.

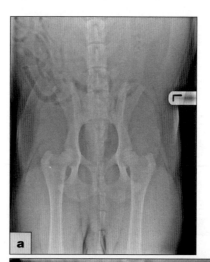

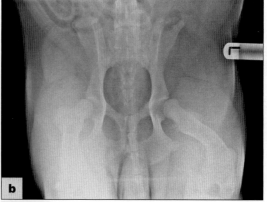

15.13 Two radiographs of a dog with hip dysplasia. **(a)** In the standard ventrodorsal view, the joint structure looks reasonable. **(b)** With the legs raised into a weight-bearing position, subluxation of the joints is obvious.

such cases should always be re-examined 10–14 days later (sooner if lameness is especially marked) and the clinician should be open-minded about reconsidering the previous diagnosis.

Osteoarthritis as a diagnosis for lameness is more common with increasing age, but can also mask other conditions. Sudden-onset lameness, or worsening of a previously noted lameness, may be associated with a flare-up of a previously diagnosed condition – or with something new. Again, radiography is the initial diagnostic tool, with the expectation that there may be signs of chronic articular changes. However, the older, arthritic patient is also more likely to be affected by problems of other body systems and the investigation of lameness may need to run hand-in-hand with the investigation of other, apparently unrelated, conditions.

Treatment

A detailed discussion of treatment for specific conditions can be found in the *BSAVA Manual of Canine and Feline Musculoskeletal Disorders*. However, it is worth emphasizing two general areas here.

Hip dysplasia

In young dogs with lameness, or breeds susceptible to joint problems, type of exercise can significantly affect the development of a condition. This is most clearly demonstrated with the hip joint. In hip dysplasia (Figure 15.14), joint laxity allows the femoral head to subluxate from the acetabulum and impact on the dorsal acetabular rim. This has two detrimental effects: damage to the acetabular rim and femoral head, due to concussive injury of weight-bearing through a reduced surface area; and failure to convey weight-bearing through the articular surfaces, which is necessary for the correct formation of the coxofemoral joint.

Increased uncontrolled boisterous exercise, which might result, for example, from an owner trying to restrict exercise by allowing a dog only to play in the garden, will lead to excessive subluxation and joint damage. Increasing controlled exercise, through lead walking, will promote appropriate weight-bearing and joint development. As a general rule of thumb for any young growing dog, lead walking is beneficial, off-lead play is not; exuberant puppy energy is best diverted to on-lead walks.

Osteoarthritis

Osteoarthritis (OA) may be the result of:

- Wear and tear on a normal joint (normal loading of normal joint)
- Normal wear of an abnormal joint (e.g. in joint incongruency)
- Abnormal wear of a normal joint (e.g. the result of injury or excessive high-performance exercise, or the increased demands placed on a joint by obesity)
- Abnormal wear of an abnormal joint (obesity, injury or excessive exercise superimposed on a joint with imperfect development).

The first of these is common in humans but very rare in dogs, whereas the other three are much more frequently encountered in the veterinary consulting room, and dogs may develop almost crippling degenerative joint disease at a comparatively young age.

There are three golden rules for the treatment of osteoarthritis.

- **Control joint inflammation to relieve pain:**
  - This is achieved primarily through the judicious use of non-steroidal anti-inflammatory drugs (NSAIDs):
    - A short course may be used to reduce inflammatory flare-up to a quiescent state
    - Lifelong medication may be needed for refractory cases.

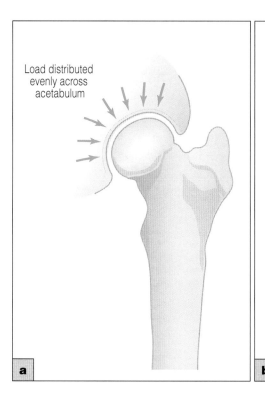
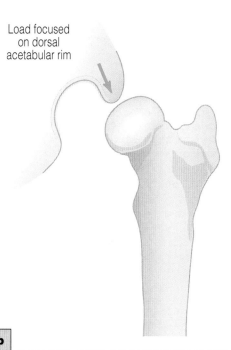

15.14 Hip dysplasia is essentially increased elasticity of the coxofemoral joint. **(a)** Whilst the joint may have the ability to be congruent, **(b)** weight-bearing allows the femoral head to subluxate so that weight-bearing is focused through a much reduced joint surface area.

Load distributed evenly across acetabulum

Load focused on dorsal acetabular rim

a

b

- **Control exercise:**
  - Thick leathery joint capsules, which are often calcified at their insertions on the bones, are much less resilient to the normal wear and tear of exercise
  - Hyperextension or sudden shearing motions (such as may be encountered in uncontrolled, vigorous exercise) may lead to tearing of fibres in the capsule due to reduced elasticity, causing pain and inflammation
  - Conversely, inactivity leads to stiffness and atrophy of supporting muscles
  - Exercise is therefore very important for arthritic patients, but should be tailored to what is appropriate for a particular condition, and varied if the condition changes (Figure 15.15).
- **Control bodyweight:**
  - The peak vertical force that passes through a joint during walking massively exceeds the weight of the dog
  - Reducing excess weight will reduce the force that a damaged joint has to sustain.

Grade of lameness	Type of exercise	Method	Patient example
7	No exercise; passive physiotherapy only	Cage rest/ hospitalization	Articular fracture pending surgery
6	Minimum, low-impact	Short toileting walks only	Immediately after articular surgery
5	Supervised, controlled	High frequency, short duration walks	Recuperation after articular surgery; arthritis flare-up
4	Lead-controlled	Decreased frequency, longer duration walks	Progression of the above, as condition improves
3	Extended, lead-controlled		
2	Supervised, off-lead	NB Warm up and wind down on the lead	
1	Supervised, free		
0	Unrestricted	Uncontrolled environment	Healthy dog
–1	Performance	Agility, etc.	Healthy high-performance dog

15.15 An exercise guide for lame dogs. This can be extremely useful to give to owners to indicate what stage exercise should have reached by the next review consultation. It may be that for a specific condition only a certain grade may ever be achievable; for example, a severely arthritic dog may only ever manage to get to grade 3 or 4. An owner who understands the limitations is likely to be more compliant and more satisfied than one with unrealistic expectations.

This is the 'Holy Trinity' of arthritis treatment; although there may be many other treatment options (e.g. physiotherapy, acupuncture) they remain as adjuncts to the above and should never be substituted for any of those three. This can require tactful discussions with clients. Controlling exercise and weight management in their dog requires significant input by the owner and often a lifestyle change. Also, NSAIDs can be perceived as 'nasty' drugs and clients may be keen to look for a 'safer, natural' alternative. Nutraceuticals may have a role in the treatment of arthritis in dogs, but research has shown little benefit over placebos in many trials (Vandeweerd *et al.*, 2012). The ability to rebuild the structure of damaged articular cartilage will be limited in many canine arthritic patients, which often have severe erosion of the cartilage due to focused weight bearing on a small joint surface due to incongruency (Figure 15.16).

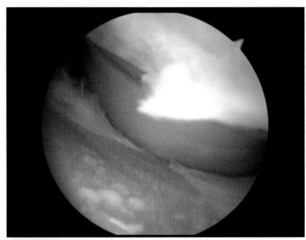

15.16 Arthroscopic view of the elbow in a 6-month-old Labrador Retriever, showing joint incongruency with severe cartilage destruction.

References and further reading

Coughlan A and Miller A (2006) *BSAVA Manual of Canine and Feline Fracture Repair and Management* [*revised reprint*]. BSAVA Publications, Gloucester

Holloway A and McConnell F (2014) *BSAVA Manual of Canine and Feline Radiography and Radiology: A Foundation Manual.* BSAVA Publications, Gloucester

Houlton JEF, Cook JL, Innes JF and Langley-Hobbs SJ (2006) *BSAVA Manual of Canine and Feline Musculoskeletal Disorders.* BSAVA Publications, Gloucester

Lindley S and Watson P (2010) *BSAVA Manual of Canine and Feline Rehabilitation, Supportive and Palliative Care: Case Studies in Patient Management.* BSAVA Publications, Gloucester

Vandeweerd J-M, Coisnon C, Clegg P *et al.* (2012) Systematic review of efficacy of nutraceuticals to alleviate clinical signs of osteoarthritis. *Journal of Veterinary Internal Medicine* **26**, 448–456

QRG 15.1 Assessment of anterior cruciate instability

This is achieved by demonstrating cranial translocation of the tibia (i.e. movement of the tibia cranially with respect to the femur) with the joint held at a fixed degree of flexion. It should be performed with the joint at varying angles, but the joint should neither flex nor extend during the test. This can usually be carried out with the dog conscious, but in painful, tense or fractious animals may be facilitated by sedation. There are two techniques.

Cranial drawer test

This test should be performed with the joint in varying degrees of flexion, but the joint should always be static during the test.

1 With the dog in lateral recumbency, hold the distal femur firmly with one hand by placing the thumb behind the lateral fabella, the forefinger on the patella, and supporting the distal femur and thigh with the rest of the hand.

2 Use your other hand to hold the proximal tibia firmly, placing the thumb behind the head of the fibula, the forefinger on the tibial tuberosity and supporting the proximal tibia and crus with the rest of the hand.

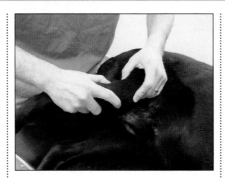

3 With the joint held such that it will neither flex nor extend, attempt to move the tibia cranially with respect to the femur, as if pulling a drawer forwards. In normal joints there is a small amount of movement and an abrupt stopping point as the cruciate ligament becomes taut. When there is damage to the ligament there will be excessive movement, which will gradually become tighter as the joint capsule becomes taut to limit the movement.

Anterior tibial thrust

1 Use one hand to hold the stifle joint to prevent flexion or extension, by seating the patella in the cup of the hand, supporting the joint with the fingers and thumb, but extending the forefinger down the tibial tuberosity.

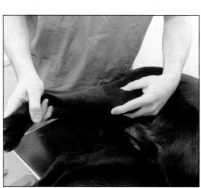

2 Grasp the foot with your other hand, and gradually flex the hock (whilst always holding the stifle in a fixed degree of flexion).

3 With a normal joint there will be no movement in the stifle during attempts to flex the hock. With anterior cruciate instability there will be cranial translocation of the proximal tibia (detected by the forefinger on the tibial tuberosity) when the hock is flexed.

QRG 15.2 Assessing hip laxity

This is best performed with the dog sedated and can be combined with radiography of the hips.

1 With the dog in lateral recumbency, flex the stifle to allow the distal femur to be grasped in one hand.

2 Rest your other hand over the pelvis, with the thumb over the greater trochanter of the femur.

3 Lower the stifle towards the table and push the femur proximally (the hand on the pelvis preventing movement of the dog). These actions allow abduction of the femoral head so that it rides up on to the dorsal acetabular rim.

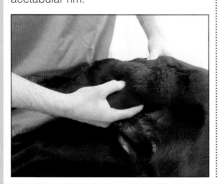

4 Maintaining the proximal thrust on the femur, rotate the limb away from the plane of the table until the femoral head slips back over the dorsal acetabular rim and reduces into the acetabulum. This sudden reduction is accompanied by a palpable, and often audible 'thud', which is referred to as the Ortolani sign.

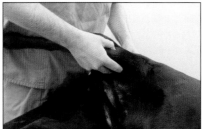

Notes:

- This laxity and the Ortolani sign can also be demonstrated bilaterally with the dog in dorsal recumbency and the femurs forced perpendicularly towards the table.
- However, the benefit of assessing each joint individually is that the degree of laxity when the femoral head abducts from the acetabulum can be felt with the overlying thumb.
- With experience this measurement, whilst still subjective, can be quite accurate.

Paralysis and spinal pain

Alex Gough

Spinal disease is a common presentation in practice. Dogs with spinal disease can present with a range of signs, including pain (which can sometimes be quite difficult to localize), ataxia, and paresis or paralysis.

Definitions

- Ataxia refers to a failure of muscle coordination, and can be vestibular, cerebellar or proprioceptive (due to lesions in the forebrain, brainstem, spinal cord or peripheral nerve)
- Paralysis, or the suffix -plegia, refers to an inability to initiate movement
- Paresis refers to a reduced ability to initiate movement
- Monoparesis or monoplegia involves only one limb
- Hemiparesis or hemiplegia involves one side of the body
- Paraparesis or paraplegia involves the pelvic limbs
- Tetraparesis, quadriparesis or quadriplegia involves all four limbs

---

Presentations that require emergency attention include:

- Severe pain
- Paralysis or marked paresis
- Trauma that is known to or might involve damage to the vertebrae.

Obtaining a detailed history and a careful physical examination are essential in formulating a differential diagnosis, localizing the lesion and giving a prognosis. Some cases of inability or reluctance to move will be due to weakness (see Chapter 17) or pain rather than neurological conditions.

History

History-taking should include the recent general health of the animal (e.g. appetite, thirst, weight loss, exercise tolerance, cough, breathing difficulties, vomiting, diarrhoea) as well as previous ill health, vaccination status and parasite control. Any history of foreign travel or exposure to toxins should be ascertained. Historical data important in the investigation of the suspected spinal patient include urinary function, such as continence and ability to void consciously. Episodes of crying out for no apparent reason, or unusual behaviour, may suggest that pain is a feature of the condition. Speed of onset and progression of the disease are important in compiling a differential diagnosis list. For example, degenerative conditions such as degenerative myelopathy tend to be chronic and progressive, whereas a vascular event such as a fibrocartilaginous embolism is more likely to be acute, with slow improvement.

Clinical examination

A full neurological examination should be undertaken, including cranial nerve assessment (see also Chapters 11 and 21).

Notes on handling

- A dog with a suspected spinal cord injury should be handled sympathetically. Many cases will be in marked pain, and there is a risk of injury to owners and clinicians from aggressive behaviour
- Every effort should be made to prevent movement of the spinal column, but it is accepted that moving a patient for investigation and treatment is necessary, and can be carried out using a spinal board (if the patient will tolerate this without struggling), stretcher or blanket
- Once a patient is sedated or anaesthetized, intrinsic immobilization of the spinal column from the musculature is abolished, and it is vital at this stage that movement of the spinal column is minimal. Therefore the patient should only be sedated or anaesthetized once it has been transferred to a flat surface or a stretcher

---

Observation

Specific examination of the patient with suspected spinal disease should include assessment of posture (e.g. there may be a wide-based stance) and gait. Lameness, paresis/paralysis and ataxia should be differentiated by observation of the dog walking:

- A dog with lameness due to pain will exhibit a shortened stride or even carry the affected limb
- A dog with paresis will often drag the limb.

Occasionally, lameness can be due to a neurological lesion affecting the nerve root ('nerve root signature', i.e. referred pain causing lameness or elevation of the limb). Bilateral lameness can cause signs that mimic neurological disease. Ataxic patients lack co-ordinated movement (see also Chapter 11). Patients with gait problems due to orthopaedic problems are discussed in Chapter 15.

Testing proprioception

After observation, the patient should be assessed for conscious proprioception. This can be done in a number of ways, including:

- Placing the dog's foot on a piece of paper and sliding it sideways
- Hopping (picking up three of the dog's feet to make it hop)
- Hemi-walking (picking up two feet on the same side and letting it hop sideways)
- 'Wheelbarrowing' (picking up the hindlegs and walking the dog forwards)
- Tactile placing (letting the dorsal part of the dog's feet touch the side of a table while its eyes are covered).

The author's preferred first method is to turn each foot over in turn so that the dorsal foot is in contact with the ground or table top (the knuckling test). It is important that this is done gently, so as not to elicit a withdrawal response, and that only the foot is moved, to avoid stimulation of receptors in other joints.

PRACTICAL TIP

It is important to make an allowance for the reluctance of a lame animal to return its foot to a normal position because of pain. Supporting the animal's weight while performing the knuckling test (Figure 16.1) can help reduce this problem

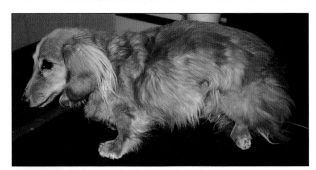

16.1 Delayed placing reaction due to reduced conscious proprioception in a 4-year-old Dachshund with intervertebral disc disease, demonstrated using the knuckling test.

In all of these tests, a normal dog will return its leg to a normal position under its centre of gravity. A dog with poor proprioception will show a delayed response, leading to a slow or absent return to a normal position after knuckling (Figure 16.1) or the paper-slide test, or the limb moving a significantly long way beyond the centre of gravity on hopping and hemi-walking tests. Multiple tests of proprioception may be necessary, especially in equivocal cases.

Testing spinal reflexes

The spinal reflexes can be assessed next.

The most important reflex is the **pedal withdrawal reflex**. Pinching firmly between the pads with thumb and forefinger should lead to a firm withdrawal, involving flexion of all the joints. The amount of pressure and the strength of withdrawal can be assessed in this way. This is a useful test for sciatic nerve function.

The **panniculus (cutaneous trunci) reflex** is tested by pinching the skin just lateral to the spine on both sides with artery forceps, starting from the lumbosacral region and working cranially, one vertebra at a time. A normal reaction is a skin twitch. The sensory pathways of this reflex are the spinal nerves from T11 to L1, so any lesion caudal to L1 will display a normal reflex. Note: The efferent arm of this reflex is the lateral thoracic nerve, so an absence of motor function of the panniculus reflex can be due to a lesion at the level of cord segments C8 to T1, which can mislead as to the localization.

The **patellar reflex** is easily performed: with the animal in lateral recumbency, the upper limb is tested. The patellar ligament is struck briskly with a reflex hammer (Figure 16.2). A normal response is a single, quick extension of the stifle. Absence may indicate a spinal lesion at L4–L6, or the femoral nerve root, but dogs over the age of 10 years and dogs with stifle pathology may also have an absent patellar reflex (Levine *et al.*, 2002).

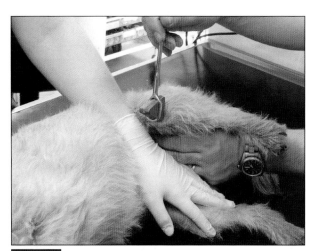

16.2 Evaluating the patellar reflex.

The **perineal reflex** is assessed by gently stroking the perineum on the right and the left. A normal response is contraction of the anal sphincter and flexion of the tail.

Other reflex tests such as triceps and gastrocnemius can be performed, but are less important. Although specific reflex tests can accurately localize a lesion, what is more important in the initial assessment of a case is deciding whether the reflexes are generally reduced, reduced in one specific limb, or are normal. This can help localize a lesion to one of four spinal locations (see Figure 16.3), but also helps to differentiate central from peripheral lesions.

PRACTICAL TIPS

- Reduced spinal reflexes in all four limbs is suggestive of a polyneuropathy, but it is important to distinguish muscle weakness from neurological disease
- A dog with muscle weakness and no neurological disease may have weak spinal reflexes, but will have normal conscious proprioception

---

Pain assessment

Once non-painful procedures have been concluded, the next step is to assess the dog for neck and spinal pain. This can be done by firmly palpating the vertical and lateral spinal processes to assess for an aversive reaction.

Neck pain should also be assessed by flexing the neck. A young dog without neck pain should be able to put its nose flat along its flank. Although the dog should not be forced into this position, some reasonable pressure to overcome the dog's natural resistance to performing this task is acceptable. Some dogs, particularly those with a history of previous neck pain, will not tolerate this procedure. In these cases, assessing their ability to move their head in all directions as they track a piece of food can be a useful substitute.

WARNING

It is important not to ventroflex the neck of young, small-breed dogs, because this could be dangerous in the presence of atlantoaxial subluxation

---

PRACTICAL TIP

In older dogs, spinal arthritis and spondylosis may limit the range of neck motion

---

Lumbosacral pain can be difficult to differentiate from hip pain. One slightly awkward method of assessing the presence of lumbosacral pain is for the vet to elevate both hindlegs off the ground while using their chin to press down on the lumbosacral region. Another, easier, method is to elevate the tail firmly, which puts pressure on the lumbosacral joint.

Palpation and manipulation of the dog's limbs and spine also allows assessment of bony deformities, strength and muscle tone, and whether there is any evidence of atrophy. Palpation and manipulation of the tail should be performed to assess for pain. An orthopaedic assessment should also be performed to rule out conditions that might mimic neurological disorders, such as bilateral cruciate rupture or bilateral luxating patellas.

Finally, **deep pain** can be assessed. This is not necessary in a dog that has a good superficial pain response or voluntary motion in all four limbs; deep pain is expected in these cases and it is not necessary to inflict a painful test. However, in cases where there is paralysis, the deep pain test gives important prognostic information. The test for pain can be started with a relatively gentle aversive stimulus to the distal extremity of a foot, such as a pinch, and progressed in the face of a negative response with increasing pressure. A true negative deep pain response can only be confirmed with the force of applying large haemostats to the metacarpals or to the periosteum of a toe. A positive response involves conscious recognition of the stimulus, such as movement of the head, vocalization, or even just a change in respiratory pattern.

PRACTICAL TIP

Withdrawal of the limb during a deep pain test is not a positive response. It is a spinal reflex, and gives no information on whether the spinal cord is intact

---

Lesion localization and severity

Establishing whether a lesion involves upper motor neurons (UMNs) or lower motor neurons (LMNs) is important to aid localization (Figure 16.3).

- UMN lesions: Damage to the upper motor neurons, which send inhibitory messages within the spinal cord, causes increased muscle tone

Spinal segments affected	Forelimb findings	Hindlimb findings	Other abnormalities
C1–C5	UMN signs	UMN signs	Ipsilateral Horner's syndrome may be present. May see urinary retention and respiratory difficulty in severe cases. Cervical pain often present
C6–T2	LMN signs	UMN signs	Ipsilateral Horner's syndrome may be present. May see urinary retention and respiratory difficulty in severe cases. Panniculus reflex may be absent if C8–T1 segment affected
T3–L3	Normal	UMN signs	Schiff–Sherrington phenomenon may be observed. Panniculus reflex reduced or absent caudal to the level of the last intact dermatome. Thoracolumbar spinal pain may be present. May see urinary retention
L4–S3	Normal	LMN signs	Lumbar spinal pain may be present. L4–L6 lesion: may see urinary retention and reduced or absent patellar reflex; intact withdrawal reflex. L6–S3 lesion: withdrawal reflex may be reduced or absent; patellar reflex may be increased; perineal reflex may be decreased; urinary incontinence may be present

16.3   Neurolocalization of spinal lesions.

and normal or hyper-reflexia, because inhibition from higher areas of the central nervous system has been removed.

- LMN lesions: Damage to the lower motor neurons causes muscle weakness and hyporeflexia, because there is interference with the motor neuron that directly supplies the skeletal muscle. In chronic cases, muscle atrophy will be more pronounced in LMN lesions.

Spinal segment numbering

There is a disparity between the spinal cord segment number and the respective vertebrae. This is because the cervical spinal cord has eight segments; and because of differences in growth between the skeletal and neurological elements of the spine during development. Thus, the cervical intumescence of C6–T2 lies within vertebrae C5–T1, and the lumbar intumescence of L4–S3 lies within vertebrae L3–L6. The spinal cord usually ends around L6–L7. Locations in most texts, including this one, refer to cord segment number, not vertebrae

---

As well as lesion localization, assessing **severity** is important because of the prognostic information it provides. Figure 16.4 shows one system for grading the severity of spinal lesions. In general, the prognosis is better for paraparesis than paraplegia, better for UMN than LMN signs, and is poor if deep pain sensation is lost.

Schiff–Sherrington phenomenon

This phenomenon (hyperextension of the forelimbs with paralysis of the hindlimbs) is due to damage to the ascending tracts of the UMNs, and is caused by a lesion caudal to the forelimbs. Proprioception is retained in the forelimbs in these cases. This phenomenon has been traditionally associated with a poor prognosis, but in fact can be observed in many cases of thoracolumbar spinal injury, and should not be taken as a poor prognostic indicator in isolation

---

Grade	Features
1	Pain but no neurological deficits
2	Ambulatory paresis
3	Non-ambulatory paresis
4	Non-ambulatory paralysis
5	Non-ambulatory paralysis with loss of deep pain sensation

16.4 Grading the severity of spinal lesions.

Differential diagnosis

Once the location and severity of a lesion has been determined, the differential diagnoses should be considered. It can be helpful to classify these according to the DAMNIT-V (VITAMIN-D) (or similar) pathological classification system.

DAMNIT-V classification of diseases

D: Degenerative
A: Anomalous
M: Metabolic
N: Nutritional, Neoplastic
I: Infectious, Inflammatory, Immune-mediated, Idiopathic
T: Toxic, Traumatic
V: Vascular

Historical clues can often help narrow the diagnosis to one of these categories. For example:

- Neoplastic or degenerative diseases tend to be slowly progressive (although they can be acute, such as in the case of spinal cord compression due to extrusion of a degenerate intervertebral disc)
- Inflammatory diseases (such as meningoencephalitis of unknown origin) tend to be progressive, but more rapidly so than degenerative conditions
- Vascular diseases (such as an intracranial infarct or haemorrhage) tend to have a sudden onset and then slowly improve.

Signalment can also help narrow the differential diagnosis list. For example:

- Small-breed chondrodystrophic dogs are prone to intervertebral disc disease
- Cavalier King Charles Spaniels are prone to syringomyelia
- Young dogs (<2 years old) are less likely to suffer from degenerative intervertebral disc disease.

Figure 16.5 lists some of the common causes of spinal pain, paresis and paralysis. Other conditions mimicking spinal disease, such as orthopaedic disease or conditions that cause weakness, ataxia or cerebellar disease should also be considered (see Chapters 15 and 17).

Degenerative
- Degenerative myelopathy
- Lumbosacral disease
- Cervical spondylomyelopathy
- Intervertebral disc disease

Anomalous
- Atlantoaxial subluxation
- Syringomyelia

Neoplastic
- Primary or metastatic tumours

Inflammatory/infectious
- Discospondylitis
- Meningoencephalitis of unknown origin

Traumatic
- Traumatic disc disease
- Spinal fracture or luxation

Vascular
- Fibrocartilaginous embolism

16.5 Common differential diagnoses for spinal pain, paresis and paralysis.

Further investigations

The clinical examination (including the neurological examination suggested above) in conjunction with the history and signalment of the patient will, in most cases, allow a reasonably accurate localization of the lesion and a list of differential diagnoses, weighted towards the most likely causes. However, in order to narrow the differential diagnosis list, and ideally achieve a definitive diagnosis, further testing is necessary.

Laboratory tests

Routine haematology and biochemistry will seldom contribute to the diagnosis in these cases, although ruling out causes of weakness such as hypoglycaemia, hypocalcaemia and anaemia can be useful, and there is value in checking blood parameters prior to general anaesthesia in an unwell animal. In certain cases more specific diagnostic blood tests might include: testing for infections such as distemper, *Toxoplasma* or *Neospora*; DNA testing for degenerative myelopathy; and endocrine function testing (e.g. thyroid status) to look for possible causes of neuropathies and myopathies. Testing for C-reactive protein, an acute-phase protein marker, can help monitor the course of an inflammatory disease such as steroid-responsive meningitis–arteritis, without the necessity for repeated cerebrospinal fluid (CSF) sampling.

Radiography

Radiography can be a useful screening test in the diagnosis of spinal disease. Spondylosis deformans may be evident, which may be a normal finding in the older dog, but can indicate areas of vertebral instability. Spinal radiography is also useful for detecting fractures/luxations (Figure 16.6) and bony neoplasia.

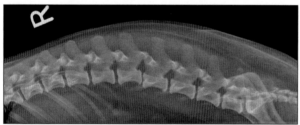

16.6   Lateral lumbar spinal radiograph showing a luxation at L3–L4. (Courtesy of Dan Ogden)

Advanced investigations

Definitive diagnosis of many spinal cord diseases will require advanced techniques, detailed discussion of which is beyond the scope of this chapter. However, it is useful to be familiar with the practicalities and limitations of these techniques in order to advise a client of the most appropriate next step.

Myelography can be used to detect spinal cord compression in the absence of the availability of advanced imaging techniques such as magnetic resonance imaging (MRI) or computed tomography (CT). Radiographs are taken after the injection of contrast medium into the subarachnoid space. Loss of the contrast medium column can help ascertain the site of a compressive lesion and can give a guide as to whether the compression is external to the cord

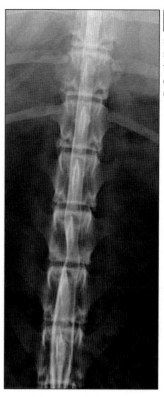

16.7   Dorsoventral myelogram showing an extradural spinal cord compression on the right side in the region of L2–L3. (Courtesy of Dan Ogden)

(e.g. an extruded disc; Figure 16.7). However, it is not possible to image in transverse planes, and the level of detail is less than with MRI or CT. Furthermore, there are some risks associated with the technique, such as neurological deterioration and myelography-induced seizures; but for many practices that perform routine surgery for disc extrusions it is a cost-effective step in planning for surgery and remains the technique of choice.

CT gives excellent bony detail. However, its ability to image the cord parenchyma is poor, so spinal cord tumours, inflammation and vascular lesions will often not be visible. CT myelography can give further information about compression.

MRI gives poorer detail of the bone, but better information about the soft tissue structures of the spine, and is generally the imaging modality of choice for suspected spinal cord lesions (Figure 16.8).

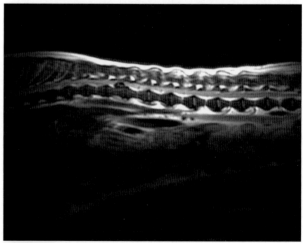

16.8   Sagittal T2-weighted MRI scan of the thoracolumbar spine, showing cord compression due to disc extrusion. (Courtesy of Dan Ogden)

Other tests that may be of use in selected neurological diseases are: nerve and muscle biopsy; nerve conduction velocity testing, to assess for peripheral neuropathy; and electromyography, which can give information on muscle disease and the innervation of the muscle. The reader is referred to the *BSAVA Manual of Canine and Feline Neurology* for more details.

Common conditions

Spinal disorders

> **WARNING**
>
> Once a spinal condition has been diagnosed, referral, or advice from a specialist neurologist or colleague with experience in managing spinal disease, should be sought

Disc disease

Most cases of spinal disease that are surgical candidates involve compressive spinal lesions (e.g. intervertebral disc disease, spinal fractures, cervical spondylomyelopathy), although some non-compressive lesions such as non-displaced fractures will also benefit from surgery. The option of surgical treatment in cases for which it is appropriate should be discussed with the owner, along with the costs, complications and risks associated with the procedure. In general, cases that are very mild can be managed conservatively, at least initially.

Conservative treatment may be the most appropriate course of action (grade 1 lesion) or may be the preferred choice for financial reasons. It consists of 4–6 weeks of strict cage rest. This means confining an animal to a small cage, such as a puppy crate. During this time the dog should only be allowed out to urinate and defecate.

It is important to monitor for, and manage, complications of recumbency such as decubital ulcers. A padded, clean bed should be provided, and the patient turned every 6 hours if recumbent. Urination and defecation should be monitored and assisted if necessary; this may involve placing an indwelling urinary catheter if urinary retention is a feature. It is important to ensure adequate nutrition and analgesia.

It is also important to monitor for deterioration. If a dog's neurological status deteriorates during conservative treatment, or if there is no improvement after 4 weeks of rest, then surgery should be reconsidered.

> **WARNING**
>
> Immobility is a form of guarding response to pain, which may be lessened with analgesic treatment. There are numerous well documented cases of acute worsening of grade 1 or 2 lesions due to extrusion of an unstable disc following movement facilitated by pain relief. It is vital to enforce strict rest

If a satisfactory response is achieved after 4–6 weeks, then a slow increase in exercise should be started. In the past, use of high-dose methylprednisolone sodium succinate within 8 hours of acute paraplegia was advocated. Some authors have also recommended the use of anti-inflammatory doses of prednisolone for the first 7–14 days after an injury. However, studies have shown little or no benefit in using corticosteroids in cervical and thoracolumbar disc disease, and they may be associated with a worse outcome (Boag *et al.*, 2001; Levine *et al.*, 2007). Consultation with a qualified physiotherapist may be useful early in the course of the disease to see at what stage physiotherapy may be of benefit. In conservatively managed cases, more intensive therapy such as hydrotherapy would not normally be started until after at least 4 weeks of cage rest. Home physiotherapy, involving passive range-of-motion exercises of the paretic or paralysed limbs for 15 minutes three times a day, will help reduce muscle atrophy.

For thoracolumbar disc disease, the most common surgical spinal disease, prognosis depends on the grade of lesion (see Figure 16.4) and whether conservative or surgical treatment was instituted:

- For grade 1 cases, conservative treatment will be successful in nearly all cases
- In grade 3 cases, conservative treatment may improve around 85% of dogs affected, while decompression might improve nearer 95%
- In cases where deep pain is absent, conservative treatment rarely leads to improvement, whereas decompression can help 50–70% of cases if performed promptly
- Surgery should be strongly recommended in grade 3 or 4 cases, and in grade 5 cases where deep pain sensation has been lost within the last 24–48 hours
- Patients that have been without deep pain sensation for >48 hours, or in which surgical treatment is not carried out, carry a poor prognosis, and euthanasia should be considered.

Non-spinal disorders

Common non-spinal causes of paralysis and paresis are listed in Figure 16.9.

- Cerebellar disease
- Brainstem disease
- Polyneuropathies: distal denervating disease; toxoplasmosis/neosporosis; endocrine disease (e.g. diabetes mellitus, hypothyroidism); idiopathic polyradiculoneuritis
- Mononeuropathies: trauma; neoplasia
- Vascular disease

16.9 Common non-spinal causes of paralysis and paresis.

Intracranial disease

Disease affecting the brainstem can cause proprioceptive deficits in all four limbs. There will often be accompanying cranial nerve deficits (see Chapter 11).

- Decerebellate rigidity occurs with severe cerebellar lesions. In these cases there is opisthotonus, the forelimbs are extended and the hips are flexed. Consciousness is usually retained.
- With decerebrate rigidity due to a brainstem lesion, all four limbs are extended, and consciousness is depressed, often to the level of coma.

Mono- and polyneuropathies

Mononeuropathies can be suspected when only a single limb is affected – with LMN signs.

- A lateralized disc extrusion would be a relatively common cause of a monoparesis/monoplegia, and may occur acutely, or over a few days to weeks.
- Nerve root tumours can lead to slowly progressive signs of paresis, reduced spinal reflexes, muscle atrophy and pain.
- Thoracic limb monoparesis or monoplegia can occur due to brachial plexus injury, which is common in road traffic accidents.
- Aortic or iliac thromboembolism is rare in dogs, but does occur, and can lead to signs of monoparesis; so checking both femoral pulses is worthwhile in these patients.

Polyneuropathies can be suspected when all four limbs are affected with LMN signs, particularly reduced spinal reflexes. Definitive diagnosis in these cases will require such diagnostic procedures as nerve conduction velocity testing, electromyography and nerve/muscle biopsy.

References and further reading

Bagley RS (2005) *Fundamentals of Veterinary Clinical Neurology.* Blackwell, Iowa

Boag AK, Otto CM and Drobatz KJ (2001) Complications of methylprednisolone sodium succinate therapy in dachshunds with surgically treated intervertebral disc disease. *Journal of Veterinary Emergency and Critical Care* **11**, 105–110

Jaggy A (2010) *Small Animal Neurology.* Schlütersche, Hannover

Levine JM, Hillman RB, Erb HN and DeLahunta A (2002) The influence of age on patellar reflex response in the dog. *Journal of Veterinary Internal Medicine* **16**, 244–246

Levine JM, Levine GJ, Johnson SI *et al.* (2007) Evaluation of the success of medical management for presumptive cervical intervertebral disk herniation in dogs. *Veterinary Surgery* **36**, 492–499

Platt SR and Garosi L (2012) *Small Animal Neurological Emergencies.* Manson, London

Platt SR and Olby NJ (2012) *BSAVA Manual of Canine and Feline Neurology, 4th edn.* BSAVA Publications, Gloucester

Lethargy and weakness in endocrine disease

Sarah Packman

> **Definitions**
> - Lethargy is a state of dullness and listlessness with a lack of energy
> - Weakness is a lack of muscle strength

Lethargy and weakness are common presenting signs in first-opinion practice but can be difficult to distinguish for both the owner and clinician. They may be primary signs but are more commonly secondary to another disease process. Many conditions can result in lethargy and/or weakness, and in order to determine the exact cause of the signs, a full history should be obtained and clinical examination and diagnostic work-up performed. This chapter will concentrate in detail on endocrine causes of lethargy and weakness. Other causes, such as myopathies and orthopaedic causes are discussed in Chapter 11 and 15, respectively.

Some causes of lethargy and weakness can occasionally present as emergency situations, e.g. endocrine collapse due to hypoadrenocorticism (Addison's disease). In these cases emergency treatment, such as intravenous fluids to support the circulation, must be instigated before embarking on a diagnostic work-up.

History

A good history is vital when determining the cause of lethargy or weakness and helps to narrow the list of differential diagnoses. As weakness and lethargy are very common in any disease process, the history-taking aims to distinguish between primary conditions and secondary signs.

It is important to consider the signalment of the patient: age, sex, whether the patient is neutered, and vaccination status can help to narrow down the differential list. For example: pyometra should be on the differential list for an older entire bitch, whereas a portosystemic shunt should be considered for younger dogs. Enquiries should also be made as to foreign travel and ectoparasite control, as vector-borne infections such as *Babesia* and *Leishmania* may result in lethargy.

The owner should be asked to describe the clinical signs the dog is showing. Sometimes, asking the owner to film the episodes can be very enlightening. Further questions to ask the owner include:

- How long has the lethargy/weakness been present?
- Is the weakness constant, or are there times when the dog is normal?
- Is the dog gradually deteriorating, or do signs wax and wane?
- When was the dog last normal?
- Has anything changed in the environment recently or at the time of the onset of lethargy and/or weakness?
- Is there anything that exacerbates the clinical signs? Does the weakness get worse/improve with exercise?
- Is the dog taking any medication? (In addition to sedative drugs, other medications/preparations (e.g. antihistamines, phenobarbital, skullcap and valerian) can have sedative effects; other drugs (e.g. glucocorticoids) can cause muscle weakness.)
- Has the dog had access to toxins?
- Has there been a diet change or change in appetite?
- How much does the dog drink?

Questions should then be asked relating to organ systems. As disease in every organ system can result in lethargy and/or weakness, this line of questioning should include questions relating to gastrointestinal, urogenital, neurological, cardiopulmonary and musculoskeletal health. Examples of such questions include:

- Is the dog passing urine normally – frequency/amount/associated pain?
- Is the dog continent?
- Does the dog maintain bladder function overnight?
- Are the faeces normal – any changes in the frequency/consistency/colour?

It should be remembered that concurrent disease may make identification of the primary cause of the lethargy and/or weakness difficult to achieve.

Physical examination

A thorough clinical examination, whether head to toe or using a body systems approach, should be undertaken. In addition a neurological examination should be performed (see Chapters 11 and 16 and the *BSAVA Manual of Canine and Feline Neurology*).

- Head:
  - Examine for signs of symmetry, inflammation and muscle wastage
  - Examine the oral cavity, including the mucous membranes to look for redness, pallor, icterus, cyanosis, petechiae and to allow assessment of the dog's hydration status. Note any evidence of halitosis and check the teeth for tooth root infections
  - Assess cranial nerve function (see Chapter 16).
- Eyes:
  - Examine the retina for any evidence of hypertensive damage, or inflammation
  - Examine the lens for evidence of cataract development.
- Thorax:
  - Auscultate the chest and upper respiratory tract, paying special attention to laryngeal noise, cardiac abnormalities and abnormal lung sounds
  - Additionally, the chest should be percussed for evidence of dullness.
- Abdomen:
  - Palpate for evidence of organomegaly (e.g. hepatic enlargement), pain and effusions.
- Body condition: Examine for symmetry and for evidence of muscle atrophy.
- Gait: Observe gait at a walk and after more intensive exercise. Look for evidence of lameness or a stiff gait. Note whether the lethargy or weakness gets worse with exercise.

- Skin: Examine for abnormalities including alopecia and dry flaky skin.
- Temperature, pulse and respiration (TPR):
  - Assess body temperature for hypothermia or pyrexia
  - Assess pulse quality and rate. Record any abnormalities such as pulse deficits.

> **WARNING**
>
> If any obvious abnormalities are detected at this stage – such as dehydration or hypothermia – they should be treated promptly before any further diagnostic work-up is attempted

Differential diagnosis

There is a vast list of conditions that can cause lethargy and/or weakness (Figure 17.1).

When investigating a dog that presents with weakness or lethargy, investigating the other clinical signs present can significantly narrow the differential diagnosis list. For example: a dog with hyperadrenocorticism will often be weak and lethargic, but it will also be likely to have polyuria/polydipsia, polyphagia, panting and, possibly, symmetrical alopecia. A problem list approach is best applied in more complex cases.

It can be difficult to distinguish between orthopaedic disease, endocrine disease and myopathies as the cause of lethargy and weakness. Additionally, in older dogs orthopaedic conditions may occur concurrently with endocrine diseases such as hypothyroidism and osteoarthritis. These cases can be difficult to manage if the underlying cause for the lethargy or weakness is overlooked, or not identified and treated. Figure 17.2 presents an algorithm to help the clinician distinguish between myopathies, endocrine and orthopaedic disease.

Body system/disease type	Potential conditions
Neuromuscular/neurological	Myasthenia gravis. Polymyositis. Malignant hyperthermia. Toxin exposure – botulism/tetanus. Thiamine deficiency. Lysosomal storage disease. Epilepsy. Vestibular disease. Meningitis
Endocrine	Hyperadrenocorticism – pseudomyotonia. Hypoadrenocorticism. Hypothyroidism. Diabetes mellitus/diabetic ketoacidosis. Hypoparathyroidism. Hyperparathyroidism
Cardiac	Aortic stenosis; pulmonary stenosis. Heart failure – dilated cardiac myopathy; mitral valve disease. Cardiac arrhythmia – bradycardia; tachycardia. Pericardial effusion; constrictive pericarditis
Respiratory	Hypoxia. Tracheal collapse. Laryngeal paralysis. Pleural effusion. Pulmonary hypertension
Haematological	Acute blood loss. Anaemia. Polycythaemia
End-stage disease	Hepatitis. Chronic renal disease/failure
Gastrointestinal	Severe inflammatory bowel disease. Parvovirus infection
Neoplasia	Lymphoma. Insulinoma. Phaeochromocytoma. Neoplasia in any body system
Pyrexia	Infection – pyelonephritis; pyometra; prostatitis; leptospirosis. Pancreatitis. Exercise-induced hyperthermia
Immune-mediated disease	Immune-mediated haemolytic anaemia. Immune-mediated polyarthritis. Systemic lupus erythematosus
Orthopaedic	Osteoarthritis. Polyarthritis. Spinal disease – congenital or acquired. Myopathies
Vector-borne infections	*Ehrlichia. Babesia. Leishmania*
Miscellaneous	Inadequate nutrition. Pregnancy. Pain. Hepatic encephalopathy. Portosystemic shunts/vascular shunting. Obesity. Cachexia

17.1 Differential diagnoses for lethargy and weakness.

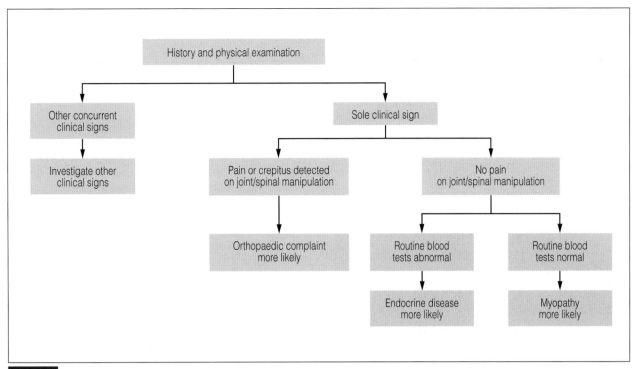

17.2   Differentiating orthopaedic, endocrine and muscular disorders in dogs presenting with lethargy and/or weakness.

Diagnostic tests

Diagnosing the cause of lethargy and weakness can be very time-consuming and expensive. From the history and physical examination the clinician should have a good idea as to where to direct the investigation.

Initially a full biochemical profile to include creatine kinase and total thyroxine (T4) is needed. A full blood count and white cell differential count should be obtained, looking for evidence of (or lack of) a stress leucogram. Additionally, urinalysis should be performed and blood pressure measured. From the results of these tests, the clinician can determine the best next step in the investigation, e.g. further biochemical testing, abdominal/thoracic imaging, electrocardiography, echocardiography, or endoscopy.

Electroencephalography, muscle and nerve biopsy, and an edrophonium response test are more specialized tests that may be performed, but these tests are more often done when other tests have not led to a diagnosis.

Endocrine disorders causing lethargy and weakness

Hypothyroidism

The pituitary gland releases thyroid stimulating hormone (TSH) which acts on the thyroid gland to release thyroxine (T4) and, to a lesser extent, tri-iodothyronine (T3 – the active form). These thyroid hormones control their own release, as they have a negative feedback effect on the pituitary gland that prevents further release of TSH (Figure 17.3). Hypothyroidism is caused by reduced production and release of T3 and T4 from the thyroid gland.

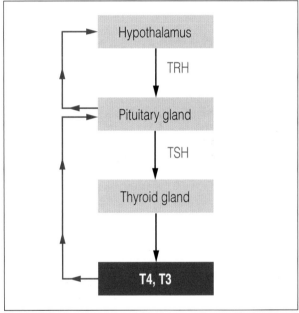

17.3   Control of thyroid hormone release. Red arrows = negative feedback. TRH = thyroid releasing hormone; TSH = thyroid stimulating hormone.

The most common form of hypothyroidism is acquired; congenital hypothyroidism, although very rare, is recognized most commonly in German Shepherd Dogs with panhypopituitarism caused by a cyst in Rathke's pouch. Acquired hypothyroidism may be caused by lymphocytic thyroiditis or idiopathic thyroid atrophy. Rarely, thyroid neoplasia may cause hypothyroidism.

Signalment

Hypothyroidism most commonly affects middle-aged dogs (mean 7 years). Predisposed breeds include the Boxer, Miniature Schnauzer, Cocker Spaniel, Poodle, Golden Retriever and Irish Setter.

Clinical signs

The most common presenting complaint is progressive lethargy, inactivity and weight gain. Additionally, some dogs develop muscle weakness, myopathy, bradycardia, seizures and infertility. Skin complaints, such as non-pruritic bilateral flank alopecia (Figure 17.4), hyperpigmentation, seborrhoea and recurrent skin infections, are common, and are often the most obvious signs to the owner.

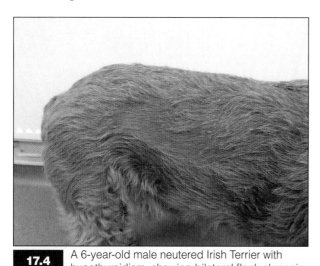

17.4 A 6-year-old male neutered Irish Terrier with hypothyroidism, showing bilateral flank alopecia.

Diagnosis

The diagnosis is supported by performing routine biochemistry and haematology on a blood sample. Hypercholesterolaemia is detected in 80% of cases, with hyperlipidaemia and mildly elevated creatine kinase seen less commonly. A non-regenerative anaemia (normocytic, normochromic) is seen in 50% of cases.

A subnormal thyroid hormone level is required for diagnosis. This can result from thyroidal or nonthyroidal illness (such as stress, or exogenous glucocorticoid or potentiated sulphonamide administration within the last 4 weeks).

In order to confirm hypothyroidism, the T4:TSH ratio must be calculated. Low T4 in conjunction with high TSH is supportive of hypothyroidism. However, TSH can occasionally be high in sick euthyroid syndrome or perversely low in hypothyroid dogs, so it is important to consider the findings in conjunction with the clinical signs. Additional tests which can be performed in order to confirm the diagnosis of hypothyroidism are: free thyroxine level; recombinant human TSH (rhTSH) or thyroid releasing hormone (TRH) stimulation tests; or anti-T3 and anti-T4 antibody assays. These additional tests are expensive, however, and may not provide reliable results.

A treatment trial with levothyroxine, noting the response to therapy, can be a more cost-effective approach for confirming the diagnosis in equivocal cases.

Treatment

Treatment is with levothyroxine (11–22 μg/kg orally q12h). An improvement in mentation is usually seen within 2–6 weeks. Peripheral neuropathies take 8–12 weeks to resolve, and alopecia may take up to 3 months. Serum T4 levels should be monitored. The author's protocol for monitoring is as follows: 4 weeks after starting the treatment, 4–6 hours after the dose of levothyroxine has been administered; thereafter, every 2 months for 6–8 months whilst the thyroid levels stabilize; then twice yearly.

Prognosis

The prognosis for treated dogs is good.

Hyperadrenocorticism

Hyperadrenocorticism (HAC; Cushing's disease) is one of the most common endocrine diseases seen in dogs. It is caused by the excessive production of cortisol by the adrenal cortex. The majority of cases (>80%) result from a microadenoma on the pituitary gland (pituitary-dependent HAC (PDHAC)). A smaller number of cases (<20%) have a tumour on the adrenal gland (adrenal-dependent HAC (ADHAC)); this tumour may be benign or malignant. Iatrogenic HAC results from exogenous administration of glucocorticoids.

Signalment

PDHAC is found in middle-aged to older dogs (median 7–9 years). Poodles and small terriers are at increased risk and there is no sex predisposition. ADHAC occurs more commonly in older (11–12 years) larger breed dogs; bitches are at greater risk of developing the disease.

Clinical signs

Dogs will present with one or a combination of the following: polyuria, polydipsia, polyphagia, weakness, lethargy, panting, a pot-bellied appearance, and symmetrical alopecia/poor hair regrowth/'rat-tail' appearance (Figure 17.5). Smaller breeds often present with many of the clinical signs described above, but larger breeds often present with just polydipsia/polyuria. Rarely, dogs may present with seizure activity due to the growth of a pituitary mass.

PRACTICAL TIP

Remember that the 'rat-tail' appearance of the tail is not specific for hypoadrenocorticism, and is a common finding in both hyperadrenocorticism and hypothyroidism

---

Diagnosis

On physical examination the dog may have evidence of thinning skin or comedones, muscle wastage (especially around the temporal muscles), and/or chronic infections.

The most common abnormality detected on routine biochemistry is a raised level of alkaline phosphatase (ALP), which may be raised when there are few or no changes in other liver enzymes. Other common causes of an increase in ALP, such as exogenous steroid administration, should be excluded. Other abnormalities may include hypercholesterolaemia, raised levels of other liver enzymes, and mild hyperglycaemia. A stress leucogram is often present. On urinalysis the most common finding is hyposthenuria (the kidneys are actively diluting the urine); in HAC this is due to antidiuretic hormone (ADH) acting on the collecting duct of the kidney. Other urine abnormalities include pyuria/bacteriuria and proteinuria.

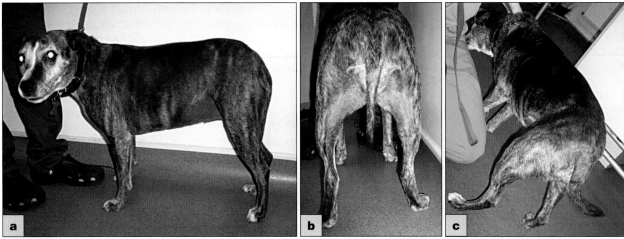

17.5 An 8-year-old neutered Staffordshire Bull Terrier bitch with hyperadrenocorticism, showing **(a)** flank alopecia and **(b)** 'rat-tail'. **(c)** The same bitch following treatment with trilostane for 6 months; there is hair regrowth on the body and tail.

HAC is confirmed by performing an adrenocortico-trophic hormone (ACTH) stimulation test or a low-dose dexamethasone suppression (LDDS) test (Figure 17.6); for protocols see the *BSAVA Guide to Procedures in Small Animal Practice*.

■ The ACTH test is less time-consuming and is a good test when used to confirm HAC.
■ The LDDS test is a good test to perform when trying to **rule out** HAC. However, if the test is positive for HAC, it can then help to differentiate between PDHAC and ADHAC.

■ Another measure that is useful when trying to **rule out** HAC is the urine cortisol:creatinine ratio. This is best obtained using urine collected at home from a non-stressed patient over several days.
  • A negative result, i.e. a urine cortisol:creatinine ratio <13.5, can reliably exclude HAC as a diagnosis.
  • A positive test result, i.e. a urine cortisol:creatinine ratio >13.5, cannot on its own confirm the diagnosis. A positive test only indicates that there is an elevated serum cortisol level; this may be caused by adrenal or non-adrenal illness.

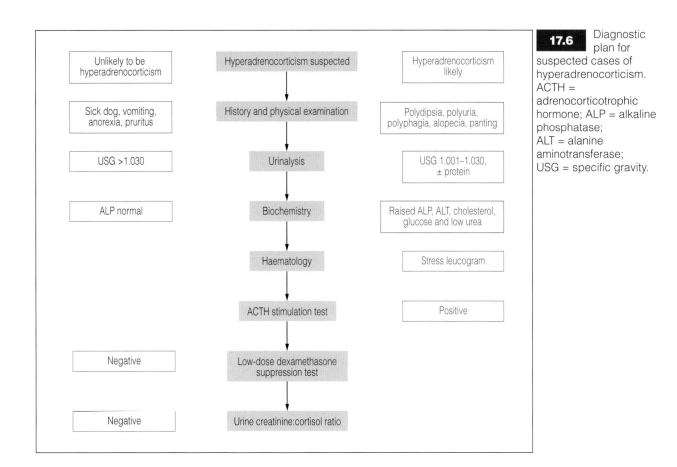

17.6 Diagnostic plan for suspected cases of hyperadrenocorticism. ACTH = adrenocorticotrophic hormone; ALP = alkaline phosphatase; ALT = alanine aminotransferase; USG = specific gravity.

Treatment

The only drug authorized for treating HAC in dogs in the UK is trilostane.

- The starting dose is 2–5 mg/kg/day given orally once daily with food. Sometimes twice-daily dosing is required.
- In order to check that the right dose of medication is being given, regular monitoring of blood biochemistry, electrolytes and haematology, is needed. An ACTH stimulation test should also be performed 4–6 hours after dosing.
- It is important that the clinical signs of HAC are well controlled and that the adrenal glands are not oversuppressed by a high dose of trilostane.
  - An excessive dose of trilostane may lead to signs of *hypo*adrenocorticism (e.g. lethargy, anorexia, vomiting, diarrhoea, cardiovascular signs, collapse). Monitoring of blood levels of cortisol (pre- and post-stimulation), liver enzymes and electrolytes to detect hypoadrenocorticism is therefore very important and should be performed after starting treatment at: 10 days; 4 weeks; 12 weeks; and thereafter every 3 months.
  - If the dose of trilostane is found to be incorrect, the dosage should be changed and monitoring repeated at the above intervals.

Additional treatments are available, such as mitotane (unauthorized), and surgical removal of the mass (see the *BSAVA Manual of Canine and Feline Endocrinology*).

PRACTICAL TIP

When treating HAC there is a possibility of unmasking concurrent steroid-responsive diseases such as osteoarthritis or atopy

---

Prognosis

Untreated, the clinical signs of HAC become progressively worse, although most dogs maintain an acceptable quality of life. When treated, the prognosis in dogs with PDHAC is good, but for dogs with ADHAC the prognosis is less good. For most dogs the clinical signs of polyuria, polydipsia, polyphagia and lethargy resolve within days to weeks. The muscle weakness and skin changes often take several months to resolve. Dogs who present with neurological signs have a poor prognosis; seizure activity can be controlled with antiseizure medications, but the side effects of some of these medications can exacerbate the lethargy and weakness.

Hypoadrenocorticism

Hypoadrenocorticism, deficient adrenal gland production of glucocorticoids and/or mineralocorticoids, can be categorized as primary (Addison's disease) or secondary (atypical Addison's).

Addison's is an uncommon disease, which results in glucocorticoid and mineralocorticoid deficiency and is suspected to be caused by immune-mediated destruction or atrophy of the adrenal cortex. Aldosterone is the major mineralocorticoid in the body; its loss results in an inability to conserve water and sodium, and a failure to excrete sodium. Loss of >85% of the adrenocortical cells is required before clinical signs of hypoadrenocorticism are seen.

Atypical Addison's is rarer still, and results from pituitary ACTH deficiency. Glucocorticoid production is deficient, but often mineralocorticoid production is preserved.

Signalment

Hypoadrenocorticism has been reported in young to old dogs, but most are between 2 and 7 years old at the time of diagnosis. There is a genetic predisposition in Standard Poodles and Bearded Collies, and the disease is over-represented in some breeds, including the West Highland White Terrier, Great Dane and Rottweiler. Bitches are twice as likely as males to have hypoadrenocorticism.

Clinical signs

Acute hypoadrenocorticism presents as hypovolaemic collapse, bradycardia, vomiting, diarrhoea, abdominal pain and/or hypothermia. Chronic signs may involve intermittent vomiting and diarrhoea, lethargy, weakness, megaoesophagus, or muscle cramping.

Diagnosis

Findings include the absence of a stress leucogram on haematology, and azotaemia, hyponatraemia, hyperkalaemia, hypochloraemia and hypoglycaemia on serum biochemistry. Hypercalcaemia is present in 30% of cases with unknown aetiology. A reduced sodium:potassium ratio is a common feature, but cannot be used as a diagnostic tool. Urinalysis often shows reduced urine specific gravity, reflecting a reduced renal medullary sodium concentration resulting in medullary washout. Survey radiographs may show a reduced cardiac silhouette, and adrenal ultrasonography may be abnormal. Electrocardiogram (ECG) abnormalities confirm hyperkalaemia (peaked T waves, prolonged P–R interval; Figure 17.7) but not the cause.

An ACTH stimulation test confirms the diagnosis. Administration of supraphysiological doses of ACTH (250 micrograms) normally produces significant increases in plasma cortisol levels, especially in

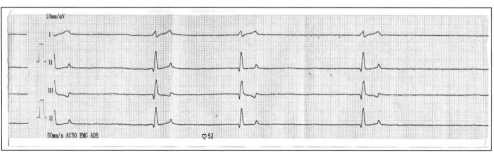

17.7 An ECG from a 5-year-old male neutered German Shepherd Dog with hypoadrenocorticism. The marked hyperkalaemia in this case is shown on this ECG as an absence of P waves (atrial standstill) and peaked T waves.

sick animals; however, in hypoadrenocorticism this increase is minimal or absent. Plasma ACTH concentrations are required to differentiate primary from secondary disease.

Treatment

Acute treatment involves fluid resuscitation, correction of electrolyte imbalances, glucocorticoid supplementation, and correction of life-threatening cardiac arrhythmias. Rapid initiation of shock boluses (20–30 ml/kg) of crystalloid fluids is essential to reduce the hyperkalaemia and improves renal perfusion. Compound sodium lactate-containing fluids help to correct the metabolic acidosis. Fluid supplementation alone will often correct hyperkalaemia; however, some cases require either a combination of intravenous glucose and insulin, or calcium gluconate administration to correct the hyperkalaemia. Glucocorticoids should be initiated early in the acute crisis.

Maintenance therapy includes fludrocortisone and prednisolone supplementation.

- Fludrocortisone, a synthetic adrenocortical steroid, has potent mineralocorticoid and mild glucocorticoid activity. The dose is 15–30 µg/kg orally q24h, although sometimes much higher doses are required.
- Prednisolone has good glucocorticoid and minimal mineralocorticoid activity. Dogs are stabilized on 0.2–0.5 mg/kg orally q24h. After stabilization this dose is reduced, and may be discontinued. If discontinued, prednisolone must be reinstated during periods of physiological stress. Side effects of treatment include iatrogenic hyperadrenocorticism; if this occurs, the dosage of prednisolone must be reduced.

Therapeutic success is monitored by measuring electrolytes whilst the dog is hospitalized, then at 1 week after discharge, and 2 weeks later, then monthly to bi-monthly. Additionally, it is important to assess levels of azotaemia.

Prognosis

Overall, the prognosis for dogs with hypoadrenocorticism receiving hormone replacement therapy is excellent provided there is good owner education about the disease and the importance of regular treatment and monitoring. One aspect that must be discussed in depth with the owner if prednisolone therapy is to be discontinued, is that of physiological stress. Owners understand that a visit to the vet's might be stressful, but not that a change in environment, such as temperature, diet or exercise, might also apply a stress to the dog.

Diabetes mellitus

Diabetes mellitus is a common disease in dogs. Insulin is normally secreted by the pancreas in response to hyperglycaemia and reduces the blood glucose concentration by promoting the uptake of glucose by the peripheral tissues. In insulin-dependent diabetes mellitus (IDDM) there is an absolute lack of insulin; this can be idiopathic or a consequence of end-stage pancreatitis. Diabetes mellitus may also arise due to insulin resistance. IDDM is the more common form in dogs.

Signalment

Samoyeds, Tibetan Terriers and Yorkshire Terriers are over-represented, while Boxers, Golden Retrievers and German Shepherd Dogs are under-represented. Middle-aged to older dogs (>7 years) and entire bitches (8–10 years) are much more likely to develop diabetes mellitus.

Clinical signs

The common clinical signs that dogs present with are polyphagia, polyuria/polydipsia, and weight loss. Additionally, dogs can present with lethargy, depression, collapse and vomiting. Physical examination may reveal hepatomegaly and diabetic cataracts.

Diagnosis

Serum biochemistry findings include hyperglycaemia, hypercholesterolaemia, hypertriglyceridaemia and, commonly, raised ALP and alanine aminotransferase (ALT) levels. If diabetic ketoacidosis is present, serum biochemistry may reveal abnormalities in electrolytes, urea and creatinine. In-house urinalysis will show glucosuria if the blood glucose concentration exceeds the renal threshold for glucose (>10 mmol/l); ketonuria, haematuria, and proteinuria can additionally be tested for. As bacterial urinary tract infections are more frequent in diabetic patients, it is important to check the sediment for evidence of whole blood and white blood cells. In order to confirm the diagnosis of diabetes, blood fructosamine should be assayed; measuring this glycosylated serum protein gives a mean blood glucose level for the past 1–3 weeks. This test can confirm the diagnosis of diabetes and is useful in monitoring the response to treatment. Additional imaging can be performed to check for evidence of pancreatitis, but this is not required for the diagnosis.

Treatment

IDDM treatment always requires insulin (Figure 17.8). This can be administered once or twice daily; the frequency of injections depends on owner compliance and the dog's response to treatment. The starting dose rate depends on bodyweight but is usually in the range of 0.5–1 IU/kg s.c. q12–24h. (This author usually starts dogs on a dose range

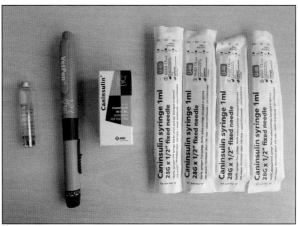

17.8 There are two types of insulin authorized for use in dogs: Caninsulin and Prozinc. Caninsulin is the more widely used and is available in two formulations: the VetPen; or with specific insulin syringes. Owners may find it easier to inject insulin with the VetPen.

from 10–20 IU per dog s.c. q12–24h.) The dose should be adjusted according to the dog's response to treatment. The dog's response to insulin should be monitored initially using blood glucose curves, urinalysis and fructosamine levels. The dog will take 3–7 days to respond to any change in insulin levels so a curve is best to perform a week after initiating therapy and changing a dose. Blood pressure may also be measured.

Another important aspect to consider when treating the disease is diet. Daily feeding should be consistent in terms of volume, timing and composition of the diet. A high level of complex fibre in the diet is recommended, as it slows digestion and absorption, therefore reducing postprandial glucose spikes. Exercise levels should also be kept stable. For more detail on management of diabetes in dogs see the *BSAVA Manual of Canine and Feline Endocrinology* and the *BSAVA Manual of Canine and Feline Rehabilitation, Supportive and Palliative Care*.

Prognosis

Diabetes is a life-limiting disease but, with effective treatment and regular monitoring, dogs with diabetes can be managed well. It must be remembered that diabetes remains an expensive disease to treat and some owners will not have the necessary funds. In these cases euthanasia may need to be considered.

Complications that may arise include insulin resistance in entire bitches, infections, diabetic cataracts and diabetic ketoacidosis (see the *BSAVA Manual of Canine and Feline Endocrinology* and the *BSAVA Manual of Canine and Feline Emergency and Critical Care*).

- Entire bitches: Immediately following 'heat', the ovaries produce the hormone progesterone (see Chapter 5). Progesterone has a negative influence on the role of insulin. Ovariohysterectomy removes the source of progesterone and helps normalize insulin requirements. Bitches diagnosed with diabetes mellitus should be spayed as soon as possible to make their diabetes easier to manage (see QRG 5.1).
- Infections: Any infection can induce insulin resistance (though the mechanism is still not fully understood); thus a higher dose of insulin will be required to produce the same effect. The most common site for an infection is the urinary tract, hence the importance of urinalysis monitoring and of treating any infection found (ideally after culture and sensitivity testing).
- Diabetic cataracts: When there is excess sugar in the eye fluid, excess sorbitol is produced. Sorbitol pulls water into the lens, which in turn disrupts lens clarity. A hypermature cataract can induce uveitis, which can be very painful. If uveitis develops, cataract surgery or enucleation is recommended to remove the source of the pain.

Hypoparathyroidism

Hypoparathyroidism may be primary (inadequate production and secretion of parathyroid hormone (PTH)) or, rarely, secondary (a failure of response to PTH (pseudohypoparathyroidism)). Primary disease is caused by idiopathic destruction or atrophy of the parathyroid gland, which is thought to be immune-mediated.

Signalment

Hypoparathyroidism is a rare disease of middle-aged dogs, although dogs of any age can develop the disease. There is no breed predisposition. A female bias has been reported.

Clinical signs

The clinical signs of hypoparathyroidism relate to hypocalcaemia. They include muscle weakness, ataxia, muscle fasciculations, a stiff gait, lethargy, seizures, focal trembling and panting. The clinical signs seem to be exacerbated by exercise, excitement or stress, and may wax and wane.

Diagnosis

Routine biochemistry shows profound hypocalcaemia and severe hyperphosphataemia, with normal urea and creatinine levels. When presented with a low calcium level it is important to check the blood albumin level and, ideally, to obtain an ionized calcium level (where available). The calcium measured in a routine test is total calcium (the portion bound to albumin plus the unbound calcium); only the ionized calcium (unbound) is the active molecule. Low albumin levels may result in low measured total calcium although normal levels of ionized calcium are present.

Differential diagnoses include eclampsia, pancreatitis, chronic renal disease and intestinal malabsorption. A PTH assay is required to confirm the diagnosis of primary hypoparathyroidism, shown by an inappropriately low PTH level in response to low blood calcium.

> **PRACTICAL TIP**
>
> PTH assay samples need to be sent on ice to specialist laboratories, as PTH is heat-labile. Consult the laboratory for detailed requirements

Treatment

Treatment is with calcium supplementation. For hypocalcaemic tetany, parenteral administration of 10% calcium gluconate is required. For maintenance, calcium and vitamin D must be supplemented and tailored to the correct dosage depending on the serum calcium level.

Prognosis

With regular monitoring of patients the long-term prognosis is good.

Hyperparathyroidism

Hyperparathyroidism may be primary (excessive PTH secretion) or secondary (an adaptive response of increased PTH secretion due to a reduced ionized calcium level – commonly secondary to chronic renal disease). Primary hyperparathyroidism is uncommon and it is often caused by a small adenoma of the parathyroid gland, although adenocarcinomas can, very rarely, be the cause.

Signalment

Hyperparathyroidism usually affects middle-aged to older dogs. Keeshonds appear to be over-represented. German Shepherd Dogs, Poodles, Golden Retrievers, Labrador Retrievers and Cocker Spaniels can get the disease, but no genetic link has been found in these breeds. There is no sex predisposition.

Clinical signs

Clinical signs vary from asymptomatic mild disease to severe systemic illness. Polyuria and polydipsia are the most common signs, but dogs may present with anorexia, vomiting, muscle weakness, lethargy, constipation and weight loss.

Diagnosis

Serum biochemistry in primary hyperparathyroidism reveals hypercalcaemia and hyperphosphataemia, with normal renal function. If renal failure is present, primary and secondary hyperparathyroidism can be difficult to distinguish (Figure 17.9). Circulating PTH levels are inappropriately high in cases of primary hyperparathyroidism. An important differential to consider when investigating a patient with hypercalcaemia is hypercalcaemia of malignancy. In these cases PTH concentrations are low, but PTH-related protein (PTHrP) is high.

Ultrasound examination of the parathyroid gland by an experienced ultrasonographer can help to distinguish between hyperplastic glands and parathyroid adenomas.

Treatment

Treatment of mild hypercalcaemia involves intravenous fluids to promote calcium excretion, and furosemide administration at 2–4 mg/kg i.v. q12h. For treatment of hypercalcaemic crisis see the *BSAVA Manual of Canine and Feline Emergency and Critical Care*. Bisphosphonates may be used to control the hypercalcaemia, and are good options for dogs with hypercalcaemia of malignancy.

Primary hyperparathyroidism may be treated by surgical removal of the parathyroid gland. Postoperative complications include hypocalcaemia, which is usually transient and easily controlled.

Prognosis

The prognosis following surgical removal of the parathyroid gland is good. Development of additional neoplastic nodules is rare.

References and further reading

Bexfield N and Lee K (2014) *BSAVA Guide to Procedures in Small Animal Practice, 2nd edn*. BSAVA Publications, Gloucester

King LG and Boag A (2007) *BSAVA Manual of Canine and Feline Emergency and Critical Care, 2nd edn*. BSAVA Publications, Gloucester

Lindley S and Watson P (2010) *BSAVA Manual of Canine and Feline Rehabilitation, Supportive and Palliative Care: Case Studies in Patient Management*. BSAVA Publications, Gloucester

Mooney CT and Peterson ME (2012) *BSAVA Manual of Canine and Feline Endocrinology, 4th edn*. BSAVA Publications, Gloucester

Platt S and Olby N (2013) *BSAVA Manual of Canine and Feline Neurology, 4th edn*. BSAVA Publications, Gloucester

Disease	Serum calcium	Ionized calcium	Phosphate	Urea and creatinine	PTH	PTHrp
Primary hyperparathyroidism	↑ or ↓	↑	↓	Normal or ↓	↑	↓
Hypercalcaemia of malignancy	↑	↑	↓	Normal or ↑	↓	↑
Renal failure	10–20% ↑ Normal or ↓	Normal or ↓	↑	↑	↑	↓
Hypoadrenocorticism	↑	Normal or ↑	Variable	↑	Normal or ↑	↓
Hypervitaminosis D; granulomatous disease	↑	↑	↑	Normal or ↑	Normal or ↓	↓

17.9 Differentiating causes of hypercalcaemia. PTH = parathyroid hormone; PTHrP = parathyroid hormone-related protein.

Hyperthermia and pyrexia

Sarah Packman

A raised rectal temperature is a common finding on physical examination. It is important for the clinician to determine the cause of the raised rectal temperature and to differentiate pyrexia from hyperthermia.

The thermoregulatory centre is located in the hypothalamus and is composed of two parts: the rostral region, which is involved with heat loss and is under parasympathetic control; and the caudal region, which controls heat production and is under sympathetic control. Thermoreceptors in the skin, abdomen and central nervous system help to maintain the body temperature via the thermoregulatory centre. Most internal body heat is generated via oxidative reactions in the liver; however, muscle activity can rapidly produce a lot of heat.

Hyperthermia results from increased muscle activity, increased ambient temperature, or an increased metabolic rate. Hyperthermia can be further subcategorized into heat exhaustion/heat stroke, exercise-induced hyperthermia, and malignant hyperthermia (Figure 18.1).

Pyrexia in a dog is defined as having a rectal temperature >39.2°C at rest. Pyrexia occurs when the hypothalamus resets the body's thermoregulation to a higher point than normal, resulting in physiological mechanisms that increase the body temperature. Inflammatory mediators such as cytokines (primarily IL-1) that are released from leucocytes in response to exogenous and endogenous pyrogens (released in bacterial, viral, neoplastic and immune-mediated disease) alter this thermoregulatory set point.

History

Severe cases of hyperthermia often have an acute presentation; the history taken is usually brief and may be taken after treatment has been instigated.

With pyrexia, the signs may be acute or chronic, and may be intermittent, occurring over the preceding few weeks. Chronic cases of pyrexia often have vague signs and can be difficult to diagnose unless the dog is presented during a pyrexic episode. The breed, age, sex and neutering status can help to narrow the differential list. For example: younger dogs are more likely to develop steroid-responsive meningitis–arteritis, whilst older dogs are more likely to develop neoplastic conditions. Autoimmune disease is more common in bitches.

The owners should be asked about:

- The dog's environment in recent hours:
  - What was the ambient temperature?
  - Has it been shut in a car recently?
  - Has it had access to water?
  - Has it had any access to toxins?
- Do any other dogs, animals or people in the house have signs of illness? (Many causes of pyrexia are transmissible diseases)
- Is the dog vaccinated, and when was the last vaccination given? (Immune-mediated diseases have been linked to recent vaccination; unvaccinated dogs need to be barrier-nursed; infections such as leptospirosis and parvovirus need to be excluded from the differential list)
- Has the owner given any medications recently?
- Has the dog been exercising, and what has its recent exercise tolerance been?
- Is there a history of foreign travel? (Leishmaniosis can present with pyrexia)
- What products, if any, have been used for tick control?

Heat exhaustion/stroke

Marked increase in body temperature caused by exercise and/or environmental temperature rise that overwhelms the body's normal thermoregulation. Examples: healthy dog shut in a hot car; dog with status epilepticus

Exercise-induced hyperthermia

Body temperature rises excessively in response to moderate exercise. Example: exercise-induced hyperthermia in collies

Malignant hyperthermia

Abnormal calcium metabolism caused by medications or anaesthetics (e.g. halothane). Causes a rapid, often fatal increase in body temperature through uncoupled metabolic heat production

Pyrexia

Increase in body temperature due to a resetting of the thermoregulatory set point in the hypothalamus. Examples: infectious and immune-mediated diseases

18.1 Causes of raised rectal temperature and the mechanism of action.

- Has there been a recent tick bite or exposure? (Lyme disease, *Ehrlichia* and *Babesia* are spread by ticks)
- Has there been a recent skin injury which might have allowed a foreign body to enter under the skin?
- Has there been any recent surgery or illness?

The owner should then be questioned about body systems to help narrow the differential list. Questions should relate to the gastrointestinal tract, urinary tract, neurological system, respiratory tract, pancreas, cardiac system, and orthopaedic system.

Clinical signs

Owners will report either one of or a combination of:

- Lethargy
- Inappetence or anorexia
- Panting
- Shivering
- Collapse.

The most common reason for dogs to present to the clinician with hyperthermia is heat stroke due to being locked in a car (Figure 18.2). Even on mild days the temperature in a car can rise very high; owner education is therefore vital to prevent recurrence. Dogs with heat stroke may present with blindness, ataxia, disorientation or collapse.

> **WARNING**
>
> Severe cases of hyperthermia often have an acute presentation as the dog has not had time to adjust to the high body temperature. This is especially true in cases of heat stroke, and rapid cooling is needed in order to prevent ongoing damage

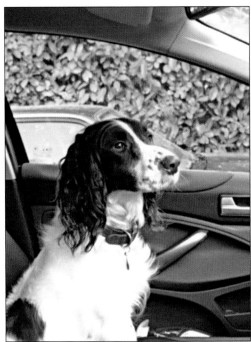

18.2 A dog's body temperature can increase rapidly if it is locked in a car, even on relatively cool days.

Physical examination

Marked pyrexia is an obvious clinical sign for the clinician to detect. Taking the rectal temperature is a quick, easy and reliable procedure and should be done routinely for any sick dog and at pre- and post-operative checks. A wide range of rectal thermometers is available (Figure 18.3), providing a reliable reasonable approximation for core body temperature. Additionally, with marked pyrexia, the dog will feel hot to the touch.

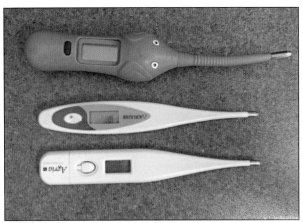

18.3 Examples of digital rectal thermometers with rigid and soft tips.

Once pyrexia is detected a full physical examination should be performed.

- Head:
  - Examine for signs of injury, inflammation and symmetry
  - Examine the nose for discharge and abnormalities of the mucocutaneous junction
  - Look for evidence of hypersalivation
  - Examine the oral cavity, including the mucous membranes to look for redness, pallor, icterus, cyanosis, petechiae and to allow assessment of the dog's hydration status. Note any evidence of halitosis and check the teeth for tooth root infections. Examine under the tongue for abscesses and salivary duct abnormalities, and the roof of the mouth for pathology and symmetry.
- Eyes:
  - Look for redness and record any discharges
  - The sclera is the best area to check for evidence of jaundice/icterus
  - Examine the retina for signs of inflammation.
- Neck:
  - Examine for evidence of a dilated oesophagus
  - Perform a tracheal pinch for evidence of coughing.
- Thorax:
  - Auscultate the chest and upper respiratory tract, paying special attention to laryngeal noise, cardiac abnormalities and abnormal lung sounds
  - Additionally, the chest should be percussed for evidence of dullness
  - Assess pulse quality and rate, and record abnormalities such as pulse deficits.

- Abdomen: Palpate for evidence of organomegaly (e.g. hepatic enlargement), pain and effusions.
- Skeleton: Manipulate the joints and spinal column, watching for evidence of pain, swelling or weakness.
- Skin: Examine for abnormalities including alopecia and dry flaky skin, infections, urticarial reactions, and tick bites.
- Lymph nodes: Palpate all peripheral lymph nodes and record any enlargement.
- Rectum/anus:
  - A rectal examination should be performed in male dogs to assess for prostate gland size and whether any pain is elicited on palpation
  - In males and females, examine the anal sacs for infection/masses.

Diagnosis and differential diagnoses

Heat stroke, exercised-induced hyperthermia and malignant hyperthermia should be treated by reducing the body temperature as a matter of urgency (see later), as ongoing organ damage continues when the body temperature is >41.1°C.

With pyrexia, it is more important to diagnose the underlying condition. The differential diagnosis list for pyrexia is vast (some possibilities are listed in Figure 18.4), but with a good history and clinical examination this can be narrowed down.

For dogs presenting with pyrexia that is attributable to a known cause, the reader should refer to the relevant chapter of this book for diagnostic work-up, which may include performing one or many of the following: a full blood count, serum biochemistry, urinalysis, faecal analysis, imaging, endoscopy, electrocardiography or serum testing for vector-borne diseases.

When pyrexia is the only abnormality detected and the pyrexia lasts for longer than 3 weeks without a diagnosis, then it is classified as pyrexia of unknown origin (PUO). For cases of PUO, the following diagnostic work-up is suggested (see also Figure 18.5):

- Haematology: to include a full blood count, white cell differential count and smear examination for evidence of anaemia, intracellular red cell inclusions, platelet numbers, and leucocyte abnormalities
- Serum biochemistry: including electrolytes and thyroid testing. Specific biochemical tests on the serum, such as canine pancreatic lipase immunoreactivity (cPLI) and serum protein electrophoresis, should be performed only if indicated
- Urinalysis: to include chemistry, specific gravity, sediment examination, urine protein:creatinine ratio, culture, and cytology if indicated from previous urine results
- Faecal analysis: should be performed if gastrointestinal signs are present
- Imaging: survey thoracic and abdominal radiography and abdominal ultrasonography to rule out infection foci, masses, organ abnormalities, and the presence of fluid. *The prostate gland should be examined in male dogs*
- If the above have not yielded a diagnosis, then the following tests are advised (for details of techniques see *BSAVA Guide to Procedures in Small Animal Practice*):
  - Bone marrow biopsy if abnormalities in the full blood count are detected
  - Echocardiography if a diastolic aortic murmur is indicated (to check for evidence of endocarditis)
  - Antinuclear antibody (ANA) testing if two of the major signs of systemic lupus erythematosus (polyarthritis, glomerulonephritis, haemolytic anaemia, thrombocytopenia, polymyositis, skin lesions) and two of the minor signs (e.g. PUO, oral ulceration, lymphadenopathy, seizures) are detected
  - Bronchoscopy if lower respiratory tract disease is suspected
  - Cerebrospinal fluid sampling and cytology (for steroid-responsive meningitis–arteritis, granulomatous meningioencephalitis and infectious meningitis)
  - Cytology of fine-needle aspirates from enlarged lymph nodes (avoid the submandibular nodes unless these are the only lymph nodes that are enlarged) (see Chapter 28)
  - Coombs' test (for immune-mediated haemolytic anaemia)
  - Serology for *Borrelia*, *Toxoplasma*, *Neospora*, *Ehrlichia*, *Babesia*, *Dirofilaria*
  - Arthrocentesis (for polyarthritis)
  - As a last resort, an exploratory laparotomy to search for neoplastic changes or abscessation may be performed, although this is seldom done due to its invasive nature.

Disease type	Potential conditions
Immune-mediated	Immune-mediated haemolytic anaemia. Immune-mediated thrombocytopenia. Immune-mediated polyarthritis. Steroid-responsive meningitis–arteritis. Granulomatous meningoencephalitis. Glomerulonephritis. Polymyositis. Systemic lupus erythematosus. Vasculitis
Bacterial infection	Abscesses and cellulitis. Discospondylitis. Bacterial bronchopneumonia. Infectious tracheitis. Prostatitis. Pyometra. Pyothorax. Bacterial peritonitis. *Leptospira*. *Bordetella bronchiseptica*. *Brucella*. *Borrelia* (Lyme disease). Pyelonephritis. Endocarditis. Bacterial cholangiohepatitis. Septic arthritis. Cystitis. Dental infections
Viral infection	Parainfluenza. Parvovirus. Distemper. Canine infectious hepatitis
Fungal infection	*Aspergillus*. *Cryptococcus*
Parasitic infection	*Babesia*. *Ehrlichia*. *Leishmania*. *Toxoplasma*
Neoplasia	Any neoplastic condition including: lymphosarcoma, multiple myeloma and myeloproliferative disorders
Sterile inflammatory	Pancreatitis. Pansteatitis/postsurgical fat necrosis. Nodular panniculitis
Miscellaneous	Pain. Drug reaction (e.g. tetracycline). Hypocalcaemic tetany

18.4   Differential diagnoses for pyrexia.

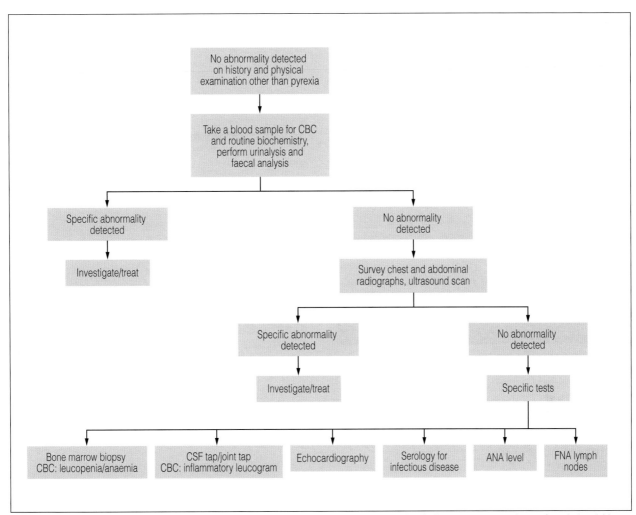

18.5 Suggested diagnostic work-up in a dog with pyrexia of unknown origin. If all tests are negative, referral should be considered. ANA = antinuclear antibody; CBC = complete blood count; CSF = cerebrospinal fluid; FNA = fine-needle aspiration.

Treatment

Treating hyperthermia

Simple hyperthermia will often subside if the dog is allowed to rest in a cool environment. Therefore, if a raised rectal temperature is found during an otherwise normal examination, re-measuring the temperature in 20 minutes can help to diagnose hyperthermia. Offering cool water by mouth if the dog is not collapsed is useful. Often no further treatment is required.

Severe cases of hyperthermia should be treated as a matter of urgency. Treatment focuses on whole body cooling. This aims to reduce the body temperature rapidly to prevent ongoing damage. Wetting the dog with cold water is the simplest and fastest way to reduce its body temperature.

- Cold water baths are very effective.
- Additionally, cool water enemas, spirit on the paw pads, placing wet towels over the dog (Figure 18.6), and using fans (with a wet dog) can be helpful.
- Administering intravenous fluids at room temperature is also an effective way of reducing core body temperature.

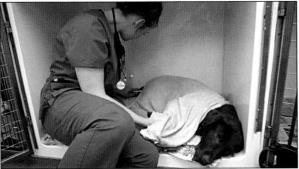

18.6 A 6-month-old Labrador Retriever being rapidly cooled with wet towels after being trapped in a hot car.

> **WARNING**
>
> - It is important to reduce the body temperature quickly, but not *too* rapidly, as normal thermoregulatory mechanisms are usually disrupted and as the animal cools, its heat-generating mechanisms may be impaired
> - Active cooling should be stopped when the rectal temperature reaches 39.4°C to prevent hypothermia. Any condition associated with ongoing muscular activity and heat generation should be treated (e.g. antiseizure medication for status epilepticus; see Chapter 11)

Once the dog has been stabilized, serum biochemistry should be performed to monitor for organ damage and to detect acidosis and electrolyte abnormalities in need of correction. Reduced cholesterol, low albumin, low total protein, raised creatinine, and raised total bilirubin levels are all associated with a poorer prognosis.

Dogs may develop kidney damage due to a combination of direct thermal damage to the renal tubular epithelium, hypotension, and thrombosis associated with disseminated intravascular coagulation. Hypotension can also lead to liver damage and gastrointestinal ulceration. Brain damage may result from thermal damage to neurons.

The prognosis with heat stroke is variable, and depends on the amount of organ damage present before the body is cooled down. Some cases may be fatal; others can make a full recovery. Long-term damage can be assessed by repeating serum biochemistry 1 week after the episode.

WARNING

The use of non-steroidal anti-inflammatory drugs (NSAIDs) is contraindicated in cases of heat stroke. They may contribute to iatrogenic hypothermia and may worsen gastrointestinal ulceration and ischaemic renal damage

Treating pyrexia

Because pyrexia results from a change in the thermoregulatory set point, whole body cooling is not advised; the body will increase its metabolic rate to try and keep the body temperature at the higher level set by the hypothalamus.

There is some controversy about treating mild pyrexia as it is thought to be a protective process (Figure 18.7), although there is no conclusive evidence to support this.

Dogs with rectal temperatures >41.1°C *should* be treated, as prolonged severe pyrexia can interfere

Proposed result of fever	Protective mechanism
Release of proteolytic enzymes by lysosomes	Destructive to viruses
Reduces the ability of bacteria to trap iron. Pyrogens released in pyrexia may cause iron sequestration in hosts	Iron stores less available to bacteria
Interferon production increases	Affects viral growth
Leucocyte mobility, phagocytic activity and bactericidal activity increased	Better immune response

18.7 Protective mechanisms thought to be produced by pyrexia.

with cellular metabolism and lead to brain damage, organ damage and disseminated intravascular coagulation. Many cases of pyrexia need supportive treatment with intravenous fluids and nutritional support. Treating the primary condition will often result in resolution of pyrexia within 2–3 days.

- Confirmed cases of bacterial infection must be treated with appropriate antibiotics, ideally based on the results of culture and sensitivity testing.
- Immune-mediated diseases will often respond to prednisolone, alone or in combination with other immunosuppressants.
- Pain is usually best controlled with NSAIDs (as long as they are not contraindicated) or with opioid medications.
- Antifungals should be used: topically for local disease, or systemically for systemic cases of disease. Note: Before systemic antifungals are used it is important to take baseline liver parameters and also to monitor liver function during treatment.
- Antivirals may be used; however, due to the expense of these medications, supportive treatment is often the only treatment used.
- Neoplastic conditions need to be treated specifically (see the *BSAVA Manual of Canine and Feline Oncology*).
- Parasitic diseases, such as the vector-borne diseases, need to be treated specifically.

Referral to a canine medicine specialist should be considered for cases of PUO where, despite a thorough investigation, a diagnosis cannot be determined.

It must be remembered that pyrexia can result in significant morbidity, lethargy and inappetence and therefore symptomatic treatment must sometimes be instigated. The two main classes of medications used to treat pyrexia are NSAIDs and glucocorticoids, but the latter are usually contraindicated unless there is a specific diagnosis and indication (e.g. a glucocorticoid-responsive immune-mediated disease). Additionally, sedatives such as acepromazine can be used to reduce body temperature via peripheral vasodilation for severe persistent cases that are unresponsive to treatment, but care must be taken to correct fluid deficits before using these.

References and further reading

Bexfield N and Lee K (2014) *BSAVA Guide to Procedures in Small Animal Practice, 2nd edn*. BSAVA Publications, Gloucester

Dobson J and Lascelles DX (2011) *BSAVA Manual of Canine and Feline Oncology, 3rd edn*. BSAVA Publications, Gloucester

King LG and Boag A (2007) *BSAVA Manual of Canine and Feline Emergency and Critical Care, 2nd edn*. BSAVA Publications, Gloucester

Epistaxis, sneezing and nasal discharge

Robert Williams

Disorders of the nose and associated structures often present with similar signs. Epistaxis, sneezing and nasal discharge are three of the most common and consistent signs associated with nasal disease, and all three signs are often present in one condition (Figures 19.1 and 19.2). This chapter will outline a simple initial approach for a dog presenting with these signs and also how to investigate the more complicated or recurrent case.

- Clotting disorders
- Neoplasia
- Trauma (acute)
- Aspergillosis
- Foreign body
- Dental/oral disease (e.g. tooth root abscess, oronasal fistula)
- Elevated blood pressure
- Hyperadrenocorticism

19.1 Common differential diagnoses for epistaxis.

- Neoplasia
- Foreign body
- Inflammatory disease (e.g. allergic rhinitis, nasopharyngeal polyps)
- Infection (e.g. fungal, viral, secondary bacterial)
- Dental disease
- Cleft palate

19.2 Common differential diagnoses for nasal discharge and sneezing.

Emergency treatment of epistaxis

In an emergency situation (i.e. severe blood loss) there are several simple things that can be done:

- Cage rest and keeping the animal quiet. This may necessitate the use of sedatives (e.g. acepromazine, diazepam, butorphanol) at low doses
- The application of direct pressure to the nares or ice packs on the nose
- In severe cases it may be necessary to anaesthetize the animal and pack both the nasopharynx and nasal cavity with saline-soaked swabs.

Initial approach to nasal disease

The initial approach to nasal disease should focus on: history; general clinical examination; and a specific examination of the nose, face and mouth. A standardized approach should be used for every case.

History

Pertinent areas to focus on include:

- Duration and incidence of signs:
  - Are they acute or chronic, constant or intermittent?
  - Are there any temporal associations, such as sneezing after walking through a corn field?
  - Is this a recurrent problem, and is it seasonal?
- Character of the discharge:
  - Serous, mucoid, purulent, bloody, mixed?
  - Unilateral or bilateral?
  - Has the discharge changed over time?
  - Is there also an ocular discharge present?
  - Has there been a progression over time; if so, is this change acute or chronic?
- Sneezing:
  - Present or absent?
  - Frequency?
  - Are there other respiratory noises present (stridor, stertor, cough, etc.)?
  - What type of material is produced on sneezing?
- Has the dog had any treatment for nasal disease (recent or historically) and has it been effective? (A course of anti-inflammatory drugs is likely to have resolved signs associated with simple rhinitis, but a course of antibacterials will, in the vast majority of cases, only have masked signs related to a tumour or fungal infection.)
- Are other body systems affected (e.g. appetite, exercise tolerance)?

> **PRACTICAL TIP**
>
> Always consider a clotting disorder as a cause of epistaxis

General clinical examination

> **PRACTICAL TIP**
>
> The initial examination should avoid the nose and face and concentrate on gathering information from the rest of the animal first. It is often the case that dogs resent examination of their nose and face, or of any area that is painful. Concentrating on the area of interest at the outset of the examination can therefore result in a poor clinical examination due to lack of cooperation

Following the systematic examination of the rest of the body (see Chapter 3), the area of interest can be investigated.

Examination of the nose, face and mouth

Observation: Key points include:

- Observe the dog breathing: are there signs of increased respiratory effort or respiratory distress? (See Chapter 8 for emergency procedures)
- Is the dog's face symmetrical? (For example, tumours can occasionally cause distortion of facial symmetry through destruction or proliferation of tissue)
- Are there changes to the orbit?
- Are there any signs of skin involvement (e.g. depigmentation of the nasal planum, periocular dermatitis)?
- Is there a discharge present (Figure 19.3), and if so of what type?
- Is the dog sneezing or coughing?
- Does the dog appear to be in discomfort?

- Can you make any judgement with regards to unilateral or bilateral involvement (e.g. based on unilateral *versus* bilateral discharge, discoloration of the nasal planum)?
- Are there any signs of a bleeding disorder (e.g. petechiae, ecchymoses)?

Palpation/manipulation: The aim of the hands-on examination is to feel for structural changes, changes in normal anatomical consistency and any foci of pain.

- Palpate the nasal and maxillary bones (muzzle), face, zygoma, globes, sinuses and submandibular lymph nodes, feeling for asymmetry, swellings and pain.
- Open the mouth; note whether it will open fully or not, and any obvious resistance. Inspect the teeth, especially the canines, molars and fourth upper premolar, for signs of dental disease (see Chapter 20). Look at the hard (and soft) palate; are there any palate deficits (Figure 19.4)? Is there an oronasal fistula, or is severe periodontal disease present?
- With the mouth closed, use a thumb to occlude the nasal opening on one side. Can the dog still breathe through its other nostril? Repeat for the other nostril.
- Airflow can also be checked by holding a microscope slide in front of each nostril and watching for fogging of the slide (indicating airflow).

Information gleaned from this approach should narrow the list of differential diagnoses.

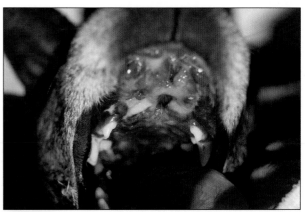

19.4 A rostral cleft in the hard palate following a dog fight. There is a circular communication between the oral and nasal cavities and extensive loss of the oral mucosa covering the hard palate.

Diagnostic investigations

For a thorough and systematic investigation of nasal disease, further investigation under general anaesthesia is mandatory.

Blood tests

Haematology and biochemistry are useful, as they may highlight an underlying systemic illness or evidence of a bleeding disorder. A coagulation profile will similarly highlight any deficiency of the clotting system and is also useful prior to nasal biopsy. Serological tests for *Aspergillus* are available, but results are unreliable and must be interpreted carefully in the context of other clinical findings.

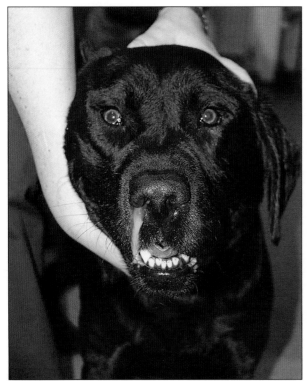

19.3 Typical appearance of a nasal discharge. This unilateral (right-sided) purulent nasal discharge was associated with nasal aspergillosis.

Oral examination

A thorough dental examination (see Chapter 20) is useful to rule out periodontal disease (this involves probing the lingual and labial gingival margins of all teeth). The soft palate should be palpated; it is relatively soft and should deform when pressure is applied. Any change in expected texture should be considered significant (e.g. tumour, nasopharyngeal polyp). Figure 19.5 shows surgical removal of a nasal polyp that was identified initially on palpation of the soft palate by finding a firm swelling on the nasal side.

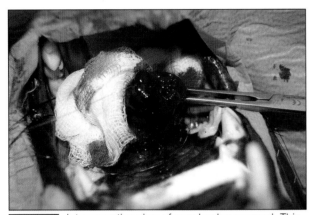

19.5 Intraoperative view of nasal polyp removal. This polyp was responsible for a chronic bilateral mucoid nasal discharge that was partially responsive to NSAID therapy. The polyp was identified on palpation of the soft palate (firm object palpated through the soft palate), and retrograde rhinoscopy whilst the dog was anaesthetized.

Radiography

Radiography may be helpful in adding to an index of suspicion, although it can be of limited value. Two views are commonly used: dorsoventral intraoral (DVIO) and skyline frontal sinus. A lateral view of the nasal passages is rarely useful, due to superimposition of the two sides of the skull. If it is easily available, computed tomography (CT) is extremely useful as an aid to diagnosis, but may be beyond the means of many clients.

Rhinoscopy

Rhinoscopy is the ideal tool for the investigation of nasal disease as it allows direct visualization of the nasal passages. Two types of endoscope may be used: flexible bronchoscopes can be retroflexed to examine the nasopharynx and choanae and can be passed a moderate distance into the nasal passages through the external nares; a 2.7 mm rigid endoscope is used to examine the nasal passages (and frontal sinus). For a thorough description of the technique, readers are directed to the *BSAVA Manual of Canine and Feline Endoscopy and Endosurgery.*

Samples can be collected for cytology, histology and fungal culture. Foreign bodies identified can often be removed under endoscopic guidance.

Bacterial culture

Bacterial culture and sensitivity testing of the nasal discharge or a swab sample from the nasal passages are rarely useful. Primary bacterial rhinitis is very rare and any bacterial infection present is usually secondary to one of the other causes of nasal disease.

Antibiotics in nasal disease

The use of antibiotics in cases of nasal disease can often lead to frustration and dissatisfied clients. Primary bacterial rhinitis is extremely rare, so any effect the antibiotics have is almost always due to treating a secondary bacterial infection. This may be entirely appropriate in a case of viral rhinitis with a concurrent secondary bacterial infection. However, for most other common causes of nasal disease (foreign body, inflammatory rhinitis, aspergillosis, neoplasia) there will be only temporary improvement whilst a secondary bacterial infection is controlled. Once the antibiotics are stopped, signs will recur relatively quickly. It is always worth counselling clients when prescribing antibiotics that signs of nasal disease are very likely to recur and will need further investigation

---

Common conditions and presentations

Epistaxis

Epistaxis can initially be a difficult problem to deal with. It is important to distinguish between: epistaxis as a reflection of primary nasal disease; and bleeding due to a systemic disorder. A broad database should be gathered, paying particular attention to evaluating haemostasis (complete blood count including platelet count and morphology, a clotting profile), blood pressure (systemic hypertension can cause epistaxis), biochemistry and urinalysis. Systemic diseases such as hyperadrenocorticism and neoplasia (e.g. haemangiosarcoma) may also cause epistaxis. Treatment is directed at removing the underlying cause, if possible.

Seasonal allergic rhinitis

While not very common, seasonal allergic rhinitis ('hay fever') does occur in some dogs, usually in the warmer months of the year. It presents with sneezing and a serous oculonasal discharge (Figure 19.6). It can often be managed with combinations of antihistamines, steroids and avoidance of any suspected

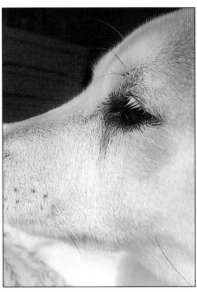

19.6

Serous ocular discharge in a 10-year-old neutered Shiba-Inu bitch with seasonal allergic rhinitis. (Courtesy of Emma-Leigh Craig)

allergens (usually pollen). There may be a variable response to treatment, and signs usually start to resolve spontaneously once environmental pollen load subsides or as the season changes.

Inflammatory rhinitis

Inflammatory rhinitis (lymphocytic/plasmacytic rhinitis) is a reasonably common and often frustrating cause of chronic nasal discharge in dogs. Several rounds of symptomatic treatment may have been tried with variable success, but signs will often return within 1–2 weeks of treatment ceasing. The nasal discharge is usually bilateral and mucoid. Sneezing is also common, as is stridor. Definitive diagnosis relies on endoscopic biopsy (and elimination of all other causes of nasal disease). A diagnosis of inflammatory rhinitis requires careful client counselling as it may not be possible to 'cure' the problem.

Systemic steroids form the cornerstone of treatment. Prednisolone at a high dose (1 mg/kg orally q12h) may be required (note that it is judicious to prescribe gastroprotectant medication at this dose). There is unfortunately a variable response to treatment. Other options include topical application of steroids, either instilling steroid drops directly into the nose or by use of a nasal inhaler spray. Hypoallergenic diets have also been suggested, as the nasal disease might be an unusual presentation of a food allergy.

Viral rhinitis

Viral rhinitis presents as sneezing and a serous nasal (or oculonasal) discharge. These dogs will also be pyrexic, lethargic and inappetent. Viruses involved include: adenovirus type 1 and 2 and parainfluenza virus. Signs will usually resolve in 5–7 days with appropriate supportive care (non-steroidal anti-inflammatory drugs (NSAIDs), mucolytics, ± antibiotics if a purulent discharge is present).

> **WARNING**
>
> It is important to caution owners to avoid contact with other dogs and to practice good hand hygiene after feeding/playing with the dog, washing food and water bowls

Severe periodontal disease (and/or oronasal fistula)

These may occasionally present with a purulent nasal discharge and/or epistaxis. If there is severe periodontal disease or an oronasal fistula in a dog with signs of nasal disease, the oral lesion should be treated first; this will often lead to resolution of the signs that suggested nasal disease. Readers are directed to an appropriate surgical or dental textbook for details of treatment for these problems (e.g. *BSAVA Manual of Canine and Feline Dentistry*; *BSAVA Manual of Canine and Feline Head, Neck and Thoracic Surgery*).

Foreign bodies

Nasal foreign bodies will present in one of two ways: acute or chronic.

Acute presentations are characterized by sudden onset of sneezing, head shaking and pawing at the nose. Foreign bodies may be lodged within the nasal passages or stuck in the nasopharynx/choanae. Such foreign bodies are typically grass awns, corn heads, thorns or small twigs. Dogs presenting in this way should be examined endoscopically under general anaesthesia. If an endoscope is not available, then drawing the soft palate rostrally and using a bright light and dental mirror will allow examination of the nasopharynx. The narrow speculum of an otoscope can also be passed into the external nares of larger dogs. It is possible to flush each nasal cavity with a 60 ml catheter tip syringe filled with saline (remember to inflate the endotracheal (ET) tube cuff and pack the pharynx) to try and dislodge the foreign body (Figure 19.7).

1. Anaesthetize the dog.
2. Inflate the cuff on the ET tube.
3. Pack the nasopharynx with moist swabs.
4. Fill a 60 ml catheter tip syringe with saline.
5. Introduce the tip of the syringe into one of the nasal openings. Apply lateral-to-lateral pressure across the nares, such that a tight seal is formed around the catheter tip syringe and the contralateral naris is sealed.
6. Depress the syringe plunger forcefully. Hopefully, this will dislodge any foreign body, which may be found in the nasopharynx or within the nasopharyngeal swab.
7. This process may be repeated several times for each nasal chamber.

19.7 Using a catheter tip syringe to flush the nasal cavity.

Chronic foreign bodies usually present as mucopurulent nasal discharges and intermittent sneezing. The patient may initially respond to symptomatic treatment (e.g. NSAIDs ± antibiotics), but signs are likely to recur once medication is stopped.

Aspergillosis

Aspergillosis is a relatively common cause of nasal disease in dogs. It is usually found in young to middle-aged dogs of particular dolichocephalic breeds (e.g. German Shepherd Dog, Border Collie); brachycephalic breeds are rarely affected.

Profuse nasal discharge is present and is usually of mixed type, either mucopurulent or sanguineopurulent; or epistaxis may be present. There is often pain on palpation of the nose and sinuses and, as chronicity develops, ulceration and depigmentation of the nasal planum occurs.

Diagnosis is made by accumulating evidence that fungal disease is present, as it is easy to make both false-positive and false-negative diagnoses. Several of the following should be present:

- Characteristic clinical signs: mixed nasal discharge; pain on palpation; depigmentation of the nasal planum; chronicity
- Radiographic findings suggestive of fungal nasal disease: loss of ethmoturbinates (Figure 19.8)
- Rhinoscopy: visualization of fungal plaques and destruction of turbinates (Figure 19.9)
- Histology/cytology: large numbers of fungal hyphae seen
- Positive culture of *Aspergillus* spp.
- Positive serological test for *Aspergillus* (not to be used alone).

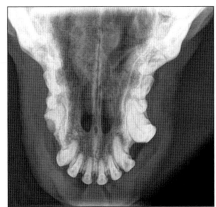

19.8
Radiographic appearance suggestive of *Aspergillus* infection. There is turbinate destruction, with increased radiolucency within the nasal chambers.

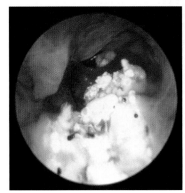

19.9 In this rhinoscopic image, turbinate destruction has exposed the frontal sinus, and classic white plaques of *Aspergillus* can be seen within the sinus cavity. (Reproduced from *BSAVA Manual of Canine and Feline Endoscopy and Endosurgery*)

Treatment involves instilling a liquid or ointment preparation of clotrimazole into the nasal cavity (and frontal sinus if indicated) for 1 hour under general anaesthesia. This is the most successful treatment described, with an initial success rate of approximately 85% (Sissener *et al.*, 2006). A more detailed description of the treatment is available in most surgery textbooks.

Neoplasia

Neoplasia is a common cause of nasal discharge in older dogs. Initially the discharge tends to be unilateral but can become bilateral as the disease advances. Other common signs include epistaxis, facial deformity/swelling, ocular discharge, exophthalmos, involvement of the hard palate and maxillary teeth, sneezing and dyspnoea.

Squamous cell carcinoma, adenocarcinoma, chondrosarcoma and osteosarcoma are all possible, though adenocarcinoma is most common in dogs.

Diagnosis involves imaging:

- Radiography: generally the DVIO view is the most useful, revealing either increased soft tissue opacity and/or loss of turbinate detail. As the disease progresses there may be loss of the bony nasal septum. The tumour may also extend into the frontal sinus with increased soft tissue density filling one or both sinuses
- Rhinoscopy (Figure 19.10): allows direct visualization of the tumour (or area of abnormality on radiographs) and allows for collection of biopsy samples.

Nasal tumours are often slow growing and slow to metastasize but carry a poor prognosis. Metastasis is usually to the brain, local lymph nodes and lung. There are treatment options available for nasal tumours; however, in most cases the mean survival time is only 3–5 months. This may be increased with combined therapies such as surgical debulking and radiation therapy, or laser ablation of the tumour. Early discussion with an oncologist for up-to-date advice on the treatment of nasal tumours is recommended.

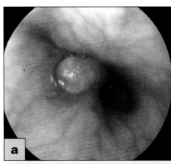

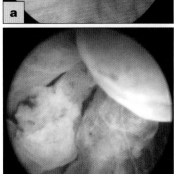

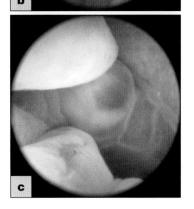

19.10 **(a)** Adenocarcinoma at the choanae, viewed in air. **(b)** Opaque irregular pale adenocarcinoma, with swelling and erythema of the surrounding turbinates. **(c)** Same dog as in (a), showing the appearance under irrigation. The tumour is pale and smooth, giving the appearance of a polyp. (Reproduced from *BSAVA Manual of Canine and Feline Endoscopy and Endosurgery*)

References and further reading

Cooke K (2005) Sneezing and nasal discharge. In: *Textbook of Veterinary Internal Medicine, 6th edn*, ed. SJ Ettinger and EC Feldman, pp.207–211. Elsevier Saunders, St. Louis

Gieger T (2005) Bleeding disorders: epistaxis and hemoptysis. In: *Textbook of Veterinary Internal Medicine, 6th edn*, ed. SJ Ettinger and EC Feldman, pp. 225–232. Elsevier Saunders, St. Louis

Hedlund CS (2007) Surgery of the upper respiratory system. In: *Small Animal Surgery, 3rd edn*, ed. TW Fossum, pp.817–866. Mosby, St. Louis

Lhermette P and Sobel D (2008) Rigid endoscopy: rhinoscopy. In: *BSAVA Manual of Canine and Feline Endoscopy and Endosurgery*, ed. P Lhermette and D Sobel, pp. 109–130. BSAVA Publications, Gloucester

Schmeidt CW and Creevy KE (2012) Nasal planum, nasal cavity and sinuses. In: *Veterinary Surgery: Small Animal*, ed. KM Tobias and SA Johnson, pp.1691–1707. Elsevier Saunders, St. Louis

Schmiedt C, Danova N, Bjorling D, Brockman DJ and Holt DE (2005) The nose and nasopharynx. In: *BSAVA Manual of Canine and Feline Head, Neck and Throat Surgery*, ed. DJ Brockman and DE Holt, pp.44–55. BSAVA Publications, Gloucester

Sissener TR, Bacon NJ, Friend E, Anderson DM and White RA (2006) Combined clotrimazole irrigation and depot therapy for canine nasal aspergillosis. *Journal of Small Animal Practice* **47**, 312–315

Tutt C, Deeprose J and Crossley D (2007) *BSAVA Manual of Canine and Feline Dentistry, 3rd edn*, BSAVA Publications, Gloucester

Oral and dental problems

20

Robert Williams

Signs of disease originating in the oral cavity are a common cause for presentation in general practice. The initial reason for presentation is often vague, such as a smelly or painful mouth or difficulty with eating (see also Chapter 14). There is often a simple explanation for what the owner has identified as a problem; however, it pays to keep an open mind and to have a thorough approach to dealing with these cases, as there can sometimes be a more serious or sinister cause (Figures 20.1–20.3).

- Abscess
- Chronic oronasal fistula or cleft palate
- Dental disease
- Foreign body
- Lip-fold dermatitis
- Tumour (infected/necrotic)
- Uraemia/ketones (not strictly halitosis but detectable smell can be present)

20.1 Common causes of halitosis.

- Abscess
- Craniomandibular osteopathy
- Dental disease
- Foreign body
- Otitis media
- Temporomandibular joint disease
- Tongue laceration
- Trauma

20.2 Common causes of a painful mouth.

- Abscess
- Craniomandibular osteopathy
- Foreign body (interarcade)
- Severe periodontal disease
- Tooth fracture
- Trauma
- Trigeminal neuritis
- Tumour

20.3 Common causes of difficulty in eating.

The mouth can also act as a sentinel to the general health of the animal, as colour changes in the oral mucous membranes are often readily noticed by owners and are important features during a veterinary examination.

Trauma

Trauma to the head and mouth is often the result of dog fights, road traffic accidents, or a kick from a large animal (or human). Animals usually present in obvious distress and pain and often with a very distressed owner.

> **WARNING**
>
> As when dealing with any case of trauma, it is important to remember the obvious injury may not be the most important. First assess the neurological, respiratory and circulatory status of the animal and treat any abnormalities prior to any further examination or treatment (see Chapters 8 and 10)

Once the dog has been stabilized, a more thorough examination of the mouth is possible. Pay particular attention to the temporomandibular joint (TMJ), mandible, and hard and soft palates, as injuries in these sites are likely to require repair. Fractures of the maxilla usually cause minimal displacement, are stable, and seldom require repair.

> **Approach to oral trauma**
>
> 1. Assess breathing, circulation, central nervous system (CNS)
> 2. Stabilize the patient
> 3. Provide multimodal pain relief
> 4. Restore normal anatomy and function
> 5. Appropriate supportive care, such as intravenous fluids and assisted feeding (oesophageal feeding tube, percutaneous endoscopic gastrostomy (PEG) tube)

The prognosis for most traumatic oral injuries is good, provided they are treated appropriately, after a thorough and systematic work up have been performed.

Initial approach to the non-emergency presentation

The initial approach should focus on: history; general clinical examination; and specific examination of the head and mouth. A standardized approach should be used for every case.

History

Pertinent areas to focus on include:

- Duration and incidence of signs:
  - Are they: acute or chronic; constant or intermittent?
  - Are there any temporal associations, e.g. difficulty or pain when eating, altered preference for soft over hard food?
  - Recent trauma
  - History of dog carrying sticks or owner throwing objects for the dog to retrieve
  - Does the owner feed the dog bones?
- General clinical signs of illness:
  - Alterations in appetite or water intake
  - Lethargy or reduced exercise tolerance
  - Are other body systems affected (e.g. is there ascites, coughing, vomiting)?
- Has the dog had any treatment for oral disease (recent or historically) and has it been effective?

General clinical examination

> **PRACTICAL TIP**
>
> The initial examination should avoid the nose and face and concentrate on gathering information from the rest of the animal. It is often the case that dogs resent examination of their nose and face, or of any area that is painful. Concentrating on the area of interest at the outset of examination can therefore result in a poor clinical examination due to lack of cooperation

Following the systematic examination of the rest of the body (see Chapter 3), the area of interest can be investigated.

Examination of the head and mouth

Observation may reveal asymmetry of the head (Figure 20.4). When examining the head, palpation, manipulation and some specific examinations should be carried out. It is generally possible to do this initially without general anaesthesia. The examination is repeated under general anaesthesia to reveal more information, as the dog is not then fearful or in pain. Details of dental examination are given in QRGs 20.1 and 20.2.

Palpation/manipulation: The aim of the hands-on examination is to feel for structural changes, changes in normal anatomical consistency and any foci of pain. This is initially performed with the animal conscious, but then repeated in the anaesthetized animal.

- Palpate the nasal and maxillary bones (muzzle), face, zygoma, globes, sinuses and submandibular lymph nodes, feeling for asymmetry, swellings and pain.

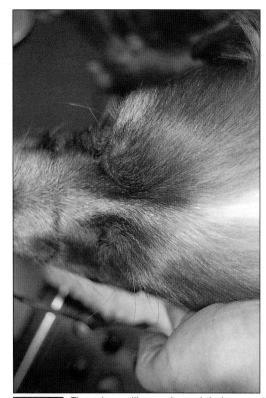

20.4 There is swelling and exophthalmos on the right-hand side of the head of this dog with an intraoral abscess.

- Open the mouth; note whether it will open fully or not, and any obvious resistance. Inspect the teeth, especially the canines, molars and fourth upper premolar, for signs of dental disease. Look at the hard (and soft) palate; are there any palate deficits? Is there an oronasal fistula, or severe periodontal disease present?
- Apply gentle digital pressure to the orbits, checking for disparity in size, pain, exophthalmos.
- Check airflow down each nostril.
- Examine the oral cavity: inspect the mucous membranes, teeth (see QRGs 20.1 and 20.2), tongue, pharynx, hard and soft palates, nasal planum and lip-folds.
- Perform otoscopy (see Chapter 22): what may seem to the owner like a mouth problem (difficulty with eating) may in fact be due to pain from one of the ear canals.

In most cases this examination will elicit what the most likely problem is (e.g. severe periodontal disease causing halitosis in an elderly terrier) or where further investigation should be focused (e.g. a painful mandible on manipulation requires analgesia, examination under anaesthesia plus imaging). Further tests or examinations (Figure 20.5) will usually require general anaesthesia.

> **PRACTICAL TIP**
>
> Spending time palpating and gently manipulating the mandible in cases of fracture can be invaluable in helping to generate a mental image of the fracture configuration and which segments of the mandible are affected

Procedure	Comment
Manipulation	Check range of motion of the TMJ Check for bony instability of the mandible, maxilla and zygoma
Palpation	Bony structures of face/mouth Hard and soft palates Submandibular lymph nodes Orbit Tongue
Probing	Tooth–gingival margins Any oral wounds or fistulas
Biopsy	Any obvious mass present or detected by imaging: incisional biopsy (multiple); fine-needle aspiration of lymph nodes
Imaging	Appropriate views as indicated for: trauma; TMJ disease; craniomandibular osteopathy; suspected tumour (especially bone involvement); dental problems

20.5 Further examination of the oral cavity under general anaesthesia.

Further diagnostic investigations

Imaging: The skull has complex bony anatomy which makes imaging specific lesions challenging. Oblique views are often required to try and highlight an area of interest. It is worthwhile consulting an imaging text such as the *BSAVA Manual of Canine and Feline Radiography and Radiology* or the *BSAVA Manual of Canine and Feline Musculoskeletal Imaging* from the outset.

Useful views include:

- A true dorsoventral (DV) view of the skull centred on the TMJ, which provides a good view of the TMJ (Figure 20.6)
- A DV intraoral view, if looking for fractures of the hard palate/maxilla or evidence of nasal neoplasia
- A 45 degrees (or greater) lateral oblique view of the mandible, to highlight the TMJ and fractures/tumours of the mandible (Figure 20.7).

Biopsy: The need to biopsy masses in the oral cavity is relatively common; in many cases the mass will be a tumour. If the mass is fluctuant on palpation (or appears to be fluid-filled) then needle drainage may be appropriate initially (see Chapter 28). Biopsy should

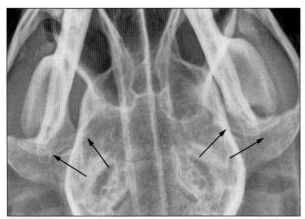

20.6 DV radiograph of the skull, showing the normal appearance of the temporomandibular joints (TMJs; arrowed). In the absence of CT imaging, this is a very useful view for highlighting the TMJs.

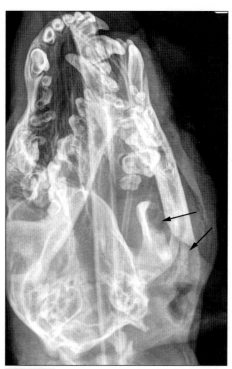

20.7 Right lateral oblique radiograph of the mandible, showing a caudal mandibular fracture (arrowed).

be performed on any mass that has the appearance of abnormal tissue (e.g. any raised firm pink, red, grey or black mass, whether smooth, rough, pedunculated, ulcerated or bleeding) or alters normal anatomy. The following should be borne in mind.

- Multiple biopsy samples increase the likelihood of a diagnosis – there is often a significant inflammatory reaction around oral tumours.
- Remember that the biopsy site (and any approach to the biopsy site) should be included in the body of tissue to be resected in the event that there is a malignant tumour.
- It is often worthwhile raising a mucoperiosteal flap directly over the area of interest, as sampling through the mucosa often reveals inflammation but not the underlying neoplastic process. Sometimes it is possible to take a superficial tissue sample and further (deeper) tissue samples through that initial site.
- Use skin biopsy punches, rongueurs, bone biopsy needles or soft tissue cup biopsy forceps as appropriate to retrieve samples (see *BSAVA Guide to Procedures in Small Animal Practice*). Skin biopsy punches are useful for obtaining a core of tissue from a mass, particularly once a mucoperiosteal flap has been raised.
- Fine-needle aspiration of oral lesions does not reliably yield diagnostic samples. However, fine-needle aspiration should be performed on draining lymph nodes as part of a tumour staging process.

Common problems

Figure 20.8 lists common clinical conditions associated with the presenting signs of halitosis, oral pain and difficulty in eating. These are discussed further below.

Clinical condition	Causes halitosis?	Causes a painful mouth?	Causes difficulty in eating?
Abscess	✓	✓	✓
Dental disease (excluding periodontal disease and fractures)	✓	Variable	Unlikely
Severe periodontal disease	✓	✓	Variable
Fractured tooth	Acute: no Chronic: possible if also infected	Acute: yes Chronic: probably not	Variable
Fractured mandible/maxilla	✓ if an open fracture	✓	✓
Lip-fold dermatitis	✓	Variable	✗
Foreign body	Variable; yes with chronicity/infection	Variable	Variable
Trauma	✗	✓	✓
Tongue laceration	✗	✓	✓
Craniomandibular osteopathy	✗	✓	Often
Temporomandibular joint disease	✗	✓	✓
Tumours	✓ if infected/necrotic	Variable; more likely if bone involved	Variable; depending on location/tissue involved
Trigeminal neuritis	✗	✗	✓
Otitis media	Occasionally	Variable	Variable

20.8 Association of clinical conditions and common presenting signs.

Dental disease

Dental disease is a very common presentation in canine practice. A very brief summary of common conditions is given in Figure 20.9. Tooth extraction is described in QRG 20.3. More detail of specific problems and their treatment can be found in the *BSAVA Manual of Canine and Feline Dentistry*.

Foreign bodies

Oral foreign bodies are a reasonably common finding in canine practice.

Sites affected include:

- Ventral to the tongue or the base of the tongue (e.g. stick injuries)
- Wedged transversely across the hard palate between the maxillary PM3 teeth
- Wedged between adjacent teeth, especially premolars and molars
- Tonsillar crypts and fauces
- Oropharynx (may present in acute respiratory distress especially if the object is large such as a tennis ball).

Objects retrieved include: bone, sticks, grass seeds, balls, thorns, hedgehog spines and fishing hooks (see also Chapter 23).

Dogs may present:

- Acutely: in obvious distress, with oral discomfort and often gagging and pawing (often frantically) at their mouth. They are usually reluctant to allow examination of the mouth. There is often a history of chewing a bone or stick or retrieving sticks
- Chronically: with halitosis, oral pain or dysphagia. The foreign body usually incites an inflammatory reaction and an abscess develops, which leads to the presenting signs. Abscesses are usually within the soft tissues (fauces (see Figure 20.12), tongue, oropharynx) but foreign bodies can occasionally be the cause of a tooth root abscess if the object is wedged between two teeth.

Whatever the presentation, general anaesthesia is usually required to allow thorough examination of the oral cavity. In obvious cases, such as a bone wedged across the hard palate or a ball stuck at the

Clinical problem	Comment	Treatment
Tartar/gingivitis (mild)	Very common presentation in dogs >2 years old	Scaling (see QRG 20.2), preventive treatment (e.g. tooth brushing, appropriate diet)
Periodontal disease (Figure 20.10)	Very common presentation, particularly in older dogs	Scaling, tooth extraction (see QRG 20.3), antibiotics as appropriate
Fractured teeth	Can be secondary to trauma or severe dental disease. Teeth usually either fracture in the sagittal plane (Figure 20.11) or lose the tip of the crown	If the pulp cavity is not exposed the tooth may remain *in situ*. If it is exposed it may need extraction or root canal treatment. Sagittal fracture: the tooth should be extracted (see QRG 20.3). Analgesia should be provided in cases of acute fracture and where the pulp cavity is exposed
Tooth root abscess	Either a progression of periodontal disease or secondary to a foreign body. Can also result from an untreated tooth with exposed pulp	Extraction of the affected tooth (or teeth) (see QRG 20.3). Appropriate antibiotics and analgesia

20.9 Common dental problems in dogs.

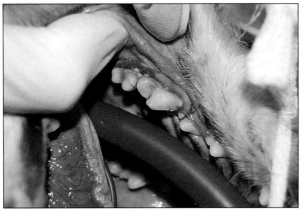

20.10 This 11-year-old Cocker Spaniel bitch showed some typical signs of periodontal disease. There is tartar on PM4 and M1, with associated gingivitis. Pus is also evident between the teeth.

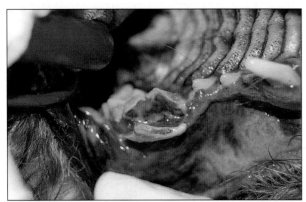

20.11 Sagittal fracture of PM4 resulting in periodontal disease. This tooth should be extracted (see QRG 20.3).

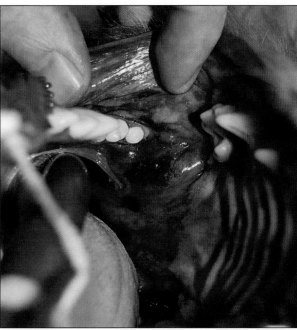

20.12 An intraoral abscess due to a stick foreign body, shown after lancing.

Benign
■ Epulides
■ Fibroma
■ Lipoma
■ Odontogenic tumours
■ Osteoma
■ Papillomatosis

Malignant
■ Chondrosarcoma
■ Fibrosarcoma
■ Haemangiosarcoma
■ Lymphoma
■ Malignant melanoma
■ Mast cell tumour
■ Osteosarcoma
■ Squamous cell carcinoma

20.13 Examples of benign and malignant oral tumours.

oropharynx, this may be very straightforward. In cases with a less obvious cause and more chronic history, a systematic exploration (digital palpation, good light source, blunt probe) of the mouth and pharynx will usually reveal the source of the problem.

Treatment is directed at retrieving the foreign body. A foreign body lodged across the hard palate (i.e. wedged transversely between the maxillary PM3 teeth) may be dislodged by gentle levering or pushing it caudally. Any associated abscess should be lanced (Figure 20.12), debrided and lavaged. Appropriate antibiosis and analgesia should be given. If there is tooth root involvement, tooth extraction may be necessary (see QRG 20.3). The prognosis is generally good following removal, but in cases where the foreign body cannot be retrieved, signs may recur.

Oral tumours

Tumours affecting the oral cavity are relatively common in canine practice; examples of tumour types are listed in Figure 20.13.

Gingival hyperplasia

As the name implies, this is not strictly a tumour, but it can have the appearance of one. It is thought to be a degenerative process secondary to periodontal disease and is common in some breeds (e.g. Boxer). Multiple firm (sometimes mineralized) lesions are present at the gingival margin. Treatment is by excision and attention to underlying problems.

Papillomatosis

Papillomas may develop on the lips, gingival margin and tongue in young dogs. They are caused by a papillomavirus and will regress spontaneously.

Epulis (peripheral odontogenic fibroma)

Epulides (Figure 20.14) are benign gingival proliferations arising from the periodontal ligament and are the most common tumour of the oral cavity. They usually affect older, large-breed dogs. They are usually pedunculated with a smooth shiny surface (unless ulcerated through self-trauma) and although they are firmly attached to the alveolar bone they are not invasive. Treatment is by excision – including the bony attachment. The acanthomatous epulis is malignant, with aggressive invasion into the underlying bone (though it does not undergo distant metastasis).

Malignant melanoma

This is the most common malignant tumour of the mouth, presenting as ulcerated masses often on the gingival margin, often with invasion of bone. They

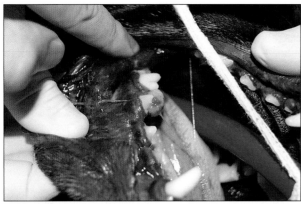

20.14 Typical appearance of an epulis: a firm, pink to red mass originating on the gingival margin.

are not always pigmented and are more common in older male dogs, especially breeds with pigmented mucosae (e.g. Cocker Spaniel, German Shepherd Dog). Growth, local invasion and metastasis to local lymph nodes (and lungs) are rapid and prognosis is poor.

Squamous cell carcinoma

Squamous cell carcinoma (SCC) may present as discrete masses or there may just be areas of ulcerated gingiva, often with bone involvement. The rostral mandible is the most common site, though SCC may also be found in any part of the oral mucosa, tonsils and tongue. Caudal sites are often painful and affect eating. The metastatic rate is low and prognosis is good for very rostral lesions, but the prognosis worsens with more caudal sites, and tonsillar SCC is highly metastatic.

Fibrosarcoma

These tumours usually affect the gingiva and hard palate, and the area between the canine tooth and PM4 is over-represented, especially in large-breed males. Fibrosarcoma often affects younger dogs (<7 years). It presents as firm, smooth masses, often with ulceration, but is locally invasive and will recur after excision unless a wide (compartmental) excision can be achieved. Thus, although slow to metastasize, the prognosis is poor, especially for very young dogs.

Osteosarcoma

Flat bone osteosarcomas are less common than the long bone variety and usually less aggressive, though prognosis remains poor. They generally affect older dogs.

Palate defects

Congenital palate defects

Congenital defects are usually midline on the hard and/or soft palate. They are easily identified and all puppies should be checked at birth (e.g. after caesarean or assisted whelping) or when first presented to the practice; a severe defect (see Figure 5.12) may prompt consideration of euthanasia. Cases that have not been identified (Figure 20.15) may present with nasal regurgitation of food, nasal discharge, gagging, coughing and ill-thrift. Repair is not straightforward and is prone to failure if performed incorrectly; details of the procedure are given in the BSAVA *Manual of Canine and Feline Head, Neck and Thoracic Surgery.*

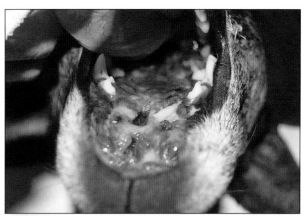

20.15 A 2-year-old male Patterdale Terrier with a chronic congenital cleft palate. The dog presented with intermittent mucopurulent nasal discharge and halitosis. A rostral premaxillectomy was used to deal with the abnormal tissue and small cleft at the rostral extent of the lesion, and a bilateral mucoperiosteal flap technique was used to close the large defect of the hard palate.

Acquired palate defects

Acquired defects (e.g. oronasal fistula; Figure 20.16) are usually caused by trauma or secondary to severe dental disease. They predominantly present as cases of nasal discharge (see Chapter 19). Treatment consists of debridement of the fistula and closing the defect with a mucoperiosteal flap (see *BSAVA Manual of Canine and Feline Head, Neck and Thoracic Surgery*).

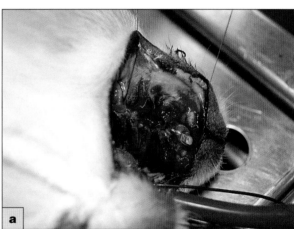

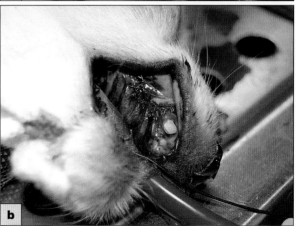

20.16 A 9-year-old Jack Russell Terrier bitch with an acquired oronasal fistula secondary to the loss of a canine tooth. **(a)** Elevation of a mucoperiosteal flap. **(b)** Appearance following repair.

Temporomandibular joint disease and loss of function

TMJ disease can be very debilitating, causing considerable pain and difficulty in eating. Conditions may be challenging to treat (e.g. TMJ ankylosis) or transient (e.g. craniomandibular osteopathy). Some common causes of TMJ loss of function are outlined in Figure 20.17. Cases often present as either open-mouth or closed-mouth 'lock jaw'.

Condition	Clinical signs	Treatment and prognosis
TMJ luxation	Isolated injury or in combination with other trauma. Inability to close mouth, with mandible deviated to affected side	Radiography to check for other injuries (e.g. articular fractures). Reduction under general anesthesia
TMJ fracture	Often associated with multiple trauma	Treatment is often conservative as the fractures can be relatively inaccessible and it is difficult to place implants. Immobilizing the jaw using a tape muzzle may be helpful. Variable outcome depending on injury to joint
TMJ ankylosis	? Post trauma/ craniomandibular osteopathy. True = affects joint. False = affects zygoma/ coronoid. Unable to close mouth (or open the mouth)	Excision of all affected tissue. Variable outcome
Trigeminal neuropathy	Bilateral temporary paralysis affecting mandibular branch of the trigeminal nerve. Dropped lower jaw. Non-painful on manipulation	Symptomatic and supportive care. Usually resolves spontaneously after several weeks

20.17 Some causes of loss of function of the temporomandibular joint (TMJ).

Craniomandibular osteopathy

Whilst craniomandibular osteopathy is commonly associated with juvenile West Highland White Terriers, it is also seen in other terrier breeds, Labradors, Great Danes and Boxers. It is idiopathic but is thought to have a genetic component. Presentation is usually in young dogs (4–8 months of age), who have difficulty in eating and pain on opening the mouth. The mandibles are often palpably enlarged, due to the non-neoplastic bilaterally symmetrical proliferation of bone affecting the mandibles, bullae and zygomatic arches. Damage to the TMJ may result in ankylosis. The condition is self-limiting and bone proliferation usually regresses, although analgesia and supportive care are vital. Corticosteroids may provide better analgesia than non-steroidal anti-inflammatory drugs (NSAIDs). The prognosis is good if the TMJ remains functional but some owners may opt for euthanasia in extreme cases due to the dog's distress.

Masticatory muscle myositis

This can occur in any breed, although spaniels and German Shepherd Dogs may be over-represented. Presentation may be acute (pain, difficulty in eating, swelling of the masticatory muscles) or chronic (difficulty in opening the mouth and atrophy of the masticatory muscles). Diagnosis can be enhanced by muscle biopsy. Treatment is with immunosuppressive doses of steroids.

Lip-fold dermatitis

Lip-fold dermatitis (see also Chapter 27) is a common cause of halitosis. It is most often seen in spaniels and setters but can occur in any dog that drools excessively or has a pronounced lip fold. Chronic exposure of the lip fold to saliva and food debris causes cheilitis and dermatitis. Mild cases may be controlled by basic hygiene (regular bathing with chlorhexidine) and occasionally topical antibiotics, but many cases only resolve after excision of the fold (Figure 20.18).

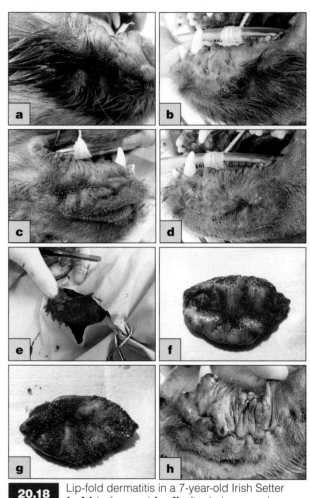

20.18 Lip-fold dermatitis in a 7-year-old Irish Setter **(a,b)** before and **(c,d)** after hair removal. **(e)** An ellipse of skin **(f,g)** is sharply dissected to remove the ulcerated tissue. Haemorrhage from superficial vessels may appear considerable, but is controlled by swabbing and closure of the incision. **(h)** The incision has been closed with a continuous subcutaneous suture.

Tongue lacerations

These are usually the result of trauma. The dog may be presented because of difficulty in eating or halitosis (chronic cases), or because the owner has noticed that the dog is bleeding or in pain. Treatment is by debridement and suturing. Double-layer suturing is necessary; 1 or 1.5 metric (5/0 or 4/0 USP) polyglactin 910 or poliglecaprone 25 in a simple interrupted pattern is appropriate.

Burns

Oral burns may be chemical or electrical and usually cause ulceration of the palate and dorsal surface of the tongue. Treatment is with supportive care: intravenous fluids, analgesia and assisted feeding.

Changes in oral mucous membranes

There are many causes for changes in the appearance or colour of the mucous membranes. These changes can often be accompanied by other serious signs such as collapse or respiratory distress, although there may be minimal clinical signs. Until proven otherwise, all cases should be viewed as potentially serious, and most dogs presenting with marked changes will need to be admitted for further investigation.

In general, the normal appearance of the oral mucous membranes is pink and moist. Changes include: pallor; injected or 'brick-red'; yellow (jaundiced); and bluish (cyanosis).

PRACTICAL TIP
Some breeds normally have pigmented membranes (e.g. Chow Chow)

Initial approach

The approach when presented with altered mucous membranes should be the same as for any potentially serious medical problem:

- Obtain a good history
- Perform a thorough clinical examination
- Obtain a minimum database, including urinalysis, haematology and biochemistry
- Other tests may be needed, depending on initial suspicions: e.g. clotting profile, Coombs' test, blood film cytology, thoracic and abdominal imaging, systemic blood pressure measurement, blood-gas analysis (if available), bone marrow biopsy and echocardiography.

Jaundice

Jaundice is characterized by hyperbilirubinaemia and deposition of bile pigment in the skin, mucous membranes and the sclera, causing the typical yellow appearance of these tissues. Jaundice can be pre-hepatic, hepatic or post-hepatic in origin (Figure 20.19).

Cyanosis

Cyanotic, bluish mucous membranes occur due to increased amounts of reduced haemoglobin within the bloodstream. Central cyanosis (Figure 20.20) is due to unsaturated arterial blood or the presence of a specific haemoglobin derivative, whereas peripheral cyanosis is due to desaturation of blood due to a regional reduction in blood flow.

Pale mucous membranes

Pale mucous membranes originate from either shock (see Figure 9.2a) or anaemia (Figure 20.21).

The approach to a dog with pale mucous membranes is summarized in Figure 20.22.

Primary problem	Subcategory	Causes
Anaemia	Haemolytic anaemia	Immune-mediated anaemia Infectious (e.g. leptospirosis) Toxic (e.g. onions, propylene glycol, lead) Disseminated intravascular coagulation Haemangiosarcoma
Hepatic and/or biliary disease	Hepatobiliary disease	Cholangiohepatitis Cirrhosis Diffuse neoplasia Copper toxicity
	Post-hepatic biliary obstruction	Pancreatitis or severe enteritis Trauma Neoplasia Cholelithiasis Biliary duct stricture or rupture

20.19 Common causes of jaundice.

Central cyanosis
- Cardiac (right-to-left shunt, e.g. reverse patent ductus arteriosus) - Hypoventilation - Pneumothorax, pleural effusion - Laryngeal paralysis - Airway obstruction - Pulmonary thromboembolism - Pulmonary infiltration - Methaemoglobinaemia

Peripheral cyanosis
- Central cyanosis - Decreased arterial supply - Peripheral vasoconstriction - Obstruction of venous drainage

20.20 Common causes of cyanosis.

Primary problem	Subcategory	Causes
Shock	Hypovolaemic	Severe blood loss Severe dehydration Hypoadrenocorticism
	Distributive	Sepsis Endotoxaemia
	Cardiogenic	Dilated cardiomyopathy Hypertrophic cardiomyopathy Myocarditis Cardiac tamponade Severe arrhythmia
Anaemia	Regenerative	Haemolysis Blood loss Oxidative injury Copper toxicity Fragmentation
	Non-regenerative	Anaemia of chronic disease Kidney failure Endocrine disorders Aplastic anaemia Myelodysplasia Myeloproliferative disorders

20.21 Common causes of pale mucous membranes.

Treatment

The initial approach to treatment should be to stabilize the patient, especially dogs that are in shock, collapsed (see Chapter 9) or systemically unwell. This should include:

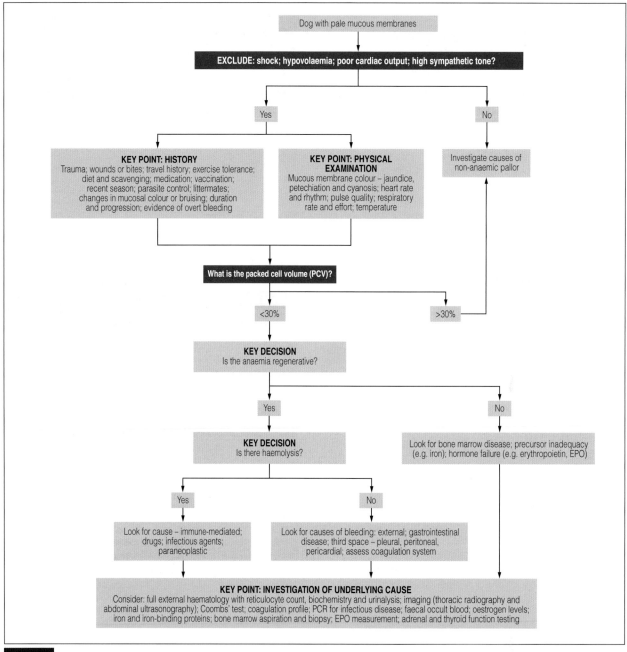

20.22 An approach to the dog with mucous membrane pallor. (Courtesy of L Holm and K Sturgess)

- Restoring circulating blood volume and/or maintaining blood pressure using crystalloids, colloids or blood products as appropriate
- Arrest any obvious source of haemorrhage (e.g. splenectomy if ruptured spleen)
- Provide supplemental oxygen (see Chapter 8)
- Monitor vital signs as an indicator of response to first aid treatment.

References and further reading

Barr F and Kirberger R (2006) *BSAVA Manual of Canine and Feline Musculoskeletal Imaging.* BSAVA Publications, Gloucester

Bexfield N and Lee K (2014) *BSAVA Guide to Procedures in Small Animal Practice, 2nd edn.* BSAVA Publications, Gloucester

Eddlestone SM (2005) Jaundice. In: *Textbook of Veterinary Internal Medicine, 6th edn,* ed. SJ Ettinger and EC Feldman, pp. 222–225. Elsevier Saunders, St. Louis

Hedlund CS and Fossum TW (2007) Surgery of the oral cavity and oropharynx. In: *Small Animal Surgery, 3rd edn,* ed. TW Fossum, pp. 339–367. Mosby Elsevier, St. Louis

Holloway A and McConnell F (2013) *BSAVA Manual of Canine and Feline Radiography and Radiology: A Foundation Manual.* BSAVA Publications, Gloucester

Holm L and Sturgess K (2013) How to...approach a dog with pale mucous membranes. In: *How To...Collected Articles from BSAVA companion,* ed. M Goodfellow, pp. 50–9

Liptak JM and Withrow SJ (2007) Oral tumours. In: *Withrow and MacEwen's Small Animal Clinical Oncology, 4th edn,* ed. SJ Withrow and DM Vail, pp. 455–476. Saunders Elsevier, St. Louis

Morrison WB (2005) Pallor. In: *Textbook of Veterinary Internal Medicine, 6th edn,* ed. SJ Ettinger and EC Feldman, pp. 211–215. Elsevier Saunders, St. Louis

Petrie J-P (2005) Cyanosis. In: *Textbook of Veterinary Internal Medicine, 6th edn,* ed. SJ Ettinger and EC Feldman, pp. 219–222. Elsevier Saunders, St. Louis

Reiter AM and Smith MM (2005) The oral cavity and oropharynx. In: *BSAVA Manual of Canine and Feline Head, Neck and Thoracic Surgery,* ed. DJ Brockman and DE Holt, pp. 25–44. BSAVA Publications, Gloucester

Tutt C, Deeprose J and Crossley D (2007) *BSAVA Manual of Canine and Feline Dentistry, 3rd edn.* BSAVA Publications, Gloucester

White RAS (2003) Tumours of the oropharynx. In: *BSAVA Manual of Canine and Feline Oncology, 2nd edn,* ed. JM Dobson and BDX Lascelles, pp. 206–214. BSAVA Publications, Gloucester

QRG 20.1 Examining the mouth in a conscious dog

by Lisa Milella

Oral examination in the conscious dog is limited to visual inspection and some digital palpation. Some dogs resent examination of the mouth, especially if there are painful areas. The aim of the conscious oral examination is to obtain a tentative diagnosis that can help formulate a treatment plan. As good practice, owners should be advised that it is only under a general anaesthetic that the mouth can be fully examined and the true extent of oral disease evaluated.

1 Approach the dog from the side or from behind. Gently make contact with the dog and stroke its head prior to examining the mouth. Gentle technique is essential as some dogs may have dental pain or discomfort.

> ### PRACTICAL TIP
> It is important always to have good lighting when examining the mouth

2 Examine the head externally:

■ Check visual symmetry. In cases of a tooth root abscess, for example, the area of the nose below the eye may be swollen, or in cases of an oral tumour, a swelling may be obvious on one side

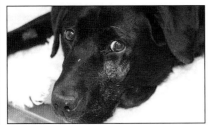

A draining sinus is present in this Labrador Retriever, with cellulitis of the left maxilla secondary to a fractured maxillary carnassial tooth with pulp exposure.

■ Gently palpate the facial muscles, facial bones and salivary glands.

3 Palpate the lymph nodes:

■ The mandibular and retropharyngeal lymph nodes at the angle of the jaw
■ The cervical chain extending down the neck to the prescapular lymph node
■ The retropharyngeal lymph nodes may only be palpable if enlarged.

> ### PRACTICAL TIP
> An enlarged lymph node may indicate infection or inflammation

4 Perform a closed mouth examination. Gently hold the jaws closed and retract the lips. *Do not pull on the fur to retract the lips.* Examine the soft tissues and buccal aspects of the teeth.

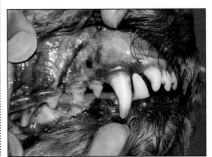

Mild gingivitis and calculus accumulation can be seen on the buccal surfaces of the teeth.

Examine:

■ Occlusion:
  • Is this normal for the breed or are there any signs of soft tissue trauma?
  • Check the incisor relationship: the lower incisors should occlude palatal to the upper incisors
  • Check the canine interlock (the lower canine should occlude in the diastema between the upper canine and third incisor
  • Check the premolar alignment (the teeth should interdigitate) and the distal occlusion should be that the mandibular premolars and molars occlude on the palatal surface of the maxillary premolars
  • Check the position of individual teeth.

> ### PRACTICAL TIP
> The above may vary with brachycephalic head shapes

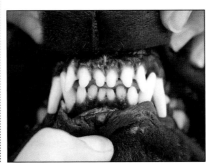

Correct incisor occlusion.

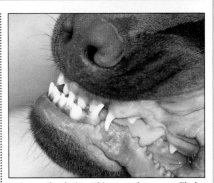

Incisor malocclusion. This puppy has a mandibular prognathism, with the maxillary incisors biting into the oral soft tissues lingual to the mandibular incisors, causing trauma to the soft tissue.

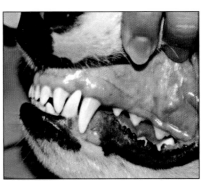

Correct canine interlock.

■ Mucous membranes: Check for inflammation, ulceration or any swelling of the buccal mucous membranes, gingival tissues and oral mucosa.

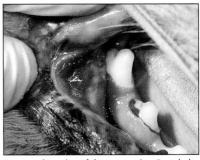

Contact ulceration of the mucosa in a Bearded Collie with chronic ulcerative paradental stomatitis.

■ Teeth:
  • Check for missing teeth or extra teeth
  • Look at the gingival margin – is it inflamed, swollen or receded?
  • Check the crown for defects such as fractures
  • Check to see whether any of the teeth are mobile by digital manipulation ▶

QRG 20.1 *continued*

- Check the calculus coverage on individual teeth *versus* the whole mouth.

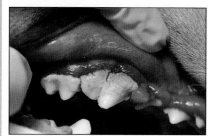

Severe inflammation of the gingiva (gingivitis) with hyperplasia of the maxillary fourth premolar and molar.

5 Perform an open mouth examination.

i. Approach the dog from the side.
ii. Place one hand over the muzzle, with the forefinger and thumb placed just behind the upper canine teeth. Gently press the lips into the oral cavity while tilting the dog's head slightly upwards.

iii. Place a finger from the other hand on the lower incisors, and exert gentle pressure. In larger dogs, the thumb and forefinger are placed behind the lower canines to open the mouth.

Do not use the fur under the mandible to try to pull the jaw down.

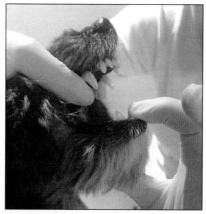

The correct way to open a dog's mouth.

Examine:

- The mucous membranes of the hard palate: check for foreign bodies lodged across the palate

- The oropharynx (soft palate, palatoglossal arch, tonsillary crypts, tonsils and fauces)
- The lingual and palatal surfaces of the teeth (brief evaluation)
- The occlusal surfaces of the maxillary and mandibular molars for caries decay (discoloration seen on examination)

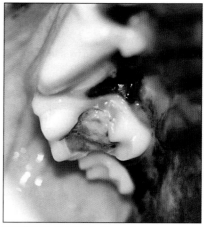

Maxillary molar affected by caries.

- The tongue: gently place pressure externally between the mandibles to lift up the tongue.

QRG 20.2 Scaling and polishing teeth
by Lisa Milella

Professional periodontal treatment is carried out to deal with plaque-retentive surfaces and to reduce areas of plaque stagnation, ensuring the mouth is then in the best condition to enable the client to provide ongoing plaque control.

Patient preparation

General anaesthesia is always required in order to perform a scale and polish because areas in the mouth may be painful, the dog may resist examination of the mouth and a secure watertight airway is needed to prevent aspiration of the water used for cooling equipment, or aspiration of debris and blood from the procedure itself.

The dental chart

Dental charts are a diagrammatic representation of the dentition, where information (findings and treatment) can be entered in a pictorial and/or notational form. The chart should be completed and filed following any dental examination and treatment. The canine dental chart shown here uses the modified Triadan tooth numbering system, where individual numbers are assigned to individual teeth to ensure

accurate recording of the clinical findings and treatment. The numbers correspond to the 42 teeth found in the permanent dentition of dogs.

	Incisors	Canines	Premolars	Molars	TOTAL
Maxilla	3	1	4	2	X2 = 42
Mandible	3	1	4	3	

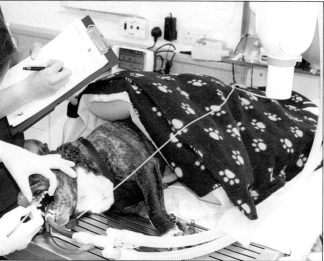

The dog is examined and findings are recorded on a dental chart by an assistant.

▶

QRG 20.2 *continued*

Your practice details here

Canine Dental Chart

Date	
Animal's name	Age
Owner's name	Sex
Breed	Client ref.

Buccal

Buccal R **MAXILLA** L

Palatal 110 109 108 107 106 105 104 103 102 101 201 202 203 204 205 206 207 208 209 210

CI																			
GI																			
Other																			

Buccal

Buccal R **MANDIBLE** L

Lingual 411 410 409 408 407 406 405 404 403 402 401 301 302 303 304 305 306 307 308 309 310 311

CI																					
GI																					
Other																					

Treatment	Recommendations

GI (Gingivitis index)
0 = Normal; no inflammation
1 = Marginal gingivitis; red line/oedema
2 = Bleeds on gentle probing. Swollen
3 = Severe inflammation. Spontaneous bleeding

CI (Calculus index)
0 = No calculus either side tooth
1 = Up to 25% cover bucally above/below gingiva
2 = From 25%–75% cover on buccal crown
3 = From 75%–100% cover on buccal crown

M (Mobile Tooth)
0 = Normal
1 = Slight
2 = Moderate
3 = Severe

CODE KEY
	Missing tooth	FX	Fractured tooth	RD	Persistent deciduous tooth (draw position)
X	Extracted tooth	PE	Pulp exposure	XR	X-ray of tooth taken
P (mm)	Periodontal pocket	CA (class)	Carious lesion	AT	Attrition
GH	Gingival hyperplasia	F	Furcation exposure (F₁, F₂, F₃)	OM	Oral mass
GR	Gingival recession	R	Restoration (Rc, Ri or Ra)	OD	Odontoplasty
	(Draw line to indicate exact buccal location)	ED	Enamel defect	GVP	Gingivoplasty
		3°D	Tertiary dentine		

© BSAVA 2010
British Small Animal Veterinary Association, Woodrow House, 1 Telford Way, Waterwells Business Park, Quedgeley, Gloucester GL2 2AB
Tel: 01452 726700   Fax: 01452 726701   Email: administration@bsava.com   Web: www.bsava.com

🔱 **BSAVA**
BRITISH SMALL ANIMAL
VETERINARY ASSOCIATION

Full-size downloadable chart available to BSAVA members at www.bsava.com

Equipment

Periodontal probe

The periodontal probe is a thin, rounded, blunt-ended graduated instrument. The blunt end allows the probe to be inserted into the gingival sulcus without causing trauma.

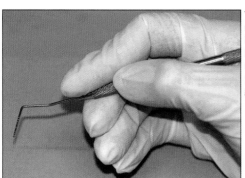

The periodontal probe is held in a modified pen grip, as with all dental instruments except elevators and luxators. Graduations (millimetres) are marked on the end of a periodontal probe to enable measurements of the gingival sulcus.

Explorer probe

The dental explorer probe is a sharp-ended instrument.

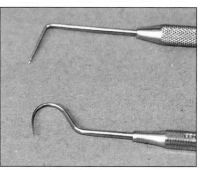

Differently shaped dental explorer probes.

Other hand instruments

- Hand scaler: the sharp point means that this can be used supragingivally only, to avoid damaging the periodontal tissues.
- Subgingival curette: the rounded blunt toe allows this instrument to be used subgingivally. A Gracey curette pattern 5/6 is a useful size to clean below the gingival margin in dogs.

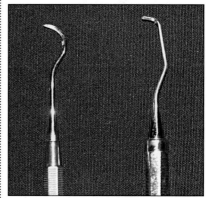

Hand scaler (left) and Gracey curette (right).

- Extraction forceps (e.g. 76N, with small narrow beaks).

Scaler

An ultrasonic scaler with a sickle-shaped tip is recommended.

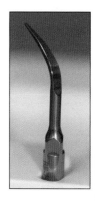

Make sure that the tip is water-cooled. The water setting should be that which produces a fine mist when in motion and a fine droplet off the point. The water reduces the heat generated by the tip and also aids calculus removal by the process known as cavitation. ▶

QRG 20.2 *continued*

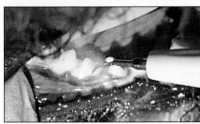

Cavitation is the formation of partial vacuums in the water, resulting in the pitting and wearing away of the calculus as a result of the collapse of these vacuums in the surrounding liquid.

The power setting of the scaler should be set according to the manufacturer's recommendations, but ideally at the lowest possible setting to avoid excessive heat generation.

Procedure

1 Prior to scaling and polishing, examine the mouth using a periodontal probe and explorer probe.

- Use the periodontal probe to check for: bleeding of the gingival tissues; periodontal probing depths around all teeth; tooth mobility; and exposed furcations (the areas between two roots).

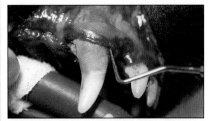

Periodontal probe being used to check for gingivitis and probing depths on the maxillary right canine.

- Use the explorer probe to check for defects of the crown, such as pulp exposure in fractured teeth, or worn teeth.

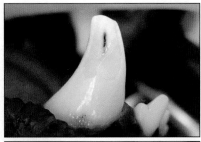

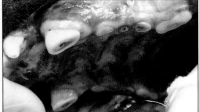

Pulp exposure in fractured and worn teeth. The explorer probe is used to check for defects in the crown.

2 Rinse the mouth with a proprietary chlorhexidine mouthwash (e.g. Hexarinse). This reduces the bacterial aerosol created by ultrasonic scaling.

3 Remove any large pieces of calculus using extraction forceps, without contacting or traumatizing the gingiva.

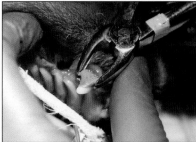

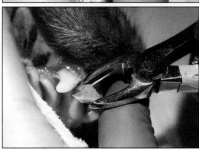

4 Using the ultrasonic scaler, start by scaling the crowns of the teeth above the gingival margin (supragingival scaling). Clean all the buccal surfaces of the dental arcades that are uppermost, and then all the lingual and palatal surfaces of the opposite arcades.

PRACTICAL TIP

Always use the side of the scaler tip and never the point, as this damages the tooth enamel

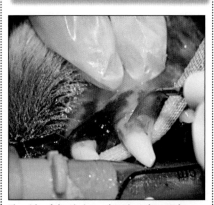

The side of the tip is used against the tooth surface. The fine water spray can also be seen.

5 If calculus is present below the gingival margin, use a hand curette to remove it and any diseased cementum.

- The instrument is positioned below the gum margin, with the working edge against the tooth surface to be cleaned, and then pulled towards the crown.

- The instrument is moved circumferentially around the tooth, using overlapping vertical strokes.
- Oblique or horizontal strokes are also used, particularly in the furcation area of multi-rooted teeth.

PRACTICAL TIP

Use an explorer probe to check that all calculus has been removed, or gently puff some air under the gingival margin using the air/water syringe from the dental unit

6 Polish the teeth to remove any remaining plaque and small bits of calculus.

WARNING

Immense iatrogenic damage can be caused by polishing incorrectly

- Always use a fine grit polishing paste with a soft rubber cup.
- Use plenty of polishing paste to reduce friction between the rotating cup and the tooth surface.
- Use enough pressure to flare the cup gently against the tooth surface. The cup can be gently flared below the gingival margin to clean any subgingival plaque.
- The speed of rotation should be set so that the cup just slows down when it contacts the tooth surface. Too much pressure, too much friction or too high a speed rotation will result in excess heat being produced that can ultimately cause pulpitis (inflammation of the pulp – usually irreversible, leading to pulp necrosis). *This can be appreciated by performing the same action against your thumb nail to feel the heat generated.*

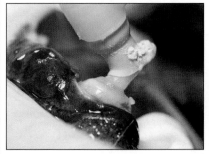

7 Rinse the dog's mouth with water, followed by a chlorhexidine mouthwash. Any further treatment such as extractions (see QRG 20.3) can then be carried out.

QRG 20.3 Tooth extraction
by Lisa Milella

Indications

- Severe periodontal disease (mobility, furcation exposure, periodontal probing depths) or teeth with moderate periodontal disease where homecare is not going to be provided.
- Complicated crown fracture (pulp exposed).
- A tooth where a fracture extends subgingivally, to involve the root, whether the pulp is exposed or not.
- Teeth affected by caries.
- Teeth involved in a jaw fracture.
- Unerupted teeth causing clinically significant disease.
- Teeth causing malocclusions.
- Supernumerary teeth.
- Chronic ulcerative paradental stomatitis.

Equipment

- Luxator 3 mm and 4 mm straight and curved (not essential).
- Elevators: Couplands 1 (3 mm) and Couplands 3 (4 mm).
- Periosteal elevator.
- Scalpel handle and blades.
- Extraction forceps: pattern 76N.
- Selection of burs for bone removal and sectioning the teeth. The author recommends: friction grip round 2 and 4 to remove bone; 701 tapered fissure bur to section teeth; and a large round diamond bur to smooth bone edges following the extractions.
- High-speed turbine water-cooled handpiece on a dental unit with a three-way syringe.
- Soft tissue protector, such as a plastic spatula.
- Surgical kit for closure of oral flaps.
- Monofilament absorbable suture material.

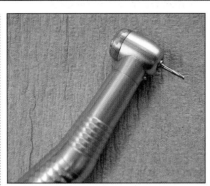

High-speed turbine, water-cooled handpiece.

Patient preparation

- The dog should always be anaesthetized with a cuffed endotracheal tube in place. Care must always be taken to ensure that the tube is securely fastened, to minimize any movement when manipulating the head during dental treatment.
- Appropriate pain relief should be given (pre-, intra- and post-operatively). Consideration should be given to the use of opioids, NSAIDs and local anaesthetic techniques (see specific dental texts).
- Ideally, the teeth should be scaled and polished (see QRG 20.2) prior to extraction, to ensure that the oral surgery is performed in a clean mouth. As a minimum, the mouth should be rinsed with a chlorhexidine mouthwash and gross calculus removed prior to extraction.
- Pre-extraction radiographs should be taken to assess the tooth, its roots and the disease present.

Procedures

Non-surgical or 'closed' technique

This technique is used for all single-rooted teeth or teeth that have been sectioned into individual roots.

Multi-rooted teeth

- To section multi-rooted teeth into individual roots, use a tapered fissure friction grip bur (701) on a high-speed handpiece with water cooling
- The furcation must first be identified. The furcation is the area between the roots and generally lies below the main cusp. It can be identified by raising some of the gingival tissue away from the bone or by gently using a puff of air from the three-way syringe

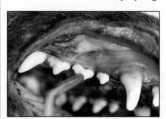

- Start sectioning the tooth from the furcation towards the cusp, from the buccal to the lingual/palatal aspect of the tooth. *Care should be taken not to damage the gingival attachment at the furcation*

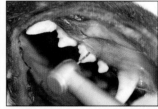

- To check that the tooth has been adequately sectioned, place an elevator between the two sections of the tooth and gently rotate – both parts of the crown should move independently
- Each tooth root is then extracted individually as described below

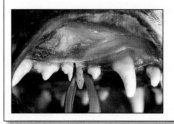

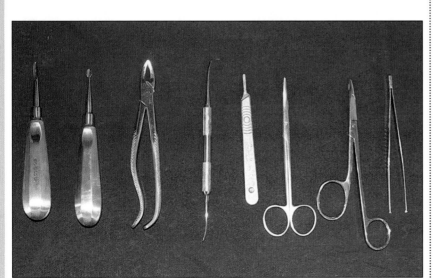

From left to right: Couplands 1 elevator; winged elevator; extraction forceps pattern 76N; Goldman Fox periosteal elevator; scalpel handle; scissors; needle holders; rat-toothed forceps.

QRG 20.3 *continued*

1 The gingival attachment is cut around the whole circumference of the tooth, using a No. 11 scalpel blade or a sharp luxator. A sharp elevator can also be used.

2 Either a luxator or elevator of appropriate size (e.g. Couplands 1 for incisors, premolars and molars in small dogs; Couplands 3 for carnassials and molars in large dogs) is then inserted into the periodontal ligament space to cut the periodontal ligament fibres.

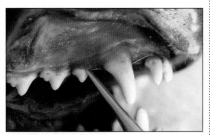

Couplands 1 elevator being used on the maxillary right first premolar.

3 The elevator is used to work circumferentially around the tooth, applying some apical and rotational pressure at an acute angle to the tooth root. The rotational pressure should be applied for 10 seconds at a time to break down the periodontal ligament fibres.

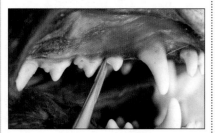

4 Once the tooth is mobile it can be removed from the socket using either fingers or extraction forceps. The forceps should be applied as low down the root as possible. They are initially used in a rotational manner to break down any remaining fibres prior to the tooth being lifted out of the socket.

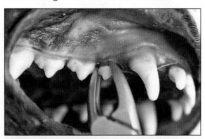

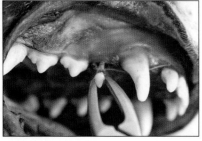

Surgical or 'open' technique

This technique should be used for extraction of canine teeth, for retrieval of root remnants and if any abnormal tooth morphology exists. It may also be the surgeon's preference to use a surgical technique if multiple adjacent teeth need to be extracted or for challenging extractions, such as the carnassial teeth in larger dogs.

1 Vertical releasing incisions are made mesial and distal to the tooth/teeth to be extracted.

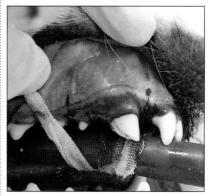

2 A mucoperiosteal flap is raised using a periosteal elevator.

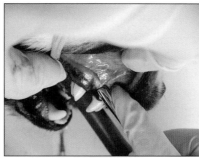

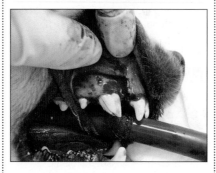

3 The overlying buccal bone is removed using a round friction grip bur on a high-speed handpiece with water cooling.

4 For a canine tooth, grooves can be made along the mesial and distal aspects of the root to create space for placement of a dental elevator using a small gauge bur. An elevator of an appropriate size is placed in the groove and gently rotated to tear the periodontal ligament fibres.

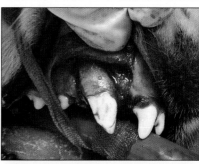

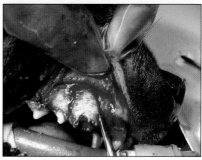

5 Once the tooth is mobile it can be extracted from the socket using either forceps or fingers. Forceps are used to twist the tooth gently without levering the root, to break down any remaining fibres and lift the tooth from its socket.

6 The edges of the socket are then smoothed using a large round diamond bur.

7 The mucoperisoteal flap is then replaced and sutured, with no tension, using a fine (1 metric; 5/0 USP) monofilament absorbable suture material. Simple interrupted sutures are placed.

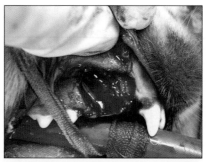

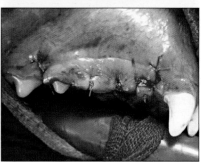

▶

QRG 20.3 *continued*

Extraction of deciduous canine teeth

Indications for extraction of deciduous teeth include malocclusion in puppies and persistent deciduous teeth in adult dogs.

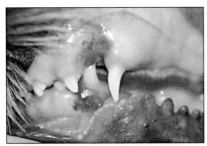

Mandibular canine malocclusion in a 10-week-old puppy.

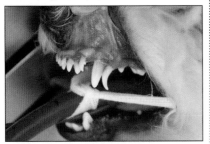

Persistent deciduous teeth (maxillary incisors, maxillary canine and mandibular canine) in a 6-month-old Yorkshire Terrier.

1 A dental radiograph is taken to assess where the permanent tooth bud is positioned or, in the case of persistent deciduous teeth, whether the root is being resorbed. With resorption there is loss of density of the dentine and periapical resorption. In cases where the root is being resorbed, a simple non-surgical extraction technique as detailed above can be used.

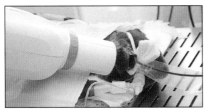

Positioning for radiography of the mandibular canine teeth.

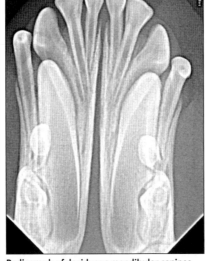

Radiograph of deciduous mandibular canines, showing relative position to secondary canines and incisors.

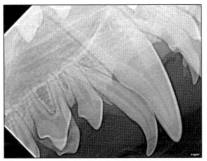

This radiograph shows a persistent deciduous canine tooth, with no evidence of root resorption.

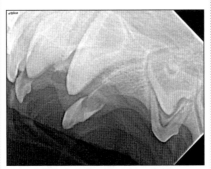

This radiograph shows a resorbing deciduous canine root.

2 In young puppies or dogs with persistent deciduous teeth where the root is not being resorbed, raise a small mucoperiosteal flap: use a No. 11 scalpel blade to make the releasing incisions; then a periosteal elevator to raise the flap.

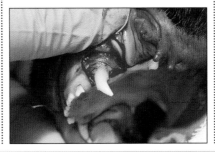

3 Use a small round bur to remove the buccal bone. Care must be taken not to damage the root of the permanent or adjacent teeth.

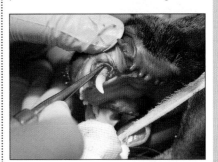

4 Use a small elevator (e.g. Super Slim which is 1.3 mm wide) to luxate the tooth gently, taking care not to position the elevator in a position where the permanent tooth could be damaged.

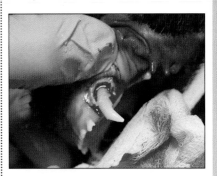

PRACTICAL TIPS

- If extracting *mandibular* deciduous canines, no instrument should be placed on the lingual (inner) aspect of the tooth, as this will damage the permanent developing mandibular canine and probably also the third incisor

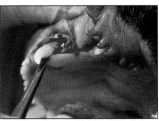

Avoid placing the elevator in this position, as there is a risk of damage to the developing permanent canine tooth.

- If extracting *maxillary* deciduous canines, take care placing any instrument on the mesial (front edge) aspect as the permanent tooth bud develops in front of the deciduous tooth

QRG 20.3 *continued*

5 Gently rotate and luxate the deciduous tooth. Once there is some mobility, use extraction forceps with a small beak (pattern 76N) in a rotational manner to break down any remaining fibres prior to the tooth being lifted out of the socket.

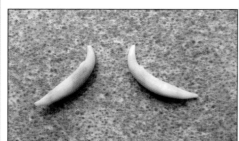

Extracted deciduous mandibular canines, showing the length of the crown relative to the length of the roots.

6 Suture the flap closed using a fine (1 metric; 5/0 USP) monofilament absorbable suture material with simple interrupted sutures, ensuring that there is no tension on the sutures.

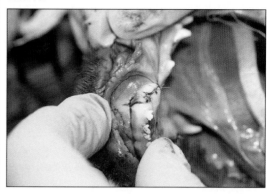

Ocular problems

21

Gary Lewin

Ocular problems are commonly encountered in general practice and can range from conjunctivitis to sight-threatening emergencies. This chapter describes how to conduct a thorough ophthalmic examination, as well as how to recognize and manage common ocular problems. The clinician needs to evaluate each individual case, the situation of the owners, any financial constraints, and the first-opinion facilities available to them. Referral is not an option in every case, but if the appropriate facilities are not available to the first-opinion clinician, referral should be considered and discussed with the owner at an earlier rather than later opportunity.

The ophthalmic examination

Examining the eye can place the examiner's face in close proximity to that of the dog, and care should always be taken. If there is any doubt the patient should be muzzled (see Chapter 1) or sedated as appropriate. However, the vast majority of dogs are very tolerant of procedures on and around the eyes, and a full examination, including procedures such as nasolacrimal duct irrigation, can usually be carried out with only minimal restraint and topical anaesthesia.

The patient is often best restrained, as for many other procedures, held against the body of the handler with the patient's head resting on one arm of the handler and the handler's other arm over the patient's back (Figure 21.1). This is usually sufficient to restrain the head and is more effective than holding the chin and nose, since this often creates more resentment and movement by the patient.

It is helpful to bring the patient and examiner to the same eye level, either by elevating the examination table, or with smaller dogs, by carrying out the examination seated. Illumination is then directed along the central visual axis, to greatest effect.

Although sedation may, rarely, prove necessary to facilitate an examination, chemical restraint is not a substitute for thorough examination. If a diagnosis cannot be reached with the patient conscious, referral should be considered for a full examination with appropriate equipment, rather than resorting to examination under anaesthesia which, in itself, is unlikely to yield further information.

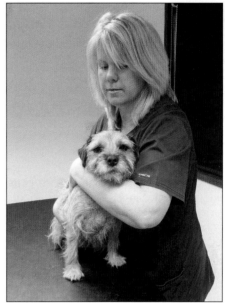

21.1
Restraining a patient for an ophthalmic examination.

Examination equipment and techniques

The majority of ocular conditions can be diagnosed with very little equipment. An effective examination of the eye can be carried out with no more than a bright focal light source, some means of magnification and an examination room that can be darkened.

- **Light source:** This can be as simple as a pen torch giving a focused light beam or illumination provided by the direct ophthalmoscope. Of equipment readily available in the consulting room, the otoscope (auroscope) is often the brightest source of illumination.
- **Magnification:** A 20 Dioptre (20 D) lens gives a magnified view of the lens, cornea and anterior chamber and, when used as an indirect ophthalmoscope, enables visualization of the fundus.

Direct ophthalmoscopy

The ophthalmoscope provides a light beam along which the examiner looks to visualize the intraocular structures (see later). The image is real and magnified (approximately 2 optic disc diameters). However, due to the magnification and small field of view, it is often of limited use for locating fundic lesions or appreciating fundic topography. Many lens settings are available on most direct ophthalmoscopes, but only the zero setting is required for viewing the fundus.

Distant direct ophthalmoscopy: With the ophthalmoscope on the zero setting, the fundus is viewed at arm's length (Figure 21.2). Any opacities are silhouetted against the fundic reflection and appear black. This is the simplest means of identifying the presence of cataracts, which appear black, and differentiating them from nuclear sclerosis (age-related hardening of the lens) through which the fundic reflection can be readily appreciated.

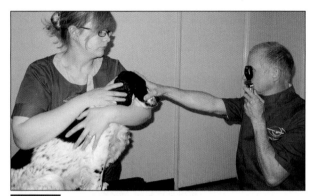

21.2 Distant direct ophthalmoscopy.

Indirect ophthalmoscopy

The examiner looks along the light beam while holding a condensing lens (usually 20 D) at arm's length in front of the dog's eye. The light is focused into the eye by the condensing lens and the image of the fundus is viewed immediately in front of the condensing lens. This gives a less magnified but wider view of the fundus and is the technique of choice for general fundic examination.

Although binocular indirect ophthalmoscopes (Figure 21.3) can represent a considerable investment, monocular indirect ophthalmoscopy can be carried out using an inexpensive 20 D lens with a focal light source (Figure 21.4). A pen torch can be held to the side of the clinician's head, while viewing the image with the eye adjacent to the penlight, or the image can be viewed through an otoscope (without the otoscope lens or speculum) held up to the clinician's eye.

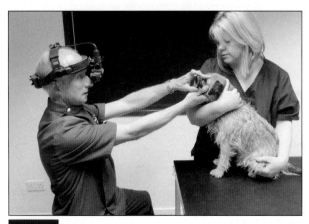

21.3 Binocular indirect ophthalmoscopy.

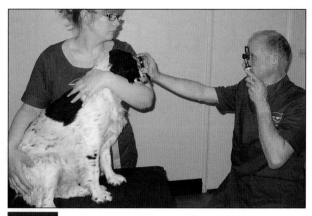

21.4 Monocular indirect ophthalmoscopy.

Assessing vision

Obstacle course: A simple obstacle course can be readily constructed from items in the consulting room (e.g. the legs of the consulting table, chairs, bin) to assess whether the patient has functional vision. Poor performance in low-level lighting can indicate impaired rod function, such as in generalized progressive retinal atrophy (see later).

Menace response: The menace response can be the simplest and most effective means of determining whether an eye is visual. It is best elicited by advancing a hand across the field of view from beyond the lateral canthus (Figure 21.5). Advancing a hand or finger directly towards the dog's eye is less likely to elicit a response, and may create a draught resulting in a false-positive result.

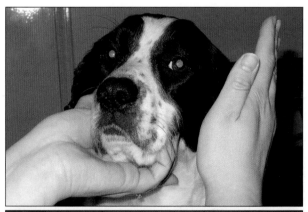

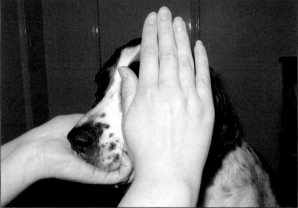

21.5 Eliciting a menace response by advancing a hand in front of the eye.

Pupillary light reflex:

- Direct: The pupil constricts in response to illumination of the eye.
- Indirect: The pupil constricts in response to illumination of the contralateral eye.

Swinging flashlight test: The light source is shone from one eye to the other. Both pupils should normally be constricted and remain constricted. This enables the examiner to distinguish between blindness and impaired pupil mobility (Figure 21.6).

Condition	Direct response		Indirect response	
	Affected eye	*Contralateral eye*	*Affected eye*	*Contralateral eye*
Blindness	✗	✓	✓	✗
Impaired pupil mobility	✗	✓	✗	✓

21.6 Swinging flashlight test results.

Assessing ocular structures

A methodical examination is required, starting with the globe as a whole and then progressing from the eyelids rostrally through to the fundus caudally, as appropriate.

PRACTICAL TIPS

- Try to adhere to an examination routine: starting at the front of the eye and working systematically to the back
- Try to avoid being drawn immediately to an obvious lesion to the exclusion of all else

---

Globe: Both globes should be compared with regard to position and size. Ease of retropulsion and third eyelid mobility are assessed by pressing firmly on the globe through the upper lid.

Schirmer tear test

If there is any mucoid or mucopurulent discharge, a Schirmer tear test (STT) should be carried out at the beginning of the examination. Fold the STT paper strips over at the notch while still in the packet to avoid touching the ends, and then apply the test strip over the central lower eyelid for 60 seconds. Tear production of <9 mm on a STT is consistent with keratoconjunctivitis sicca (KCS)

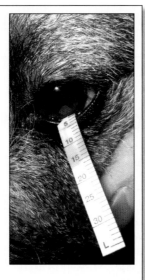

Eyelids: Eyelid innervation is assessed using the menace response (mediated by cranial nerve (CN) II and CN VII; see Figure 21.5) and the palpebral reflex (the blink elicited when the eyelid is touched; mediated by CN V and CN VII). The eyelids should be assessed for size, shape and position of the palpebral aperture, and regularity and position of the eyelid margins. The presence of distichia should be noted (the extra lashes may be more readily identified by silhouetting them against the sclera; see Figure 21.16) and the eyelids everted to check for ectopic cilia (see Figure 21.17).

Cornea: Assessing corneal reflection gives an indication of the regularity of the corneal contour and its lubrication; any irregularities and opacities should be noted (Figure 21.7 and 21.8). Fluorescein instilled on to the cornea highlights any ulceration by staining exposed corneal stroma; the cornea should be irrigated with sterile saline after application to prevent fluorescein retention by mucus.

Anterior chamber: This is assessed for depth, clarity and abnormal contents. Uveitis may create an aqueous flare, evident as haziness in the anterior chamber.

Iris and pupil: The iris and pupil are assessed for mobility by observing constriction of the pupil on exposure to a light source and dilation of the pupil after the application of topical tropicamide. Pupillary distortion may be seen in cases of iris adhesions to the anterior lens capsule or cornea, or in cases of iris neoplasia.

Lens: Cataracts are most readily identified using distant direct ophthalmoscopy.

Mydriasis

Mydriasis with tropicamide facilitates examination of the whole lens and the identification of lens subluxation. The eye is assessed before mydriasis and then afterwards, allowing 20–30 minutes for the pupil to dilate. It is important to explain to the owner that it is essential to wait for mydriasis to occur before completing the examination; it may be necessary to ask them to wait or to send them away until the end of a busy surgery. Sometimes it may be preferable to admit the patient to allow for examination later

---

White

- Lipid: crystalline
- Scarring: diffuse, milky
- Oedema: diffuse, blue-white, denser if pressure applied to the globe through the upper lid

Vascularization

- Superficial: branching. Indicates superficial corneal lesion
- Deep: straighter. Indicates deeper corneal lesion or intraocular disease

Pigmentation

- Usually superficial in response to chronic inflammation

21.7 Corneal opacities.

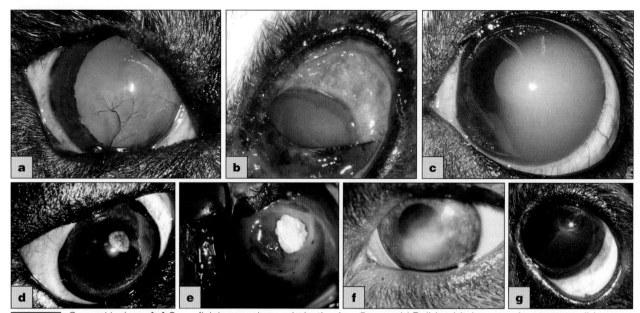

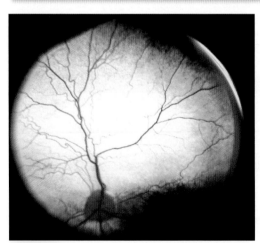

21.8 Corneal lesions. **(a)** Superficial corneal vascularization in a 5-year-old Bulldog bitch, secondary to upper lid distichiasis. The keratitis responded to removal of the extra lashes and symptomatic topical dexamethasone and ciclosporin. **(b)** Deep vascularization, evident as a purple brush border, in a 14-year-old Cocker Spaniel with uveitis. (Courtesy of Chris Dixon) **(c)** Corneal oedema is evident as a diffuse blue-white opacification of the cornea in this 7-year-old male Boston Terrier with primary endothelial degeneration. (Courtesy of Chris Dixon) **(d)** Corneal lipidosis in a 5-year-old male Boxer; the lesion was non-progressive and clinically insignificant. **(e)** Corneal calcification in a 12-year-old Yorkshire Terrier bitch. The associated ulceration resulted in corneal perforation and necessitated enucleation. **(f)** Corneal scarring in a 6-year-old Springer Spaniel bitch, as a result of an alkali burn. The ulceration healed with conservative management and the scarring, although dense, did not cause a significant visual impairment. **(g)** Superficial corneal pigmentation in a 4-year-old male Pug due to chronic exposure keratitis caused by the large palpebral aperture and the exophthalmic conformation.

Posterior segment (vitreous and fundus): The vitreous is examined for any opacities. The fundus is assessed for colour, tapetal reflectivity (increased with retinal necrosis), vascularization (attenuated with retinal degeneration) and the size and colour of the optic disc (smaller and darker with optic nerve degeneration). A normal fundus is shown in Figure 21.9.

> **PRACTICAL TIP**
>
> A fundic examination is not always necessary in cases of surface ocular disease, and significant intraocular disease can usually be ruled out simply by assessing the pupillary light reflex and fundic reflection

21.9 Normal canine fundus. Note the branching retinal vascularization, coloration of the tapetal fundus and irregular myelinated margin of the optic disc.

> **Surgical equipment**
>
> - For the majority of ophthalmic surgical procedures, correct instrumentation, illumination and magnification are necessary, along with appropriate experience
> - Head loupes, particularly those with an attached light source, can be invaluable when carrying out eyelid surgery and corneal surgery
> - Operating microscopes provide greater magnification and also coaxial illumination, and are mandatory for virtually all intraocular procedures
> - A surgical kit containing small strabismus or tenotomy scissors, Foster needle-holders and Adson forceps will facilitate eyelid and adnexal surgery, but for corneal and intraocular procedures microsurgical instruments are required

Conditions of the eyelids

Entropion

Entropion is the inversion of the eyelid causing the palpebral hairs to contact the cornea or bulbar conjunctiva (Figure 21.10). It may be seen as a localized eyelid abnormality or may occur in conjunction with abnormalities of facial conformation. The clinical signs are those of corneal abrasion (discomfort and epiphora, with or without ulcerative or non-ulcerative keratitis).

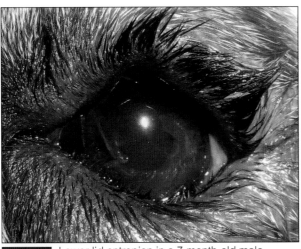

21.10 Lower lid entropion in a 7-month-old male Bulldog.

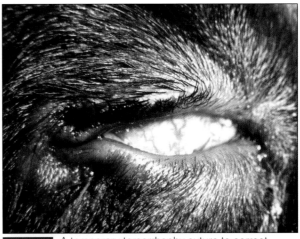

21.12 A temporary tarsorrhaphy suture to correct lateral lower lid entropion in a 14-week-old Labrador Retriever bitch.

Lateral lower lid entropion
This can occur in a dog of otherwise normal facial conformation and is usually encountered in the first months or years of development. It may also occur in cases of spastic entropion, where ocular discomfort results in hypertrophy of the orbicularis oculi muscle and secondary inversion of the eyelid. Some cases may be intermittent and not readily apparent, but may be indicated by tear wetting and staining of the lateral lower lid. A Hotz–Celsus resection along the affected eyelid margin, combined where necessary with a lateral lid-shortening wedge excision, is usually sufficient to correct the majority of these cases (Figure 21.11). In juvenile cases (<4 months of age) a temporary lateral tarsorrhaphy suture (Figure 21.12), left *in situ* for up to 4 weeks may be sufficient to give permanent correction.

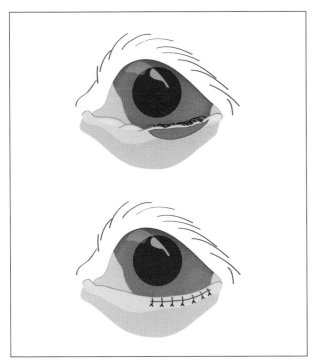

21.11 Lower lid entropion is most readily corrected by excising a crescent from the affected lower eyelid (Hotz–Celsus resection). Keeping the incision close to the lid margin (ideally within 2 mm) turns the eyelid out instead of pulling it down, and reduces the risk of iatrogenic ectropion.

Lateral upper lid entropion
This is usually associated with a conformation of excessive facial skin (e.g. St Bernard, Shar Pei) or ageing dogs with pendulous, low set ears (e.g. Cocker Spaniel). A Hotz–Celsus resection may be insufficient to alleviate the entropion or, in cases of progressive facial droop, may provide only temporary relief. More extensive eyelid resection may be necessary and, in pronounced cases where the globe is largely obscured by the upper lid, a facelift procedure may be required.

Medial lower lid entropion
Entropion of the medial lower lid is typically seen in brachycephalic dogs, often associated with a macropalpebral aperture. The entropion and macropalpebral aperture can both be addressed simultaneously by carrying out a permanent medial tarsorrhaphy.

Ectropion
Ectropion is an eversion of the eyelid, most commonly seen as eversion of the central lower lid in conjunction with lateral lower lid entropion in the 'diamond eye' conformation of breeds such as the St Bernard (Figure 21.13). Ectropion may be corrected by a simple lid-shortening wedge excision of the lower lid, but more often surgery needs to address the overall eyelid conformation.

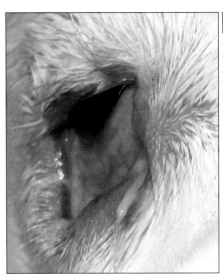

21.13 Diamond eye conformation in a 6-year-old Clumber Spaniel bitch.

Trauma

Eyelids are well vascularized and heal readily. When repairing traumatic lacerations it is important to re-create the smooth eyelid margin (see later). Debridement of any tissue of questionable viability should be minimal, since even heavily contused tissues may prove to be viable.

Neoplasia

Eyelid neoplasms (see Chapter 28) are, in the vast majority of cases, benign and rarely present a risk of metastatic disease. They can present a surgical challenge if occupying a significant proportion of the eyelid margin, and early removal is indicated to avoid the need for complex eyelid reconstruction. If the tumour is occupying <20% of the eyelid margin, the mass may be removed by full-thickness wedge excision. Repair of the defect is readily achieved by direct closure using 1 or 1.5 metric (5/0 or 4/0 USP) swaged-on suture material, taking care to re-form a smooth, regular eyelid margin while avoiding corneal abrasion by the suture material (Figures 21.14 and 21.15). Soluble material such as polyglactin 910 can be used to avoid the need for suture removal.

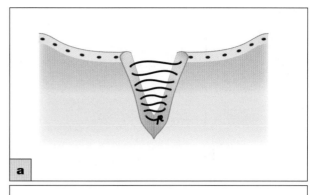

a

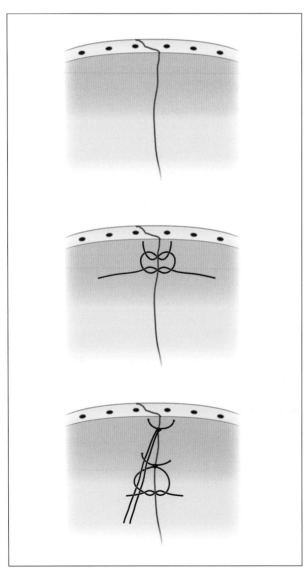

21.14 Small eyelid defects can be closed with simple interrupted sutures, entrapping the ends of the suture material at the eyelid margin within the adjacent suture to prevent corneal abrasion.

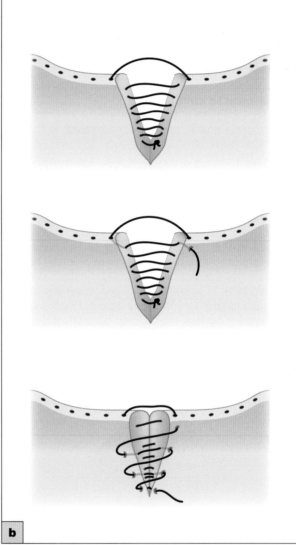

b

21.15 **(a)** A more secure closure, suitable for larger defects, is achieved with a 2-layer continuous suture starting from the eyelid margin and progressing within the subconjunctival stroma up to the margin, and returning to close the cutaneous layer. **(b)** Exiting and entering the eyelid margin through the meibomian gland openings helps to ensure accurate closure of the eyelid margin.

Distichiasis

Distichia are extra eyelashes that arise from the meibomian glands and emerge from the meibomian gland openings on the eyelid margin (Figure 21.16). These lashes may be single or multiple, usually emerging over the first 18 months of life, and can be of varying clinical significance. They may cause ocular discomfort, keratitis and, rarely, corneal

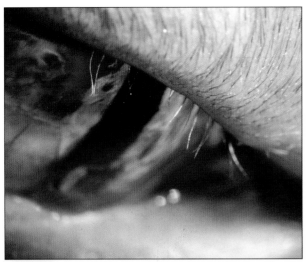

21.16 Distichiasis. The extra lashes arising from the meibomian glands are readily identified when silhouetted against the sclera.

ulceration, but they can be clinically silent. Clinical signs may be temporarily alleviated by plucking the extra lashes, and this can be of use in determining their significance. Permanent removal requires destruction or excision of the follicles, which can be variously achieved by cryosurgery, electrolysis or surgical excision. These surgical procedures require specific instrumentation and magnification and should not be attempted in their absence due to the risk of significant distortion of the eyelid margin.

Ectopic cilia

Ectopic cilia also arise from the meibomian glands, more commonly of the upper eyelid, but emerge directly through the conjunctiva and therefore impinge directly on the cornea (Figure 21.17). They are almost invariably associated with ocular discomfort, which can be acute in onset, and characteristically presents as unremitting ocular discomfort in the juvenile. Secondary ulceration, typically focal, central and progressive, can occur. Do not forget to look under the upper lid in cases of ocular discomfort, with or without ulceration, in juvenile dogs. Treatment of ectopic cilia is as for distichiasis.

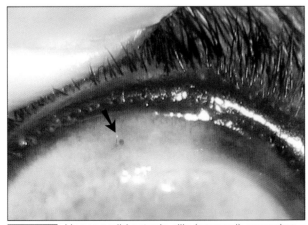

21.17 Upper eyelid ectopic cilia (arrowed), emerging through the palpebral conjunctiva adjacent to a small pigmented focus.

Conditions of the nictitating membrane (third eyelid)

Prolapse of the third eyelid gland ('cherry eye')

Prolapse of the gland of the third eyelid presents as a pink regular mass, protruding from behind the third eyelid (Figure 21.18). The gland produces a proportion of the precorneal tear film and its preservation is advocated. The prolapsed gland may be repositioned into a pocket deep to the bulbar conjunctiva, which is then closed over the gland while leaving ports at either end of the closure to allow the egress of tears from the gland.

Excision of the gland is indicated in the Neapolitan Mastiff in which pronounced granulomatous reactions can occur in response to suture material buried within the conjunctiva.

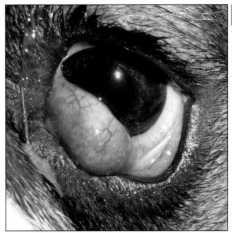

21.18 Third eyelid gland prolapse in a 4-month-old male Bulldog.

Scrolled third eyelid cartilage

This can present with some similarity to prolapse of the third eyelid gland, but is caused by eversion of the free margin of the third eyelid due to distortion of the cartilage. It may not be clinically significant but can result in exposure and inflammation of the third eyelid (nictitating membrane). The condition is corrected by excision of the deviant portion of the cartilage, approached from the bulbar aspect of the third eyelid. The conjunctiva is left unsutured.

In the Great Dane, surgery to correct a scrolled third eyelid cartilage can be followed by prolapse of the third eyelid gland, and prophylactic surgery to prevent gland prolapse should be considered.

Neoplasia

Neoplasia of the third eyelid may present as protrusion of the lid and a space-occupying lesion of the third eyelid may be appreciated on inspection and/or palpation under topical anaesthesia. Such a mass is usually readily accessible for biopsy. If neoplasia is confirmed histologically, excision of the third eyelid may be indicated.

WARNING
The third eyelid plays an important role in protecting the cornea and its excision is indicated only in cases of neoplasia

Conditions of the conjunctival sac

Conjunctivitis

Primary conjunctivitis may be caused by infection, allergy or environmental irritants (e.g. cement or plaster dust from building work). It presents as hyperaemia of the conjunctiva and an ocular discharge (serous, mucoid or mucopurulent), and is not normally associated with ocular pain. Most cases respond to symptomatic treatment with topical antibiotics and/or steroids. Conjunctival swabs may be taken for bacterial culture and sensitivity testing but may yield only opportunistic bacteria of doubtful significance. It is important to check for, and treat, any underlying diseases such as KCS or eyelid abnormalities, and to eliminate any environmental causes.

Foreign body

Remarkably large foreign bodies, such as grass awns, may reside within the conjunctival sac, particularly beneath the third eyelid. They can result in non-responsive cases of ocular discharge, conjunctivitis, discomfort and/or corneal ulceration, particularly medially. It is important to examine the conjunctival sac and beneath the third eyelid under topical anaesthesia.

Conditions of the sclera

Limbal melanoma

This is a benign melanoma, which sits astride the limbus. It is well circumscribed and slow-growing in older dogs but can progress more rapidly in younger individuals. It should be monitored to assess its rate of progression, and, if progressing significantly, surgical excision or laser ablation, with corneoscleral reconstruction, may be indicated.

Nodular granulomatous episclerokeratitis

The sclera and episclera may be affected by inflammatory conditions, often idiopathic, categorized by the structures affected (scleritis, episcleritis, episclerokeratitis). The most common inflammatory condition is nodular granulomatous episclerokeratitis (NGEK), which presents, as the name suggests, as one or more inflammatory nodule(s) overlying the sclera, with associated conjunctival hyperaemia and variable corneal involvement. Symptomatic treatment is indicated and some or all of topical corticosteroids, oral corticosteroids, subconjunctival corticosteroids and oral azathioprine may be required to control the inflammation. The condition may resolve, or long-term treatment may prove necessary to maintain control.

Conditions of the nasolacrimal system

Dacryocystitis

Dacryocystitis is inflammation of the nasolacrimal duct and is characterized by a mucopurulent discharge in the presence of normal tear production. It may resolve with nasolacrimal duct irrigation (which may need to be carried out on more than one occasion), but if a foreign body is present (often characterized by blood on irrigation) surgical exploration is indicated.

Keratoconjunctivitis sicca

KCS typically presents as a dry tenacious mucopurulent ocular discharge (Figure 21.19). As the condition progresses, a keratitis with varying degrees of corneal vascularization develops, typically in the dorsolateral quadrant of the cornea. Tear production of <9 mm on a STT (see above) is consistent with KCS. The underlying cause in the majority of cases is lacrimal gland adenitis, which may respond to topical ciclosporin. Adjunctive treatment with topical corticosteroids to control any keratitis, and topical lacrimomimetics, may be indicated. KCS can be induced by oral sulphonamide medication, particularly sulfasalazine, and such drugs should be withdrawn if a concurrent KCS develops.

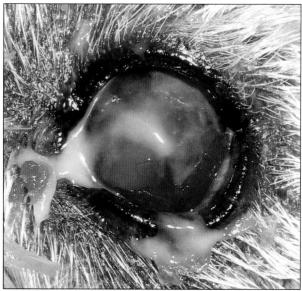

21.19 Keratoconjunctivitis sicca showing the characteristic tenacious ocular discharge.

PRACTICAL TIP

Always perform an STT in any case of ocular discharge or non-responsive conjunctivitis

---

Treatment

- Topical ciclosporin q12h to restore tear production.
- Topical ocular lubricants q6h or as needed.
- Topical corticosteroids to control any keratitis (e.g. dexamethasone and neomycin q6h initially).
- Treat as above for 6 weeks. If there is no improvement, medication with an increased concentration of ciclosporin, or with tacrolimus, may be indicated; however, neither drug is authorized for this use in the UK.
- Parotid duct transposition (PDT) (to be considered if all medical options have been exhausted):
  - Can be very effective in providing lubrication but can be associated with side effects such as corneal opacification and blepharitis
  - If a PDT does prove necessary, it is best carried out before an extensive keratitis has developed.

Conditions of the cornea

Ulceration

Corneal ulceration is usually traumatic in origin but may be complicated by secondary infection, or a failure of the cornea to heal appropriately.

Ulcers may be defined by their depth:

- Superficial: affecting only the epithelium
- Stromal: involving the stroma to a varying depth
- Descemetocele: extending down to Descemet's membrane.

PRACTICAL TIP

Remember to check for underlying disease, such as ectopic cilia or entropion, in cases of corneal ulceration

---

Simple traumatic ulceration can be expected to heal if the underlying cause is no longer present or removed (e.g. a conjunctival sac foreign body) and secondary infection is controlled with a topical antibiotic. Oral non-steroidal anti-inflammatory drugs (NSAIDs) should also be considered to control any discomfort and reflex uveitis. It is very important that stromal ulceration is monitored regularly at the veterinary surgery (e.g. every 3–5 days depending on the depth and extent) until it is fluorescein-negative; it should not be left to the owner to 'see how it goes'.

Corneal vascularization may develop with significant or long-standing ulcers and may facilitate healing but will also result in corneal scarring. Vascularization persisting *when the ulceration has healed* may be encouraged to regress with the administration of topical corticosteroids.

WARNING

Topical steroids impede corneal healing and if applied to an ulcerated cornea can result in progression of the ulcer and possible perforation of the globe. Always check for corneal ulceration with fluorescein before prescribing a topical steroid

---

Epithelial dystrophy

Also known as spontaneous chronic corneal epithelial defect (SCCED), this presents as a non-healing, superficial ulceration with under-running of the epithelium. It can occur in any dog, but is typically seen in the Boxer, while Corgis, Staffordshire Bull Terriers and Border Collies are also predisposed. The characteristic appearance is of a shallow ulcer with a margin of loose epithelium (Figure 21.20), which should be removed under topical anaesthesia by gentle abrasion with a cotton bud. Sclerosis of the superficial corneal stroma can prevent healing by direct re-epithelialization. The ulcer may heal by granulation if corneal vascularization develops, but surgical intervention may prove necessary.

Treatments that have been advocated include: keratotomy, using either a hypodermic needle or mechanical burr to penetrate the affected superficial stroma; keratectomy; chemical cautery with liquefied

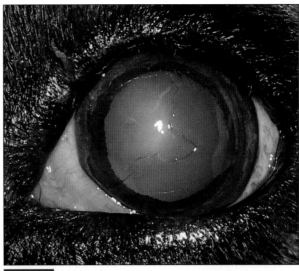

21.20 Epithelial dystrophy in an 8-year-old Boxer bitch.

phenol; bandage contact lens; and third eyelid flap. Topical antibiosis (to prevent secondary infection) and analgesia are also indicated.

Healing of a superficial ulcer may be protracted and the owner should be advised that it can take a few weeks. In cases of non-progressive superficial ulceration the patient may only need to be re-examined every 1–2 weeks and surgical intervention may need to be considered only if the ulcer is failing to heal over a period of 2–4 weeks.

Descemetocele

A descemetocele (Figure 21.21) is a deep ulcer exposing Descemet's membrane, which appears as a dark area at the base of the ulcer which fails to stain with fluorescein, in contrast to the adjacent oedematous fluorescein-positive corneal stroma. Descemetoceles carry a significant risk of corneal perforation. Small, non-progressive descemetoceles may heal by granulation and may be managed conservatively if there is a significant vascular response. The majority of cases, however, are preferably managed by surgical repair with a conjunctival graft or corneoscleral transposition, for which adequate magnification and appropriate instrumentation are essential.

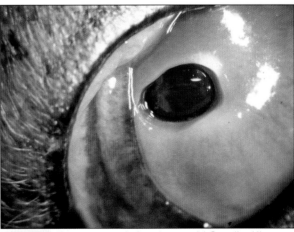

21.21 Descemetocele in a 6-year-old Cavalier King Charles Spaniel bitch with concurrent keratoconjunctivitis sicca. The cornea was repaired successfully with a conjunctival pedicle graft.

Keratomalacia

Keratomalacia (melting ulcer) occurs in the presence of collagenase, typically seen with *Pseudomonas aeruginosa* infections, and is characterized by a rapidly progressive corneal ulceration with a gelatinous appearance of the corneal stroma (Figure 21.22). **It is a sight-threatening disease, which requires immediate, intensive medication to preserve the globe.** Once the keratomalacia has been controlled, surgical repair of the cornea may be contemplated, or the cornea may heal uneventfully by granulation. In either case significant corneal scarring can be anticipated.

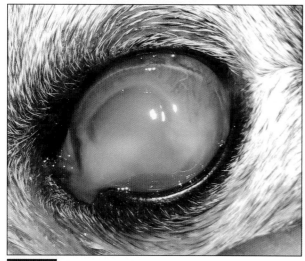

21.22   Melting ulcer.

Medical management:

- Topical serum:
  - Autogenous serum
  - Inhibits collagenase, provides antibodies and growth factors
  - Applied q2h; stored in the refrigerator, keeps for 48 hours.
- Topical antibiotics:
  - Active against *Pseudomonas aeruginosa* (e.g. aminoglycosides, fluoroquinolones).
- Oral oxytetracycline:
  - Effective against matrix metalloproteases when administered orally.
- Uveitis treatment:
  - Mydriasis and NSAIDs.

Topical plasma/serum and antibiotics should be applied 2-hourly for 48 hours or until the keratomalacia is under control. Thereafter, treatment is as for a deep stromal ulcer.

Pannus

Pannus (chronic superficial keratitis) is seen typically in German Shepherd Dogs, sight hounds and Border Collies. It is associated with corneal exposure to ultraviolet light and is more prevalent in the summer months. It presents as superficial vascularization and/or superficial corneal pigmentation (Figure 21.23), characteristically bilateral and originating at the ventrolateral limbus, and can progress to affect the entire cornea. Treatment is aimed at controlling the inflammation with topical steroids and/or ciclosporin and

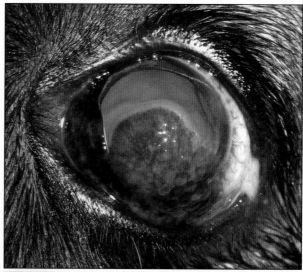

21.23   Pannus in a 6-year-old German Shepherd Dog bitch.

minimizing the exposure to ultraviolet light. In advanced cases, subconjunctival depot steroid injections may be of benefit. Once the inflammation is controlled, the frequency of topical medication may be reduced, but lifelong medication, once or twice daily, is necessary to prevent recurrence or progression of the keratitis.

Lipid keratopathy

The most common cause of corneal lipid deposits is corneal lipid dystrophy, an idiopathic condition, which presents as a crystalline lipid deposit, approximating to an oval shape, usually immediately ventral to the central visual axis. The deposit is characteristically bilateral and non-progressive, and is rarely clinically significant. Lipid deposits in the corneal stroma may also be seen in cases of hypothyroidism and hyperlipidaemia.

Endothelial dystrophy

The corneal endothelium maintains the cornea in a transparent, dehydrated state. Impaired endothelium function, allowing the ingress of aqueous into the corneal stroma, can occur due to endothelial dystrophy. The resulting corneal oedema can present bilaterally symmetrically or unilaterally, and may result in corneal ulceration and keratitis, eventually causing significant visual impairment. The oedema and associated keratitis may be controlled with long-term topical hyperosmotic medication such as topical 5% sodium chloride 3–4 times daily.

Foreign bodies

Corneal foreign bodies (typically thorns) may be non-penetrating, embedded in the corneal stroma, or may penetrate into the anterior chamber. Clinical signs of ocular discomfort, corneal oedema/keratitis and uveitis will vary, depending on the size of the foreign body and degree of penetration.

If it is proud of the corneal surface, a foreign body can be removed by impaling it on a 25 G hypodermic needle. To avoid pushing the foreign body further into the cornea or anterior chamber the needle is advanced at a tangent to the corneal surface and perpendicular to the long axis of the foreign body.

Dermoid

A dermoid is an island of ectopic skin, most commonly situated superficial to the cornea at the lateral limbus. It is a congenital condition but often only becomes apparent at 2–4 months of age, when hair growth from the dermoid is evident and results in ocular discomfort and discharge. The dermoid is excised by lamellar dissection of the affected tissues, and at a sufficient depth to ensure excision of all hair follicles.

Conditions of the iris

Cysts

Iris cysts arise from the posterior surface of the iris, from where they detach, floating through the pupil and settling in the ventral anterior chamber (Figure 21.24). The cysts are spherical, fluid-filled and usually slowly progressive; as they enlarge, they come to be positioned more centrally in the pupil. Occasionally they rupture, leaving a pigment deposit on the corneal endothelium. Removal of an iris cyst is indicated if the cyst is encroaching on the pupil and obstructing the central visual axis. Cysts can be removed by aspiration or can be ablated using a laser delivered transcorneally.

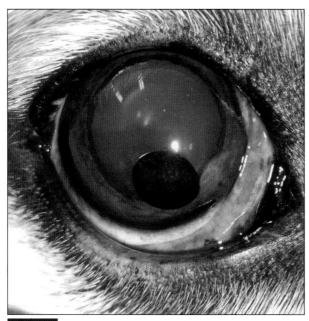

21.24 Iris cyst in a 7-year-old male Labrador Retriever.

PRACTICAL TIP

Iris cysts can be distinguished from melanomas as free-floating structures that can be transilluminated

Neoplasia

Melanoma

Most iris melanomas in dogs are benign. They present as dark, circumscribed space-occupying lesions of the iris and can be differentiated from benign iris pigmentation by elevation of the surface contour of the iris and/or distortion of the pupil (which may only be evident with mydriasis). The rate of progression of the melanoma can be an indicator of its malignant potential.

- A slowly growing melanoma is unlikely to be malignant and may not prove to be clinically significant for many years. While still circumscribed the melanoma may be amenable to curative transcorneal laser ablation. Left untreated, the melanoma may ultimately occupy the anterior chamber or may progress around the filtration angle (ring melanoma) and can result in glaucoma or globe perforation necessitating enucleation.
- A rapidly progressing melanoma is more likely to be malignant, and the risk of metastasis may be high. Early enucleation in such cases is indicated, and the patient should be monitored for signs of any subsequent metastatic disease.

Ciliary body adenoma

Ciliary body adenomas are benign, non-pigmented tumours arising immediately caudal to the iris and presenting as pale, sparsely vascularized masses visible at the pupil. The risk of metastatic disease is very low and the tumour may be amenable to local excision, with or without adjunctive laser ablation. If local excision is not appropriate, enucleation can be expected to be curative.

Atrophy

Atrophy of the iris musculature can be seen in ageing dogs, resulting in a poorly responsive pupil but with no associated visual impairment. This can manifest as an irregular and/or dilated pupil, and occasionally full-thickness defects in the iris, but is rarely clinically significant.

Uveitis

Uveitis is inflammation of the uvea, the vascular layer within the eye that comprises the iris, ciliary body and choroid. It may affect the iris and ciliary body (anterior uveitis), the choroid (posterior uveitis), or the iris and choroid (panuveitis). Clinically these different categories may not be easily differentiated, and the term uveitis is typically used to refer to anterior uveitis, with or without involvement of the choroid.

Uveitis may be caused by ocular trauma, or by inflammatory corneal disease, particularly deep cornea ulceration. It may be seen in cases of intraocular disease, or can arise due to the presence of a systemic inflammatory condition.

The cardinal sign of uveitis is miosis (constriction of the pupil), which may be associated with protein exudate into the anterior chamber (aqueous flare) condensing on the ventral corneal endothelium as keratic precipitates, and perilimbal vascular congestion. There may be signs of ocular discomfort, and responses to vision tests may be attenuated or absent. If the cause of the uveitis is not readily apparent, initial investigations should include serum biochemistry and haematology. Serology for specific infectious causes (e.g. *Neospora, Borrelia*) can be carried out, but symptomatic medication should be initiated while awaiting laboratory results.

Treatment

Prompt treatment to relieve the ciliary spasm and achieve mydriasis is imperative, while also controlling the inflammation and identifying and treating any underlying cause.

- **Mydriasis:**
  - Topical atropine ± topical phenylephrine, q30min until full mydriasis has been achieved. Subsequently, tropicamide should be used q12h until the uveitis has fully resolved.
- **Systemic anti-inflammatory medication:**
  - NSAIDs provide analgesia in addition to anti-inflammatory activity, but corticosteroids may have a greater anti-inflammatory effect
  - Initially, in cases of intense inflammation, NSAIDs and soluble dexamethasone can be administered simultaneously, in conjunction with an H1 antagonist (e.g. cimetidine) to protect the gastric mucosa
  - *Systemic or oral steroids should be used with care in cases of corneal ulceration (see above) but are unlikely to compromise corneal integrity in the short term.*
- **Topical steroid medication:**
  - Prednisolone acetate applied q4h can help to control intraocular inflammation, but must only be used in the absence of corneal ulceration.
- **Topical antibiotics:**
  - Should be used if corneal ulceration is present.
- **Systemic or oral antibiotics:**
  - Of limited benefit, but will penetrate the anterior chamber in the presence of uveitis and are indicated if there has been penetration of the globe.

Glaucoma

Glaucoma usually manifests as increased intraocular pressure (IOP). It can occur as a primary condition, or may be secondary to other intraocular disease. Primary glaucoma most commonly arises due to pectinate ligament dysplasia, resulting in occlusion of the iridocorneal angle. Primary open-angle glaucoma, where there is no gross abnormality of the iridocorneal angle, has been studied extensively in a colony of Beagles but is rarely encountered in practice. Secondary glaucoma occurs as a result of other intraocular diseases such as uveitis, lens luxation and neoplasia.

In the majority of cases, primary canine glaucoma presents as an acute condition. Typical signs of elevated IOP include:

- Absence of response to vision tests
- Generalized corneal oedema
- Episcleral vascular congestion (Figure 21.25)
- Mid-sized or dilated pupil, sometimes irregular
- Megaloglobus

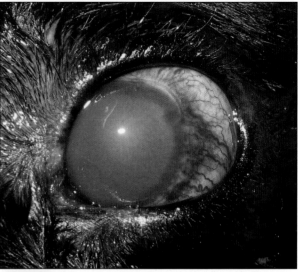

21.25 Glaucoma with episcleral vascular congestion and corneal oedema.

- Lens subluxation: the lens is displaced but not unstable and may be displaced other than ventrally (in contrast to lens instability and ventral displacement seen in primary lens luxation).

The clinical signs of episcleral vascularization, congestion, corneal oedema, dilated non-responsive pupil and loss of vision should arouse a high suspicion for glaucoma. Definitive diagnosis relies on the accurate measurement of IOP by applanation or rebound tonometry.

> ### PRACTICAL TIP
>
> If a tonometer is not readily available, IOP can be gauged by assessing the ease with which the globe can be indented with a blunt probe (such as a thermometer bulb) and comparing this with the contralateral eye. A glaucomatous eye will be tense, whereas a uveitic eye will be soft and easily indented

Treatment

Immediate treatment of increased IOP is essential to preserve vision of the affected globe; however, once gross changes to the eye are evident the vision has usually already been irreversibly lost due to optic disc atrophy. Management of glaucoma should aim to ensure that the first affected eye, if blind, is not a source of discomfort, while monitoring the contralateral eye to identify any increase in IOP and treating this promptly.

Effective treatment of glaucoma requires accurate measurement of IOP. In the absence of accurate tonometry, glaucoma treatment can only be of dubious benefit.

Medical treatment

This may include:

- Topical prostaglandin analogues (latanoprost, travoprost):
  - Increase uveoscleral outflow

- Administer 1–2 times daily
- Reduce IOP by up to 50%.
- Topical carbonic anhydrase inhibitors (e.g. acetazolamide):
  - Reduce production of aqueous humour
  - Reduce IOP by approximately 7 mmHg.
- Intravenous mannitol:
  - Hypertonic infusion reduces the volume of the vitreous by osmosis to achieve a rapid reduction in IOP but carries some risk of acute renal compromise
  - Topical prostaglandin analogues may be equally effective.

Surgical treatment
This may include:

- Increasing aqueous outflow:
  - Drainage tubes have been developed to drain aqueous variously into the subconjunctival space, retrobulbar space and frontal sinus
  - This is often confounded by the development of fibrosis, which ultimately occludes the outflow.
- Reducing aqueous production:
  - Endoscopic laser cyclophotocoagulation to partially ablate the ciliary epithelium and reduce the production of aqueous
  - The technique has a significant complication rate but can achieve long-term control of the IOP.
- Enucleation:
  - If a glaucomatous eye is blind and a potential source of persistent discomfort, enucleation is indicated.

Conditions of the lens

Cataract
A cataract is an opacity of the lens. Cataracts may vary in their position within the lens, their rate of progression and their clinical significance. In particular breeds (e.g. Labrador Retriever; Figure 21.26), cataracts may be inherited and may be of a characteristic appearance. Cataracts may be seen in cases of uveitis and lens trauma and may develop secondary to retinal degeneration or secondary to diabetes mellitus. They may also arise due to senile lens changes, or can be apparently spontaneous.

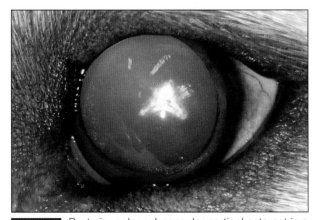

21.26 Posterior polar subcapsular cortical cataract in a 4-year-old male Labrador Retriever, characteristic of inherited cataracts in this breed.

Cataracts are most readily diagnosed by distant direct ophthalmoscopy. If the cataract is small and progressing only slowly, no action need necessarily be taken. If the cataract is extensive, bilateral or progressing rapidly, referral at this stage is indicated (even if a lendectomy is not currently necessary) while at least one fundus can be visualized and assessed for the presence of any underlying retinal degeneration. In cases of rapidly developing cataracts a lens-induced uveitis (phacolytic uveitis) may occur. This may be subtle and can easily be mistaken for conjunctivitis. Such cases require symptomatic medication to control the uveitis, and prompt referral if cataract surgery is being contemplated.

PRACTICAL TIP

Nuclear sclerosis, an age-related hardening of the lens, appears as a bilateral bluish-grey haziness and can readily be mistaken for a cataract. These are most readily differentiated by distant direct ophthalmoscopy. The fundic reflection is unobstructed by nuclear sclerosis, while a cataract will obscure the reflection and appear black

---

Luxation
Primary lens luxation (PLL) is the result of an inherited weakness of the zonular fibres. It is typically seen in terriers but can occur in a variety of breeds. It is usually encountered in 'middle-aged' dogs (4–6 years old).

WARNING

In a terrier breed with an acute onset painful eye, suspect lens luxation and treat accordingly until the position of the lens has been identified

---

Genetic testing

The gene responsible for PLL in many breeds has been identified, and genetic testing is now readily available. This is advisable in any susceptible dog intended for breeding. If an individual is identified as being at risk of PLL, prophylactic lens extraction surgery, before any lens instability has developed, can be considered

---

The degeneration of the zonular fibres may allow vitreous to pass into the anterior chamber and this may be seen as a smoke-like wisp or plume extending through the pupil. As zonular fibre degeneration progresses, the lens becomes more unstable, although still supported on the anterior face of the vitreous. The anterior chamber becomes deeper and a tremor of the iris (iridodenesis) may be apparent. Ventral subluxation of the lens may be evident, with an aphakic crescent visible dorsally, but this can only be appreciated with mydriasis. (If a case presents with a readily evident aphakic crescent, a mydriasis will already be present, suggestive of a primary glaucoma.) Referral for lens extraction surgery should be considered at this stage.

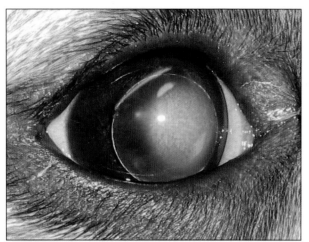

21.27 Anterior lens luxation in a 4-year-old Lancashire Heeler. The lens equator can be seen refracting the light, and focal corneal oedema is present due to the endothelial decompensation where the lens is contacting the corneal endothelium.

Anterior lens luxation

If sufficiently unstable, the lens may luxate anteriorly, occupying the anterior chamber and coming into contact with the cornea (Figure 21.27). The attached vitreous can occlude the pupil, obstructing the flow of aqueous from the ciliary body to the iridocorneal angle and causing a pupil-block glaucoma.

The clinical signs of an anterior lens luxation are an acutely painful eye, corneal oedema and episcleral vascular congestion. The clinician should have a high index of suspicion of lens luxation in an acutely painful eye in a middle-aged dog of a susceptible breed.

Prompt management of an anterior luxation is critical to preserve vision in the affected eye. The administration of a topical mydriatic and systemic NSAID should alleviate a pupil block. With the concomitant reduction in IOP, the corneal oedema should reduce and the position of the lens may become apparent. A residual localized ventral corneal oedema may then be appreciated due to the contact of the lens against the corneal endothelium. With effective mydriasis, a lens luxation is no longer an ocular emergency but prompt referral is indicated for lens extraction surgery.

Posterior lens luxation

If, in a case of subluxation, the vitreous degenerates and liquefies, the lens is no longer supported at the pupil and will migrate to the floor of the posterior segment. In such a case there is low risk of anterior luxation and pupil-block glaucoma but there is a significant risk of the development of chronic glaucoma. Surgical intervention before a posterior luxation has developed is preferable.

Conditions of the retina

Progressive retinal atrophy

Generalized progressive retinal atrophy (gPRA) is a blanket term, referring to a number of inherited retinal degenerations and dysplasias, which present with an ophthalmoscopically similar appearance. gPRA presents as a progressive blindness, becoming apparent over a period of months or years, initially evident as night blindness with poor vision in low-light conditions

and then progressing to reduced visual acuity in daylight and, ultimately, a total loss of vision. The ophthalmoscopic appearance is characterized by attenuation of the retinal vasculature, hyper-reflectivity of the tapetal fundus, demyelination and atrophy of the optic disc, and depigmentation of the non-tapetal fundus (Figure 21.28). Secondary cataracts commonly develop but, in such cases, cataract surgery will be of limited benefit.

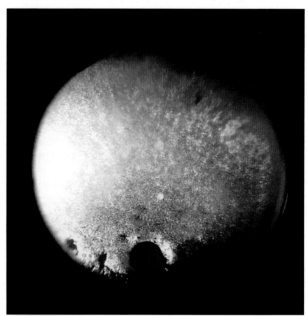

21.28 Advanced retinal degeneration characterized by retinal vascular attenuation, tapetal hyper-reflectivity and optic disc demyelination.

Genetic testing

gPRA is untreatable and inexorably leads to blindness. Owners need to be counselled on managing the blindness and should be advised not to breed from an affected dog, or from offspring that might be carriers. Many of the PRAs can now be identified on genetic testing and this is advisable for any dog of a susceptible breed intended for breeding

Collie eye anomaly

Collie eye anomaly (CEA) is a condition seen in collie breeds and some others. It is characterized by the presence of an optic disc coloboma (a ballooning of the globe at the optic disc) and/or choroidal hypoplasia (presenting as a choroidal defect lateral to the optic disc). It has largely been eliminated from working collies as a result of testing under the BVA/KC/ISDS examination scheme. In other breeds, most notably the Shetland Sheepdog, the condition is very prevalent. CEA may be associated with retinal detachment and retinal haemorrhage, but this is encountered rarely in affected dogs and most cases are clinically silent.

Retinal detachment

The neurosensory retina lies in apposition to the underlying retinal pigment epithelium (RPE) and is held in position by the vacuum within the potential space between the two layers. Any material occupying that potential space, or any lesion destroying the vacuum within it, will create a retinal detachment.

- **Effusive retinal detachment** may be seen in cases of retinitis and can present as bilateral retinal detachments, sometimes idiopathic. The detachment may respond to oral prednisolone at 1–2 mg/kg q24h in conjunction with treatment of any underlying systemic disease.
- **Rhegmatogenous detachment** is caused by a retinal tear that allows the vitreous, if liquefied, to pass into the subretinal space. The prognosis for restoring vision in such cases is very guarded. Treatment necessitates surgical access to the posterior segment to reposition the retina and to create adhesions between the neuroretina and RPE using an ophthalmic laser.

Conditions of the globe and orbit

Retrobulbar space-occupying lesions
Neoplasia and cellulitis/abscessation are the most commonly encountered retrobulbar space-occupying diseases. The cardinal signs of a retrobulbar space-occupying lesion are rostral displacement of the globe accompanied by protrusion of the third eyelid, to be distinguished from globe enlargement in cases of glaucoma where protrusion of the third eyelid does not occur. Clinical suspicions may be confirmed by ultrasonography, identifying a lesion of soft tissue density (neoplasia) or a fluid focus (retrobulbar abscess).

Cellulitis
Retrobulbar cellulitis can occur due to traumatic inoculation of infection into the orbit or by extension from an adjacent septic focus such as a tooth root abscess, but many cases are idiopathic and are presumed to be due to haematogenous spread of infection. The condition often presents acutely, with swelling of the conjunctiva, and characteristically with pain on opening the mouth.

Most cases of retrobulbar cellulitis will respond to broad-spectrum systemic/oral antibiosis. Rarely, in refractory or peracute cases, drainage via the oral mucosa caudal to the caudal upper molar is necessary, but this carries some risk of trauma to the optic nerve.

Neoplasia
Retrobulbar neoplasia typically has a less acute onset than cellulitis and is non-painful. Displacement of the globe other than rostrally may be appreciated, depending on the position of the neoplasm. Magnetic resonance imaging (MRI) and computed tomography (CT) are the methods of choice for accurately localizing a retrobulbar neoplasm. Fine-needle aspiration of an orbital neoplasm may be attempted, but the cells harvested may not be representative and results can be misleading.

Since the majority of the orbit is encased in bone, orbital neoplasia is rarely amenable to *en bloc resection* with clear surgical margins. Enucleation and tumour excision is rarely curative but may be indicated to alleviate pain associated with the corneal desiccation and ulceration that may accompany globe displacement. A clear margin of dissection may be achieved with a medial orbitectomy, but this may entail entry into the cranial vault.

Traumatic globe proptosis
Typically seen in road traffic accident cases, traumatic globe proptosis is characterized by rostral displacement of the globe and entrapment of the eyelids behind the globe equator. The proptosis is alleviated by drawing the eyelids in front of the globe (facilitated by a lateral canthotomy if necessary) and suturing them in apposition to protect the globe while the retrobulbar swelling resolves over the next few days with anti-inflammatory medication. Often, in such cases, optic nerve trauma renders the globe blind. Rupture of the medial rectus muscle can occur, causing lateral deviation and rostral displacement of the globe, and may necessitate enucleation.

Horner's syndrome
Horner's syndrome is caused by a lesion affecting the sympathetic innervation of the eye. It can result from brachial plexus avulsion or otitis media, but most cases are idiopathic. The clinical syndrome comprises enophthalmos, third eyelid protrusion, drooping of the upper lid, miosis and conjunctival hyperaemia. This needs to be distinguished from similar clinical signs that may be seen with corneal pain. Horner's syndrome is confirmed by resolution of the clinical signs following the instillation of topical phenylephrine into the conjunctival sac.

The ocular signs are rarely clinically significant and idiopathic cases often resolve in 6–8 weeks. Any underlying disease (e.g. otitis media, see Chapter 22) should be identified and managed. Topical phenylephrine may be applied to the eye twice daily to control the clinical signs and prevent the third eyelid obstructing the central visual axis.

References and further reading

Bexfield N and Lee K (2014) *BSAVA Guide to Procedures in Small Animal Practice, 2nd edn.* BSAVA Publications, Gloucester
Gould D and McLellan G (2014) *BSAVA Manual of Canine and Feline Ophthalmology, 3rd edn.* BSAVA Publications, Gloucester

Ear problems and head tilt

Robert Williams

Disorders of the ears are some of the most common presentations in first-opinion canine practice; rarely will a day go by when a practitioner doesn't need to deal with a case of ear disease. They can often be a source of frustration for the vet and owner, and a source of much discomfort for the dog.

Ear disease can present in a variety of ways including:

- Ear scratching, head shaking, face rubbing
- Aural malodour, otorrhoea
- Erythema of the pinna
- Nystagmus, ataxia, paresis
- Head tilt
- No signs.

There are few, if any, true emergencies arising from ear problems, but owners may perceive that urgent attention is required if there is:

- An acute onset: ear problems that present acutely (e.g. vestibular syndrome or aural haematoma) can cause significant anxiety for owners
- Acute worsening of a pre-existing problem: the dog may become extremely distressed, scratching repeatedly at the ear (e.g. otitis externa)
- A foreign body in the ear canal, such as a grass awn.

Prompt examination is warranted in all these cases.

Clinical examination of the ear

Clinical examination of the ear should be preceded by a thorough general examination of the skin looking for signs of inflammatory skin disease, multifocal lesions or signs of parasitic infestation (fleas, mites, lice).

Once this has been performed, examination of the ear can begin. Each clinician will develop their own way of doing this, but a systematic approach is often useful.

1. Palpate the external ear canal and periauricular tissues.
2. Examine and palpate the pinna.
   - Examine the outer edges of the pinna for crusting associated with scabies.
   - Note whether the concave section of the pinna is erythematous (a strong indicator of allergic disease).
3. Use a fine comb to brush the pinna, looking for parasites such as lice.
4. Using a cotton swab, obtain a cytology sample from the ear canal. If infection is suspected, obtain a sample for culture and sensitivity testing.
5. Cytology (see QRG 22.1) allows the characterization of inflammatory cells and any microbes present (e.g. Gram-positive cocci, Gram-negative rods, yeast). If Gram-negative

---

Top tips for ear problems

1. Adopt a consistent approach to each case
2. Client education is vital in medicine, and particularly when dealing with ear disease
   - Ear disorders are often slow to resolve and may be indicative of a more generalized problem – if a client appreciates this from the outset they may be more patient
   - If the client understands what is wrong with their dog and how it can be managed, they are more likely to be understanding of the particular difficulties of treating ear disease
   - Owner compliance is often poor, as medicating painful ears is difficult
   - Owners can also get disheartened, as they may feel that the problem is never-ending
   - It is important to explain to the client what is happening in the dog's ear, to provide a clear demonstration of how to clean and medicate the ear, and to outline the objectives of the treatment
3. Repeat examinations are vital for treatment success. Retaining these cases and seeing them repeatedly until they resolve is of paramount importance. Successful conclusion of a case is more likely when both vet and client work together to achieve a result
4. A consistent approach, involving several members of the practice as a team, will give good results

rods are found, culture and sensitivity testing should be performed.
6. Perform otoscopy (see QRG 22.2). It is very important to examine the entire length of the external ear canal and the tympanic membrane. This may not be possible in conscious animals with severe aural pain, canal stenosis or an uncooperative temperament. Such dogs are likely to require examination under deep sedation or anaesthesia.

Mites

Ear mites are a relatively common presentation, particularly in juvenile dogs.

Otodectes cynotis mites (Figure 22.1) cause acute inflammation of the external ear canal. The mites activate the ceruminous glands, which produce copious amounts of dark brown cerumen. The mites are white and easily visible moving around on the wax. Multiple drugs can be used, but moxidectin and selamectin are particularly useful. They are available as topical spot-on treatments; a second dose should be applied after 4 weeks. It is also necessary to clean the ears and to treat any secondary otitis externa. Infection is contagious, so in-contact dogs (and cats) should also be treated.

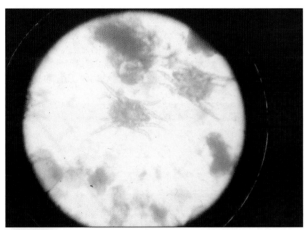

| 22.1 | *Otodectes cynotis* ear mite. (Original magnification X80) (Courtesy of Ken Robinson) |

PRACTICAL TIP

The activity of ear mites increases as the temperature of the ear canal rises. So, if you are unsure, patience with the otoscope in position usually pays off

---

Demodex mites can cause disease of the ear canal. The pinna is also one of the predilection sites for the scabies mites (*Sarcoptes scabiae* var. *canis*; see Chapter 27).

Aural haematoma

On presentation, the concave surface of the pinna is swollen and distended, with a variably sized fluid accumulation in the subcutaneous space. The skin of the pinna overlying the swelling is usually erythematous (Figure 22.2), often causing irritation. The exact

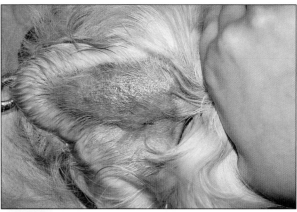

| 22.2 | Typical appearance of an aural haematoma, showing a bulging fluid-filled mass on the concave surface of the pinna. |

pathophysiology of aural haematoma formation is not fully understood, though owners usually report a period of vigorous head shaking prior to noticing the typical fluid-filled swelling of the pinna. It is thought that shear forces are established by the head shaking and that these disrupt blood vessels within or overlying the cartilage plate of the pinna. The vessels subsequently bleed into the subcutaneous space, tearing the loose fibrous connections between the skin and the underlying cartilage.

PRACTICAL TIPS

- It is very important to check for an underlying cause of the head shaking that usually precedes the haematoma
- The pinna should always be examined for signs of disease (including ectoparasites), and otoscopy performed to look for otitis externa or a foreign body
- If any underlying problem is found, this will need treating concurrently

---

Treatment
Many treatments for aural haematoma have been described; the following is the author's preferred approach. Whichever drainage technique is used, it is usually necessary also to treat the underlying otitis externa.

Non-surgical drainage
The haematoma can be drained using a 19 G butterfly needle and 10 ml syringe (Figure 22.3).

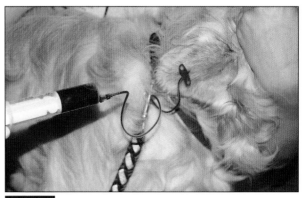

| 22.3 | Needle drainage of an aural haematoma. |

An alternative is to apply local anaesthetic cream (e.g. EMLA) to the lowermost section of the swollen concave aspect of the pinna (distal to the ear canal opening) and then to create an opening using a biopsy punch (8 mm). This leaves a permanent drainage hole, allowing sustained drainage. Antibiotic cover is recommended.

Surgical treatment

Surgery may be necessary in cases refractory to needle drainage, so it is important to advise clients from the outset that this may ultimately be required. The technique is straightforward (see QRG 22.3).

Laceration of the pinna

Lacerations of the pinna are most often caused during dog fights or by dogs running free and snagging an ear on a sharp object, such as barbed wire. Torn ears bleed profusely (Figure 22.4).

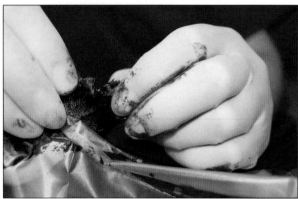

| **22.4** | Laceration of the pinna; note the profuse bleeding. |

Treatment of small tip lacerations is often achieved most easily by amputating the tip and suturing over the exposed end of the pinna. Larger lacerations should be repaired: a two-layer closure is best, suturing both skin surfaces separately with a fine-gauge suture material (1.5 metric; 4/0 USP).

Local anaesthetic cream (e.g. EMLA) may be applied topically over the repair. It is important to pay attention to pain relief as these dogs are often quite sore in the first 1–2 days after the operation. Bandaging ears postoperatively, particularly after pinna surgery, is often advocated. If done incorrectly, however, this may cause ischaemic damage to the pinna. The author prefers not to bandage ears as it rarely appears to be necessary, and head bandages are often poorly tolerated.

Foreign bodies

The foreign bodies encountered most commonly in the ear canal are grass awns, and the condition is thus more common in summertime. Dogs present with acute-onset vigorous head shaking and ear scratching, often following a period of outdoor activity. The proximal ear canal is visibly inflamed and dogs resent (strongly) palpation or manipulation of the external ear canal. It is preferable to examine the external ear canal under heavy sedation (or light anaesthesia). The

foreign body can be anywhere in the external ear canal but is usually distal, close to the tympanum.

Once located, the easiest way to remove the foreign body is to grasp it using crocodile forceps under otoscopic guidance, and to use gentle traction to remove the foreign body, forceps and otoscope from the ear canal *in one movement*. All foreign material should be removed. It is very important to examine the ear canal once the foreign body has been removed, and to check the state of the tympanum. Most tears will resolve in a number of weeks; however, it would be advisable to avoid topical medication if the tympanum is not intact. Most dogs will benefit from a short course of anti-inflammatory drugs to reduce the discomfort associated with the foreign body. These can be delivered topically *if the tympanic membrane is intact*.

Otitis externa

Otitis externa (OE) is defined as inflammation and/or infection of the external ear canal and associated structures. OE may be acute or chronic, and may be associated with other diseases of the ear (aural haematoma or otitis media), or can be a part of generalized skin disease. The disease process is often thought of in terms of predisposing factors, primary factors and perpetuating factors (Figure 22.5). Cases will have a combination of several of these factors present; it is important to identify each factor and manage or eliminate it as appropriate. All breeds of dog can be affected by OE, although certain breeds are more commonly affected (e.g. spaniels, Boxer, Labrador Retriever, West Highland White Terrier).

Predisposing factors
▪ Ear canal conformation
▪ Excess cerumen
▪ Obstructive ear disease
▪ Systemic diseases
▪ Excess moisture
Primary factors
▪ Parasites
▪ Foreign body
▪ Hypersensitivity diseases
▪ Autoimmune diseases
▪ Disorders of keratinization
▪ Cutaneous (ceruminal gland hyperplasia)
Perpetuating factors
▪ Bacteria
▪ Yeast
▪ Pathological changes (skin)
▪ Otitis media
▪ Inappropriate treatment

| **22.5** | Predisposing, primary and perpetuating factors in otitis externa. |

Clinical signs

Dogs presenting with *acute* OE tend to display head shaking and scratching, with erythema of the pinna and proximal external ear canal (Figure 22.6). There can be variable amounts of discharge present (Figure 22.7).

Chronic OE may have few signs other than a malodorous ear discharge (with soiling of the proximal external ear canal and pinna); head shaking and

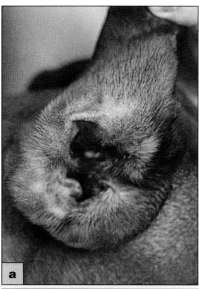

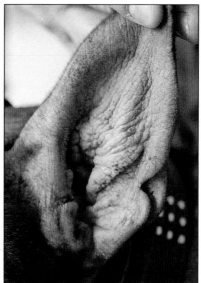

Chronic otitis externa, showing thickening of the skin lining the ear canal and narrowing of the canal, in a middle-aged Staffordshire Bull Terrier.

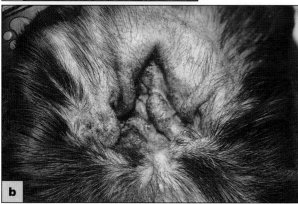

22.6   **(a)** Young cross-breed dog with early otitis externa, showing erythema of the outer canal.
(b) Typical gross appearance of otitis externa.

Discharge colour/ type	Likely cause
Dark brown/black	*Staphylococcus, Streptococcus*, Gram-positive cocci, ear mites, *Malassezia*
Yellow/cream/ green	*Pseudomonas, Proteus, Klebsiella*, Gram-negative rods
Blood	Neoplasia, trauma

22.7   Types and likely causes of aural discharge in otitis externa.

scratching are variable and may be absent. There may also be thickening of the external ear canal (Figure 22.8), and pain on palpation.

Treatment of a simple case (first presentation)
In most cases the following is appropriate:

- Ear cleaning (see below) once daily
- Topical medicated eardrops effective against cocci and *Malassezia*, and with some anti-inflammatory steroid present
- It may also be useful to use steroids orally to reduce severe inflammation of the ear canal, especially if the canal is too narrow (due to inflammation) to allow full examination; subsequent re-examination may allow a better inspection of the ear canal
- Cases should be checked after 7–10 days, repeating cytology and otoscopy. Treatment and checks should continue until the ear canal has

returned to normal on visual inspection, and cytology fails to demonstrate inflammatory cells or microbes. It is always worth checking whether the owner is cleaning and medicating the ears correctly. Compliance may be poor for a variety of reasons, including a poor understanding by the owner of the condition, and patient factors such as aural discomfort.

It is useful to employ adjunctive treatments, such as tris-EDTA in cases of *Pseudomonas* infection. Where topical treatment is not possible (e.g. it would be too painful), oral antibiotics and steroids can be used. It is also helpful to treat any underlying inflammatory or immune-mediated skin disease (see Chapter 27).

The prognosis for OE is variable, and should be excellent for cases caused by parasites such as *Otodectes*, or in simple cases with minimal inflammation and sparse cocci seen on cytology.

Ear cleaning

- Ear cleaning is very important as it can dramatically improve treatment outcomes
- It allows for a thorough evaluation of the ear canal and tympanum
- It removes pus and debris, which can inactivate certain antibiotics; this also reduces some of the stimuli to the inflammatory process
- There are many ear cleaning products available. Ceruminolytic products containing docusate sodium, propylene glycol, gylcerine or mineral oil work particularly well. Further information on specific ear cleaners can be obtained by consulting a dermatology text such as the *BSAVA Manual of Canine and Feline Dermatology*
- In severely soiled ears, or where a severe infection is present, lavage of the ear canal is also beneficial. A ceruminolytic agent should be used first, followed by copious lavage of the canal with sterile saline. Various methods of lavage are possible (e.g. fluid bag, three-way-tap, intravenous cannula and syringe, nasogastric feeding tube and syringe, or specific ear lavage systems; all require deep sedation or, ideally, general anaesthesia)

Chronic or complex cases

In severe cases, long-standing chronic cases, cases associated with underlying skin disease or intractable cases, it may only be possible to manage the condition rather than cure it. In these situations, it is important to discuss this fact with the owner and explain why the treatment will aim to manage and not to cure. Surgery such as lateral wall resection, total ear canal ablation (TECA) or lateral bulla osteotomy (LBO) is an option, though this surgery is not for all cases and not for the inexperienced surgeon.

Otitis media

Otitis media (OM) is inflammation of the middle ear and is often secondary to otitis externa (see above). The inflammation may be secondary to infection, neoplasia or foreign bodies. In cases of infection the pathogens are usually similar to those encountered in OE and may have spread across the tympanic membrane or along the auditory tube. Cases may progress to otitis interna.

Clinical signs are similar to those of OE and there may also be pain on opening the mouth, during eating or on palpation of the ear canal or bulla. Facial nerve paralysis and Horner's syndrome may also be present.

Otoscopy should be performed under general anaesthesia and may show the tympanic membrane to be: ruptured; intact (in which case it may appear opaque due to pus accumulation in the middle ear); or bulging into the ear canal. Samples should be taken for cytology and culture; myringotomy may be required if the membrane is intact (see *BSAVA Guide to Procedures in Small Animal Practice*). Radiography (using a skyline bulla view) may show fluid in the bulla or sclerosis of the bone.

Treatment may be successful with lavage and antibiotics, but surgery (ear canal ablation and bulla osteotomy) may be required in some cases, especially if there are chronic changes in the external ear canal.

Vestibular disease

Head tilt is a common presentation, particularly in geriatric dogs (Figure 22.9) and is a manifestation of dysfunction of the vestibular system. *Peripheral* vestibular disease (PVD) is due to dysfunction of the peripheral vestibular system, which consists of the semicircular canals, the utricle and saccule, vestibular neurons and the vestibular portion of cranial nerve VIII. *Central* vestibular disease is due to

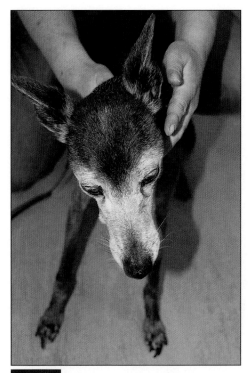

22.9   Head tilt in a geriatric dog.

abnormalities of the central vestibular structures, including the brainstem vestibular nuclei and cerebellum. It is important to distinguish between central and peripheral disease (see Chapter 11).

Common causes of PVD include:

- Geriatric vestibular syndrome
- Otitis media/interna (see earlier)
- Neoplasia/polyps of the middle ear
- Trauma
- Ototoxic drugs
- Hypothyroidism(?).

Geriatric vestibular syndrome

This is the most common form of peripheral vestibular disease, predominantly affecting dogs >10 years of age. It is an acute idiopathic syndrome that presents as an emergency and is often erroneously referred to as a 'stroke'. The neurological signs are head tilt, ataxia, vomiting/nausea, horizontal/rotatory nystagmus and strabismus with Horner's syndrome or facial nerve deficits. It is important to perform a thorough clinical examination and to perform otoscopy on both ears (geriatric vestibular syndrome is a diagnosis of exclusion).

This idiopathic disease is self-limiting; a large proportion of affected dogs will have started to improve by the time they reach the clinic and will continue to do so over the next 48–72 hours. The prognosis is excellent. There is no specific treatment for this syndrome. The dog should be confined indoors until the signs resolve. In first-opinion practice a number of medications are commonly prescribed, including:

- Anti-emetic drugs (e.g. maropitant, metoclopramide), as vomiting and nausea are common signs

- Steroids (for their anti-inflammatory effects)
- Propentofylline (often used in geriatric patients with central nervous system signs).

To the author's knowledge there is no evidence for the use of the latter two.

Aural neoplasia/polyps

Tumours sited in the bullae may damage or involve the peripheral vestibular structures, or there may be extension from a tumour affecting the external ear canal after it has crossed the tympanic membrane. Inflammatory polyps (Figure 22.10) may also cause vestibular dysfunction if similarly involving the bulla.

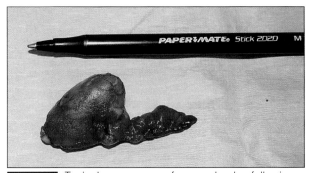

22.10 Typical appearance of an aural polyp following removal. This is a relatively large, smooth, pale pink/purple mass with an obvious 'stalk'.

Ototoxic drugs

Many drugs and chemicals are described as ototoxic. If vestibular signs develop after topical administration of a drug or chemical into the ear canal, the agent should be stopped. Signs will generally resolve over time.

Hypothyroidism

Hypothyroidism has been implicated in many cases of peripheral neurological dysfunction, although the exact pathophysiology is not known and the response to thyroid hormone supplements often has a poor effect on improving the vestibular dysfunction.

References and further reading

Bacon NJ (2012) Pinna and external ear canal. In: *Veterinary Surgery: Small Animal*, ed. KM Tobias and SA Johnston, pp. 2059–2077. Elsevier Saunders, St. Louis

Bensignor E and Forsythe PJ (2012) An approach to otitis externa. In: *BSAVA Manual of Canine and Feline Dermatology, 3rd edn*, ed. H Jackson and R Marsella, pp. 110–120

Bexfield N and Lee K (2014) *BSAVA Guide to Procedures in Small Animal Practice, 2nd edn*, BSAVA Publications, Gloucester

Fossum TW (2007) Surgery of the ear. In: *Small Animal Surgery, 3rd edn*, ed. TW Fossum, pp. 289–316. Mosby, St. Louis

Scott DW, Miller WH and Griffin CE (2001) Diseases of eyelids, claws, anal sacs and ears. In: *Muller & Kirk's Small Animal Dermatology, 6th edn*, ed. DW Scott *et al.*, pp.1185–1235. Saunders, Philadelphia

Tobias KM and Morris D (2005) The ear. In: *BSAVA Manual of Canine and Feline Head, Neck and Thoracic Surgery*, ed. DJ Brockman and DE Holt, pp. 56–72. BSAVA Publications, Gloucester

White RAS (2012) Middle and inner ear. In: *Veterinary Surgery: Small Animal*, ed. KM Tobias and SA Johnston, pp. 2078–2090. Elsevier Saunders, St. Louis

QRG 22.1 Ear cytology

This should be done prior to cleaning the ear.

Most dogs will allow sample collection without sedation. An experienced handler, such as a veterinary nurse, should be available to help restrain the dog's head.

1 Introduce a sterile sample collection swab into the ear canal, under direct visualization. Gently roll the swab against the ear canal wall. The cotton tip of the swab will become covered in a representative sample of the external ear canal contents, including cerumen and pus, if present.

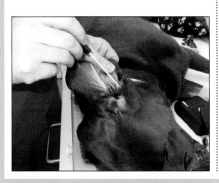

2 Gently roll the cotton tip along a clean microscope slide to transfer some of the sample to the slide. It is usually possible to make two or three smears per sample.

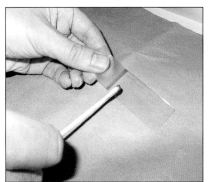

3 Stain the slide using Gram's stain or a bench-top stain such as Diff-Quik.

4 Examine the slide using light microscopy. Depending on the underlying disease process, smears may include epithelial cells, neutrophils, rods, cocci or yeast.

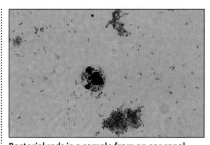

Bacterial rods in a sample from an ear canal. Some bacteria are being phagocytosed by neutrophils, showing that the infection is active. (Original magnification X1000)

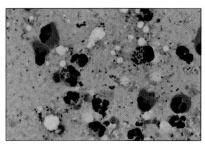

Bacterial cocci in a sample from an ear canal. Some bacteria are being phagocytosed by neutrophils, showing that the infection is active. (Original magnification X1000)

QRG 22.2 Otoscopy

Patient preparation and positioning

- Most dogs will require some level of restraint to enable otoscopic examination. This can range from relatively minimal hand restraint to hold the dog's head still, to full anaesthesia for a particularly fractious and/or painful dog. The level of restraint that is required is a matter of clinical judgement.
- Heavily haired ears may require some hair plucking; this may be possible with the dog conscious, but judging the temperament of the dog is important.
- Heavily soiled ears should be lavaged with sterile saline warmed to body temperature. Often a 10 ml syringe and soft intravenous catheter will suffice. Allowing the dog to shake its head afterwards will aid in drying the ear canal.
- The conscious patient is best examined in a sitting position with the head held in a neutral position (i.e. looking straight ahead). Lateral recumbency, with the ear of interest uppermost, is the position if the dog is anaesthetized.

Procedure

1 Grasp the most proximal part of the external ear canal and gently pull it laterally and ventrally. This action helps to bring the vertical and horizontal canals into a straight line.

2 Whilst looking through the otoscope, introduce the speculum into the external ear canal, always under direct visual guidance.

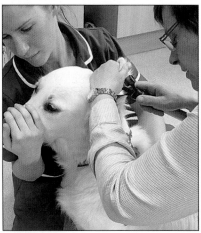
© Sue Paterson

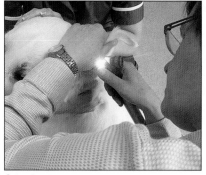
© Sue Paterson

WARNING

Never advance the otoscope unless you can visualize where it is going

3 The ear canal is then visualized by moving the otoscope ventrally, dorsally and laterally (small movements).

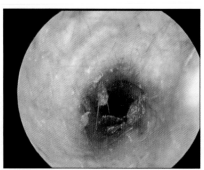
Normal ear canal, with a small amount of wax.
© Sue Paterson

4 Advance the otoscope slowly along the ear canal to view the tympanum. It is important to try and view the tympanum in every case. It is divided into two areas: the pars tensa, which has a greyish-blue striated appearance; and the dorsal pars flaccida, which has a pinkish appearance. The manubrium of the malleus is visible in the pars tensa; there are blood vessels visible along the manubrium.

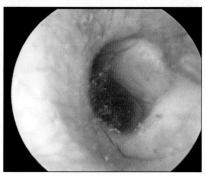
Normal tympanic membrane. © Sue Paterson

Video-otoscopy

Video-otoscopy is becoming more widely available

- It is an invaluable diagnostic aid and is also extremely useful in client education, as it allows the client to see the condition of the dog's ear canal
- It allows visualization under lavage in soiled ears, and the collection of samples under direct visualization
- It can also be used to document the response to treatment

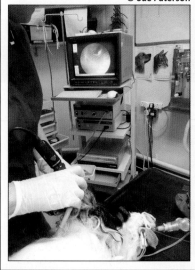
© Sue Paterson

QRG 22.3 Surgical treatment of aural haematoma

by Tim Hutchinson

Patient preparation and positioning

With the dog under general anaesthesia, place it in lateral recumbency, with the affected ear uppermost.

PRACTICAL TIP

It is essential to perform otoscopy (see QRG 22.2) prior to preparation of the pinna for surgery, as it is important to assess the external ear canal for underlying pathology

- Both surfaces of the pinna should be clipped and prepared aseptically.
- Once the pinna has been prepared, it is draped such that both surfaces of the pinna are accessible.

Procedure

1 Make an incision on the concave surface of the pinna, through the skin along the length of the haematoma swelling.

2 Drain the haematoma. The fluid component will drain freely through the incision, but it is also important to remove any clots and fibrous tissue by swabbing inside the haematoma cavity (grasping a swab in mosquito forceps to push it into the space is helpful).

3 Using monofilament suture material and starting on the concave surface, pass the needle full-thickness through the pinna. Pass the needle back through the convex surface of the pinna and tie a knot on the concave surface, such that a simple mattress suture is formed.

- 2 or 3 metric (3/0 or 2/0 USP) nylon or polypropylene would be appropriate; or pseudomonofilament (e.g. 3 metric (2/0 USP) sheathed polyamide).
- The sutures are started about 1 cm away from the incision edge and staggered in rows separated by 10–15 mm. The orientation of the sutures is vertical rather than horizontal.
- The incision is not sutured closed. This allows free drainage of any fluid postoperatively.

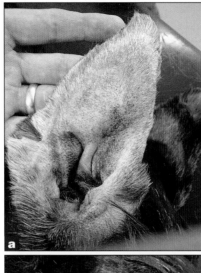
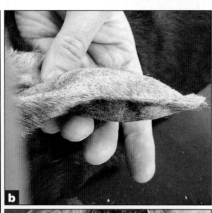
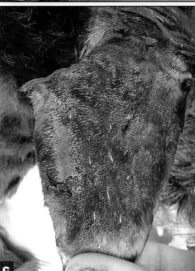
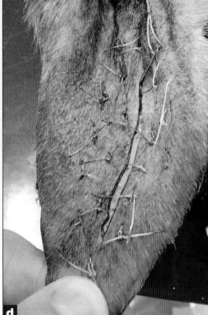

(a,b) Preoperative views, showing the extent of the haematoma. (c) Sutures on the convex surface of the pinna. (d) The concave surface, showing the sutures and drainage channel. The postoperative photographs were taken after removal of the drapes, but before final clean (the sutures continue to ooze for some time afterwards).

Postoperative care

- An Elizabethan collar is fitted, and non-steroidal anti-inflammatory drugs and antibiotics dispensed.
- Sutures are removed after 14 days.

PRACTICAL TIPS

- Ensure that the whole blood clot is removed prior to placing sutures
- Leave a drainage hole for further fluid to escape. Remember to warn the owners that this could be messy
- Do not tie sutures too tightly, as this will cause irritation if they cut into the skin
- Leave sutures in place for at least 2 weeks. Contrary to popular belief, the aim of suturing is not to compress the skin back to the cartilage, but to promote fibrous reactions around the suture material and effectively 'spot-weld' the tissues together

Abbnormalities of the throat and neck

Robert Williams

Abnormalities of the throat and neck are among the less common presentations in general canine practice; however, they can be a cause of frustration as many of them are difficult to deal with. This chapter will highlight some of the more common presentations and how to avoid some of the pitfalls in dealing with these cases. Clinical signs affecting the throat and neck may include:

- Swellings and lumps (see also Chapter 28)
- Wounds (NB may be an emergency presentation, see Chapter 10)
- Abnormal function (e.g. laryngeal paralysis (see Chapter 24); gagging/retching)
- Pain (e.g. sore throat due to infection; cervical spine-associated pain, see Chapter 16).

Swellings and lumps

Soft tissue swellings and lumps that affect the neck include:

- Salivary gland disease (sialoceles predominantly)
- Lymphadenopathy
- Thyroid neoplasia
- Foreign body
- Abscess.

Salivary gland disease

Sialoceles, sialoliths and salivary gland tumours are all described in dogs, but the sialocele (salivary mucocele) is by far the most common salivary gland disorder.

A sialocele is the collection of saliva within the subcutaneous tissues. Leakage of saliva occurs either from rupture of the salivary gland itself or, more commonly, from the draining salivary duct. The saliva incites an inflammatory reaction within the surrounding tissue and the sialocele has a lining composed of mostly fibrous tissue (a pseudocapsule). The majority of cases are idiopathic, though reported causes include sialoliths, trauma, foreign body and neoplasia.

Breeds commonly affected include poodles, German Shepherd Dogs, spaniels and Dachshunds, and dogs are typically young. Presentations and clinical signs vary depending on the gland affected, but include:

- Zygomatic gland: exophthalmos; third eyelid protrusion; painless orbital swelling
- Pharyngeal gland: laboured breathing; swelling in the region of the epiglottis
- Sublingual gland: dysphagia; tongue deviation
- Cervical gland: affects the submandibular and sublingual glands and most commonly presents as an intermandibular/ventral neck swelling.

Cervical gland sialocele

This presents as an acute, non-painful, fluctuant swelling of the intermandibular and ventral cervical region (Figure 23.1). Diagnosis is made by aspirating the swelling to reveal a thick, viscous fluid which is yellow to pink in colour. Cytology will demonstrate small numbers of lymphocytes, macrophages, neutrophils and red blood cells within a proteinaceous background.

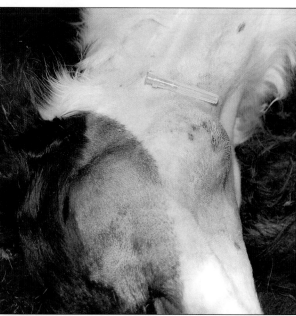

23.1 Typical gross appearance of a cervical (submandibular) mucocele. (The needle is for size comparison.) The head is towards the bottom of the photograph.

Two points are critical for success:

- Do not be tempted to treat the sialocele conservatively: this is a surgical disease and although drainage of the mucus will lead to short-term improvement there will, inevitably, be a return of the mucocele
- It is important to establish which side is affected (remember the salivary glands are paired). When the dog is placed in dorsal recumbency, the swelling will typically fall to the affected side. If there is doubt, then contrast sialography or exploration of the swelling and following the tract cranially can also aid diagnosis.

Treatment is through excision of the affected glands, which in most cases involves removing the submandibular and sublingual glands on the affected side (Figure 23.2). Prognosis is excellent, provided the affected glands are removed entirely; recurrence is reported to be about 5%.

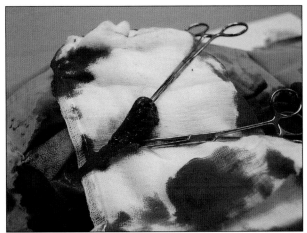

23.2 Intraoperative view of sialocele dissection. The head of the dog is to the left. Allis tissue forceps are placed on the submandibular gland and dissection is proceeding towards the sublingual gland.

Lymphadenopathy

Lymphadenopathy of the submandibular lymph nodes is a common finding on clinical examination. These lymph nodes are the major draining lymph nodes for the head and thus any disease process affecting the head (e.g. dental disease, otitis externa, rhinitis) is likely to cause lymphadenopathy. The approach to masses, including abnormal lymph nodes, is discussed in more detail in Chapter 28. Finding enlarged submandibular lymph nodes should provoke a more thorough examination of the head, looking for signs of infection, inflammation or neoplasia. As with any abnormal swelling or mass, it is worthwhile obtaining a fine-needle aspirate to characterize the enlarged node cytologically.

> **WARNING**
>
> Do not rush to a hasty diagnosis of lymphoma based on palpating enlarged submandibular lymph nodes. In general (though not always) you would expect other lymph nodes (i.e. prescapular, popliteal, inguinal) to be enlarged and easily palpable in a dog with lymphoma

Thyroid neoplasia

Tumours of the thyroid gland can also present as a ventral neck mass. They generally affect middle-aged and older dogs, without sex predilection. Thirty to fifty percent may be benign adenomas and well encapsulated, but the majority of thyroid tumours are adenocarcinomas. These can be large, extremely vascular, poorly encapsulated and locally invasive. Presentation is usually because the owner has noticed a firm, painless, ventral cervical swelling, although occasionally there may be clinical signs associated with dysfunction of cervical structures, e.g. coughing, gagging, dysphonia, dysphagia, retching or regurgitation. Thyroid neoplasms in dogs are almost exclusively non-functional; hyperthyroidism in this species is very rare indeed.

Further investigation involves fine-needle aspiration or biopsy (ultrasound guidance is preferred, due to the vascular nature of the tissue). Well encapsulated masses can be excised, but any highly vascular or invasive tumour should be discussed with an experienced oncologist.

Foreign bodies

Foreign bodies affecting the neck occur commonly, often secondary to pharyngeal stick injuries. Clinical signs most frequently reported include cervical swelling, discharging sinus, oral pain and dysphagia.

- With acute stick injuries, the dog is usually very quiet and guarded, exhibiting pain around the head and neck and resenting movement of the head and opening of the mouth. Drooling is often present, and the dribbling saliva may be blood-tinged.
- Cervical swelling and a discharging sinus are more typical of chronic foreign bodies.

Cases suspected of having a cervical foreign body can be imaged in a variety of ways. A plain lateral-to-lateral radiographic view of the cervical region is one of the most useful images, and cervical emphysema will indicate the extent of a penetrating wound. Advanced imaging may also be useful.

With acute stick injuries it is important to examine the wound thoroughly, with the dog under general anaesthesia. There may be no foreign body apparent, in which case flushing of the wound, antibiosis and analgesia are employed. However, if a cervical foreign body is identified, surgery should be considered. There are three approaches that are commonly employed to resolve the problem:

- Ventral midline cervical exploration to identify the disrupted fascial plane and remove the foreign body
- Exploration and debridement of a cervical discharging tract
- Debridement and lavage of any oropharyngeal wound.

In chronic cases an abscess will have formed around the foreign body. This should be lanced and flushed, explored for any foreign material, and left open to drain. It is often worthwhile to debride as much inflammatory tissue as possible. Owners should be warned that signs may recur in spite of appropriate management.

Wounds

Dog bite wounds and draining sinus tracts are common presentations affecting the neck. Further information on wound management is given in Chapter 10.

Bite wounds

Dog fights are common occurrences; although bite wounds can occur anywhere on the body, the ventral neck is particularly vulnerable to attack (Figure 23.3).

The following points offer a quick guide to dealing with dog bite wounds.

■ Remember ABC – Airway, Breathing, Circulation (see Chapter 10).

■ It is easy to get carried away with the stress of the situation, particularly as the owner is likely to be very distressed. It is important to stay calm.

■ *The skin wounds are often **not** the most important problem for the dog.*

- Dog bite wounds can be described as 'iceberg' wounds, as the skin wound often conceals far more sinister damage to vital structures beneath the skin, which are the result of teeth tearing through deeper tissues during the struggle.

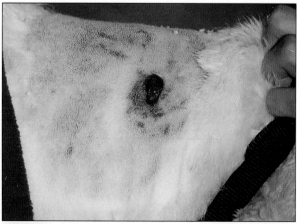

23.3   A bite wound on the neck. It is always worth remembering that the visible skin wound often gives no indication as to the severity of underlying wounds. Fortunately in this case, other than muscle damage no vital structures were affected.

- The overlying skin usually moves with the teeth, so small puncture wounds can conceal significant deeper damage.

■ Treat shock, give pain relief and antibiotic cover initially, and stabilize any major problems (i.e. respiratory distress) (see Chapter 8). The initial goal should be to stabilize the animal prior to any invasive procedure (this includes imaging).

■ Once the animal is stabilized and any life-threatening issues have been dealt with, it is then possible to perform imaging and/or exploratory surgery as required.

■ In dogs that have purely superficial wounds and no damage to vital structures the wounds are often best cleaned and left open, with the animal prescribed antibiotics and pain relief. Repair, if needed, should be delayed for 48–72 hours and until after any discharge has ceased. A light absorptive bandage may be applied to keep the wounds clean.

Draining sinus tracts

Draining sinus tracts occasionally occur in the neck and are typically caused by a foreign body or previous surgery.

Draining sinus tracts can be extremely difficult to deal with. It is important to be up front with clients when dealing with a sinus tract that there are no easy answers to this problem. Conservative treatment will almost certainly fail.

Close questioning regarding previous history is important:

■ Has the dog had surgery on the neck or associated structures (e.g. total ear canal ablation, lateral/ventral bulla osteotomy, salivary gland removal)?

■ Does the dog chew/carry sticks, or does the owner throw sticks for the dog to retrieve?

■ Is the dog a working dog (e.g. gundog)?

■ How long has the draining tract been present?

■ Has there been any previous treatment?

A draining sinus tract can be dealt with in two ways. Ideally, advanced imaging such as magnetic resonance imaging (MRI) can be employed to try and locate the source of the draining tract prior to surgery, but this may not be feasible for the client, so thorough careful and meticulous dissection of the tract can be followed from the skin to its source, removing all abnormal tissue encountered. Whatever approach is adopted it is probably not a surgery for the novice surgeon. It is often suggested that injecting contrast medium into the tract to outline it is useful; in most cases, however, the radiographs are of very limited value.

Abnormal function

Abnormal function of structures in the throat and neck can have profound consequences for the affected animal (e.g. laryngeal paralysis; see Chapter 24).

Gagging and retching are two common presenting complaints in first opinion practice.

■ Gagging is the reflex contraction of the muscles of the throat, generally caused by stimulation of the pharynx, that may induce retching.

■ Retching is a strong involuntary and unproductive effort to vomit.

The approach to both complaints should be as for every other condition:

■ Obtain a good history
■ Perform a thorough clinical examination
■ Perform localized examination/tests as indicated by the initial examination
■ Keep a simple approach to these cases initially, as most of the time the answer may be straightforward (e.g. simple gastritis)
■ If a case is a repeat presentation or has very obvious systemic involvement or intractable signs, then a more proactive approach is required.

As can be seen from these lists, there is no pre-scriptive way of approaching these cases other than being thorough and methodical.

Common causes of gagging

■ Pharyngitis/laryngitis
■ Pharyngeal/laryngeal foreign body
■ Trauma
■ Elongated soft palate
■ Tracheal collapse
■ Laryngeal paralysis
■ Neoplasia (caudal oral cavity, pharynx, larynx)
■ Smoke inhalation
■ Chemical burn (following ingestion)
■ Myasthenia gravis

Common causes of retching

■ Oesophageal/gastric foreign body
■ Oesophagitis/gastro-oesophageal reflux/chemical irritation
■ Recent anaesthesia
■ Hiatal hernia
■ Gastric dilatation/gastric dilatation–volvulus
■ Any other cause of vomiting

References and further reading

Dobromylskyj MJ, Dennis R, Ladlow JF and Adams VJ (2008) The use of magnetic resonance imaging in the management of pharyngeal penetration injuries in dogs. *Journal of Small Animal Practice* **49**, 74–79
Doran IP, Wright CA and Moore AH (2008) Acute oropharyngeal and oesophageal stick injury in forty-one dogs. *Veterinary Surgery* **37**, 781–785
Gengler W (2005) Gagging. In: *Textbook of Veterinary Internal Medicine, 6th edn*, ed. SJ Ettinger and EC Feldman, pp.126–128. Elsevier Saunders, St. Louis
Griffiths LG, Tiruneh R, Sullivan M and Reid SW (2000) Oropharyngeal penetrating injuries in 50 dogs: a retrospective study. *Veterinary Surgery* **29**, 383–388
Nicholson I, Halfacree Z, Whatamough C, Mantis P and Baines S (2008) Computed tomography as an aid to management of chronic oropharyngeal stick injury in the dog. *Journal of Small Animal Practice* **49**, 451–547
Reiter AM and Smith MM (2005) The oral cavity and oropharynx. In: *BSAVA Manual of Canine and Feline Head, Neck and Thoracic Surgery*, ed. DJ Brockman and DE Holt, pp.25–44. BSAVA Publications, Gloucester
Ritter MJ and Stanley BJ (2012) Salivary glands. In: *Veterinary Surgery: Small Animal*, ed. KM Tobias and SA Johnston, pp.1439–1447. Elsevier Saunders, St. Louis
Twedt DC (2005) Vomiting. In: *Textbook of Veterinary Internal Medicine, 6th edn*, ed. SJ Ettinger and EC Feldman, pp.132–137. Elsevier Saunders, St. Louis

Cardiorespiratory problems

24

Mark Maltman

Cardiorespiratory signs are a common reason for presentation in canine practice, and in acute situations involving collapse (see Chapter 9) or dyspnoea (see Chapter 8) can be a source of stress to clinician and owner alike. This chapter will present a clinical approach to the following signs: cough; dyspnoea; heart murmur; and arrhythmia. In doing this, attention will not be paid to the specific aetiology, pathogenesis and treatment of each individual condition, and the reader is referred to the *BSAVA Manual of Canine and Feline Cardiorespiratory Medicine* for more specific information. Further reading for more detail on diagnostic modalities is suggested at the end of the chapter.

General approach to cardiorespiratory signs

The equipment necessary to investigate cardiorespiratory disease is now present in most veterinary practices, but the ability to take an accurate history and carefully examine the animal remains essential.

History

Common clinical signs associated with cardiorespiratory disease include:

- Coughing
- Dyspnoea
- Exercise intolerance
- Abdominal distension
- Syncope (see Chapter 9).

Other non-specific signs, such as weight loss and anorexia, may also occur. The vet should consider the signalment of the patient and how likely it would be for any particular dog to be affected with certain types of disease. For example, a Cavalier King Charles Spaniel with cough and dyspnoea or a Dobermann with syncope are most likely to be affected by cardiac diseases; while a young terrier with a chronic honking cough may well be suffering from tracheal collapse. Gough and Thomas (2010) have thoroughly reviewed breed predispositions.

Clinical examination

Careful observation of the patient prior to physical examination can elicit important information such as: whether the dog can walk; the pattern of respiration; and whether there is spontaneous coughing. A general examination should be carried out, paying particular attention to the following:

- Mucous membrane colour
- Capillary refill time
- Presence or absence of jugular vein distension, with or without ascites
- Size of submandibular and prescapular lymph nodes
- Pulse rate and quality
- Perfusion of the extremities.

> **PRACTICAL TIP**
>
> Gentle compression of the trachea should produce just a single cough: induction of a bout of repeated coughing suggests tracheobronchial disease

Thoracic auscultation

- Respiratory auscultation is performed across the top of the chest and, to a lesser extent, in the cranioventral thorax.
- Different heart valves may be heard in specific locations. Rather than attempting to identify the position of valves relative to specific intercostal spaces at a designated level, a more straightforward approach allows for individual variation (Figure 24.1).
  - Normal resting heart rates in dogs are generally accepted to be 70–160 beats per minute (depending on breed), which takes into account physiological increases associated with stress.
  - Variations in heart rate and rhythm are assessed, as well as the presence of abnormal sounds such as the turbulence associated with cardiac murmurs and the audibility of the S3 and S4 heart sounds forming a 'gallop' rhythm, which is due almost exclusively in dogs to cardiac disease rather than a variant of normal physiology.

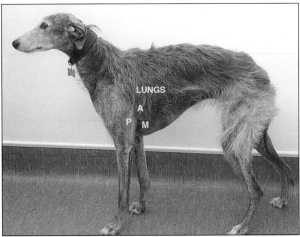

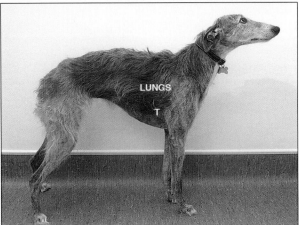

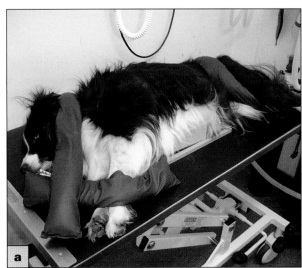

24.1 Starting on the left side of the dog, the stethoscope is placed on the chest wall just caudal to the elbow where the heart is loudest; this will approximate to the mitral valve (M) where the first heart sound (S1 or 'lub') will be most audible. In order to hear the aortic valve (A), the stethoscope is slid craniodorsally into the axilla, such that S1 fades and the lower pitched second heart sound (S2 or 'dub') becomes more notable. The pulmonary valve (P) is found by dropping slightly cranioventrally from the aortic valve to a position very close to the sternum behind the foreleg; the sounds of this valve are quieter than the other two due to the lower pressures on the right side of the heart. The tricuspid valve is found on the right side of the body (T) and represents the place where S1 is loudest on this side.

Diagnostic investigations

Radiography

The ability to produce a high-quality thoracic radiograph through good positioning, without rotation of the chest, and with exposure at peak inspiration remains the first line of investigation for all cardiothoracic disease. This can often be achieved with the patient conscious or lightly sedated, patience and plenty of sandbags (Figure 24.2). Where this is not possible, unless it is contraindicated, general anaesthesia should be used to ensure that diagnostic radiographs are obtained.

Figure 24.3 illustrates some common patterns seen on thoracic radiographs. Often the lung pattern is mixed: bronchial and diffuse interstitial patterns are frequently seen together; occasionally (e.g. with angiostrongylosis) all four lung patterns may be present on the same radiograph.

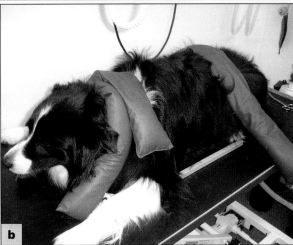

24.2 **(a)** Lateral radiographs are centred approximately at the caudal border of the scapula and two-thirds of the way down the thorax, with the forelegs drawn forward and a wedge placed under the sternum to ensure that the sternum and spine are level. Occasionally in some breeds, especially Bull Terriers, this wedge may need to be under the spine to achieve the same result. **(b)** DV radiographs are preferred for assessment of the cardiac silhouette; although if it is safe to put the animal on its back (i.e. there is no dyspnoea or pleural effusion) a VD view may offer greater information on the lung fields. The radiograph is centred in the midline at the caudal border of the scapulae, with the forelegs once again drawn forward. Effort is required to ensure that none of the body is rotated, in order to keep the thorax straight.

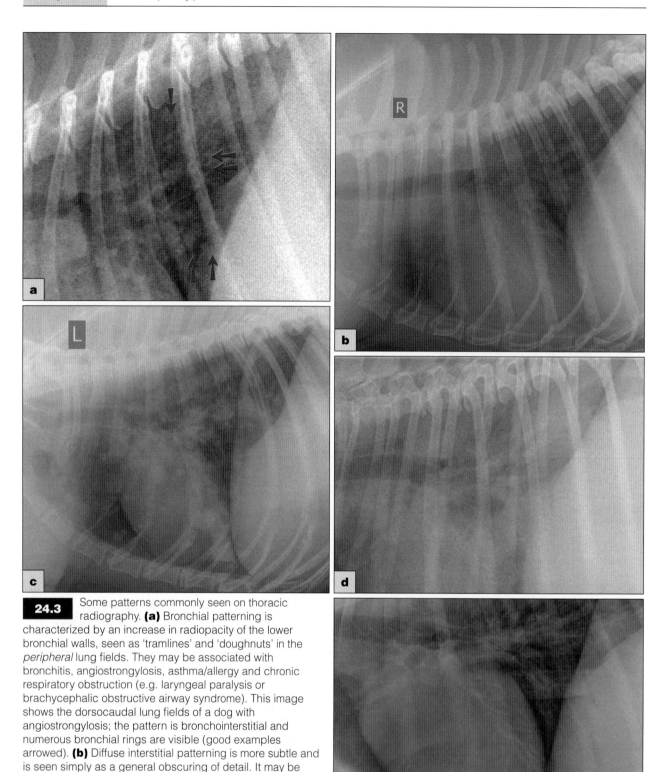

24.3 Some patterns commonly seen on thoracic radiography. **(a)** Bronchial patterning is characterized by an increase in radiopacity of the lower bronchial walls, seen as 'tramlines' and 'doughnuts' in the *peripheral* lung fields. They may be associated with bronchitis, angiostrongylosis, asthma/allergy and chronic respiratory obstruction (e.g. laryngeal paralysis or brachycephalic obstructive airway syndrome). This image shows the dorsocaudal lung fields of a dog with angiostrongylosis; the pattern is bronchointerstitial and numerous bronchial rings are visible (good examples arrowed). **(b)** Diffuse interstitial patterning is more subtle and is seen simply as a general obscuring of detail. It may be associated with pulmonary oedema, angiostrongylosis, bronchopneumonia and diffuse lymphoma in lung tissue. This image is from a dog with cardiac failure; bronchial patterning is also visible. **(c)** Nodular interstitial patterns show multiple radiopaque nodules. They may be seen with metastatic neoplasia, *Angiostrongylus*, fungal disease or pulmonary abscessation. This image is from a Boxer with pulmonary metastasis of a distant adenocarcinoma. **(d)** An alveolar pattern represents disease in the terminal bronchioles and alveoli, such as severe oedema, haemorrhage, angiostrongylosis or bronchopneumonia. Lung tissue is consolidated, showing a general increase in radiopacity so that darker bronchi are highlighted as they course through the lung lobe, so-called 'air bronchograms'. Occasionally, an entire lung lobe will be consolidated, seen as a region of marked increased radiopacity with sharp borders. **(e)** Vascular patterns are seen as increased opacity and size of the pulmonary blood vessels. They are best assessed by measuring the cranial lobar vessels as they cross the 4th rib on a lateral radiograph, where they should not be wider than the rib itself, or the caudal lobar vessels as they cross the 9th rib on a DV view, where again they should be smaller in width than the rib; on the lateral view, the artery is dorsal to the vein (separated from it by the radiolucent bronchus); on the DV view the artery is lateral to the vein (separated from it by the radiolucent bronchus). Pulmonary venous enlargement is indicative of left-sided cardiac congestion, whilst arterial engorgement is associated with obstructive disease such as angiostrongylosis or thromboembolism; an equal increase may be seen in cases of pulmonary hypertension, either idiopathic or secondary to diseases such as hyperadrenocorticism or renal insufficiency.

Electrocardiography

Electrocardiography is used to assess the rate and rhythm of the heart. Whilst measurement of components of the P–QRS–T complex (see Figure 24.17a) can be an indicator of cardiac chamber size, this is not reliable and it is advisable to combine radiography and echocardiography for this purpose. The technique is standardized by recording traces with animals in right lateral recumbency, with a 6-lead electrocardiogram (ECG) being sufficient for general practice cases. Most machines now have atraumatic clips, which are better tolerated by patients.

ECG limb lead placement
- **RED** Right forelimb
- **YELLOW** Left forelimb
- **BLACK** Right hindlimb
- **GREEN** Left hindlimb

WARNING
Surgical spirit can be applied to the clips to improve contact with the skin, but care should be taken that spirit does not run between the different clips and create a connection between them outside the patient

Echocardiography

A description of echocardiography is beyond the scope of this chapter (see the *BSAVA Manual of Canine and Feline Cardiorespiratory Medicine*). Practice is essential and the inexperienced echocardiographer should not be discouraged by failure to image certain valves or obtain certain measurements. This is part of the learning curve and one should persevere; help can be sought from a more experienced colleague on a case-by-case basis.

Other techniques

Other investigations include blood pressure measurement, bronchoscopy and bronchoalveolar lavage (BAL) (see the *BSAVA Guide to Procedures in Small Animal Practice*), and blood gas analysis. Laboratory tests provide baseline haematology and biochemistry data. Lavage fluid analysis (culture and cytology), faecal analysis (for *Angiostrongylus*) and assessment of coagulation function, as well as specific markers for cardiac size and damage (ANP, pro-BNP, troponin I; see *BSAVA Manual of Canine and Feline Clinical Pathology*), are also helpful.

A clinical approach to coughing

Coughing is a reflex triggered as a result of tracheal irritation, inflammation or compression. It is one protective mechanism by which an animal may clear its airway of foreign material (gross or microscopic) or respiratory secretions (normal or pathological). Occasional coughing is normal, but coughing may be increased in various diseases (Figure 24.4).

Emergency cases
On presentation, a rapid assessment of the dog will show whether coughing represents a life-threatening abnormality, in which case history-taking and physical examination will need to be undertaken quickly, whilst simultaneously providing oxygen and other treatment (see Chapter 8)

Organ/system affected	Conditions
Pharynx	**Non-pathogenic: reverse sneezing and cough** **Brachycephalic obstructive airway syndrome (BOAS)** Pharyngitis Trauma to pharyngeal wall: most commonly stick injury Foreign body Swallowing disorders: idiopathic, myasthenia gravis
Larynx	**BOAS** **Laryngeal paralysis** Eversion of laryngeal saccules Neoplasia Pharyngolaryngeal foreign body
Trachea	**Infectious tracheobronchitis** **Chronic tracheobronchial syndrome** **BOAS: tracheal hypoplasia** **Tracheal collapse** Tracheal hypoplasia/stenosis without BOAS Aspiration secondary to swallowing disorder and/or megaoesophagus Neoplasia: intramural or compression from extramural masses Foreign body Enlarged tracheobronchial lymph nodes Parasitic: e.g. *Oslerus*
Bronchi and lower airways	**Chronic bronchitis: idiopathic, allergic, irritant (e.g. smoke)** **Neoplasia: primary bronchial tumour, metastatic neoplasia invading or compressing lower airway** Allergic/asthmatic Bronchiectasis
Lung parenchyma	**Bronchopneumonia: secondary to megaoesophagus, ciliary dyskinesia, inhalation pneumonia, force feeding** **Idiopathic pulmonary fibrosis (West Highland White Terrier)** **Neoplasia: primary, metastatic** Eosinophilic bronchopneumopathy (formerly known as pulmonary infiltrate with eosinophils) Parasitic: *Angiostrongylus, Crenosoma, Pneumocystis, Dirofilaria, Toxocara* migration in puppies Pulmonary hypertension Pulmonary thromboembolism Pulmonary haemorrhage: trauma, coagulopathy Non-cardiogenic pulmonary oedema: e.g. near drowning, electrocution, paraquat poisoning Smoke inhalation Pulmonary abscess Pulmonary granuloma (rare in UK) Fungal pneumonia: only *Aspergillus* in UK
Heart	**Left atrial enlargement** **Pulmonary oedema secondary to left-sided heart failure**

24.4 Differential diagnoses for coughing. More common conditions are in **bold**.

History

In addition to general history-taking, information regarding the nature of the cough is required.

- Did the cough start suddenly? Or has the onset been more insidious over the preceding days and weeks?
  - Acute onset is more likely to be associated with kennel cough, inhalation of a foreign body or bronchopneumonia.
  - Cardiac disease, bronchitis, laryngeal paralysis and angiostrongylosis are usually associated with a slower onset.
- Is the patient heard to give a single cough in isolation (more often the case in chronic disease) or are there long bouts of coughing, with or without retching?
- Is the cough productive?
  - A productive cough reflects increased production of mucus in the airways or blood/oedema in the bronchioles and alveoli.
  - Drier coughs are more consistent with a foreign body in the initial stages or with external compression of the airway, such as from left atrial enlargement, tracheobronchial lymph nodes or a mass.
  - Paroxysmal coughing may be associated with a terminal retch and the expectoration of large amounts of respiratory mucus, which has the same consistency as egg whites; most owners will describe this as 'vomiting', so careful questioning is required to differentiate.
  - Regurgitation associated with oesophageal disease may also lead to coughing due to aspiration, and so the material produced may have been regurgitated.
  - It is necessary to determine whether the origin of any material is respiratory, oesophageal or gastric, to avoid pursuing the wrong diagnostic pathway.
  - The presence of blood (haemoptysis) is a notable finding. In the absence of trauma, it is usually associated with bleeding from a neoplastic lesion, damage to the airway wall from a foreign body, angiostrongylosis and/or coagulopathy.

Lungworm

With an increasing incidence of angiostrongylosis in the UK, the owner should be asked about the frequency of use of appropriate parasiticides

---

Signalment may provide useful clues:

- An aged large-breed dog is most likely to have laryngeal paralysis, neoplasia or cardiac disease
- A Cavalier King Charles Spaniel may well have endocardiosis
- An adolescent Yorkshire Terrier with a honking cough probably has tracheal collapse
- Brachycephalic dogs, especially bulldogs, may display coughing and respiratory embarrassment due to brachycephalic obstructive airway syndrome (BOAS), which comprises varying combinations of stenotic nares (Figure 24.5), soft palate elongation, laryngeal saccule eversion and/or tracheal hypoplasia.

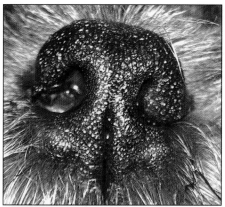

24.5 Stenotic nares is a common problem in brachycephalic breeds, as in this 1-year-old Shih Tzu cross. The photograph shows the dog after surgical correction of the right nostril. (Courtesy of Tim Hutchinson)

Physical examination

Faster intervention is required in cases where coughing is accompanied by collapse, dyspnoea or cyanosis, but generally a thorough physical examination is carried out. It is usually possible to differentiate whether the cough is cardiac or respiratory in origin.

Mucous membrane colour will usually be normal, but occasionally abnormalities will be noted. Cyanosis indicates a more severe problem of ventilation–perfusion mismatch. Pale membranes suggest anaemia or poor peripheral circulation, the latter is associated with cardiac failure or other forms of shock.

Generalized enlargement of the peripheral lymph nodes may suggest lymphoma and concurrent intrathoracic lymphadenopathy compressing the terminal trachea and bronchi. Equally, severe enlargement of the submandibular lymph nodes can lead to cough and gag, especially when eating, at the level of the pharynx.

The presence of a cardiac murmur (see later) is highly suggestive of heart disease, but care should be taken not to be misled by cases of cor pulmonale (failure of the right side of the heart brought on by long-term high blood pressure in the pulmonary arteries and right ventricle) or anaemia, which may give rise to a murmur without primary cardiac disease.

Respiratory auscultation may identify a general increase in adventitious noise, in which case one should attempt to determine whether this is of upper or lower respiratory tract origin. Auscultation of the trachea will reveal harsh movement of air in upper respiratory disease, which will also be heard, albeit more quietly, over the lung fields. The respiratory rate should be measured and the pattern of respiration noted.

Upper respiratory tract noise

- Stridor is noisy respiration associated with the upper airway that may be heard without the stethoscope; it suggests laryngotracheal disease such as laryngeal paralysis, BOAS or kennel cough
- Stertor is respiratory noise originating from the nasal passages, such as may occur with excessive nasal secretions (e.g. in hyperplastic rhinitis) or a physical obstruction (e.g. a foreign body, polyp or tumour)

Abnormal lung noises

- Crackles: the reopening of airways that have collapsed during expiration and/or the movement of air through excessive secretions/fluid in the terminal airways, e.g. in pulmonary oedema or bronchopneumonia
- Wheezing: the narrowing of airways due to the accumulation of secretions and/or the thickening of airway walls due to inflammation or infiltration, e.g. in chronic bronchitis

---

Manual compression of the cervical trachea will produce a bout of coughing in dogs with tracheal inflammation.

Abdominal palpation may reveal liver/spleen enlargement and/or ascites due to right-sided heart failure, which may be due to primary cardiac disease or to cor pulmonale (e.g. angiostrongylosis or pulmonary hypertension). The presence of one or more abdominal masses may point towards the possibility of pulmonary metastasis or multicentric lymphoma.

Rectal temperature will be normal in most cases of coughing, but pyrexia suggests an acute and deep inflammatory process in the respiratory system, such as bronchopneumonia or neoplasia.

Diagnostic investigations

Overt cardiac disease will dictate the need for radiography, echocardiography and electrocardiography (see earlier), while respiratory disease may require investigation by radiography, bronchoscopy and lavage.

Kennel cough

Cases of acute laryngotracheitis associated with kennel cough do not require immediate investigation; such cases will present with an acute-onset paroxysmal cough that usually ends in a terminal retch and expectoration of mucus, often of sufficient audibility to keep both dog and owner awake. Crucially, although they may be distressing, such cases will have no genuine respiratory embarrassment, aiding differentiation from patients that require more prompt investigation. Once a confident diagnosis of kennel cough has been made, time and supportive treatment may be employed, and most cases will resolve spontaneously. A few cases will progress to chronic tracheobronchitis, so if the dog is still coughing 2–3 weeks later, then further investigation may be required. Unless the condition is complicated by pneumonia, extremes of age, immunosuppression or significant intercurrent disease, antibiotics are not indicated in the first instance

---

Laboratory tests

Where further investigation is required, a minimum database of haematology and biochemistry should be obtained. Although this is very unlikely to offer a specific diagnosis, it may offer supportive clues (e.g. left-shifted neutrophilia in cases of broncho-

pneumonia) or promote consideration of potential intercurrent disease such as renal/hepatic compromise with implications for treatment. For example, pre-existing renal disease will be potentially compromised further if diuretics and angiotensin-converting enzyme (ACE) inhibitors are prescribed for cardiac failure.

Markers of primary coagulation (platelet count, buccal mucosal bleeding time) and secondary coagulation (prothrombin time (PT), activated partial thromboplastin time (APTT), activated clotting time (ACT) or whole blood clotting time (WBCT)) are imperative where angiostrongylosis is suspected.

Faecal examination for *Angiostrongylus*, whilst less sensitive than microscopy of bronchoalveolar lavage fluid, is a useful screening test. In addition, there is now a blood ELISA for parasitic antigen available, which is a highly sensitive, in-house test for *Angiostrongylus*.

Radiography

In cases of cardiac disease, thoracic radiographs are examined for cardiomegaly (see later) and for complications such as pulmonary oedema or pleural effusion. Abnormal lung patterns may be identified (see Figure 24.3); these often do not point to a specific disease process but they do allow a narrowing of the differential list.

PRACTICAL TIP

If coughing is due to aspiration, and megaoesophagus is suspected, this must be assessed on a radiograph taken with the dog fully conscious (Figure 24.6), as air will enter a normal oesophagus under sedation/anaesthesia and mimic the appearance. Occasionally, the same false-positive image may occur in a very 'air-hungry' dog, where air accumulates in the oesophagus and, more so, the stomach due to dyspnoeic breathing

---

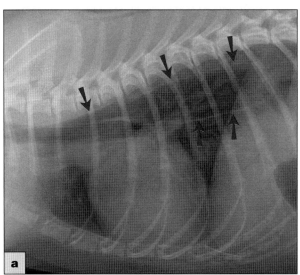

24.6 **(a)** Radiograph from a Springer Spaniel with an idiopathic megaoesophagus. The radiopaque walls of the oesophagus are seen as they course through the mediastinum (arrowed), whilst the air in the oesophagus does not change the appearance of the lung fields within these boundaries. (continues) ▶

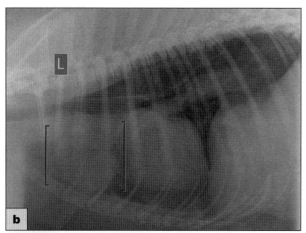

24.6 (continued) **(b)** In this Golden Retriever megaoesophagus is secondary to thymic neoplasia, visible as a radiopaque mass cranial to the heart (bracketed red).

Bronchoscopy

Bronchoscopy allows direct inspection of the bronchial lining and collection of lavage fluid for cytology and culture (see *BSAVA Manual of Canine and Feline Endoscopy and Endosurgery*).

Induction of general anaesthesia prior to bronchoscopy allows inspection of laryngeal function under light planes of anaesthesia; this is essential for confirming laryngeal paralysis. Information may be gained on: the level of inflammation/mucus; the presence of purulent exudate, which may be followed to its source; foreign bodies; blood; and neoplasia.

Lavage fluid may give a specific diagnosis in some diseases (e.g. angiostrongylosis, eosinophilic bronchopneumopathy, neoplasia) but often will only show non-specific evidence of inflammation. Most organisms cultured from canine lavage fluid will simply be opportunistic pathogens and care should be taken to avoid overinterpretation of the findings, but this still gives important information as to antibiotic sensitivity.

A clinical approach to dyspnoea

Definitions

- The term dyspnoea is taken from human medicine, where it can be experienced as a symptom and means a severe, usually acute, shortness of breath. In veterinary medicine it is used to describe the situation where the vet feels, subjectively, that an animal is having difficulty breathing. It is also termed 'respiratory distress'
- Tachypnoea is an increased respiratory rate
- Hyperpnoea is increased respiratory depth
- Orthopnoea describes the adoption of an abnormal posture to facilitate breathing, illustrated in Figure 24.7

Dyspnoea may occur due to mechanical obstruction to ventilation, failure of respiratory muscles or increased respiratory drive (e.g. in acidosis or anaemia). Differential diagnoses are shown in Figure 24.8.

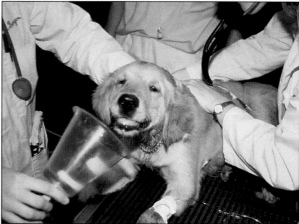

24.7 Severe respiratory distress due to neurogenic pulmonary oedema after a choking incident in a 6-month-old Golden Retriever. Notice the pale mucous membranes, extended neck, abducted elbows and reluctance to have an oxygen mask placed over the face. (Reproduced from the *BSAVA Manual of Canine and Feline Emergency and Critical Care, 2nd edn*; courtesy of Dr Ken Drobatz, University of Pennsylvania)

Organ/system affected	Conditions
Upper respiratory tract	**BOAS** **Laryngeal paralysis** Laryngeal oedema Laryngeal neoplasia Eversion of laryngeal saccules Foreign body Tracheal collapse Tracheal hypoplasia/stenosis Tracheal neoplasia Tracheal rupture Parasitic disease: e.g. *Oslerus*
Lower respiratory tract	**Bronchitis** Bronchial neoplasia Compression: enlargement of left atrium, enlargement of tracheobronchial lymph nodes, other masses Parasitic disease: e.g. *Oslerus, Pneumocystis, Crenosoma*
Lung parenchyma	**Bronchopneumonia:** e.g. aspiration, immunosuppression, ciliary dyskinesia Pulmonary thromboembolism: e.g. disseminated intravascular coagulopathy, hyperadrenocorticism, immune-mediated haemolytic anaemia, angiostrongylosis **Angiostrongylosis** Eosinophilic bronchopneumopathy (formerly known as pulmonary infiltrate with eosinophils) **Asthma/allergy** Pulmonary haemorrhage: trauma, coagulopathy Lung lobe torsion Neoplasia: primary, metastatic, lymphoma Non-cardiogenic oedema: e.g. near drowning, electrocution, central nervous system disease, paraquat poisoning Parasitic disease: e.g. *Angiostrongylus, Pneumocystis, Crenosoma, Dirofilaria* Fungal pneumonia: only *Aspergillus* in UK
Mediastinum	**Thymic disease:** thymoma, lymphoma, sarcoma Other neoplasia: e.g. oesophageal **Enlargement of tracheobronchial lymph nodes:** inflammation, lymphoma Pneumomediastinum Mediastinitis

24.8 Differential diagnoses for dyspnoea. More common conditions are in **bold**. (continues) ▶

Organ/system affected	Conditions
Heart	**Cardiac failure leading to pulmonary oedema and/ or pleural effusion** **Pericardial effusion** **Bronchial compression**
Pleural cavity and body wall	**Pneumothorax** **Pleural effusion** (see Figure 24.9) **Ruptured diaphragm** Chest wall trauma: fractured ribs, flail chest, open chest Chest wall tumour
Systemic disease	**Anaemia** **Metabolic acidosis:** e.g. ruptured bladder, renal failure, diabetic ketoacidosis Methaemoglobinaemia **Megaoesophagus leading to aspiration** Pain/fear Pyrexia **Abdominal distension:** gastric dilatation–volvulus, severe ascites, pregnancy Forced open-mouth breathing: nasal tumour, stenosis of nares Weakened respiratory musculature: hypokalaemia, peripheral neuropathy, neuromuscular disorder

24.8 (continued) Differential diagnoses for dyspnoea. More common conditions are in **bold**.

Emergency cases

The golden rule of managing dyspnoea is to avoid making the situation worse. Animals may be on the verge of a life-threatening deterioration, and stress associated with forcing clinical examination or radiography may be all that is required to precipitate this. The patient should be placed in a cool environment with supplementary oxygen until intervention is possible

History

The co-existence of coughing and dyspnoea points towards the possibility of airway, pulmonary, cardiac or mediastinal disease; history and physical examination indicators for dyspnoea will be similar to those for coughing. However, this does not rule out concurrent conditions that may be associated with diseases that also cause coughing and are directly causing the dyspnoea, but not the cough. For example: a dog with biventricular heart failure may well have a pleural effusion worsening the dyspnoea, but this effusion will not be the cause of its cough; whilst a dog with immune-mediated haemolytic anaemia secondary to lymphoma could have a cough due to mediastinal lymphadenopathy, while the dyspnoea is a consequence of anaemia or thromboembolism. Therefore, a thorough consideration of each presenting problem should be made.

Cases that started with coughing and have progressed to dyspnoea, with or without pyrexia, could be associated with aspiration pneumonia, or with an inhaled foreign body (leading to pulmonary abscessation or pneumo-/pyothorax as it migrates). A history of regurgitation may point to the former. Migrating foreign bodies will be most likely in dogs that run at speed with a wide-open glottis in crop fields or long grass.

Respiratory noise may have been recognized by the owners and is often associated with airway obstruction. Obstruction may be:

- Intraluminal (e.g. foreign body)
- Mural (e.g. tumour of the airway wall)
- Extraluminal: due to compression (e.g. left atrial enlargement, tracheobronchial lymphadenopathy, mediastinal tumour)
- Due to compromise of the structural integrity of the airway (e.g. laryngeal paralysis, tracheal collapse).

Trauma is a more likely cause of dyspnoea than it is of coughing alone, in which case the signs will be peracute in onset and the cause usually witnessed by the owner. Problems such as haemo-/pneumothorax, pneumomediastinum, pulmonary haemorrhage, fractured ribs, diaphragmatic rupture and tracheal/ bronchial tears should be considered in these cases. Urinary tract rupture may also lead to tachypnoea through metabolic acidosis.

Angiostrongylosis can cause accumulations of blood in the lungs, pleural space or mediastinum through coagulopathy, as may other disorders involving secondary coagulation (e.g. rodenticide toxicity, disseminated intravascular coagulopathy). The owner should be questioned about the regular use of parasiticides and the possibility of access to rat bait.

Signs of systemic illness may be useful indicators. For example, depression and pyrexia are most likely with severe inflammatory processes such as bronchopneumonia or pyothorax, whilst pre-existing polyuria/polydipsia would be likely with a dog now presenting with tachypnoea due to diabetic ketoacidosis. Generalized myopathy (e.g. moderate to severe hypokalaemia) or peripheral neurological disease can lead to dyspnoea through respiratory muscle failure, and owners may have noted previous musculoskeletal weakness.

Physical examination

Examination should begin with careful observation of the pattern, rate and depth of respiration and whether the animal is ambulatory or collapsed. Dyspnoea, noted as a genuine difficulty in obtaining sufficient air, points towards a disease process in the chest or larynx/trachea, whilst patients with problems due to anaemia or acidosis will be more likely to be tachypnoeic rather than 'air hungry'.

Mucous membranes should be inspected for pallor (anaemia or poor circulation associated with hypovolaemic, cardiogenic or endotoxic shock) and cyanosis. Lymph node size should be assessed.

Thoracic auscultation may reveal abnormalities associated with heart rate/rhythm/murmurs (see later) or abnormal respiratory noise as for coughing (see above) but it may also detect muffling of the heart sounds, which may be caused by a pericardial or pleural effusion. Muffling may also be created artefactually in obese animals or where there is microcardia (e.g. shock or hypoadrenocorticism). In cases where the lungs are collapsed, such as pneumothorax, heart sounds may be increased in intensity. The mediastinum does not usually remain intact in dogs and so most cases of effusion or pneumothorax are bilateral, meaning that a mediastinal shift resulting in the heart being more audible on one side is not common; however, the presence of a large tumour or other mass on one side may lead to this finding by displacing the heart. Diaphragmatic rupture may cause mixed findings; the presence of abdominal contents will muffle heart sounds on one or both sides, but if they lie unilaterally then displacement of the mediastinum may increase heart sounds on the contralateral side.

Ascites caused by cardiorespiratory disorders will most commonly reflect a modified transudate associated with reduced venous return (e.g. biventricular cardiac failure, pericardial effusion, pulmonary hypertension). Alternatively, a collapsed dyspnoeic patient with abdominal fluid may have a haemoperitoneum associated with organ rupture whilst the dyspnoea is secondary to hypovolaemic shock and anaemia. Characterization of the fluid obtained by abdominocentesis is essential (see Figure 24.12).

Peripheral pulse quality offers a good clue for narrowing the differential list: weak pulses are noted with cardiac failure or hypovolaemia; patients with respiratory or pleural disease not involving blood loss or shock, or with more chronic anaemia, should have stronger pulses due to sympathetic stimulation.

Pyrexia is likely to be associated with more severe inflammatory processes such as pneumonia or pyothorax rather than cardiac disease, but may also be a reflection of pain or inability to lose heat with laryngeal paralysis. By the time a dog with laryngeal paralysis cannot thermoregulate by panting, it is often so 'air hungry' that the larynx can be visualized in the conscious animal.

Diagnostic investigations

Radiography
Provided it can be carried out without further endangering the patient, radiography will provide the first line investigation. Changes associated with the heart and lungs may be seen, as described for coughing (see above) and heart murmurs (see below), and are indicative of those diseases.

Pleural effusion (Figure 24.9) and pneumothorax (Figure 24.10) are easily recognized on lateral radiographs.

> **WARNING**
>
> Pleural effusion is also apparent in the lateral aspects of a DV radiograph. A VD radiograph should **never** be attempted in a dyspnoeic dog or one with suspected pleural effusion even if it is not dyspnoeic

Mass lesions may cause displacement of the mediastinum to one side or other, best visualized on a DV radiograph. As radiographs from dyspnoeic patients will usually be taken with the dog conscious, an apparent megaoesophagus should not be due to intake of air during anaesthesia, but care should be taken in severely dyspnoeic patients where air may accumulate in the normal oesophagus/stomach due to gasping attempts at ventilation.

Pericardial effusions are encountered relatively commonly in first-opinion small animal practice. They may be idiopathic or associated with tumours, either

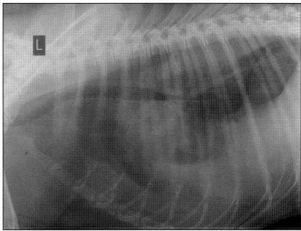

24.9 Lateral radiograph of a 9-year-old neutered Border Collie bitch with multicentric lymphoma. Pleural effusion is seen as radiopaque areas in the ventral aspect of the radiograph, causing scalloping of the lung lobes. There is dorsal displacement of the trachea in this case, though this may be due to a cranial mediastinal mass rather than to the effusion.

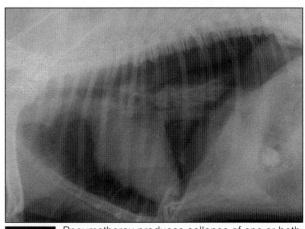

24.10 Pneumothorax produces collapse of one or both lung lobes such that their edges are no longer seen to reach the chest wall. The lungs themselves are more radiopaque than normal owing to their collapsed state. Radiolucent air is seen surrounding the lungs, giving a much darker appearance than normal, and the heart is usually raised from the sternum, with the cardiosternal ligament highlighted. This radiograph is from a German Short-haired Pointer with a ruptured pulmonary bulla; the stone in the stomach is incidental.

of the heart itself (haemangiosarcoma) or of the chemoreceptors in the aorta at the heart base (chemodectomas). Radiography shows a large globular cardiac silhouette with abnormally sharp borders, owing to the lack of movement of the stretched pericardial sac compared with the normal situation where it is closely opposed to the moving myocardial wall (Figure 24.11). Therapeutic pericardiocentesis is discussed in QRG 24.1.

Microcardia should immediately prompt consideration of hypovolaemia and, in the absence of other chest abnormalities, the possibility of haemoperitoneum. Hypoadrenocorticism may cause microcardia, but this is not likely to present with dyspnoea.

Pulmonary thromboembolism may give rise to normal radiographs and, without CT scanning, will need to be a diagnosis of exclusion in general practice. Concurrent predisposing diseases such as

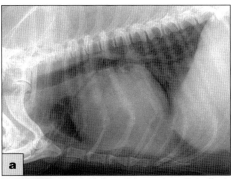 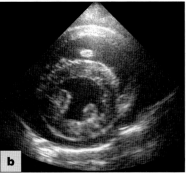 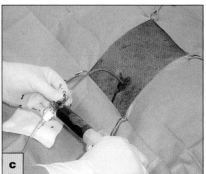

24.11 **(a)** An idiopathic pericardial effusion in a small, cross-breed terrier prior to drainage. **(b)** Echocardiogram, again prior to drainage. **(c)** Percutaneous drainage via the right 5th intercostal space, using a direct pericardiocentesis set. The effusion was drained twice percutaneously. On a third episode the dog was treated surgically with a subtotal pericardectomy via a right-sided thoracotomy, to good effect. Once the fluid can drain into the much larger pleural cavity, the patient can usually cope and the fluid can be resorbed by the pleura.

hyperadrenocorticism, immune-mediated haemolytic anaemia, loss of antithrombin III in renal disease, and angiostrongylosis may point towards thrombosis.

Thoracocentesis

Where radiography is deemed unsafe and there is a high index of suspicion of pleural effusion (muffling and inspiratory effort) or pneumothorax, diagnostic thoracocentesis may be possible. It will also allow preparation, including if necessary sedation, to drain the effusion or air, before radiographing a more stable patient to ensure that this has been achieved. Administration of oxygen to these patients may fail to stabilize them, as significant impairment will still remain. Analysis of pleural fluid (Figure 24.12) will assist in making a diagnosis. Therapeutic chest drainage is discussed in QRG 24.2.

Echocardiography

Echocardiography is indicated where there is suspicion of cardiac disease. However, in a severely dyspnoeic dog it may not be possible to hear the heart sufficiently well, due to muffling from fluid or harsh breath sounds; thus, these cases are not straightforward to identify as cardiac in origin. A basic ultrasound screen of the heart can be undertaken relatively quickly and should assess:

- Whether pericardial fluid is present (Figure 24.13)
- The sizes of the left and right atria (Figure 24.14): not likely to be normal if there is failure of one or both ventricles as the cause of dyspnoea
- The contractility of the left ventricle: poor contractility is an inappropriate response to sympathetic stimulation.

In the absence of these abnormalities, it is reasonable to move on from cardiac disease as the cause of dyspnoea for the sake of speed in a primary assessment.

Laboratory tests

It can be useful to obtain blood samples for laboratory analysis, but this should not be at the expense of inducing stress in a respiratory compromised dog. **Stabilization of an acute case should always be performed first.**

- Biochemistry and haematology are not likely to provide specific diagnoses unless the cause is increased respiratory drive, in which case anaemia or acidosis may be identified.
- Acute anaemia due to bleeding will not cause an immediate fall in red cell parameters, as proportional amounts of plasma will also be lost.

Type of fluid	Gross characteristics	Biochemistry/cytology	Differential diagnoses
Transudate	Clear; colourless	Low protein; acellular	Hypoproteinaemia
Modified transudate	Clear/slightly turbid; pale yellow, may be blood-tinged	Low protein and low cell content but slightly increased compared with true transudate	Congestive cardiac failure; neoplasia; lung lobe torsion; ruptured diaphragm
Exudate (non-septic)	Turbid; darker coloured – red/darker yellow	Higher protein; greater mixed cell content, including non-degenerate neutrophils	Neoplasia; thoracostomy tube
Exudate (septic)	Thick and turbid; variable colour; foul smelling	High protein; high mixed cell count, with numerous degenerate neutrophils and phagocytosed/free bacteria	Pyothorax
Chylous effusion	Milky white, may be blood-tinged or pinkish	Moderate protein and cell levels; small lymphocytes present	Congestive cardiac failure; neoplasia; trauma to thoracic duct; congenital; obstruction to venous return, e.g. right atrial tumour, caudal vena cava thrombosis; idiopathic; lymphangiectasia/lymphangitis
Haemorrhagic effusion	Frank blood	Similar proportions of cells to peripheral blood, but cell counts lower than peripheral blood	Neoplasia; trauma; coagulopathy; lung lobe torsion; ruptured diaphragm

24.12 Characterization of pleural fluid.

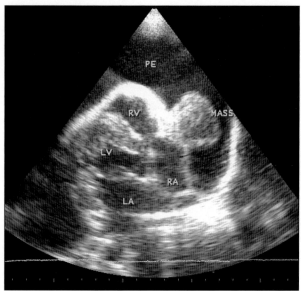

24.13 Echocardiogram of a pericardial effusion caused by a clearly apparent haemangiosarcoma of the cardiac wall in a Greyhound. Such tumours may be secondary to splenic haemangiosarcoma, but this one was not. The patient was euthanased. LA = left atrium; LV = left ventricle; PE = pericardial effusion; RA = right atrium; RV = right ventricle.

- Hypokalaemia is an uncommon finding in dogs, compared with cats, but when severe may lead to weakness of the respiratory muscles.
- Urinary tract rupture can present with profound tachypnoea due to acidosis and this should be considered in any animal where chest radiography is normal, especially in cases of trauma, as it may be the first clue; the classic triad of azotaemia, hyperkalaemia and metabolic acidosis will be noted.
- Coagulation tests (PT, APTT, ACT, WBCT) are indicated when blood is found in the pleural space or alveoli, in order to differentiate trauma from coagulopathy.

A clinical approach to heart murmurs

A cardiac murmur indicates a disturbance in the flow of blood through the heart which may occur due to:

- Cardiac disease
- Cor pulmonale and pulmonary hypertension, e.g. with *Angiostrongylus*
- Changes in blood viscosity, e.g. in anaemia/polycythaemia, hypo-/hyperproteinaemia
- Physiological murmurs, e.g. outflow tract murmurs in very athletically fit individuals, innocent murmurs in puppies
- Variants of normal anatomy, e.g. the relatively narrow aorta (even in the absence of congenital aortic stenosis) seen in Boxers compared with other breeds.

This discussion will concentrate on murmurs caused by cardiac disease.

Innocent murmurs in puppies

Innocent murmurs in puppies should be soft murmurs, graded 1/6 to 2/6 (see later), in otherwise normal individuals, and should disappear by 20 weeks of age. They are a common finding at primary vaccination appointments and need explanation to new owners in order to balance the reassurance that most cases will not be pathological with the importance of monitoring them to identify those cases that persist. Unless the murmur is loud (≥ 3/6) and/or there are clinical signs such as syncope or failure to thrive, the author's approach is to monitor the puppy monthly until 20 weeks of age and only then to recommend investigation if the murmur is still present. However, louder murmurs or those associated with clinical signs should dictate the need for immediate investigation

---

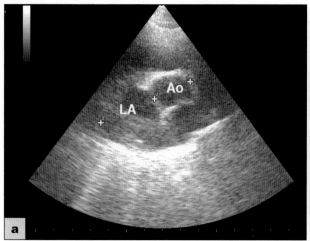

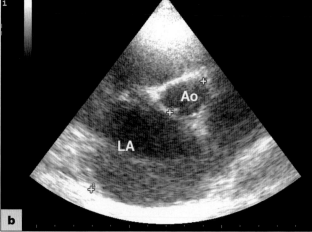

24.14 Even a quick ultrasound scan of the heart will allow assessment of left atrial size, which is not likely to be normal if cardiac failure is the cause of dyspnoea. In dogs, left atrial size (LA) is compared with the width of the aorta (Ao). Both measurements are taken at the level of the aortic valve in the right parasternal short-axis view, to allow standardization of the measurement irrespective of the size of the dog, as the aortic diameter will increase in direct proportion to bodyweight and not change with disease state. An LA:Ao ratio of ≤1.6 is considered to be normal. These images are taken from two dogs, both presenting with dyspnoea due to pulmonary congestion but with markedly different aetiologies. **(a)** Normal echocardiographic measurement of the left atrium, with an LA:Ao ratio of 1.5. This measurement quickly suggested that cardiac disease was not the cause of the problem; bronchopneumonia was subsequently diagnosed. **(b)** In this image of the Staffordshire Bull Terrier in Figure 24.16, the left atrium is clearly enlarged (LA:Ao ratio = 2.4). This allowed a cardiac diagnostic pathway and treatment plan to be promptly pursued.

History

The murmur will not be the presenting complaint unless it is severe enough to be associated with a precordial thrill and audible without a stethoscope (grade 5/6 to 6/6) or is causing clinical signs. Many murmurs remain clinically silent and will only be noted at routine examinations, usually in association with compensated cardiac disease. Where a murmur is haemodynamically significant, owners may report signs of exercise intolerance, coughing, syncope, dyspnoea/tachypnoea and cyanosis, as well as more generalized signs such as inappetence and weight loss.

Signalment will play an important role in defining a narrower list of differential diagnoses:

- Puppies <12 months of age are most likely affected by congenital heart disease
- Middle-aged to older dogs will generally have acquired heart disease
- Certain breeds are more commonly associated with congenital heart disease; for example:
  - German Shepherd Dogs and poodles with patent ductus arteriosus (PDA)
  - Golden Retrievers and Boxers with aortic stenosis (AS)
  - Bulldogs and Boxers with pulmonic stenosis (PS)
- With respect to acquired heart disease:
  - Smaller breeds (in particular Cavalier King Charles Spaniels) are likely to have mitral valve disease (endocardiosis)
  - Larger breeds are likely to have endocardiosis or dilated cardiomyopathy (DCM); valvular heart disease is also common in larger breeds.

Physical examination

The heart is assessed for rate and rhythm, as well as the presence and character of any murmur present. It is necessary to decide whether the murmur is clinically relevant to the presenting signs:

- Cardiac disease may exist for some time in a compensated state before clinical signs of cardiac failure develop and, during this time, the finding of a murmur is not likely to be haemodynamically significant
- In general, a murmur associated with slower heart rates (<100 beats/min), strong pulses and, in particular, sinus arrhythmia is not likely to be associated with heart failure and, whilst investigation may still be warranted, other differential diagnoses for the presenting complaint should be considered in these cases.

Murmur intensity is graded according to loudness and intensity (Figure 24.15).

In cases of valvular incompetence, such as endocardiosis or congenital stenosis, a louder murmur usually indicates more severe disease. Conversely, the severity of ventricular septal defects is inversely proportional to the murmur intensity because larger, more serious defects are associated with lower pressure flow. Often the murmur intensity in cases of systolic dysfunction (e.g. DCM) is deceptively low as a result of the low pressure gradient across the stretched atrioventricular value due to poor contractility of the ventricles.

Grade	Characteristics on auscultation
1	Murmur barely audible
2	Murmur audible but less intense than normal cardiac sounds (S1/S2)
3	Murmur of equal intensity to S1/S2
4	Murmur of greater intensity than S1/S2
5	Loud murmur associated with precordial thrill
6	Murmur can be heard with stethoscope held away from chest wall

24.15 Grading heart murmurs.

Almost all small animal murmurs are systolic, occurring between S1 and S2. Diastolic murmurs may occasionally be heard with incompetence of the aortic or, less commonly, pulmonic valves (usually associated with damage due to endocarditis). PDA produces the characteristic 'machinery' murmur, with both systolic and diastolic components.

The point of maximal intensity should be identified and an attempt made to relate this to the positions of the heart valves (see Figure 24.1). Left-sided murmurs may be associated with the cardiac apex (mitral valve) or heart base (aortic/pulmonic valves), whilst tricuspid murmurs and those associated with a ventricular septal defect are loudest on the right side. Pulmonary hypertension creates a cardiac murmur via tricuspid regurgitation and so this too is loudest on the right; it may also lead to a soft diastolic murmur over the pulmonic valve on the left side.

Significant regurgitant murmurs are usually long (holosystolic) and uniform (band-shaped) with harsh sounds associated with endocardiosis and softer sounds with DCM. Ejection murmurs associated with aortic or pulmonic stenosis produce crescendo/decrescendo murmurs where the intensity peaks and then tails off as systole proceeds.

The other cardiac sounds, S3 (passive ventricular filling) and S4 (atrial contraction), which create a 'gallop' rhythm are uncommonly heard in dogs, compared with cats and large animal species; when they are heard, they are almost always associated with marked cardiac failure.

Pulmonary auscultation may reveal pulmonary crackles if there is concurrent pulmonary oedema and the presence of a pleural effusion will cause heart sounds to be muffled. Ascites may be present.

The occurrence of generalized malaise and pyrexia should prompt consideration as to whether the murmur may be associated with endocarditis, which most commonly affects the valves on the left side of the heart in small animals but is still much less common than other acquired diseases.

Diagnostic investigations

A murmur deemed to be clinically significant to the presenting complaint should be investigated using chest radiography, echocardiography, electrocardiography and haematology/biochemistry.

Radiography

Cardiomegaly may be noted on thoracic radiography and may be generalized, or specific to certain chambers of the heart.

Most cases of the common acquired diseases (endocardiosis, DCM) have either the left side or both sides of the heart affected rather than the right side alone. This is seen on the lateral view as left atrial 'tenting', elevation of the tracheal bifurcation and a straight caudal border to the heart (Figure 24.16); on the DV view the left atrium pushes the mainstem bronchi apart and the left ventricle shows enlargement in the 3 to 6 o'clock positions. Enlargement of the right ventricle will increase sternal contact with the ventral border of the heart on the lateral view, whilst the right atrium will push the trachea dorsally in a position more cranial to the carina; the right ventricle and atrium occupy the 6–9 and 9–11 o'clock positions, respectively, on the DV radiograph.

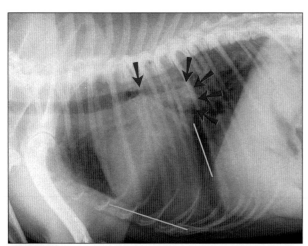

24.16 Lateral radiograph of an 8-year-old Staffordshire Bull Terrier with congestive cardiac failure due to DCM. There is left atrial tenting (red arrows), dorsal displacement of the trachea (blue arrow) and a straight caudal border to the heart (yellow line). There is also increased sternal contact (green line) suggesting that the right side of the heart is also enlarged.

Assessment of cardiac size is reviewed extremely thoroughly in the *BSAVA Manual of Canine and Feline Thoracic Imaging*. This Manual also documents the use and limitations of the vertebral heart score (VHS), in which the long and short axes of the cardiac silhouette are measured on a lateral view, summed together and then scaled against the thoracic vertebral column from the level of the T4 vertebra. While the VHS may be useful for those new to evaluating cardiac size and for sequential measurements on the same patient, it has not been proven to be superior to subjective assessment, and considerable variation has been documented between different breeds.

In addition to cardiomegaly, pulmonary oedema may be noted as patchy interstitial patterning most prominent in the perihilar regions; alveolar patterns may occur in more severe cases. Oedema represents left-sided cardiac failure. Pleural effusion (see Figure 24.9) may be seen with right-sided disease; ascites may also be documented on abdominal imaging.

Echocardiography
Echocardiography has come to be the mainstay of murmur investigation, but should be used as an adjunct to good physical examination and radiography rather than a replacement.

Two-dimensional images allow direct visualization of the heart. Measurements of chamber size can be made in both two-dimensional B-mode and one-dimensional M-mode. The size of the left atrium is measured as a ratio to the width of the aortic root in order to standardize what would be expected to be normal for the size of patient.

Spectral Doppler may be used to measure the forward and, if present, regurgitant flow through all the heart valves, as well as through abnormal apertures such as ventricular septal defects. Calculations may be made by the scanner for markers of systolic function (fractional shortening and ejection fraction). In general, forward flow velocity through valves increases in cases of stenosis and there is post-stenotic dilatation. Colour flow Doppler allows visualization of blood flow and easy identification of regurgitant jets.

Cases of cor pulmonale, including in angiostrongylosis, will usually have pulmonary hypertension that is noted and measured echocardiographically as regurgitation through the tricuspid valve in systole and through the pulmonary valve in diastole. These cases may progress to show other signs of right-sided failure.

Electrocardiography
Electrocardiography is not useful for investigating the cause of murmurs or cardiomegaly specifically. Whilst it gives valid information pertaining to the rate and rhythm of the heart, which may themselves be altered by the cardiac disease, it is unreliable for measuring cardiac chamber size. It is preferable to use radiography and echocardiography for assessing heart size.

Laboratory tests
Laboratory tests may be indicated; for example:

- Basic haematology and biochemistry will rule out changes in erythrocyte or protein levels that may alter flow patterns leading to functional murmurs
- Renal and hepatic biochemistry assesses the effect of cardiac failure on the rest of the body and provides a baseline for monitoring treatment
- Faecal parasitology may detect *Angiostrongylus* larvae or an in-house blood ELISA can be used to detect parasitic antigens
- Blood culture may be required in suspected endocarditis.

A clinical approach to arrhythmias

Cardiac arrhythmia is usually detected on clinical examination, with the owner normally reporting malaise, exercise intolerance or, in extreme cases, syncope. Some patients will be presented collapsed (see Chapter 9), though other cases may be clinically silent. Physical examination will detect a loss of the normal regular rhythm. Arrhythmias may be slow (bradyarrhythmia), fast (tachyarrhythmia) or a mixture (sick sinus syndrome). This chapter will concentrate on the most commonly encountered arrhythmias in general practice.

> **PRACTICAL TIP**
>
> Sinus arrhythmia is a variant of normal in the dog, where the rhythm slows and speeds up again in line with the animal's respiration. It is a repeated and smooth pattern, thus referred to as 'regularly irregular'

Tachyarrhythmias

The most commonly detected tachyarrhythmias in small animal first-opinion practice are:

- Atrial fibrillation (Figure 24.17b)
- Ventricular premature complexes (VPCs; Figure 24.17c), progressing in some cases to ventricular tachycardia (VT)
- Supraventricular premature complexes (SVPCs; Figure 24.17d), progressing occasionally to supraventricular tachycardia (SVT).

These abnormal rhythms are auscultated as 'extra' beats disrupting the normal rhythm and can sometimes be very chaotic. It is not usually possible to differentiate them by auscultation alone. Variations in strength of the peripheral pulse, as well as dropped pulses, may be detected when palpating concurrently with auscultation.

- **Atrial fibrillation** occurs due to left atrial enlargement, which is usually pathological in dogs. It is most commonly associated with DCM but can occasionally be seen in the normal sized left atrium of giant-breed dogs. Treatment is aimed at resolution or improvement of the underlying cause (usually cardiac failure) and reduction of the ventricular rate to <160 beats/min; restoration of normal sinus rhythm is often not possible.
- **VPCs** may be seen secondary to cardiac disease where there is stretching and subsequent poor perfusion of the myocardium but are also common secondary to a range of systemic diseases, which commonly include gastric dilatation–volvulus, splenic masses, pancreatitis, pyometra and sepsis. Treatment is aimed at abolishing the underlying cause. The recognition of runs of VPCs as ventricular tachycardia requires urgent intervention.
- **SVPCs** are less commonly observed. They are usually secondary to cardiac or non-cardiac disease and are generally haemodynamically insignificant whilst, nonetheless, giving irregularity to the auscultated rhythm. Treatment is aimed only at the underlying cause. In cases where SVPCs run together for periods, they create supraventricular tachycardia, which may need to be specifically addressed as it can be haemodynamically significant owing to the reduction in diastolic filling times.

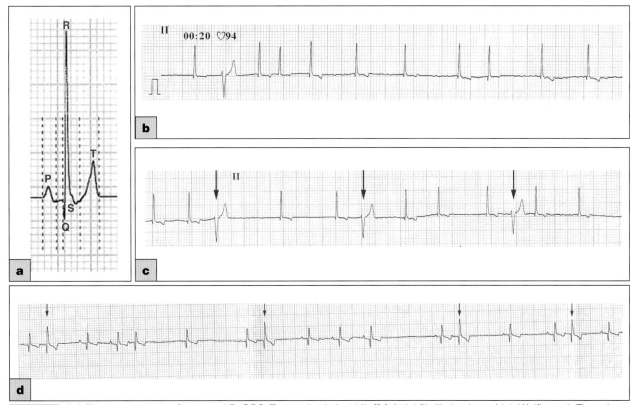

24.17 **(a)** The components of a normal P–QRS–T complex in lead II. **(b)** Atrial fibrillation in an Irish Wolfhound. There is an irregularly irregular rhythm of normally shaped, narrow and upright QRS complexes (often of differing magnitudes) without normal P waves; the P waves may be replaced by f waves associated with fibrillation of the atria, but these can be difficult to see in the baseline in many cases. A single VPC is also present. **(c)** In this ECG from the same Irish Wolfhound, VPCs are seen as wide and bizarre complexes (without P waves), which occur earlier than would be expected with the predominant rhythm (arrowed). They may be seen in runs of three or more, sometimes merging into one another so that the normal baseline is lost, and these will be defined as ventricular tachycardia. **(d)** ECG from a Boxer with kennel cough. SVPCs are recognized as a narrow, upright complex with a P wave that comes sooner than expected (arrowed). Runs of SVPCs will create supraventricular tachycardia, which is more significant. In this trace, the SVPCs interrupt an otherwise normal sinus rhythm; they resolved when the infection resolved and were not significant.

Sinus tachycardia

Sinus tachycardia is simply a faster, yet normal rhythm, seen in a variety of diseases including cardiac failure, where there is sympathetic stimulation. It may also be seen due to fear in the consulting room, pyrexia or pain

---

Bradyarrhythmias

In the author's experience, significant bradyarrhythmias are much less commonly noted than tachyarrhythmias in first-opinion practice. Bradyarrhythmia can occur as a result of: a failure or interruption of impulse generation at the sinoatrial node (e.g. sinus arrest or block); or impedance of conduction through atrial tissue or the atrioventricular node and associated tissue (e.g. atrioventricular block). Many cases are clinically silent, but where heart rates drop particularly low or there is a significant pause between beats, clinical signs such as malaise, exercise intolerance and syncope may be seen. The clinician needs to rule out systemic causes such as hypothyroidism and electrolyte disturbance; once this is done, clinically affected patients will benefit from referral for pacemaker implantation as drug therapy is usually unrewarding.

Sick sinus syndrome is an arrhythmia seen most commonly in small breeds such as terriers, where there are periods of bradyarrhythmia interspersed with tachycardia/tachyarrhythmia; these cases will also need referral.

Transient arrhythmias

Transient arrhythmias can be challenging to diagnose. Heart rhythm may normalize by the time the patient is examined or a resting ECG is recorded at the surgery, and the arrhythmia therefore remains undiagnosed. Some arrhythmias may be highly situational (e.g. associated with particular forms of exercise) and also prove hard to capture. Holter monitor recording of a continuous ECG for 24 hours (or even up to 7 days) is indicated in these cases (Figure 24.18). Such monitors

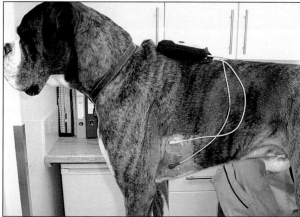

24.18 A Boxer with intermittent collapse wearing a Holter monitor. Arrhythmogenic right ventricular cardiomyopathy (a form of 'Boxer cardiomyopathy') was diagnosed.

are readily available for hire and are easy to fit to patients. Owners should be asked to keep a diary of activity, which can be interpreted in conjunction with the ECG trace.

References and further reading

Bexfield N and Lee K (2014) *BSAVA Guide to Procedures in Small Animal Practice, 2nd edn*. BSAVA Publications, Gloucester

Boon JA (2010) *Manual of Veterinary Echocardiography, 2nd edn*. Wiley–Blackwell, Oxford

Ettinger SJ and Feldman M (2010) *Textbook of Veterinary Internal Medicine, 7th edn*. Elsevier Saunders, St. Louis (Coughing pp.250–252; Dyspnoea and tachypnoea pp.253–255; Abnormal heart sounds and heart murmurs pp.259–263; Pleural effusion pp.266–268; Respiratory disease pp.1055–1142; Cardiovascular system pp.1143–1394)

Gough A and Thomas A (2010) *Breed Predispositions to Disease in Dogs and Cats, 2nd edn*. Wiley-Blackwell, Oxford

King LG and Boag A (2007) *BSAVA Manual of Canine and Feline Emergency and Critical Care, 2nd edn*. BSAVA Publications, Gloucester

Lhermette P and Sobel D (2008) *BSAVA Manual of Canine and Feline Endoscopy and Endosurgery*. BSAVA Publications, Gloucester

Luis Fuentes V, Johnson LR and Dennis S (2010) *BSAVA Manual of Canine and Feline Cardiorespiratory Medicine, 2nd edn*. BSAVA Publications, Gloucester

Murphy K (2012) How to place chest drains. *BSAVA Companion* June 2012, pp.12–18

Schwarz T and Johnson V (2008) *BSAVA Manual of Canine and Feline Thoracic Imaging*. BSAVA Publications, Gloucester

QRG 24.1 Pericardiocentesis

Pericardial effusion in dogs most commonly forms either idiopathically or secondary to neoplasia; the latter is usually either a chemodectoma at the heart base or haemangiosarcoma of the myocardium.

- Prior to drainage, echocardiography should be used to assess for the presence of cardiac or heart base tumours, as these are usually easier to image whilst there is fluid to highlight them.
- In the presence of a tumour, drainage is only likely to be palliative and it is more appropriate to consider partial pericardectomy as a longer-term management option. This is suitable for heart base tumours but not for malignant tumours of the cardiac wall (e.g. haemangiosarcoma) where the prognosis is always poor.
- In cases of malignant cardiac wall tumours, there may be a tear in the myocardium through which fresh blood can quickly replace a drained effusion. Therefore, if a larger than expected volume of effusion is drained, even if a tumour has not yet been identified, the possibility of such a tumour should be considered.

Patient positioning and preparation

- Drainage is carried out with the patient in left lateral recumbency. Removal of even small amounts of fluid will ease tamponade. Pericardiocentesis is performed from the right side of the chest, in order to take advantage of the cardiac notch between lung lobes, thus avoiding penetration of lung tissue whilst also avoiding the large left coronary artery on the left side.
- A wide area of skin is clipped and surgically prepared.

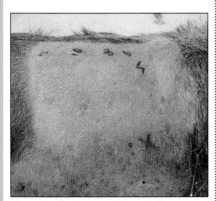

The author finds the use of a surgical pen to mark the rib numbers and incision site useful, to ensure that confusion over which intercostal space is which does not occur once drapes have been applied.

- The technique may be performed under light sedation (e.g. pethidine 2–3 mg/kg + low-dose acepromazine 0.01 mg/kg i.m.) plus infiltration of the chest wall with local anaesthetic. However, consideration should also be given to the temperament of the patient as, once one starts to drain the effusion, the dog will feel better and so may struggle or return to normal temperament before drainage is complete; some cases may warrant general anaesthesia following a careful risk/benefit analysis.

PRACTICAL TIP

An ECG should be recorded throughout to note any disturbance in rhythm, which is most likely to occur when the introduction needle is within the pericardial sac and potentially touching the myocardium

Equipment

Various types of catheter can be used but the author's preference is a veterinary pericardiocentesis catheter set, placed using the Seldinger technique. For details of the technique using an over-the-needle catheter or small-bore wire-guided drain, see the *BSAVA Guide to Procedures in Small Animal Practice, 2nd edn.*

Technique

1 The approach is made through the 5th or 6th intercostal space at the level of the costochondral junction. The wide-bore introduction needle is introduced into the chest at the designated point, through a small stab incision in the skin.

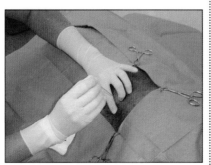

Insert the introduction needle until the typical 'scratching' sensation of the tip on the fibrous pericardial sac is felt; typically at this point, one may feel the needle tip moving with the cardiac motion. To the novice, this 'scratching' sensation may appear an enigma but one quickly becomes familiar with it, after even just one or two procedures.

PRACTICAL TIP

It is not uncommon to find *pleural* effusion coming out of the needle before the pericardium is penetrated. This is likely to be serosanguineous in nature, compared with the 'port wine' colour of a *pericardial* effusion, so should be easily differentiated to avoid inadvertently draining the pleural effusion whilst thinking one is draining the pericardial one

2 Push the introduction needle into the pericardial sac. A 'port wine' effusion will immediately emerge from the hub; advancement should stop to prevent penetration of the myocardium.

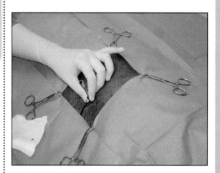

PRACTICAL TIP

The ECG should be carefully monitored in particular at this stage. The occurrence of ventricular premature complexes or runs of ventricular tachycardia at this stage would suggest the needle tip is pushing on, or is within, the myocardium and should be repositioned

3 Feed the guidewire through the needle and into the pericardial space.

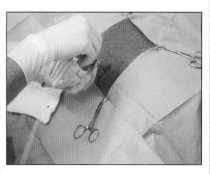

4 Withdraw the needle over the wire, taking care not to pull the guidewire out inadvertently.

▶

QRG 24.1 *continued*

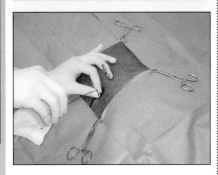

PRACTICAL TIP

Keep hold of the guidewire at all times when it is partially in the pericardium

5 Feed the catheter over the guidewire into the pericardial space.

PRACTICAL TIP

The catheter may need to be rotated slightly around its long axis at the point where the tip is being pushed through the pericardial sac in order to facilitate its entry

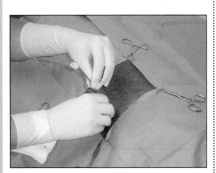

6 Remove the guidewire, taking care not to pull the catheter with it.

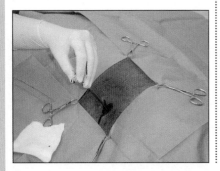

7 Attach a syringe to the catheter and withdraw a small volume of fluid that can be saved as a sample for laboratory submission.

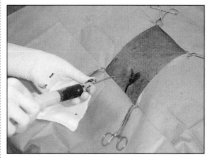

PRACTICAL TIP

Before drainage is performed, the sample can be checked to ensure that it does not clot. Clotting would give rise to concern that the sample has come from within the heart, as pericardial fluid should not clot

8 Connect a three-way tap to the catheter, and attach the syringe to one of the other arms of the tap.

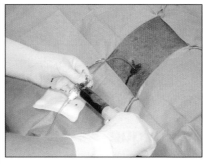

9 Connect the third arm of the three-way tap to a long giving set, to allow the effusion to be expelled into a bucket well away from the sterile area.

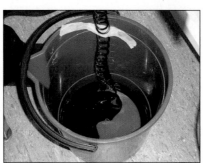

10 Once the effusion is drained, withdraw the catheter from the pericardial sac. At this stage, the catheter may be used to withdraw pleural effusion if desired, but this is not usually required unless the pleural effusion is large. Once the catheter is completely withdrawn, close the stab incision with a single nylon suture.

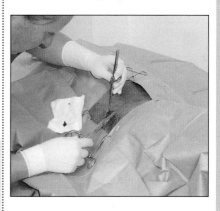

Post-drainage care

- Ascites should resolve within 24–48 hours without the need for diuretics.
- Venous return to the right side of the heart quickly increases following drainage and this can lead to increased right-sided output to the lungs, causing transient pulmonary overload. This usually passes quickly and the inexperienced clinician should not be alarmed. If signs are notable, however, then this is the one instance where a small dose of intravenous furosemide (2 mg/kg) is considered for a pericardial effusion; otherwise diuretics are avoided as they only serve to reduce preload to the heart.

QRG 24.2 Thoracocentesis and thoracic drain placement

Once the underlying cause of an effusion has been identified, and steps taken to control it, many effusions can be left to disperse without drainage, e.g. using diuresis for cardiac disease. However, if life-threatening compression of the lungs is present, the effusion should be drained. Likewise, pus associated with a pyothorax is unlikely to resolve without repeated drainage. The drainage of blood should be undertaken only in animals with severe respiratory compromise and only once clotting is known to be normal. Overzealous drainage of haemothorax risks worsening anaemia/hypovolaemia as more blood quickly replaces the drained blood in the pleural space if continued traumatic bleeding and/or coagulopathy is not addressed.

Mild pneumothorax may disperse naturally provided the ruptured lung tissue has closed over. If trauma is the aetiology and dyspnoea is mild or absent, then one may simply monitor the case. Drainage of air is indicated in more severe cases. Persistent accumulation of air associated with marked dyspnoea may be an indication for exploratory thoracotomy to identify and resect lung tissue that remains leaky due to the rupture of a neoplasm/bulla or migration of a foreign body.

Where drainage is anticipated to be needed once only, thoracocentesis using an atraumatic catheter is appropriate. Cases needing repeated drainage (of air or fluid) for prolonged stabilization will require a chest drain, as will cases of pyothorax where lavage is required.

For further details of chest drain placement, see Murphy (2012), the *BSAVA Manual of Canine and Feline Emergency and Critical Care* and the *BSAVA Guide to Procedures in Small Animal Practice.*

Preparation and positioning

■ Position the patient in sternal recumbency (or standing). Within reason, the patient should be allowed to assume the position of its choosing so that its breathing is facilitated.
■ Most dogs will tolerate thoracocentesis without sedation, but if this is not the case then sedation should be considered rather than allowing excessive movement and distress which is likely to worsen dyspnoea more than prudent selection of light sedatives. Sedation with minimal cardiorespiratory depressant effects should be chosen.

■ Clip and surgically prepare the side of the chest where the effusion is expected as judged by DV radiography. However, in most canine cases, the mediastinum will not be intact and fluid/air can often be withdrawn from either side of the chest.
■ The point of entry is at intercostal spaces 7–9, about one-third the way down the chest for draining air and two-thirds the way down (at the level of the costochondral junction) for fluid.

Equipment

■ A needle, butterfly needle or catheter is used, approximately 0.75–1.25 inches long for smaller dogs, up to 2 inches for larger dogs. Generally, 19–21 G is appropriate.
■ Ideally, a catheter is used with the stylet withdrawn after introduction as this will be less traumatic to lung tissue when the lungs reinflate as drainage proceeds. However, it can be difficult to withdraw fluid and air through a catheter, which tends to collapse, so there may be no alternative but to use a needle; if so, care should be taken to keep the needle as parallel to the chest wall as possible, and not to stab around in a perpendicular position.

Procedure

1 Using sterile gloves, introduce the needle slowly, just cranial to the rib in order to avoid the neurovascular bundle on the caudal aspect of each rib.

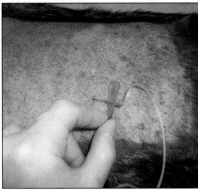

Courtesy of Nick Bexfield

2 Apply a small amount of suction to the syringe.

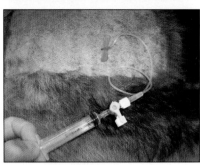

Courtesy of Nick Bexfield

■ If a small amount of blood is withdrawn or the lungs can be felt against the needle tip, reposition it.
■ If more copious blood starts to drain, stop and put 2 ml of the aspirate in a plain tube to see if it clots; blood from a haemothorax will not clot, whereas blood aspirated from inadvertent cardiac puncture will clot.

WARNING

If a haemothorax is confirmed, do not continue to drain it until careful consideration has been given as to whether there is continued bleeding in the chest which will simply replace the blood withdrawn and until clotting function has been assessed for potential coagulopathy

3 Aspirate until negative pressure is achieved and then withdraw the needle/catheter whilst maintaining suction on it with the syringe.

WARNING

■ With a pneumothorax, negative pressure may never be achieved: the withdrawn air is continually replaced in the pleural space with freshly inspired air leaking through the lung (or intrathoracic airway)
■ This is an indication that continual drainage via a thoracostomy tube is required, in the hope that the leak will seal spontaneously with time. If this is still ineffective, surgical exploration of the chest to repair the leak or remove the affected lung will be the only option. However, the latter is likely to necessitate referral to a specialist centre, and stabilization of these cases for transport can be challenging and, at times, impossible

4 Save aspirated fluid for analysis – biochemical, cytological and microbiological.

Abdominal pain and swelling

Scott Kilpatrick

An approach to the acute abdomen

Presentation of the dog with acute abdominal pain is common in veterinary practice (Figure 25.1). The general causes of abdominal pain include: distension of a hollow viscus or organ capsule; ischaemia; traction; and inflammation secondary to a variety of conditions (Figure 25.2).

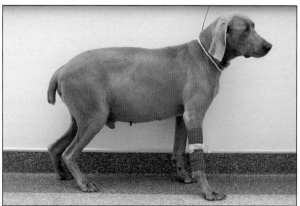

25.1 A 12-year-old male entire Weimaraner with abdominal distension due to an abdominal mass originating from a retained testicle.

PRACTICAL TIPS

- Not all life-threatening intra-abdominal problems are painful, especially in profoundly sick animals with mental depression
- Extra-abdominal sites of pain may present as an apparent acute abdomen. This happens most commonly with spinal pain

WARNING

All dogs with an acute abdomen potentially have a life-threatening condition that may require rapid surgical intervention. Although a thorough diagnostic work-up should be completed at some stage, emergency treatment must take priority

---

Gastrointestinal system
- Gastrointestinal perforation
- Gastric dilatation–volvulus
- Gastrointestinal dehiscence
- Intestinal obstruction
- Gastrointestinal neoplasia

Reproductive system
- Pyometra/uterine rupture
- Dystocia
- Ovarian cyst
- Ovarian neoplasia
- Prostatic abscess
- Prostatic neoplasia
- Testicular torsion

Hepatobiliary system
- Hepatic abscess
- Acute hepatitis
- Hepatic trauma/rupture
- Hepatobiliary neoplasia
- Cholangiohepatitis
- Biliary obstruction/rupture

Pancreatic system
- Acute pancreatitis
- Pancreatic abscess
- Pancreatic neoplasia

Urinary system
- Urinary calculi (renal, ureters, bladder, urethra)
- Pyelonephritis
- Renal neoplasia

Haemopoietic system
- Splenic mass
- Splenic rupture
- Splenic torsion

Peritoneum and abdominal wall
- Blunt trauma to abdominal wall
- Penetrating trauma to abdominal wall
- Septic peritonitis
- Chemical peritonitis (bile, urine, pancreatic)
- Mesenteric volvulus

25.2 Common causes of an acute abdomen.

Initial evaluation and stabilization

On initial presentation, a primary examination (see also Chapters 8 and 9) should include evaluation of:

- Level of consciousness
- Airway
- Breathing
- Circulation.

This should be completed within 30–60 seconds. A very brief history should be obtained at this time, but resuscitation should not be delayed in the critical patient while a complete history is obtained (Figure 25.3).

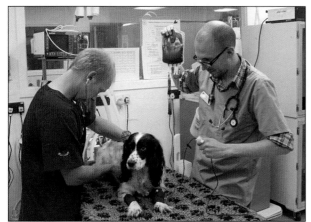

25.3 A 5-year-old male entire Cocker Spaniel receiving a blood transfusion after presenting with acute abdominal pain and abdominal distension due to a haemoabdomen (caused by a ruptured splenic haematoma). The dog initially presented collapsed, and fluid resuscitation was administered before providing transfusion support. The dog made a full recovery after surgical removal of the spleen.

The goal of any initial stabilization is to reverse the signs of shock and improve oxygen delivery to the cells.

- Oxygen and intravenous fluid therapy should be provided.
- Patients *in extremis* require rapid intubation and breathing support.
- Hypoglycaemic patients should be treated with intravenous glucose.
- Analgesia is an important part of initial stabilization. Opioids are considered the most appropriate form of analgesia; however, their dose may need to be reduced due to the fact that critical care patients are more sensitive to the sedative and negative cardiorespiratory effects of these drugs.
- The use of corticosteroids remains controversial and should be avoided until a more definitive diagnosis is made.

WARNING

Non-steroidal anti-inflammatory drugs (NSAIDs) should be avoided due to the potentially negative effects on some abdominal organs in a compromised patient

---

History

Following stabilization, a complete and detailed history must be obtained from the owner to ascertain the possible causes of the acute abdomen. Important questions to ask include the following:

- Is the dog neutered?
- Is there the potential for exposure to toxins or dietary indiscretion?
- Has there been any change in the dog's appetite or water intake in the days preceding presentation?
- Is ingestion of a foreign body a possibility?
- Does the dog have any ongoing medical problems or has it had any major medical problems in the past?
- Is the dog receiving any medication, including over-the-counter drugs (e.g. NSAIDs, aspirin)?
- Is there any possibility of trauma?
- When was the dog last vaccinated?
- Has there been any vomiting or diarrhoea? If present, characterize
- Has the dog been urinating normally? If not, characterize.

The history of a patient presenting with an acute abdomen is often vague, but reported signs will frequently include depression, anorexia and vomiting. In other instances the history may be extremely suggestive of the underlying cause. The progression of the clinical signs can also help determine the urgency of diagnosing the underlying cause. Chronic abdominal pain that has remained relatively static in its progression is not usually an emergency, although deterioration could precipitate a crisis. A dog that has a chronic problem and has deteriorated rapidly, or an animal with an acute problem, warrants a more aggressive approach to define the underlying cause.

In many cases the patient's signalment may lead to a higher index of suspicion of the aetiology. For example:

- Parvoviral enteritis may be suspected in dogs with an uncertain vaccination history
- Intussusception is more common in young animals
- Male dogs are much more likely than females to suffer from urethral obstruction
- German Shepherd Dogs and Golden Retrievers (median age of affected dogs 10 years) have a higher incidence than other breeds of haemoabdomen associated with splenic neoplasia
- Large- and giant-breed dogs have a much higher incidence of gastric dilatation and volvulus (GDV) than smaller breeds
- Entire males are at much higher risk of severe prostatitis than neutered males
- Entire female dogs may develop pyometra.

Physical examination

A full physical examination should be performed, but with initial attention to the cardiovascular, respiratory, central nervous and renal systems.

> **PRACTICAL TIP**
>
> Examination of the abdomen should occur after that of the thorax, to avoid inadvertently missing important findings that may present in other body systems. Additionally, examination of the abdomen may elicit pain and discomfort that may prevent further evaluation of the patient

Examination of the abdomen

1. **Visual inspection of the external abdomen.**
   - Abnormalities detected can include: distension (e.g. caused by effusion, gastric dilatation or organomegaly); subcutaneous swelling (e.g. resulting from cellulitis associated with urine leakage); and bruising (e.g. associated with trauma or a coagulopathy).
   - Careful observation of the periumbilical area for evidence of reddening or haemorrhage may lead to a diagnosis of haemoabdomen.
   - Any obvious wounds should also be carefully noted.

2. **Auscultation of gastrointestinal sounds.**
   - Ingestion of toxins, acute intestinal obstruction and gastroenteritis may cause an increased frequency and character of gut sounds.
   - Conditions such as ileus, anorexia, chronic intestinal obstruction and abdominal effusions can cause decreased frequency and character of gut sounds.
   - The abdomen should be listened to over a period of 2–3 minutes to determine whether gastrointestinal sounds are actually absent.
   - Abnormal sounds are not pathognomonic for any particular disease process.
   - *Note: Auscultation should precede palpation since palpation can cause gut sounds to diminish.*

3. **Percussion of the abdomen.**
   - Hands are placed lightly on either side of the abdominal wall with the animal standing. One hand is used to give a light but firm tap to one side of the abdomen, while the other feels for the presence of a ripple effect as the fluid in the abdomen is pushed towards the opposite abdominal wall.
   - This may reveal a fluid wave in dogs with abdominal effusion, or tympanic abdominal sounds in dogs with gaseous gastric distension.
   - *Note: Occasionally a fluid wave can be elicited in animals without abdominal effusion. Obese animals, as well as those with a full bladder or fluid-filled viscus (e.g. pyometra) are good examples of this.*

4. **Palpation.**
   - The abdomen should be palpated in a systematic fashion.
   - Superficial and gentle palpation should be carried out to help to localize pain.
     - Animals may react vigorously and become tense, 'guarding' their abdomen in response to superficial palpation.
     - Other more violent reactions may include vocalizing, groaning, yelping, vomiting, or attempting to bite the person performing the examination.
     - *Note: Some animals without abdominal pain will resent abdominal palpation and guard their abdomen. In these situations stroking the animal or spending some time building up the intensity of palpation will facilitate examination.*
   - The examination should, where appropriate, proceed to deeper palpation.
     - Some conditions may be associated with localized pain (e.g. cranial abdominal pain with pancreatitis and caudal abdominal pain with prostatic disease).
     - Palpation of the cranial abdomen in deep-chested dogs is improved by elevating their thoracic limbs above floor level.
     - Foreign bodies may be directly palpated and bunched up intestines may suggest a linear foreign body.
     - A thick tubular structure may indicate a foreign body or intussusception.
     - Septic peritonitis in dogs is usually, but not always, associated with severe, diffuse abdominal pain.
     - Uroabdomen and bile peritonitis may or may not be painful.
     - In many cases, sequential examination of the abdomen allows accurate assessment of the clinical condition.

Other examinations required

- Rectal temperature should always be taken, but note that in a dog with severe hypoperfusion the rectal temperature may not be elevated even if there is a raised core body temperature.
- The vulva of an intact bitch should be examined for any evidence of discharge, as seen in the case of an open pyometra.
- The oral cavity should always be examined for evidence of ingestion of caustic substances.
- Examination per rectum should always be performed to assess the caudal to middle pelvis, pelvic urethra and characteristics of the faeces. In male dogs the prostate gland should always be palpated.

Diagnostic investigations

Laboratory tests

Minimum database: Blood tests including packed cell volume (PCV), total solids (TS) via refractometer, blood urea nitrogen (BUN; by dipstick) and glucose should all be part of a minimum database (Figure 25.4). A urine sample should also be obtained at the earliest opportunity; for the measurement of specific gravity, the urine sample should be obtained before any fluid therapy.

The minimum database is unlikely to provide a definitive diagnosis, but may be helpful in prioritizing differential diagnoses and further testing. For example:

- A low TS value in the face of a normal PCV should prompt a search for haemorrhage or severe vasculitis. In acute haemorrhage, the level of TS falls but splenic contraction blunts the expected

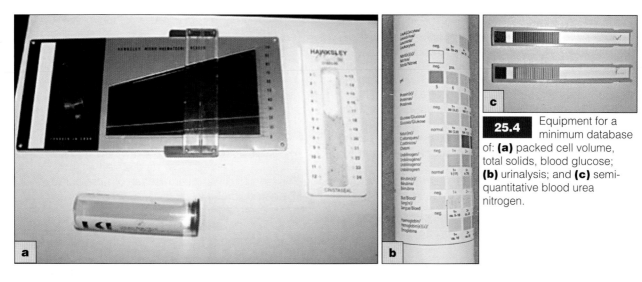

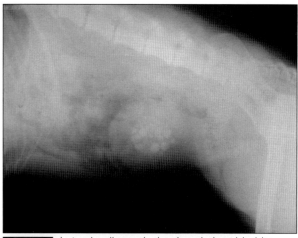

25.4 Equipment for a minimum database of: **(a)** packed cell volume, total solids, blood glucose; **(b)** urinalysis; and **(c)** semi-quantitative blood urea nitrogen.

fall in PCV. In patients with vasculitis, most commonly due to septic peritonitis, protein loss into the abdomen causes a fall in TS levels without affecting the PCV
- Decreased blood glucose is often associated with sepsis and warrants an aggressive approach to find the underlying cause of the acute abdominal pain, particularly if septic peritonitis might be present
- Dipstick BUN provides an estimate of azotaemia. Increased BUN may be due to prerenal, renal or postrenal causes. Increased BUN may also be noted in animals with acute abdominal pain caused by pyelonephritis, or urethral or ureteral obstruction.

Further tests:

- Ideally, venous blood gas and electrolyte measurements should be carried out along with serum biochemistry as part of a more extensive investigation.
- A complete blood count should be performed, with microscopic evaluation of a blood smear in order to complete a manual differential count, estimate the number of platelets, and evaluate both white and red cell morphology.
- Coagulation parameters should be evaluated in patients with suspected liver disease, systemic inflammatory response syndrome (SIRS) or sepsis.
- Serum amylase and lipase are sometimes used as indicators (albeit neither sensitive nor specific) of pancreatitis in canine patients. In cases of acute pancreatitis the preferred test that is specifically useful and sensitive is the canine pancreatic lipase immunoreactivity (cPLI) assay; the sample may be sent to a laboratory for a quantitative result, but an in-house test for positive *versus* negative is useful for an immediate answer.

Abdominal imaging

Abdominal imaging should be performed in most cases of acute abdominal pain, as soon as the patient is sufficiently stable.

Radiography: Generally, two orthogonal views of the abdomen (lateral and dorsoventral) should be taken. A systematic and detailed review of all abdominal and adjacent structures should be performed.

Radiographs should be checked for:

- Radiopaque foreign bodies
- Intestinal dilatation
- Gastric size, position and content
- Liver and kidney size
- Uterine size
- Abnormal abdominal objects (e.g. cystoliths, Figure 25.5) or masses.

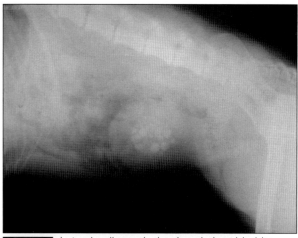

25.5 Lateral radiograph showing obvious bladder stones. This 3-year-old neutered Bichon Frisé bitch presented with dysuria and severe abdominal pain. Cystotomy was performed to remove the bladder stones that were later determined to be composed of calcium oxalate.

Loss of abdominal detail on plain abdominal radiographs may be due to lack of fat in the abdomen (in puppies or very thin animals), free abdominal fluid or a large abdominal mass. Free gas in the abdomen of a patient that has not undergone recent abdominal surgery or had a penetrating injury is consistent with bowel rupture or perforation.

Gastric distension with a normally positioned stomach is likely to be due to dilatation. If there is displacement with gastric dilatation, volvulus is likely. In cases of GDV, the stomach appears compartmentalized with band-like soft tissue opacities between gas-filled segments.

Segmental gaseous or fluid-filled distension of the small bowel suggests an intestinal obstruction. The normal diameter of the small intestine in the dog is approximately 2–3 times the width of a rib, or less than the width of an intercostal space. Additionally, all of the small intestinal loops should have a similar diameter, and it is abnormal for one segment to be 50% larger than other portions. Localized small intestinal distension is not always a definitive finding for intestinal obstruction but should prompt further investigation if an obvious foreign body is not evident (Figure 25.6). One option is to repeat radiography 3 hours later. If the intestine remains distended in the same position, this would indicate obstruction.

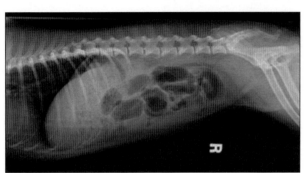

| 25.6 | Lateral abdominal radiograph showing multiple loops of distended intestine in a 2-year-old male neutered Border Terrier. No obvious obstruction was seen; however, a sock foreign body was later removed surgically. |

Contrast radiography may be necessary in some dogs with an acute abdomen, particularly those with partial gastrointestinal obstruction. Contrast radiography may be contraindicated in dogs with frequent vomiting, due to the high risk of aspiration pneumonia. The use of water-soluble contrast agents is often advocated if gastrointestinal perforation is suspected, to avoid barium contamination of the peritoneal cavity.

Ultrasonography: Ultrasound examination is more sensitive than radiography for examining abdominal masses and the presence of free fluid within the abdominal cavity. The pancreas, liver, kidneys and prostate gland can be evaluated more fully, and ultrasonography is one of the best ways of detecting pancreatitis and pancreatic masses. While pyometra may often be diagnosed radiographically, ultrasonography is a sensitive method for confirming a suspected and more subtle presentation of pyometra.

An approach to the swollen abdomen

Animals can develop a swollen abdomen for many reasons (Figure 25.7) and this can present as an emergency.

- Fluid: free fluid in abdomen; fluid inside organs; fluid in cysts
- Wear of abdominal wall muscles: hyperadrenocorticism
- Tissue: pregnancy; organ enlargement; neoplasia; fat; granuloma
- Faeces: megacolon; obstipation
- Gas: gastric dilatation–volvulus; obstruction or ileus of the gastrointestinal tract; post-surgical; rupture of the gastrointestinal tract; bacterial peritonitis

| 25.7 | Causes of abdominal distension. |

Definitions

- **Peritoneal effusion** is the abnormal accumulation of fluid in the peritoneal cavity and is not diagnostic in itself, but is a clinical sign of disease. It can result from the accumulation of transudative or exudative fluid, chylous effusions, blood, urine or bile
- **Ascites** is defined as an accumulation of serous fluid in the peritoneal cavity and is usually reserved for a transudate that is associated with liver disease or right-sided heart failure

Diagnostic investigations

As with any clinical problem, it is important to adopt a methodical approach (Figure 25.8).

Ultrasonography

One of the most straightforward ways of confirming the presence of free fluid in the abdominal cavity is with ultrasonography. Abdominal radiography is less useful in patients with large volumes of abdominal fluid, due to loss of intra-abdominal contrast. In some cases the presence of free fluid will be very obvious, and hypoechoic sharp angles will become immediately apparent once the ultrasound probe is placed on the patient (Figure 25.9).

Adopting a more structured 4-point FAST (focused assessment with sonography for trauma) scan (see QRG 25.1) will pick up on more subtle abdominal effusions (Figure 25.10). These scans can be performed very quickly and with no expert knowledge of ultrasonography needed. This is a procedure that can be carried out simultaneously with other interventions and can be repeated with little cost to the client.

Laboratory tests

Analysis of free abdominal fluid is a vital part of the evaluation of any animal with an acute/swollen abdomen. Abdominocentesis (see QRG 25.2), with or without ultrasound guidance, is a quick and easy way of retrieving abdominal fluid. It is unusual for complications to occur due to abdominocentesis and there are few contraindications to performing this procedure. Caution is advised, however, when a coagulopathy or thrombocytopenia is possible, or if there is organomegaly, or adhesions from previous surgery. A volume of at least 5–6 ml of free abdominal fluid per kilogram needs to be present for successful abdominocentesis. Diagnostic peritoneal lavage (see QRG 25.3) may be necessary in cases where fluid is not obtained.

Once abdominal fluid has been obtained, it is important to classify this to allow a more accurate diagnosis to be made. Analysis of the abdominal fluid should include: gross examination; measurement of PCV; TS by refractometer; and total nucleated cell count. Cytological examination is also very important. Biochemical and microbiological analysis are appropriate in certain cases. Classification of the main types of abdominal effusion is summarized in Figure 25.11; some further details are given below.

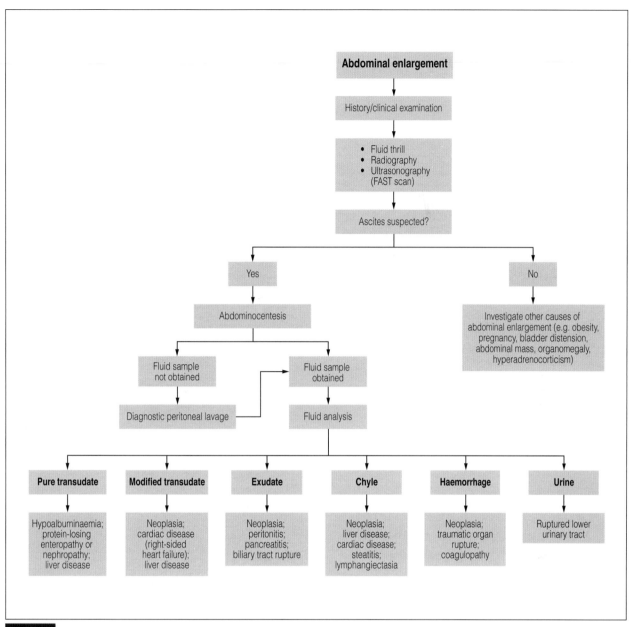

25.8 A diagnostic work-up for abdominal swelling.

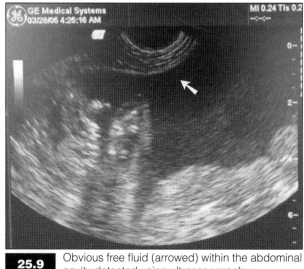

25.9 Obvious free fluid (arrowed) within the abdominal cavity detected using ultrasonography.

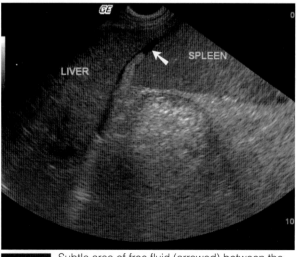

25.10 Subtle area of free fluid (arrowed) between the liver and spleen.

Characteristic	Transudate	Modified transudate	Exudate	Chylous effusion	Haemorrhagic effusion
Appearance of fluid	Clear, colourless	Clear, straw-coloured or blood-tinged	Turbid	Milky or pinkish opaque fluid	Appears similar to peripheral blood
Total protein (g/l)	<25	>25	>25	25–60	>30
Specific gravity	<1.015	1.015–1.025	>1.025	>1.025	>1.025
Nucleated cells (x10⁹/litre)	<1	1–7	>5	0.25–20	>1
Predominant cell type	Primarily mesothelial cells and macrophages	Increasing numbers of neutrophils and small lymphocytes, macrophages and possibly neoplastic cells	Primarily neutrophils (non-degenerate, or degenerate if septic)	Small lymphocytes, neutrophils, macrophages	Large proportion of red blood cells and usually without platelets
Other features	With time pure transudates will become modified due to irritation of the mesothelium	Most modified transudates are caused by neoplasia or heart failure	Can be classified as **septic** or **non-septic**	Contains high levels of triglycerides	This type of effusion does not normally clot

25.11 Classification of abdominal fluid.

■ **Transudates:**
- Usually characterized by having low cellularity, low specific gravity (SG) and low total protein
- Occur secondary to decreases in oncotic pressure due to hypoalbuminaemia (protein-losing enteropathy, protein-losing nephropathy, liver failure) or an increased hydrostatic pressure (portal hypertension, right-sided heart failure)
- Not normally associated with acute abdominal pain.

■ **Modified transudates:**
- Contain more protein and cells than pure transudates
- Usually occur due to an increased hydrostatic pressure, or increased vascular permeability in the early stages of inflammatory disease
- Often caused by neoplastic disease.

■ **Exudates:**
- Highly cellular and can be **septic** or **non-septic**:
  - The presence of toxic degenerate neutrophils with intracellular bacteria is indicative of septic peritonitis (Figure 25.12)
  - Non-septic exudates are characterized by the presence of non-degenerate neutrophils and the absence of bacteria
  - Unfortunately these cytological changes are not always present and further testing may be needed:
    o A glucose level can be taken from the effusion. An abdominal fluid glucose level of <2.8 mmol/l has been shown to indicate septic peritonitis unequivocally, since bacteria metabolize glucose present in the effusion
    o Another method is to compare the blood/effusion levels of lactate. If the lactate concentration in the peritoneal effusion is >2.5 mmol/l and higher than the blood lactate level, a septic effusion is likely.

■ **Chylous effusion:**
- Many effusions can be run through blood analysers in the same way as a blood sample

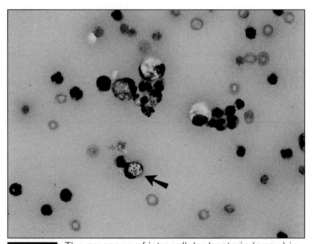

25.12 The presence of intracellular bacteria (arrow) is an indication of septic peritonitis. (H&E stain; original magnification X100)

- The triglyceride level in a chylous effusion is usually 2–3 times higher than in serum, while cholesterol is lower in the effusion than in serum
- The most common causes of chylous effusions are rupture of a lymph vessel due to neoplasia, right-sided heart failure and lymphoproliferative disease.

■ **Bilious effusions:**
- Biliary rupture will rapidly create a modified transudate that progresses to an exudate later in the disease process
- Bile effusions occur secondary to rupture of the bile duct or gall bladder. This happens secondary to trauma, cholelithiasis, pancreatitis, or necrotizing cholecystitis
- If bile peritonitis is suspected, total bilirubin should be measured. If the bilirubin concentration in the abdominal fluid is greater than that in the serum, bile peritonitis is confirmed. *Normally, there should not be any bilirubin present in abdominal fluid.* The fluid is often green and may contain bilirubin crystals.

■ **Uroabdomen:**
- Fluid from a patient with uroabdomen can range from a modified transudate to an exudate

- Uroabdomen can result from trauma or from iatrogenic causes (e.g. careless catheterization or cystocentesis). It is important to note that animals with ruptured bladders may still have palpable bladders and the ability to urinate
- If uroabdomen is suspected, the most useful abdominal fluid chemistry evaluation is creatinine. Urea nitrogen can also be measured but, because it is a smaller molecule, this diffuses rapidly and equilibrates with the plasma. A creatinine level in abdominal fluid that is twice that in serum is highly suggestive of uroabdomen
- Potassium levels are also higher in the abdominal fluid compared with blood
- *Note: If the dog has been receiving intravenous fluids, there is the potential for misdiagnosis of uroabdomen in an azotaemic patient with ascites. This is because creatinine, BUN and potassium concentrations in the plasma will be actively diluted, whereas those in the abdomen will not.*

- **Haemoabdomen:**
  - Haemorrhage into the abdomen may occur for many reasons, including trauma, neoplasia, coagulopathies and iatrogenic causes
  - A PCV of 5% or higher in diagnostic peritoneal lavage fluid is suggestive of significant haemorrhage
  - Cytologically, it may be difficult to differentiate acute haemorrhage from iatrogenically induced haemorrhage such as from inadvertent trauma of the liver or spleen. Platelets quickly aggregate, degranulate and disappear within an effusion, so their presence may be suggestive of iatrogenically induced haemorrhage.

- **Malignant effusions:**
  - Malignant effusions are often a subtype of modified transudate or exudate that contain neoplastic cells
  - Care should be taken in interpreting malignancy on cytology due to normal mesothelial cells displaying criteria that could be mistaken for neoplasia. Review by a pathologist is essential.

Surgical management

One of the most challenging decisions regarding dogs with acute abdominal pain or swelling is deciding whether *prompt* surgery is indicated.

Indications for prompt surgery

- Abdominal abscess
- Abdominal wall perforation
- Bile peritonitis
- Free abdominal gas (not associated with previous surgery or invasive procedures)
- Gastric dilatation–volvulus
- Intestinal foreign body causing pain or bowel obstruction
- Intestinal obstruction
- Ischaemic bowel
- Mesenteric volvulus
- Persistent abdominal haemorrhage
- Septic peritonitis
- Uroperitoneum

In some situations the decision to undertake surgery may not be straightforward.

WARNING

Even if prompt surgery is indicated, the immediate necessity is to stabilize the patient

References and further reading

Holt D and Brown D (2007) Acute abdominal and gastrointestinal surgical emergencies. In: *BSAVA Manual of Canine and Feline Emergency and Critical Care*, ed. LG King and A Boag, pp.174–191. BSAVA Publications, Gloucester

Kinns J (2011) Abdomen. In: *BSAVA Manual of Canine and Feline Ultrasonography*, ed. F Barr and L Gaschen, pp.72–84. BSAVA Publications, Gloucester

Lisciandro GR, Lagutchik MS, Mann KA *et al.* (2009) Evaluation of an abdominal fluid scoring system determined using abdominal focused assessment with sonography for trauma in 101 dogs with motor vehicle trauma. *Journal of Veterinary Emergency and Critical Care* **19**, 426–437

O'Brien R and Barr F (2009) *BSAVA Manual of Canine and Feline Abdominal Imaging*. BSAVA Publications, Gloucester

QRG 25.1 FAST scan

Positioning and preparation

- Right lateral recumbency is recommended, as this is also the best position for abdominocentesis, electrocardiography and echocardiography. However, this procedure can be carried out in a standing animal.
- One of the benefits of this procedure is that it can often be carried out in the conscious patient.

Technique

Placing the ultrasound probe on the four areas shown and scanning widely in both sagittal and transverse planes gives the best chance of detecting more subtle fluid accumulation (see Figure 25.10).

Limitations

- There is always the possibility of false-positive or false-negative results. For example, the gall bladder and common bile duct can

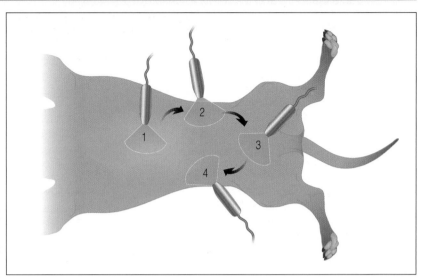

Four-point ultrasound assessment for free abdominal fluid. 1 = diaphragmaticohepatic; 2 = splenorenal; 3 = cystocolic; 4 = hepatorenal. (Redrawn after Lisciandro *et al.*, 2009)

appear as hypoechoic sharp angles, similar to free fluid, depending on the plane of imaging.
- If in doubt, the scan should be repeated on a regular basis to detect any changes.

QRG 25.2 Abdominocentesis

Positioning and preparation

- Sedation may or may not be required.
- The dog should be restrained in right lateral recumbency and it might be worth emptying the patient's bladder before the procedure.
- The abdomen should be clipped and prepared as for a non-surgical procedure.

Equipment

A 5 ml syringe, collection tubes (EDTA, plain and sterile) and some microscope slides should be prepared.

Use an 18–22 G, 2.5–3.75 cm needle or over-the-needle catheter.

Technique

Abdominocentesis can be performed by a single centesis or using a four-quadrant approach.

1 The site for single abdominocentesis is a point 1 cm lateral and to the right of the ventral midline and 1–2 cm caudal to the umbilicus.

2 Once the needle has been inserted through the skin and abdominal wall, allow fluid to drip from the needle (or catheter with needle removed) into a tube, or gently aspirate with a 2–5 ml syringe. Unless there is a large volume of free fluid it is preferable to allow it to drip from the needle hub, rather than aspirating, to avoid sucking omentum or viscera into the needle.

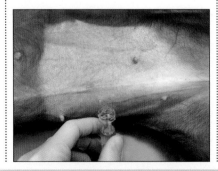

3 If fluid is not obtained from the first site, repeat the procedure in the three remaining sites.

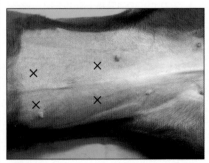

4 Collect fluid into an EDTA tube for cytology and cell count, and into a plain tube for culture and biochemical analysis.

5 Make several air-dried smears.

QRG 25.3 Diagnostic peritoneal lavage

Positioning and preparation

Positioning and preparation is as for abdominocentesis (see QRG 25.2). However, a higher proportion of patients will need to be sedated for diagnostic peritoneal lavage. Local anaesthetic is infiltrated into the ventral midline, just caudal to the umbilicus.

PRACTICAL TIP

As diagnostic peritoneal lavage introduces fluid in to the peritoneal cavity, diagnostic imaging should be carried out before this procedure

Technique

1 Using a scalpel, make a small stab incision through the skin.

2 Introduce a large-bore 10–14 G over-the-needle catheter (pre-fenestrated) through the skin and body wall, aiming caudally towards the pelvis.

3 Remove the stylet, leaving the cannula in place.

4 Attach an extension set and a three-way tap.

5 Infuse 20 ml/kg of warmed isotonic crystalloid fluid using gravity flow or gentle pressue.

6 Gently roll the patient (with the catheter in place if possible) and wait for 20–30 minutes.

7 Drain the fluid from the catheter:

- Use EDTA tubes for samples used to test total cell count and cytology
- Use plain tubes for samples for total protein and any other biochemical tests
- Fresh air-dried smears should be made

- Some fluid should be kept in a plain tube to be submitted for culture if necessary.

Notes:

- *Only a very small amount of the infused volume will be retrieved (usually only 1–2 ml). Any remaining fluid will be absorbed across the peritoneum.*
- *If the fluid obtained suggests that the gastrointestinal tract has been punctured, any hole should seal when the needle is removed.*

WARNING

Stop the procedure if blood is aspirated. Place the blood in a glass tube and monitor for clot formation. Free blood from the abdominal cavity will not clot (due to lack of platelets) but blood from a vessel or organ will clot

Urination problems; genital discharge

Angelika von Heimendahl and Julian Hoad

Disorders of the urogenital and reproductive systems are among the most common presentations at veterinary practices. There are many different disorders, and a bewildering array of investigative tests that may be applied to differentiate the disorders. This chapter suggests basic principles of thorough clinical examination, either to reach a prompt diagnosis or to decide on appropriate tests. Common disorders are discussed and recommendations for treatment are given. Further information on the diagnosis and treatment of urological disorders may be found in the *BSAVA Manual of Canine and Feline Nephrology and Urology*.

Reproductive disorders are discussed separately for males and females. Given the high rates of neutering in the UK, conditions will also depend on which reproductive organs are still in place or the age of the dog when they were removed. With a basic knowledge of normal anatomy and physiology and a detailed history of the problem, it is usually not difficult to make a diagnosis even though this does not always mean that the reproductive problem is treatable.

Emergency presentations

- Obstructed urethra; inability to pass urine
- Dystocia (unproductive straining for >2 hours, less if history of previous dystocia)
- Trauma to urinary tract or external genitalia
- Vaginal or uterine prolapse

Clinical signs and causes

Owners may have noticed the dog squatting more frequently to pass urine (pollakiuria), straining to pass urine (dysuria/stranguria), licking around the genitals, or an unusual discharge from the genitals. Although there is some overlap between the terms, dysuria is usually an observed painful or abnormal urination, whereas stranguria refers to a very diminished urine flow (usually only a few drops passed). Alternatively, the owner may be concerned about incontinence, or polydipsia. Polyuria/polydipsia (PU/PD) is discussed in Chapter 14.

Urological and genital/reproductive causes of dysuria/stranguria are listed in Figure 26.1. Neurological disorders (disc disease, spinal/pelvic injury, upper motor neuron (UMN) and lower motor neuron (LMN) disorders) may also affect micturition.

Other conditions that may mimic signs of dysuria/stranguria

- Colitis/dyschezia (straining to pass faeces may be confused with micturition)
- Perineal hernia (not involving bladder)
- Anal sac disease

Urological disorders

- Urethral obstruction: urolithiasis, neoplasia, urethritis, intrapelvic disease (constipation, obstipation, lymph node enlargement, neoplasia)
- Perineal hernia (involving bladder)
- Urinary tract infection
- Bladder/urethral neoplasia
- Neurological: urethral spasm, reflex dyssynergia

Genital/reproductive disorders

- Prostate gland enlargement: benign prostatic hyperplasia, prostatitis, prostatic abscess, prostatic cancer, squamous prostatic metaplasia
- Prostatic cysts
- Spermatic cord torsion
- Clitoral hypertrophy
- Vaginal strictures
- Vaginal hyperplasia
- Tumours of the vagina/vulva
- Vaginitis
- Occlusion of the vulva by excessive skin folds

26.1 Causes of dysuria/stranguria.

Haematuria is one of the most common causes of abnormal coloration of urine. Figure 26.2 lists common conditions associated with abnormally coloured urine or other urethral discharges. It is of prime importance to distinguish urological causes from non-urological (reproductive, haematological, extracorporeal) causes. Urological causes can often be diagnosed on the basis of history, clinical examination and examination of the discharge. Genital or reproductive disorders in the bitch are often characterized by discharge: in the male rarely so. Thorough clinical examination and history-taking will usually distinguish reproductive causes from urological ones. Non-urological causes of haematuria, haemoglobinuria and myoglobinuria are listed in Figure 26.3.

Reproductive system

- Bitch:
  - Normal: pro-oestrus, oestrus, postpartum
  - Abnormal: vaginal tumours, ulcerated polyps, vaginal foreign body, pyometra, fetal death, placental separation, subinvolution of placental sites (SIP)
- Male dog: orchitis, epididymitis, testicular tumours, balanitis, phimosis/paraphimosis, urethral prolapse, fractured os penis, penile trauma, tumours of the penis, prostatitis, prostatic cyst, prostatic abscess, prostatic neoplasia

Renal system

Nephrogenic cysts, neoplasia, pyelonephritis, trauma, nephroliths, drug-induced (cyclophosphamide), idiopathic haematuria

Urinary tract

Trauma, ureteroliths, cystitis, urolithiasis, bladder neoplasia, urethritis, urethral neoplasia

Coagulopathies

Thrombocytopenia, disseminated intravascular coagulopathy, haemolytic anaemia, drug-associated

Environmental

Heat stroke, exercise-induced

26.2 Conditions causing abnormal urine or a discharge. Haematuria is the most common abnormality but discharge can be clear or cloudy, bloody brown or green.

Haematuria

- Iatrogenic (caused by sampling)
- Coagulopathies: anticoagulant exposure, disseminated intravascular coagulation, thrombocytopenia
- Drugs: e.g. cyclophosphamide
- Strenuous exercise
- Idiopathic renal haematuria
- Hyper-reflexivity of the detrusor muscle

Haemoglobinuria

- Intravascular haemolytic anaemia
- Transfusion reaction
- Disseminated intravascular coagulation
- Postcaval syndrome (heartworm)
- Splenic torsion
- Heat stroke

Myoglobinuria

- Status epilepticus
- Crushing injury

26.3 Non-urological causes of haematuria, haemoglobinuria and myoglobinuria.

History and signalment

As with other diseases, a full clinical history should be taken. This is particularly relevant for reproductive problems, as the onset of illness may be related to a stage of the reproductive cycle. For example, a history of a 'season' 4–8 weeks prior to onset of illness in an older entire bitch may increase one's suspicion for pyometra. It is important to ask the following questions.

- For male dogs:
  - Is the dog sexually active?
  - Has it mated successfully in the past?
  - Has a recent mating resulted in any trauma?
- For bitches:
  - Are they nulliparous (have had no litters), primiparous (are gestating for the first time) or multiparous (had previous litters)? If previous matings have not been successful, then any previous test results (pre-mating progesterone levels, vaginal swabs, ultrasonography) should be reviewed
  - Have there been any previous problems with dystocia; was treatment required (oxytocin injections, caesarean section)?
- Both sexes:
  - Has a discharge been seen by the owner? If so, what colour was it? Was it odorous? Was the discharge seen during micturition, or independently (the latter is commonly seen in prostate disease)?
  - How much does the dog drink?
  - How often and how much does it urinate?
  - Is there urinary incontinence; if so how often and for what duration?
  - Has dysuria or stranguria been noted?
  - Has the owner noticed any other signs of illness (e.g. vomiting/diarrhoea, lameness, weakness)?
  - Have there been any changes in the appearance, colour and smell of the urine?

Age at onset of clinical signs is important, as problems of the reproductive tract in young animals are usually caused by anatomical and/or genetic abnormalities, whereas conditions of older entire dogs and bitches are mostly hormone-induced or neoplastic.

Examples of breed predilections

German Shepherd Dogs and Dobermanns are over-represented for prostatic disease

There are strong breed associations with various types of urolith (Adams and Syme, 2005)

Breeds at increased risk of pyometra include Golden Retriever, Rough Collie, Rottweiler and Cavalier King Charles Spaniel, with mongrels having a reduced incidence

Brachycephalic and chondrodysplastic breeds, such as the British Bulldog, Pug and French Bulldog, have an extremely elevated risk of dystocia

---

Physical examination

A full clinical examination should be carried out, paying particular attention to the size of bladder and the physical appearance of the external genitalia. A full urinalysis should also be performed: any abnormalities should be followed up by urine culture and imaging of the urinary tract. A diagnosis of urethral sphincter mechanism incompetence (USMI) is usually made on the basis of negative test results, signalment and history.

The presence and smell of any discharge should be noted: matted hairs around the prepuce or vulva may indicate that the patient has been licking the area. Urine scalding may be evident in incontinent bitches and should be distinguished from intertrigo (skin and fold infection) due to excess vulval skin folds.

Diagnostic investigations

Urinalysis

Urine collection
Urine can be collected by free catch, catheterization or cystocentesis. There are pros and cons to each method and in some instances it is appropriate to obtain urine by more than one method.

- **Free-catch** samples are the easiest to obtain.
  - Owners should be instructed to use a proprietary urine collecting bottle rather than a kitchen receptacle, as impurities (such as sugar or vinegar) can affect test results.
  - Free-catch samples are not appropriate for bacterial culture, as considerable contamination may come from environmental microbes or normal genital/skin flora. Blood may also be present if there are reproductive tract or preputial/vulval lesions.
- **Catheterization** samples are difficult to obtain with the animal conscious, especially from bitches.
  - Care must be taken to avoid microbial contamination of the catheter tip on insertion, as this could not only result in culture of contaminating bacteria but might also lead to ascending urethral infection.
  - Catheterization may be therapeutic, allowing emptying of a blocked bladder, or collection of biopsy samples in addition to urine collection (see later).
- **Cystocentesis** is a safe, convenient way of obtaining a urine sample.
  - If performed using ultrasound guidance, urine may be obtained from bladders with very low urine volumes.
  - Care should be taken if the bladder is overfull and taut, as there is an increased risk of bladder rupture.
  - Most dogs require no or only light sedation.

Cystocentesis

- The patient is held in lateral recumbency (or standing). An area of skin overlying the puncture site is clipped and basic skin preparation performed (it is not necessary to perform full aseptic skin preparation)
- The bladder is palpated and held in position close to the body wall with one hand, whilst the other hand inserts a 21–23 G, 2.5 cm hypodermic needle affixed to a 5 or 10 ml syringe through the body wall into the bladder
- Urine should be collected into a plain tube for urinalysis and a boric acid tube for bacterial culture

---

PRACTICAL TIP

In any work-up for haematuria, it is useful to obtain urine by free catch and by cystocentesis. If blood is present in the free-catch sample but not in the cystocentesis (or catheter) sample, then it is likely that the lesion is distal to the bladder

---

Urine examination
Urine should be examined as soon as possible: ideally within 30 minutes of collection. When delay is unavoidable, the sample can be stored at 4°C and brought back to room temperature just before testing. Delay can alter crystal numbers and composition, and affect morphology of casts and cells. There are five components to urine examination.

Visual inspection: The colour and clarity of the sample give clues to pathology.

Normal urine may be slightly turbid and is light yellow. Changes in colour are usually due to variations in concentration of the urine, or else the presence of pigments such as haemoglobin, bilirubin or methaemoglobin. Several drugs can also cause colour changes (e.g. metronidazole (yellow/brown); amitriptyline (blue/green); doxorubicin (red/pink)).

Changes in turbidity are usually due to haematuria, pyuria, crystalluria or lipiduria. Haematuria (frank blood in the urine) can be distinguished from haemoglobinuria (haemoglobin pigment in the urine, often a sign of intravascular haemolysis) by centrifuging the urine sample at 1500–2000 rpm for 5 minutes and looking for a cellular sediment (Figure 26.4).

Chemical analysis: This is normally carried out using multi-test dipsticks (see Figure 14.6), although most in-house laboratory analysers can determine urea and several other indices with good accuracy. The dipstick should be immersed completely in the sample and then tapped to remove excess urine.

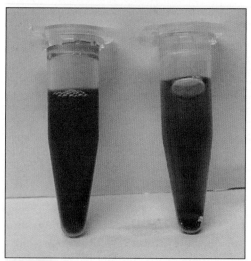

26.4 Distinguishing haematuria from haemoglobinuria. Both these urine samples have been centrifuged. The tube on the right contains a pellet of red blood cells, demonstrating haematuria; the patient was found to have cystitis. The tube on the left has no sediment, demonstrating haemoglobinuria; the patient had immune-mediated haemolytic anaemia.

The test pad colours should be compared with the colour scale at the prescribed time. Interpretation of urine dipstick test results is shown in Figure 26.5.

Measurement of urine specific gravity (USG): This should be performed using a refractometer, which should be regularly calibrated using distilled water to ensure accuracy. It is one of the most informative single tests for urine. A brief explanation of abnormal results follows, but the clinician is advised to refer to a more detailed text for further information.

- **USG <1.008 = hyposthenuria:**
  - Renal failure is unlikely in these cases, as urine must be actively diluted to be hyposthenuric
  - Diabetes insipidus (DI), primary polydipsia or medullary 'washout' may be present. DI may be central (lack of antidiuretic hormone production) or nephrogenic. Nephrogenic DI can be primary (very rare) or secondary to various conditions including: hypothyroidism, hyper- or hypoadrenocorticism, pyometra, pyelonephritis
  - Full haematology and biochemistry is indicated to investigate further.
- **USG 1.008 to 1.012 = isosthenuria:**
  - Some degree of renal failure is possible
  - Biochemistry should be performed to investigate the presence of azotaemia.
- **USG 1.013 to 1.029:** Some urine concentration is occurring.
  - Biochemistry should be investigated, or else water intake should be monitored and USG repeated.
- **USG 1.030 and above:** Normal.

Sediment microscopy: The sample should be centrifuged at 1500–2000 rpm for 5 minutes and the majority of the supernatant tipped off. A small amount of fluid will remain in the centrifuge tube, and tapping the bottom of the tube will resuspend the sediment. A drop of this fluid should be transferred to a slide and a coverslip applied. Presence of crystals, casts and cells should be noted at low power. High power should then be used to look for bacteria and to identify cells. It is not unusual to see a few crystals in urine: their significance will depend on numbers present and other clinical signs. For more details see specialist texts such as Cowell *et al.* (1999) and the *BSAVA Manual of Canine and Feline Nephrology and Urology.*

Urine culture: Samples for culture should be obtained by cystocentesis, and ideally collected into a plain tube. Any positive culture is significant, although contamination of the sample should always be borne in mind if the isolate is a common commensal.

Diagnostic imaging

Indications for further imaging of the urinary or reproductive tract include:

- Urinary outflow obstruction
- Abnormal vulval or penile discharge
- Incontinence
- Dysuria/stranguria that fails to respond to treatment or presents with abnormal test results.

Although ultrasonography enables diagnosis of many urinary tract disorders, there is still a role for radiography. At the very least, a survey study of the chest and abdomen should be carried out if neoplasia is suspected.

Radiography

Invariably, patients must be sedated or anaesthetized to allow radiographic procedures to be carried out. Radiography may demonstrate pregnancy, pyometra or masses that directly or indirectly involve the

Test	Reference value	Causes of derangement; follow-up tests
LEU (leucocytes)	Not applicable	Not a sensitive test in dogs: cytology is preferred. Microscopy should be performed on the basis of increased urine turbidity or clinical signs, or as routine
NIT (nitrites)	Not applicable	Not accurate in dogs: ignore results
PRO (protein)	Trace or 1+	Any protein seen in urine with USG <1.035 is abnormal. Proteinuria with USG >1.035 may be caused by UTI, exercise, seizures or glomerulonephropathy. To investigate further, UPC should be determined
pH	5.0–8.5	Certain drugs (e.g. thiazide diuretics, carbonic anhydrase inhibitors) can alter pH. Low (acidic) pH can be caused by metabolic or respiratory acidosis, severe vomiting or diarrhoea. High (alkaline) pH can be caused by UTI, certain diets, and respiratory or metabolic alkalosis. High pH should be followed up by urine culture and cytology
BLD (haemoglobin/haematuria)	NEG (none)	Haematuria, haemoglobinuria, myoglobinuria. Confirm haematuria by centrifugation and microscopy. Haemoglobinuria should be investigated with haematology. Should myoglobinuria be suspected, serum creatine kinase should be measured
SG.DEN (specific gravity)	>1.030	Dipsticks are inaccurate for USG and a refractometer should be used. For details about USG abnormalities refer to text
KET (ketones)	NEG (none)	Generally considered in combination with patient condition and blood glucose/urine glucose. Ketonuria with glucosuria and a weak, lethargic dog indicates ketoacidosis
GLU (glucose)	NEG (none)	A positive finding demands measurement of blood glucose. Hyperglycaemia with glucosuria usually indicates diabetes mellitus. Normal blood glucose with glucosuria may be due to proximal renal tubular disease and should prompt evaluation of BUN and creatinine. Primary glucosuria (Fanconi syndrome) can occur in some breeds (e.g. Basenji)

26.5 Interpretation of urine dipstick test results. BUN = blood urea nitrogen; UPC = urine protein:creatinine ratio; USG = urine specific gravity; UTI = urinary tract infection.

urinary or reproductive tracts. It is not possible to detect masses within the bladder on plain radiography, although some uroliths are radiopaque.

Contrast radiography, with administration of either air (negative contrast) or iodine-containing media (positive contrast), is indicated for the investigation of bladder or urethral masses, uroliths or trauma, vaginal/rectal fistulas and incontinence, and ureteral investigations (using intravenous contrast agents). For further details see the *BSAVA Manual of Canine and Feline Abdominal Imaging*.

Ultrasonography

Ultrasonography is ideally suited to examination of the bladder due to the inherently high contrast between urine and the bladder wall. It is not possible to visualize the normal ureter, nor the intrapelvic urethra; but the stretch of urethra between the perineum and the os penis of the male dog may be imaged. It is usually possible to perform ultrasound examinations with the patient conscious, or with only light sedation. A moderately full bladder is ideal; if the patient has just voided, then the bladder wall will appear naturally thicker and irregular. Bladder masses, uroliths and corrugations of the bladder mucosa can be readily identified using ultrasonography, although artefacts may cause spurious interpretations (Figure 26.6).

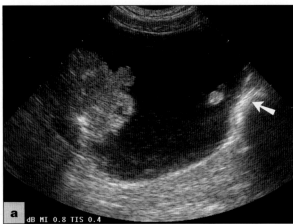

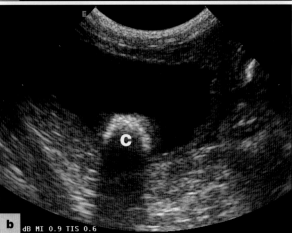

26.6 **(a)** The colon (arrowed) lies immediately adjacent to the bladder and can mimic the appearance of a large calculus. This dog also had a large bladder mass. **(b)** A genuine calculus (C) lying against the bladder wall, casting a strong acoustic shadow. The calculus moves position with gravity. (Transverse plane; right is to the left of the image.) (Courtesy of the University of Bristol; reproduced from the *BSAVA Manual of Canine and Feline Ultrasonography*)

Ultrasound investigation of the female reproductive tract can readily identify pyometra (Figure 26.7) but subtle lesions may easily be missed or confused. The aspirant sonographer is encouraged to undertake further training and to consult specialized imaging textbooks such as the *BSAVA Manual of Canine and Feline Ultrasonography*.

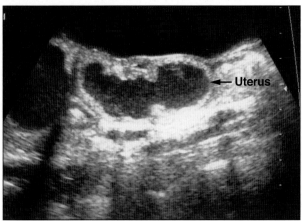

26.7 Ultrasound scan of a bitch with pyometra. The sacculated, fluid-filled uterus is labelled. The bladder is seen at the top left of the image.

Endoscopy

Endoscopy is a very useful, if expensive, tool for looking at anatomical abnormalities, infections of the vagina and uterus, and trauma in the bitch. It is also routinely used for transcervical inseminations. The endoscopes that are used are rigid and about 30 cm long, and have been specifically designed for this purpose. For more information, see the *BSAVA Manual of Canine and Feline Endoscopy and Endosurgery*.

Cytology

Vaginal cytology is used routinely to determine different stages during pro-oestrus and oestrus in the bitch. The cells that may be found will indicate whether there is any hormonal influence (see Chapter 5). Cytology is also a cheap and quick way to examine any abnormal vaginal discharge (Figure 26.8).

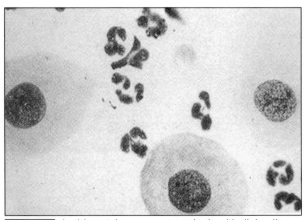

26.8 In this cytology smear, vaginal epithelial cells are small and few, but there are large numbers of polymorphonuclear leucocytes signifying vaginitis or uterine infection.

Conditions causing difficulties with urination

Urinary tract disorders

Urinary tract obstruction: emergency treatment

Signs of repeated straining with no production of urine, a hunched posture, lethargy and weakness should prompt concerns about a blocked bladder or urethra, especially if there has been a recent history of haematuria or dysuria. Palpation should readily reveal an enlarged bladder, and pain may be evident in the caudal abdomen.

Intravenous fluid therapy should be initiated and blood samples taken to evaluate hyperkalaemia and azotaemia. The immediate goal should be removal of the blockage and decompression of the bladder. In most cases a small-bore catheter can be passed up the urethra; however, in those cases where this is not possible, emergency relief can be attained by cystocentesis (although there is a small risk of rupture of the bladder). Hydropulsion may be used to dislodge a stone and flush it retrograde into the bladder.

Urethral retrograde hydropulsion

1. The patient is positioned in lateral recumbency and the penis and prepuce are flushed with dilute chlorhexidine.
2. A gloved assistant places a finger into the rectum and applies pressure to the urethra.
3. A urinary catheter is passed into the urethra to the level of the obstruction. The penis is gripped to form a seal around the catheter, and sterile saline is introduced into the urethra from a syringe attached to the catheter. This causes a pressure increase in the urethra.
4. The gloved assistant releases pressure on the urethra, resulting in a pressure wave forcing the urolith back towards the bladder.

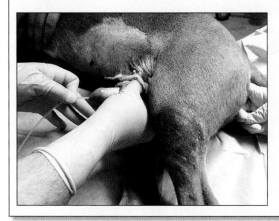

Fluid therapy should be continued for at least 24 hours to establish diuresis (which will help in the dissolution of uroliths) and any urinary tract infection must be treated on the basis of culture and sensitivity results. In cases of repeated blockage, or in rare instances where it is not possible to pass a catheter, urethrostomy should be considered.

Analgesia is mandatory and should include an opioid. Midazolam or diazepam is often added, to improve urethral muscle relaxation. Care should be exercised with non-steroidal anti-inflammatory drugs (NSAIDs) until the renal status of the patient has been ascertained or stabilized.

Urolithiasis

Palpation (especially of thin patients) may reveal the presence of uroliths in the bladder or urethra. However, imaging is usually required to confirm the presence and distribution of stones. Most uroliths are visible on radiographs: calcium oxalate (Figure 26.9) and struvite are the most radiodense; silicate and cysteine uroliths are often slightly indistinct. Urate uroliths are not visible on plain radiographs, but will show up with contrast cystography. Ultrasonography will reveal the presence of uroliths; however, many clinicians prefer radiographs, as it is easier to gain an appreciation of numbers and distribution of stones (particularly when some have passed into the urethra).

Treatment should be by surgical removal, although dissolving uroliths may be attempted if they are small (using medicated food, allopurinol or N-(2-mercaptopropionyl)-glycine, depending on the urolith type) (Figure 26.10). See also emergency treatment for obstruction, above. Analgesia should be provided; NSAIDs are appropriate and effective, provided hydration is good and there is no evidence of azotaemia.

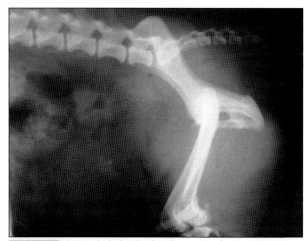

26.9 Lateral abdominal radiograph of a 5-year-old male entire cross-bred dog with a presenting history of dysuria and haematuria. The radiograph shows several small radiodense masses within the urinary bladder. The stones were removed and found to be formed of calcium oxalate.

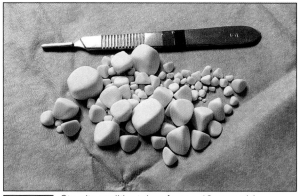

26.10 Struvite uroliths taken from a 13-year-old neutered Jack Russell Terrier bitch with a history of haematuria and dysuria.

Urinary tract infection

Urine microscopy reveals pyuria (degenerate neutrophils with phagocytosed bacteria), bacteriuria and haematuria. Urine culture should be attempted, although Gram staining of a slide may provide a good enough idea of the bacteria involved to make a rational choice of antibiotics before results are back. A good review of antibiotic selection for urinary tract infections (UTIs) is given by Grauer (2009). Antibiotic treatment should be continued for at least 2 weeks.

Dogs that fail to improve, or that have recurrent infections, should be investigated for underlying disease including pyelonephritis. Bladder ultrasonography should be performed, along with biochemistry and investigation for endocrine diseases including diabetes mellitus and hyperadrenocorticism.

Neoplasia

Transitional cell carcinoma (TCC) is the most common bladder neoplasm, although the bladder and other parts of the urinary tract can be affected by other tumours, including leiomyoma, leiomyosarcoma and transmissible venereal tumour (TVT), and through spread from prostatic carcinoma. Abnormal cells may be seen on microscopy and a mass lesion is usually readily visualized using ultrasonography (the sublumbar lymph nodes can also be examined for evidence of spread). Biopsy should be performed to rule out other tumours or inflammatory lesions. Biopsy methods include ultrasound-guided needle biopsy (although there is a small risk of iatrogenic spread along the needle tract), surgical biopsy or catheter biopsy (applying suction to a catheter placed by ultrasound guidance to lie over the mass). Cystoscopy, where available, is ideal, as biopsy samples can be taken and the bladder can be more fully assessed.

Options for treatment include surgery, chemotherapy and radiotherapy. Unfortunately, TCC shows a predilection for the trigone, ruling surgery out in these cases. The prognosis for combined surgical management and chemotherapy (e.g. doxorubicin or carboplatin) is usually <1 year. There is some evidence to suggest that COX 2-specific NSAIDs may have some efficacy in reducing tumour size (Mohammed *et al.*, 2006).

Other causes of dysuria

- Pelvic masses may be palpable per rectum, or else may be imaged radiographically or ultrasonographically.
- Perineal hernia is diagnosed on the basis of other clinical signs (see Chapter 30).
- Neurological dysuria is usually diagnosed on the basis of other clinical signs and lack of findings on urinalysis.

Genital/reproductive disorders (bitch)

Anatomical abnormalities

Occlusion of the vulva by excessive skin folds is quite common in large breeds with a lot of skin or in obese animals, or may sometimes be a feature of individual anatomy. Exudative dermatitis, vaginitis and cystitis can develop as a result. Problems during mating and, if pregnancy is achieved, during parturition are common. Surgical vulvoplasty is the treatment of choice as recurrence is very high with topical treatments.

Clitoral hypertrophy (Figure 26.11) may be caused by excessive licking, treatments with androgens (in racing Greyhounds) and, most commonly, in intersex animals. Approximately 50% of male pseudo-hermaphrodites and 100% of true hermaphrodites show clitoral hypertrophy.

Vaginal strictures are a common occurrence in bitches and can have different origins and appearances. They are usually found at the vestibulovaginal junction and are easily palpated. They can cause pruritus, vestibulitis and cystitis. In bitches that do not

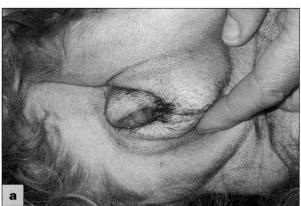

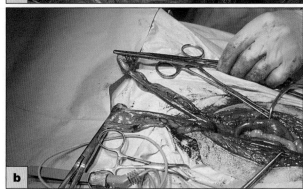

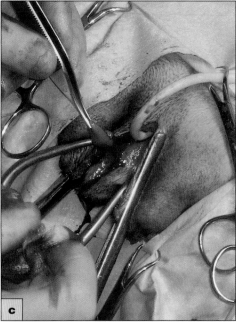

26.11 **(a)** An enlarged clitoris in a 9-month-old healthy Irish Setter. **(b)** Removal of the uterus and ovotestis. **(c)** Removal of the clitoris with the os clitoris.

show any clinical signs they may be discovered when a male dog cannot achieve intromission during mating attempts. Strictures may be circumferential or septal.

- Circumferential strictures may consist of persistent hymens or remnants thereof. These feel quite elastic and can usually be broken down digitally in oestrus bitches. More fibrous circumferential strictures are the result of inadequate fusion of the Müllerian ducts to the urogenital sinus during fetal development. Diagnosis may be made through contrast radiography or vaginal endoscopy. Treatment of choice is surgical removal of the stricture, which is not always easy.
- Septal strictures originate from the incomplete fusion of the Müllerian ducts and may vary in length from a small band, which may be broken down manually, to an elongated septum dividing the vagina.

Vaginal hyperplasia
Vaginal hyperplasia occurs during pro-oestrus and early oestrus, due to excessive oedema under normal oestrogen stimulation. It is not known why some bitches respond in this way, while others do not. Brachycephalic breeds, Staffordshire Bull Terriers and Mastiffs are more commonly affected. Bitches usually show first signs in the first 3 years of life, with a worsening of the condition with each successive oestrus.

Oedematous tissue occludes the vagina and often prolapses through the vulval lips. It is important to avoid lacerations of the prolapsed vaginal mucosa. The prolapse usually only lasts during the 7–10 days of pro-oestrus, a period dominated by oestrogen. As progesterone rises, the oedema decreases and it is sometimes possible to mate bitches. Problems can occur when oestrogen rises again towards the end of pregnancy and the oedema reappears at the time of parturition.

If the oedema becomes pronounced, the bitch should not be used for breeding. Ovariohysterectomy prevents recurrence of the problem.

Tumours of the vagina and vulva
Vaginal tumours are the second most common urogenital tumours in entire bitches after mammary gland tumours. Most of these tumours are hormone-dependent and almost 90% are benign. The most common tumours are leiomyomas, fibromas, fibromyomas and vaginal polyps. Malignant tumours are leiomyosarcomas, adenocarcinomas, haemangiosarcomas and mast cell tumours. Treatment of choice is surgical removal of the tumour with concurrent ovariectomy.

Trauma
Trauma may involve many causes and injuries.

- Trauma caused by mating is relatively rare and must be assessed in the individual patient. Repairs may be possible via the external genital opening, but sometimes an episiotomy may be necessary to gain full access.
- Foreign bodies (e.g. grass awns) are possible causes of trauma, though they usually lead to frequent micturition and a sanguineous or purulent discharge. An endoscopic examination may be necessary to identify the problem and remove the object.

Genital/reproductive disorders (male dog)

Benign prostatic hyperplasia
Benign prostatic hyperplasia (BPH; Figure 26.12) is an age-related condition of entire males. Testosterone is metabolized in the prostate gland and leads to a symmetrical increase in glandular and connective tissue. The prostate gland encircles the urethra at the neck of the urinary bladder and is surrounded by a capsule. Most entire dogs will have BPH by the time they are 5 or 6, although the majority do not have any clinical signs.

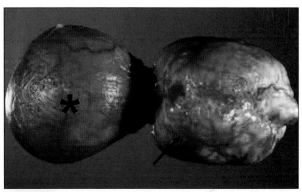

26.12 Post-mortem photograph from a dog with benign prostatic hyperplasia: the prostate gland (arrowed) was as large as the bladder (*).

Clinical signs of BPH include:

- Problems with urinating
- Faecal tenesmus
- Bloody discharge between or following micturition.

Initial assessment for BPH is by rectal digital examination, but this is not always possible, especially if the enlarged prostate gland has moved into the abdominal cavity. Ultrasonography and radiography may be more conclusive.

Treatment in older dogs not used for breeding is castration. In dogs that are still at stud, osaterone acetate is the treatment of choice.

Prostatitis
Prostatitis is an inflammation of the prostate gland that is usually secondary to other underlying problems, most commonly BPH in entire dogs or adenocarcinoma in castrated dogs. In addition to the clinical signs of prostatic disease (see above), there is usually lethargy, pyrexia and inappetence. Prostatic fluid may be collected by ejaculation, or prostatic tissue can be sampled by ultrasound-guided fine-needle biopsy, and cytology used to distinguish prostatitis from cancer. Treatment includes antibiotics, based on sensitivity testing and penetration into the prostate gland, with further therapy for any underlying causes. Fluoroquinolones, such as enrofloxacin and ciprofloxacin, diffuse readily into the prostate gland regardless of the surrounding tissue or pH. Dogs with prostatitis should be treated for 4–6 weeks to avoid recurrence.

Prostatic cysts
Prostatic cysts may be: retention cysts, originating in the tissue of the prostate gland or paraprostatic

cysts. Clinical signs depend on the size and position of the cysts. On ultrasound examination cysts can vary in size, thickness of wall, sediment or clear fluid, subdivisions and associations with other structures. Treatment of choice is surgical omentalization of the cysts.

Prostatic abscess
Prostatic infections may progress into abscesses, forming purulent pockets within the prostatic parenchyma. In acute cases dogs will present with fever and abdominal pain. In chronic cases the abscess is walled off and difficult to diagnose, unless diagnostic imaging is performed. Antibiotic treatment is rarely successful, as penetration into the abscess capsule is poor; surgical drainage and omentalization is the treatment of choice, with concurrent castration.

Prostatic neoplasia
Neoplasia of the prostate gland is uncommon. The most common prostatic neoplasm is adenocarcinoma, which tends to metastasize by direct spread into adjacent tissues and to the iliac and sublumbar lymph nodes. Clinical signs will depend on the increased size of the prostate gland and can include haemorrhagic discharge and even hindlimb lameness. Smaller breeds (terriers) are over-represented, and it may be more common in castrated than in entire dogs. Prostatic neoplasia is an extremely painful condition and prognosis is very guarded. Careful assessment of progressive illness should be made before embarking on treatments; euthanasia is almost always justified by the time the disease is clinically apparent (Figure 26.13). Osaterone acetate may provide transient relief. Analgesia should be commenced, but the response, even to strong opioids, is frequently disappointing.

Spermatic cord torsion
Spermatic cord torsion is a progressively painful event with obvious swelling of the spermatic cord, epididymis and testicle. The dog will be reluctant to move and become increasingly depressed. Removal of the engorged testicle is usually necessary (Figure 26.14).

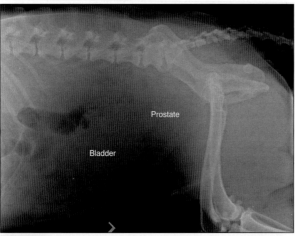

26.13 Lateral abdominal radiograph of a 10-year-old male entire Springer Spaniel with a history of lethargy, weight loss and PU/PD. Haematuria was noted on a urine sample. The radiograph shows a large abdominal prostate gland. A radiodense mass may also be seen in the sublumbar region. Ultrasonography demonstrated the presence of a heteroechoic/cystic mass in the prostate gland. Aspiration and microscopy confirmed a prostatic carcinoma. The dog was euthanased.

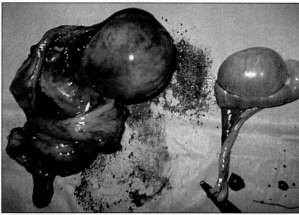

26.14 Testicles removed from a 7-year-old male entire Golden Retriever with an abdominal testicle. The dog was presented showing signs of acute abdominal pain. The testicle on the left is grossly engorged and there is torsion of the spermatic cord.

The condition is more difficult to diagnose in cases where an abdominal testicle is involved, when the pain is difficult to differentiate from other causes of abdominal pain. Analgesia should be commenced as soon as possible; an opioid is the most appropriate choice, with NSAIDs determinant on the hydration and renal status of the patient.

Conditions causing a discharge or abnormal urine

Bitch
Discharge, especially sanguineous, is a normal sign of pro-oestrus and oestrus in the bitch. This is accompanied by swelling of the vulva and behavioural changes; male dogs will show interest and the bitch may be more aggressive toward other females. The discharge, which is never purulent, changes in quantity and composition over the pro-oestrus period and ceases as metoestrus sets in.

During the postpartum period it is also normal for a bitch to produce a discharge: first, greenish-black lochia; later, ever-decreasing amounts of sanguineous discharge. This can last for up to 3 weeks but for most bitches will have subsided considerably after 1 week. Details are described in Chapter 5.

> **WARNING**
>
> Any discharge from the vulva that is not present during pro-oestrus/oestrus or the postpartum period can be considered abnormal

Vaginitis
Juvenile vaginitis, defined as vaginal discharge before the first oestrus, is not uncommon in prepubescent bitches. The causes are not known, but there is a creamy odourless discharge, with no general signs for the affected young bitch. Antibiotics may bring transient relief. The condition is self-limiting, resolving with the first oestrus, and usually does not recur. Early neutering is not recommended in these cases, as neutering prior to puberty will prevent the development of the vaginal structures that allows the condition to resolve.

Chronic vaginitis, often with transient relief from antibiotic treatment, is a condition found in neutered females. It is most probably caused by a lack of oestrogen changing the composition of the commensal vaginal flora and leading to an imbalance that gives rise to 'unwanted' bacteria. Treatment with low-dose oestrogen often brings relief.

Cystic endometrial hyperplasia

Cystic endometrial hyperplasia (CEH), a thickening of the endometrial lining and subsequent cystic enlargement of some of the uterine glands, is a normal progressive process as a result of repeated oestrous cycles. The degree of change varies between individuals but most entire bitches will have some degree of CEH once they are >8 years of age. CEH itself does not have any clinical signs but can cause reduced fertility and may allow the establishment of ascending infection in the uterus that can lead to pyometra.

Pyometra

During oestrus the cervix opens and allows the normal vaginal flora to ascend into the uterus. In a healthy uterus these can be eliminated when the season is finished, the cervix has closed again and a large influx of polymorphonuclear leucocytes is present. During the development of pyometra this does not happen: the contamination cannot be eliminated, the endometrium thickens and a purulent discharge develops inside the uterine lumen. In some cases the cervix remains closed ('closed pyometra') but in most bitches it is open and some discharge can be seen. The most common isolate is *Escherichia coli* but other bacteria may be cultured. Pyometra is most common in older nulliparous bitches that have been in season in the last 4–10 weeks.

Bitches normally present with a purulent and/or bloody discharge, which has a characteristic smell. Other clinical signs are polydipsia (about 60% of cases), inappetence, vomiting and depression. In more severe cases abdominal distension can be significant. As pyometra can develop slowly over many weeks, some of the changes are not evident to the owner.

Diagnosis of pyometra is easiest in cases with vaginal discharge and ultrasonography that confirms a filled uterus. Haematology often reveals leucocytosis with a left shift. Blood biochemistry is useful to assess kidney function.

The treatment of choice in clinically ill bitches is ovariohysterectomy (Figure 26.15; see also QRG 5.1) and fluid therapy.

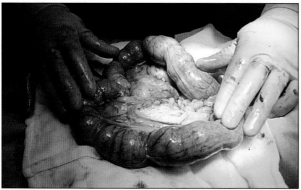

26.15 Pyometra: the fluid-filled uterus resembles a 'string of sausages'.

Non-surgical treatment of pyometra

In some cases where clinical signs are slight, and the bitch is still intended to be used for breeding, a progesterone receptor antagonist may be used:

- Aglepristone 10 mg/kg on days 1, 2 and 7 or 1, 2 and 8
- Antibiotics for 3–4 weeks (start on day 1)

An ultrasound examination should be performed at the end of treatment to ensure that there is no fluid left in the uterus. Bitches should be bred at the next season if possible, as recurrence rates of pyometra after treatment are around 30%. Pregnancy rates for these bitches are above 50%

Abnormal pregnancy

Fetal death during pregnancy will lead to various kinds of discharge, ranging from bloody to purulent to black/malodorous, depending on the stage of pregnancy and degree of maceration. The loss of one puppy does not necessarily lead to a loss of the whole pregnancy and the rest of the puppies may be carried to full term. In some cases fetuses that have died at different stages as well as live puppies may be delivered (Figure 26.16). *Utero verdin* (greenish/black discharge) in the absence of normal first-stage labour is a sign of uterine inertia and requires immediate attention. If placental separation precedes labour, or no labour is taking place, a caesarean section should be performed.

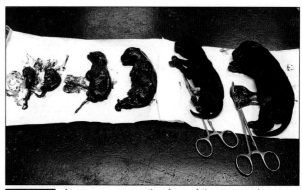

26.16 At caesarean section four of these puppies were mummified at different stages of their development, while two puppies (right) were alive.

Subinvolution of placental sites (SIP) is a condition found in bitches that keep discharging small amounts of blood, often fresh and light in colour, long after giving birth. The bitches have had a normal delivery and are healthy and well; the spotting continues for many weeks, sometimes until their next season. There is no specific treatment at this stage, although oxytocin within 24 hours of parturition may stop SIP developing. The condition does not usually recur with subsequent litters.

Male dog

Testicular neoplasia

Testicular tumours are very common, occurring in 0.9% of entire dogs (Nødtvedt *et al.*, 2011).

- Sertoli cell tumours are slow-growing and often unilateral. They usually produce oestrogen, which leads to feminization (bilateral alopecia, gynaecomastia and attractiveness to other males). Sertoli cell tumours rarely metastasize or become malignant. Removal of the affected testicle is usually curative and fertility may recover in the remaining testicle.

- Seminomas are very similar to Sertoli cell tumours and are often only distinguishable through histology.
- Interstitial cell tumours arise from the Leydig cells in the testicle and are quite small (1–2 cm); they may be multiple and present in both testicles. They are usually not hormonally active, but cause shrinkage of the testicle through atrophy of the seminiferous tubules. Spermatogenesis is arrested. Castration is the treatment of choice.

Testicular tumours are more frequent in abdominal testicles, although the incidence is not as high as previously thought and problems do not normally arise until the dog is at least 5–6 years of age. Given the position of the testicle, they are much harder to diagnose.

Phimosis

Phimosis is the inability to protrude the penis from the prepuce and is uncommon in the dog. It may be caused by a constriction of the preputial orifice, congenitally or through injury, persistent penile frenulum or anatomical abnormalities in intersex animals. Treatments include: surgical widening of the prepuce; transection of the frenulum (usually easy); or gonadectomy in intersex animals.

Paraphimosis

Paraphimosis is the inability to retract the penis into the prepuce. It occurs most commonly as a result of preputial skin rolling inwards following masturbation, but can also be caused by balanoposthitis or a small preputial opening.

Cooling and lubrication may bring transient relief, before dealing with the underlying causes. Medical or surgical castration, treatment of any infections or widening of the preputial opening may be necessary.

Fractured os penis

Fracture of the os penis is uncommon, usually caused by trauma and is very painful during urination and palpation. Radiographic imaging is helpful in diagnosis. Healing usually occurs unaided, but an indwelling urethral catheter may be necessary. In extreme cases the penis may have to be amputated.

Urinary incontinence

Incontinent dogs may be more prone to ascending urethral infection and irritation of the external urethral orifice through constant wetting and urine scalding. However, it is often the owners who suffer the most with the problem. The smell of urine, staining of carpets and furnishings, and increased cleaning costs and effort can drive a wedge into the human–pet bond and make the owner increasingly resentful towards and annoyed with their dog. The realization that the animal cannot control the leakage adds guilt to the emotions, often resulting in owners hiding their true concerns about the condition. Thus, incontinence

should be investigated as a priority and a high level of compassion should be shown.

There are several causes of incontinence, which may be roughly divided into:

- Problems of urine overflow: these are characterized by a large bladder on palpation, and include neurological lesions, reflex dyssynergia, or outflow obstruction
- Problems of urine retention: these are characterized by a small bladder, and include USMI, hyper-reflexivity of the detrusor muscle and congenital abnormalities.

It is important to establish that the problem really is incontinence: patches of urine appearing around the house may be a sign of dysuria, or increased urge to urinate, or behavioural (see Chapter 12). Incontinence is a lack of voluntary urine retention and typically results in urine being released while the dog is lying down; in some instances there is a continual leakage of urine, which may result in scalding of the vulva, prepuce or hindquarters. Occasionally, the loss of urine can be so slight that it is hardly detected, but may cause a bitch to lick the vulval area in order to clean itself. This and the leakage of urine can lead to recurring vaginitis that does not respond to antibiotic treatment. It is also important to distinguish incontinence from pollakiuria/polydipsia, which can result in reduced ability to control voiding due to large volumes of urine production (see Chapter 14).

PRACTICAL TIP

Urinalysis including specific gravity, dipstick analysis and cytology should be routinely performed in suspected incontinent cases to rule out PU/PD

Problems of urine overflow

Neurogenic disorders

Typically, dogs with neurogenic disorders of the bladder will have other neurological abnormalities on examination, such as ataxia, paresis or proprioception deficiencies. There may also be a history of spinal or pelvic trauma. However, rare neurogenic tumours or other disorders can occur. Chapters 11 and 16 discuss neurological examination in detail.

As a general oversimplification:

- If the bladder is full and easy to express, then the lesion is likely to be a LMN lesion (located at or below L5)
- If the bladder is full and hard to express, a UMN lesion should be suspected (cranial to L5).

Reflex dyssynergia (RD) is a neurological cause of incontinence seen mainly in large-breed male dogs. A typical presentation is that of a dog cocking its leg to urinate normally, passing a reasonable stream that soon diminishes into spurts. The dog then may walk off still dribbling or spurting urine. This may be difficult to distinguish from urinary outflow obstruction, but a urinary catheter is easily passed in these cases and no blockage can be found.

Urinary outflow obstruction

In these cases there is urine overflow: that is, the pressure within the bladder increases until there is sufficient pressure for urine to escape around an obstruction. Typically, the patient will be uncomfortable or in pain and may be seen frequently straining with no urine forthcoming. Urine may be seen to leak from the urethral opening. The outflow obstruction may be caused by calculi, neoplasia, pressure from extraurethral masses, urethritis or strictures. Prostatic disease in older dogs (see earlier) is a relatively common cause of outflow obstruction.

Problems of urine retention

Urethral sphincter mechanism incompetence

Although the condition can be congenital, the acquired form is much more prevalent. USMI does occur in male dogs but is uncommon.

USMI is by far the most common cause of urinary incontinence in the bitch, especially in the spayed bitch, which (due to a lack of oestrogen) may be around eight times more likely to develop the condition than the intact bitch. The onset of incontinence after spaying can vary between a few months and many years, but is not associated with the age at which a bitch is neutered, with the exception of six key breeds.

Breed predilections for USMI

The following breeds should not be spayed prior to their first season, as there is a very high risk of rapidly developing post-spay urinary incontinence:

- Old English Sheepdog
- Dobermann
- Rottweiler
- Irish Setter
- Weimaraner
- Springer Spaniel

Other factors are believed to play an important role in the development of USMI, including: length of the urethra; position of the bladder neck (intra- or extrapelvic); breed; and obesity, with larger, overweight bitches being more prone to developing or worsening USMI.

Hyper-reflexivity of the detrusor muscle

This is an inability to control voiding secondary to inflammation of the bladder or urethra stimulating the detrusor muscle. The most common cause is bacterial UTI, although tumours, calculi or chronic cystitis can also cause it. Haematuria is a common feature of this condition and the affected dog may also exhibit pollakiuria and dysuria/stranguria.

Congenital abnormalities

Puppies and immature dogs with incontinence may have ectopic ureters, persistent urachus, vaginal strictures, or congenital fistulas. Of these, ectopic ureters are the most common, and bitches are more prone. Typically a constant dribble of urine is seen, although in unilaterally affected cases urine can also be voided normally.

Treatment of incontinence

Treatment of urinary outflow obstruction is described earlier in the chapter. Neurogenic causes are best treated by addressing any underlying neurological disease, although the prognosis often remains guarded for these conditions. Surgical treatment of ectopic ureters and other congenital abnormalities is outside the scope of this book and the interested reader is directed to a surgery book such as the *BSAVA Manual of Canine and Feline Abdominal Surgery*.

USMI treatment can be divided into medical and surgical approaches. Due to the multifactorial nature of USMI, no individual treatment has been found to deal with all cases and it is necessary to adjust treatment periodically in most cases. Approximately 50% of dogs do not respond fully to treatment.

- Medical treatment: The mainstays of treatment are phenylpropanolamine and estriol. If there is a lack of response or the animal becomes refractory to treatment, it is possible to use the two drugs in combination. Recently, the gonadotropin-releasing hormone (GnRH) superagonist deslorelin has been shown to be effective in some USMI cases, possibly by stabilizing the bladder wall; however, this drug is not authorized for this use at present. Analgesia is generally not required for incontinence; however, urine scalding can occur in chronic cases. This can cause great irritation in the vulval region and is generally treated by NSAIDs and improved hygiene, including chlorhexidine washing and use of petroleum jelly.
- Surgical treatment: There are various surgical options, including colposuspension, bladder neck reconstruction, periurethral surgical slings and injection of bulking agents into the proximal urethra. The techniques are regarded as complex and require a good deal of surgical expertise. Again, the reader is encouraged to study a surgical textbook.

References and further reading

Adams LG and Syme HM (2005) Canine lower urinary tract diseases. In: *Textbook of Veterinary Internal Medicine, 6th edn*, ed. SJ Ettinger and EC Feldman, pp.1850–1874. Elsevier Saunders, St. Louis

Barr F and Gaschen L (2012) *BSAVA Manual of Canine and Feline Ultrasonography*. BSAVA Publications, Gloucester

Bexfield N and Lee K (2014) BSAVA *Guide to Procedures in Small Animal Practice, 2nd edn*. BSAVA Publications, Gloucester

Cowell RL, Tyler RD and Meinkoth JH (1999) *Diagnostic Cytology and Haematology of the Dog and Cat, 2nd edn*. Mosby, St. Louis

Elliott J and Grauer G (2007) *BSAVA Manual of Canine and Feline Nephrology and Urology, 2nd edn*. BSAVA Publications, Gloucester

England G and von Heimendahl A (2010) *BSAVA Manual of Canine and Feline Reproduction and Neonatology, 2nd edn*. BSAVA Publications, Gloucester

England GCW (1998) *Allen's Fertility and Obstetrics in the Dog*. Blackwell Science, Oxford

Fieni F (2006) Clinical evaluation of the use of aglepristone, with or without cloprostenole, to treat cystic endometrial hyperplasia-pyometra complex in bitches. *Theriogenology* **66**, 1550–1556

Grauer G (2009) Urinary tract infections. In: *Small Animal Internal Medicine, 4th edn*, ed. RW Nelson and CG Couto, pp.660–666. Mosby Elsevier, St. Louis

Hagman R and Kuhn I (2002) *Escherichia coli* strains isolated from the uterus and urinary bladder of bitches suffering from pyometra. Comparison by restriction enzyme digestion and pulsed field gel electrophoresis. *Veterinary Microbiology* **84**, 143–153

Holt P (2012) Sphincter mechanism incompetence. In: *Veterinary Surgery: Small Animal*, ed. K Tobias and S Johnston, pp.2011–2018. Elsevier Saunders, St. Louis

Johnston SD, Root Kustritz MV and Olson PN (2001) *Canine and Feline Theriogenology*. WB Saunders, Philadelphia

Lhermette P and Sobel D (2008) *BSAVA Manual of Canine and Feline Endoscopy and Endosurgery*. BSAVA Publications, Gloucester

Mannion P (2006) *Diagnostic Ultrasound in Small Animal Practice*. Blackwell, Oxford

Matthews K (2012) Ureters. In: *Veterinary Surgery: Small Animal*, ed. K Tobias and S Johnston, pp.1962–1977 Elsevier Saunders, St. Louis

Mohammed SI, Dhawan D, Abraham S *et al.* (2006) Cyclooxygenase inhibitors in urinary bladder cancer: *in vitro* and *in vivo* effects. *Molecular Cancer Therapy* **5**, 329–336

Nødtvedt A, Gamlem H, Gunnes G *et al.* (2011) Breed differences in the proportional morbidity of testicular tumours and distribution of histopathologic types in a population-based canine cancer registry. *Veterinary and Comparative Oncology* **9**, 45–54

O'Brien R and Barr F (2009) *BSAVA Manual of Canine and Feline Abdominal Imaging*. BSAVA Publications, Gloucester

Smith J (2008) Canine prostatic disease: A review of anatomy, pathology, diagnosis and treatment. *Theriogenology* **70**, 375–383

Williams JM and Niles JD (2005) *BSAVA Manual of Canine and Feline Abdominal Surgery*. BSAVA Publications, Gloucester

Skin problems: a clinical approach

Ken Robinson

The main presenting signs of skin disease are: pruritus; alopecia (symmetrical, localized, diffuse, patchy); scaling and crusting; erosions and ulceration; papules, pustules and vesicles; lumps and nodules; and pigmentation disorders. Solving each dermatological conundrum requires an ability to listen, observe, feel and smell. Using all the information gathered through these senses, the cause of most dermatological presentations can be ascertained. When presented with a dog with a skin problem, a thorough history should first be obtained. Following the history-taking and physical examination, a basic differential diagnosis list can be drawn up and may indicate further diagnostic tests. The investigations noted here, coupled with a logical approach derived from the history and physical examination, should allow most cases to be diagnosed and suitable treatment selected. It is useful to divide cases on presentation into **pruritic** and **non-pruritic** (or pruritus not being the primary sign) cases, and algorithms are provided for both types of presentation. Should a case not resolve, it is necessary to go back to the beginning and review the case again, as new lesions or historical facts may be present. It is also important to check that therapy has been administered properly. Common conditions are discussed in approximate order of prevalence. Details of specific tests and drug doses, along with details of uncommon conditions listed, can be found in the *BSAVA Manual of Canine and Feline Dermatology*.

There are few true emergencies in canine dermatology. Toxic epidermal necrolysis probably constitutes the only one in the UK and is rare, while in other countries venomous bites would be considered an emergency.

History

The time invested in getting a good history can prevent wasting time doing unnecessary diagnostic investigations and also avoid unnecessary expense for the owner. It is helpful to develop a basic line of questioning to avoid missing any information. A questionnaire can be used (an example is given at the end of the chapter), but it is possible to memorise a sequence of questions that can be asked during the physical and dermatological examination, for efficient use of time. The following questions should be asked:

- How old was the dog when the problem started? For example: an early age of onset could indicate demodicosis or a congenital or hereditary condition; between 1 and 3 years of age could suggest atopic dermatitis; older than 6 years could suggest endocrine, metabolic or neoplastic disease
- What did the skin problem look like originally? For example: atopy is often merely pruritic initially, with few or no skin lesions
- Where on the body did the first lesions appear, and what did they look like?
- Is the dog itchy and, if so, how severe is the itch? Itching, scratching, licking, chewing, biting or rubbing are all signs of pruritus and may not be volunteered by the owner
- Is the diet of good quality and is there any relation to the onset of skin signs when it is fed?
- Are in-contact animals or people affected?
- Has the dog recently been acquired from or visited kennels?
- What percentage of time is spent indoors? Do clinical signs vary with the amount of time spent outdoors or indoors?
- Is there any seasonality? This may be seen with atopy or parasitism
- Are siblings or other relatives of the dog affected?
- Is there effective flea control on all the animals in the house, and in the environment?
- What medications (dermatological and others, including supplements) is the dog taking? Has the condition responded to medication? Uncomplicated atopy is very steroid-responsive, while food allergy, scabies and forms of pyoderma can be poorly responsive
- Is there a recent history of foreign travel?

Non-dermatological information can also be used to direct investigation of a dermatosis:

- Bouts of vomiting and diarrhoea may indicate food intolerance

- Polydipsia and polyuria may indicate an endocrinopathy, e.g. hyperadrenocorticism
- Lethargy and thermophilia may indicate hypothyroidism
- Abnormalities of the oestrous cycle can be associated with endocrinopathies
- Changes in biochemistry profiles, particularly hepatic, could indicate hepatocutaneous syndrome or endocrinopathies.

Physical examination

> ### PRACTICAL TIP
>
> A physical examination of *all* major body systems should be carried out. General signs such as anaemia (systemic disease), lymphadenopathy (demodicosis, juvenile cellulitis, lymphoma), bradycardia and being overweight (hypothyroidism), swollen abdomen and hepatomegaly (hyperadrenocorticism) help point the clinician towards a diagnosis

A thorough examination of *all* the skin is required, not just the affected areas presented by the owner. Particular attention should be paid to the interdigital skin, paws, nails, mucocutaneous regions and ears. Areas such as the ventrum, dorsum, face, axillae and groin are examined by parting the coat to find lesions that might not be obvious on initial inspection. It may be necessary to clip areas to show lesions. An illuminated magnifying glass is very useful. Some

dermatological lesions are illustrated in Figure 27.1; a fuller description of individual lesions can be found in the BSAVA *Manual of Canine and Feline Dermatology*. Lesions can be categorized as primary or secondary, although some can be either. All lesions should be carefully recorded in the clinical notes.

The distribution of lesions can point towards certain problems:

- Lesions involving the face, ears, axillae, groin and feet strongly suggest atopy or food allergy
- Lesions involving the lumbosacral area strongly suggest flea-allergic dermatitis
- Lesions involving the elbows and pinnae suggest scabies.

The nature of the lesions may suggest the cause:

- Papules may indicate pyoderma, scabies, ectoparasitism or hypersensitivity
- Pustules might suggest pyoderma, but also demodicosis or pemphigus foliaceus
  - Large pustules may be associated with endocrine disease complicated by pyoderma
- Follicular casts may be seen with pyoderma, demodicosis, dermatophytosis or keratinization disorders
- There may be a malodour, possibly suggesting a *Malassezia* infection.

The skin should be palpated to detect thickening (lichenification) or thinning (suggesting hyperadrenocorticism). The haircoat should also be examined; chewed hair has a rough feel when brushed backwards with the fingers.

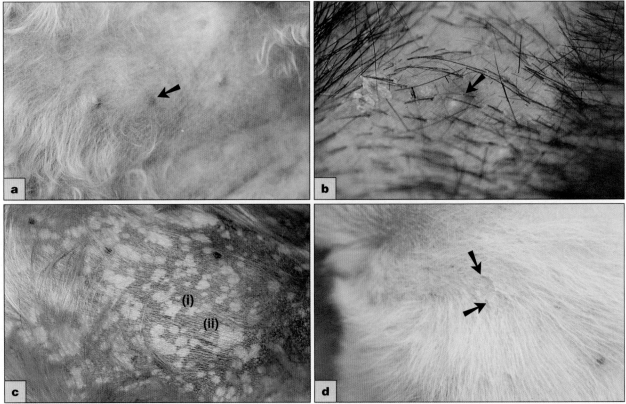

27.1 Examples of dermatological lesions. **(a)** Papule: a solid elevated lesion, <1 cm diameter (arrowed). **(b)** Pustule: a circumscribed elevation of the skin, which contains pus (arrowed). **(c)** Hypopigmentation: (i) <1 cm macule; (ii) >1 cm patch. **(d)** Scale: an accumulation of loose fragments of the cornified layer of the skin (arrowed). (continues) ▶

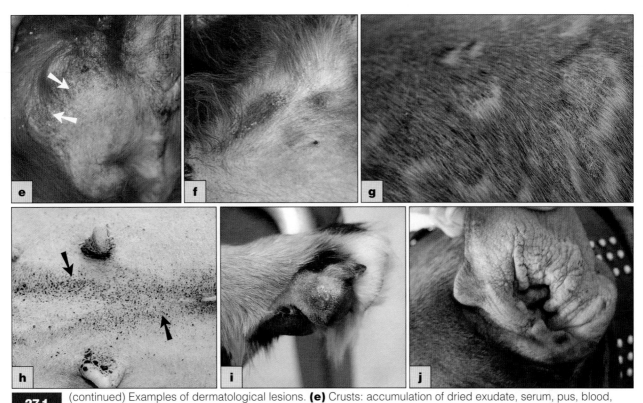

27.1 (continued) Examples of dermatological lesions. **(e)** Crusts: accumulation of dried exudate, serum, pus, blood, cells or scales (arrowed). **(f)** Epidermal collarette: circular arrangement of scale. **(g)** Alopecia: loss of hair. **(h)** Comedones: dilated hair follicles filled with cornified cells and sebaceous material (arrowed). **(i)** Nodule: a circumscribed solid elevation, >1 cm in diameter). **(j)** Lichenification: thickening and hardening of the skin.

Diagnostic techniques

More information on these techniques can be found in the BSAVA *Manual of Canine and Feline Dermatology*.

PRACTICAL TIP

In a busy clinic it can be difficult to perform these tests during a consulting session, so if time is limited collect the samples and look at them after the appointments have finished; then ring the owners to discuss the findings

---

Parasite collection and identification

All dermatological cases should have skin scraping performed (see QRG 27.1) to avoid missing a parasite problem. Superficial parasites can also be checked for by using an acetate strip (e.g. for *Cheyletiella*) or a flea comb. It is useful to have a chart with diagrams of parasites adjacent to the microscope, to help identification (obtainable from some pharmaceutical companies, or one can be made).

Cytology

Cytology of adhesive tape or direct smear samples (see QRG 27.2) is an inexpensive and much underused diagnostic technique available in practice. It can be used to detect infective agents, immune-mediated cells, inflammatory infiltrate, acanthocytes and neoplastic cells. Establishing whether cocci, rods or *Malassezia* are present can direct appropriate antimicrobial therapy.

Trichograms

Trichograms (see QRG 27.3) are another underused and inexpensive diagnostic aid. Anagen and telogen hairs can be identified and the anagen:telogen ratio calculated. If telogen hairs predominate, then an endocrine or nutritional disorder is likely. Shaft deformities (trauma, congenital) and melanin clumping (colour dilution alopecia) may be seen. Broken hair shaft ends suggest trauma. Fungal hyphae can be seen on hairs infected by dermatophytes.

Bacteriology, fungal culture and Wood's lamp examination

If a bacterial or fungal cause is suspected, samples can be sent for bacterial culture and sensitivity testing (particularly indicated if bacterial rods are present) and/or fungal culture.

Wood's lamp examination

- Wood's lamp examination can demonstrate yellow/green fluorescence in *Microsporum canis*-infected hair shafts in about 30–80% of isolates. Some rare dermatophytes may also fluoresce
- Care should be taken to avoid falsely identifying fluorescence due to medications or debris
- Allow the lamp to heat up adequately (5–10 minutes) before use

---

Skin biopsy

Skin biopsy (see QRG 27.4) can identify some specific conditions, but most often helps in ruling out others. Samples may be used for histopathology or culture. Biopsy should never be used as a short cut to diagnosis in place of the basic work-up.

Further tests

Blood can be collected for haematology, biochemistry and serology where indicated, e.g. endocrinopathies and systemic diseases. Allergies can be investigated further by intradermal skin testing or serology, but these must not be used as the sole means of diagnosis. Other tests include diascopy (a glass slide applied to reddened skin will blanch if the redness is due to vascular engorgement, but remain red with haemorrhage) and the Nikolosky sign (gentle rubbing of the skin causes peeling in conditions such as pemphigus, toxic epidermal necrolysis and erythema multiforme).

Pruritic conditions

Pruritus is the most common dermatological presentation in practice, and often the most stressful for practitioners. Owners will not tolerate pruritus in their pets, so there is pressure to apply a 'quick fix', but this will usually only result in postponing the problem. Common causes of pruritus are listed in Figure 27.2; other conditions may present with pruritus (e.g. pemphigus, seborrhoea) but their primary signs are more important (see later).

- **Fleas**
- **Atopic dermatitis**
- **Food hypersensitivity**
- **Pyotraumatic dermatitis**
- **Acral lick dermatitis**
- **Scabies**
- Superficial pyoderma
- *Malassezia*
- *Cheyletiella*
- *Demodex*
- Pediculosis
- *Neotrombicula*

27.2 Causes of pruritus. The most common causes are in **bold**.

A logical step-by-step approach is required (Figure 27.3). In dealing with pruritic cases, the concept of *pruritic threshold* should be considered: several skin conditions can collectively exceed the threshold; clearing one or two of these dermatoses can often bring the animal below the threshold and thus reduce the itch.

> **PRACTICAL TIP**
>
> Some form of assessment scale can be used (score 1–10) to review response to therapy, as the comment 'It is no better' can be very misleading. The itch may be 50% reduced but still present, as may often be the case if a pyoderma has cleared but there was an underlying allergy

Fleas

Fleas are still the commonest ectoparasite seen in practice, despite all the insecticide products available. This is largely because of poor advice and improper use of preparations. Animals may have large

numbers of fleas and yet very few clinical signs or, in the case of flea-allergic dogs, severe signs with only a few fleas. Animals of any age can be affected.

Flea hypersensitivity is rare in animals <6 months of age but usually developed by 1–3 years. Lesions commonly involve the lumbosacral region, caudal thighs and groin. There may be papules, erythema and alopecia. Some cases can present as pyotraumatic dermatitis.

The coat should be examined for evidence of fleas, flea eggs and flea dirt (Figure 27.4). It is important to check whether there are other animals in the house, especially cats, and if they or the people in the household have lesions.

> **PRACTICAL TIP**
>
> The type of flea or its life stage may indicate the source. Mainly small juvenile fleas would suggest poor environmental control

The owner should be asked about flea control in order to establish whether they are using an effective preparation in an appropriate way. It is also necessary to ascertain how often the dog is bathed or goes swimming, as this could decrease the efficacy of topical treatments.

- Treat *all the animals in the household* with a topical monthly preparation that has a good duration of activity, or with oral spinosad. Alternatively, in the case of dogs, one of the new isoxazolines (fluralaner, afoxolaner) can be used.
- Treat the environment with an insecticide and insect growth regulator (IGR) spray.
- Lufenuron is an oral IGR that can be given to *all animals in the household* to inhibit fleas breeding.
- Vacuum the house and dispose of the contents of the vacuum cleaner.
- Treat the outside environment and the car with an insecticide. *Note that some preparations are affected by exposure to UV radiation.*

> **PRACTICAL TIP**
>
> A common mistake is to treat only the affected animal. Treat all animals in the house and the environment

Atopic dermatitis

Atopic dermatitis is a common cause of pruritus in dogs. Initially there are few if any skin lesions, but lesions develop later due to self-trauma. Areas commonly affected include the face (Figure 27.5), eyelids, ears (especially the convex surface of the pinna, often without initial involvement of the horizontal canal), axillae, groin, interdigital region, perineum, and carpal and tarsal regions. Pruritus can be severe (scratching, licking, biting, chewing or rubbing) and can be exacerbated by secondary flare factors like fleas and other parasites, bacteria, *Malassezia* or diet. Atopic dogs are particularly prone to secondary microbial infections. The condition is often seasonal initially, but in most cases progresses to occurring all year round. Relatives can be affected.

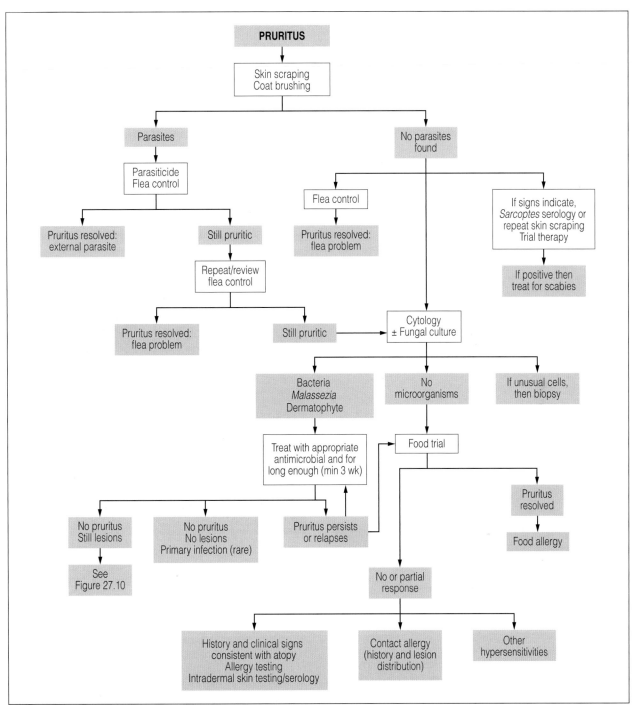

PRURITUS

↓

Skin scraping
Coat brushing

Parasites | No parasites found

Parasiticide
Flea control

Pruritus resolved: external parasite | Still pruritic

Flea control

Pruritus resolved: flea problem

If signs indicate, *Sarcoptes* serology or repeat skin scraping Trial therapy

If positive then treat for scabies

Repeat/review flea control

Pruritus resolved: flea problem | Still pruritic

Cytology ± Fungal culture

Bacteria *Malassezia* Dermatophyte | No microorganisms | If unusual cells, then biopsy

Treat with appropriate antimicrobial and for long enough (min 3 wk)

Food trial

Pruritus resolved

Food allergy

No pruritus Still lesions | No pruritus No lesions Primary infection (rare) | Pruritus persists or relapses

See Figure 27.10

No or partial response

History and clinical signs consistent with atopy Allergy testing Intradermal skin testing/serology | Contact allergy (history and lesion distribution) | Other hypersensitivities

27.3   An approach to the dog with pruritus. Prior to embarking on using the chart, a thorough clinical history should be taken and a physical examination carried out.

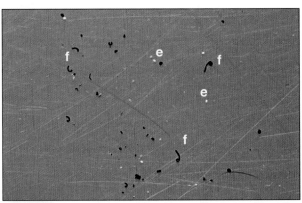

27.4   Comma-shaped flea faeces (f), along with white flea eggs (e) are visible in these haircoat combings on an examination table.

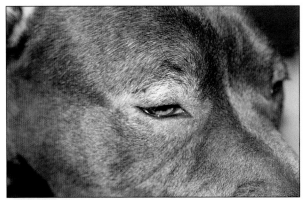

27.5   Alopecia, erythema and papules on the eyelids in an early case of atopic dermatitis in a young Staffordshire Bull Terrier.

A successful diagnosis depends on careful history-taking. The condition is rarely seen before 6 months of age (though some breeds can present very young, e.g. Golden Retriever or Shar Pei); most cases present at between 1 and 3 years of age. There is a breed predisposition that can vary with country and region, and includes the Boxer, Labrador Retriever, Golden Retriever, setters, terriers (Scottish, West Highland, Cairn, Staffordshire), Lhasa Apso, Shih Tzu, Bulldog, Cocker Spaniel, Shar Pei, German Shepherd Dog and Dalmatian. Favrot *et al.* (2010) proposed a series of criteria from which a combination of five would be highly suggestive of atopic dermatitis (Figure 27.6).

- Onset of signs at <3 years of age
- Predominantly indoor lifestyle
- Pruritus responds to glucocorticoids
- Initially pruritus without lesions
- Forefeet involvement
- Pinnae of ears involvement
- Ear margins not affected
- Dorsolumbar region not affected

27.6 Criteria for diagnosing atopic dermatitis. A combination of five of these criteria would be highly suggestive of atopic dermatitis (Favrot *et al.*, 2010).

Atopic dermatitis is regarded as a steroid-responsive disease: proven effective treatments include steroids (prednisolone 1.1 mg/kg orally q24h, reducing later), ciclosporin (5 mg/kg orally q24h), oclacitinib (0.4–0.6 mg/kg orally q12h, reducing to q24h after 14 days) and immunotherapy. Therapies with variable responses include antihistamines, essential fatty acids and Chinese herbs. Topical therapy is also very important in management, especially to restore the skin barrier function. Where there is secondary infection, antimicrobials are essential. Regular check-ups are required to monitor progress.

Pyotraumatic dermatitis (acute moist dermatitis)

In this condition lesions are produced by self-trauma in response to a painful or pruritic insult. Lesions appear as red, moist and exudative close to the cause, with a sticky surface discharge, and radiating out from the initial lesion (Figure 27.7). The surface is contaminated with bacteria. The classic appearance of the lesions suggests the diagnosis. The condition is more common in densely coated breeds (Golden and Labrador Retrievers, Collies, German Shepherd Dogs, St Bernards and Newfoundlands), due to the poor ventilation at skin level. It is more common in hot humid weather. There is an acute onset, often within hours, as a result of an itch–scratch–itch cycle. Underlying causes include ectoparasites, allergy, anal sac disease, otitis externa, an unkempt coat, a painful orthopaedic problem, or behavioural disorders.

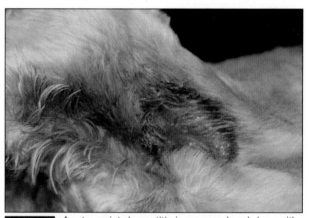

27.7 Acute moist dermatitis in a cross-bred dog, with an exudative lesion behind the axilla.

The affected area should be clipped and cleaned with an antiseptic solution. Sedation is often needed, as the condition is painful. Steroids are required to break the itch cycle, and should be used until there is total resolution. Topical ointments can be used but are often not as effective as oral steroids. Some cases require oral antibiotics, in particular if there is evidence of papules developing associated with a folliculitis.

There is a high risk of relapse. Even successful cases can take time to heal, with regression due to contracture of the associated scab formation over the lesion causing further irritation. It is important to inform the owner about the anticipated course of this disease to avoid frustration when these setbacks occur.

Acral lick dermatitis (lick granuloma)

In this condition a raised ulcerated lesion is seen, usually on the limbs. It is important to differentiate behavioural from organic causes. Other behavioural problems seen include flank sucking and anal licking. Organic causes (e.g. bacteria, fungi, demodicosis, allergy, joint disease) should be treated or eliminated before assigning a behavioural cause. A thorough behavioural investigation should then be carried out to identify the initiating causes (see Chapter 12). Certain breeds have been associated with behavioural causes, often being anxious individuals (Dobermann, Great Dane, German Shepherd Dog, Irish Setter, Labrador and Golden Retrievers).

PRACTICAL TIP

If access to the lesion is prevented and the dog begins to lick elsewhere, this is strongly indicative of a behavioural problem

The lesion is treated using combinations of topical steroids (take care, as this may focus the dog's attention on the lesion), oral or intralesional steroids, surgery, laser therapy, acupuncture and sometimes antibiotics. The area can be bandaged but some dogs may just extend their chewing to the bandage edges. Behavioural therapy may be indicated.

Sarcoptic mange

The burrowing mite *Sarcoptes scabiei* causes an intensely pruritic dermatosis. Lesions affecting the pinnae, especially the edges (Figure 27.8), elbows, hocks and ventrum are strongly suggestive of scabies. There is scaling, crusting, erythema and alopecia. Rubbing the edge of the pinna commonly elicits an itch response. There may be a history of contact with infected animals in a kennel, or indirect contact with foxes. *This is a contagious disease for animals and humans.*

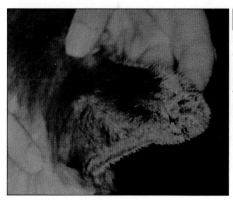

27.8

Scaling and crusting lesions on the pinna of a dog with sarcoptic mange.

Diagnosis is by identifying the mite in deep skin scrapings (see QRG 27.1), although negative results are not uncommon. Multiple deep scrapings taken from the pinnal edges and elbows will improve yield, and using potassium hydroxide solution (KOH) instead of liquid paraffin on the slide will dissolve the keratin to allow better visualization. Serology can be used where skin scrapings are negative but suspicion is high (care must be taken in interpreting results as there is cross-reaction with housedust mites). Sometimes trial therapy is required.

Treatment is with amitraz or a spot-on insecticide (the latter at an 'off-label' frequency of every 2 weeks). A poor response to treatment may require 'off-label' use of avermectins (ivermectin/milbemycin). The reader is referred to the *BSAVA Manual of Canine and Feline Dermatology* for further discussion.

Superficial pyoderma, folliculitis and furunculosis

These can be very pruritic conditions. Most infections are staphylococcal, mainly involving *Staphylococcus pseudintermedius*. Lesions seen include papules, pustules, patchy alopecia, erythema and epidermal collarettes, later extending to oedematous purulent/haemorrhagic exudate when infections are deeper.

Most cases are complications of other conditions, e.g. atopic dermatitis, but lesions can be primary (e.g. short-haired breed folliculitis presenting as a 'moth-eaten' coat). The *BSAVA Manual of Canine and Feline Dermatology* has a very good flowchart illustrating the approach to bacterial skin infections.

Cytology is performed on material gathered from intact pustules or papules, by opening them with a needle and then swabbing. Degenerative neutrophils are seen, with active phagocytosis of bacterial cocci (see QRG 27.2) or, rarely, rods. Furunculosis lesions may yield less and contain a mixed cell population with macrophages, lymphocytes and plasma cells as well as neutrophils. Culture and sensitivity testing is indicated in recurrent infections.

Superficial infections require a minimum of 3–4 weeks treatment with an antibiotic appropriate for the skin (e.g. co-amoxiclav, first-generation cephalsporin, clindamycin) and should be continued until 1 week past lesion resolution. Potentiated sulphonamides may still be useful, where finance is an issue for owners; although there is a relatively high incidence of resistance, an improved response can be achieved at higher doses.

WARNING

Do not prescribe potentiated sulphonamides for Dobermanns

Deep infections require culture and sensitivity testing to identify the most appropriate antibiotic. This should be administered for a minimum of 6–8 weeks, and be continued for 2 weeks beyond clinical cure.

PRACTICAL TIP

A very common mistake is not using antibiotics for the long periods required. This will result in relapses and the potential development of antibiotic resistance

Antimicrobial topical ointments (e.g. containing fusidic acid or mupirocin) can be used for both superficial and deep infections.

Food hypersensitivity/intolerance

This condition presents with lesions very similar to those of atopic dermatitis and can often be found in association with it. Food hypersensitivity may also present as relapsing pyoderma or urticaria. Lesions involving predominantly the ears, feet or perineum are strongly suggestive. Onset can be at any age, including <6 months (in contrast to atopic dermatitis, see above). There may be a history of gastrointestinal signs, and a poor response to steroid therapy may have been observed.

A variety of foodstuffs may be responsible, so a careful diet history must be taken. Some foods seem to feature more commonly, e.g. dairy produce, beef, fish and cereals, and the offending food may have been fed for some time.

Diagnosis is through an elimination diet trial, avoiding any previously fed foods. A home-cooked diet is preferable but commercial hydrolysed diets can be used if the owner is not prepared to cook food for the dog. Ideally, the elimination diet should be fed for 6–8 weeks, followed by challenging again with the original diet to demonstrate relapse, usually occurring within 24 hours to 2 weeks. Serology cannot currently be recommended for diagnosis.

Management consists of avoiding the food(s) responsible, and treatment of any secondary changes and pruritus.

Malassezia infection

This yeast infection can complicate many dermatoses, especially allergic disease. There is a high prevalence in certain regions of the body: perioral, ears, axillae, feet (interdigital and nail folds), groin and perineum/anus. There is a musty malodorous smell, with greasy skin and coat, and erythema. Pruritus is common and there is a brown discoloration of the skin and coat. Chronic cases become alopecic, with lichenification and hyperpigmentation. Basset Hounds are predisposed to infection. Cytology is performed on samples taken from lesions using acetate tape impressions or superficial scrapings with a moistened blunt scalpel blade. *Malassezia pachydermatis* is a peanut-shaped yeast (see QRG 27.2). Culture can also be performed. Treatment is with topical antifungals (e.g. miconazole 2%/chlorhexidine 2% shampoo, selenium sulphide shampoo) or with oral ketoconazole (5–10 mg/kg orally q8–12h) or itraconazole (5 mg/kg orally q24h).

Contact dermatitis (irritant or hypersensitivity)

The distribution of lesions reflects those areas in contact with the offending substance. Seasonal reactions to vegetation can occur. Pruritus can be very intense, leading to significant self-trauma. There is often a history of a poor response to steroids (in contrast to atopic dermatitis, see above). The owner should be asked whether there has been a change in bedding, washing powder, carpet, walking routes, etc. Diagnosis can be through avoidance or by patch testing with samples of suspected materials. Management is ideally through avoidance of the offending material, but some cases will require symptomatic therapy.

PRACTICAL TIP

Never ask owners to make radical changes to their house, such as changing carpets, based on supposition

---

Cheyletiellosis

The surface-dwelling parasite *Cheyletiella* mainly affects the dorsum, with scaling, erythema and variable pruritus (more severe in young animals). *It is contagious and can affect both humans and animals.* The dog may have been recently acquired from, or stayed at, kennels. Acetate strip samples or superficial skin scrapings are examined for mites or eggs attached to hairs. Treatment is with a topical insecticide. The environment should also be treated.

Pediculosis

Louse infestation may involve *Linognathus setosus* (sucking louse) or *Trichodectes canis* (biting louse); the latter is an intermediate host for the *Dipylidium caninum* tapeworm. These lice are specific to the canine host. They are more common in young, old or debilitated individuals. Affected animals are pruritic. Direct observation of the coat will reveal the parasite, and then identification of species can be performed by microscopy. Treatment is with an appropriate insecticide for 3–4 weeks.

Demodicosis

Demodicosis can present as a pruritic problem, especially when there is secondary pyoderma. For details on *Demodex* see Alopecia, below.

Neotrombiculosis

Larval stages of the harvest mite *Neotrombicula* can affect the ventral abdomen (Figure 27.9), as well as the more usual sites involving the feet and pinnae. For more details, see Chapter 29.

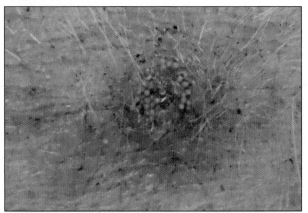

27.9 Orange *Neotrombicula* mites are visible on the ventral abdomen of this terrier.

Non-pruritic conditions

An approach to non-pruritic conditions, and conditions where pruritus is not the major clinical sign, is given in Figure 27.10.

Alopecia

Alopecia can be primary or can result from hair loss as a result of other lesions. The distribution pattern can help to differentiate causes (symmetrical, localized, diffuse/patchy).

Symmetrical alopecia

Causes of symmetrical hair loss are listed in Figure 27.11.

Hyperadrenocorticism: Hyperadrenocorticism (HAC; see also Chapter 17) is a relatively common endocrine condition; 85–90% of canine cases are pituitary-dependent, with the rest associated with adrenal neoplasia. A breed predisposition makes the Poodle, Boxer, Dachshund, Beagle, Boston Terrier and other terriers more commonly affected. HAC affects middle-aged to older animals.

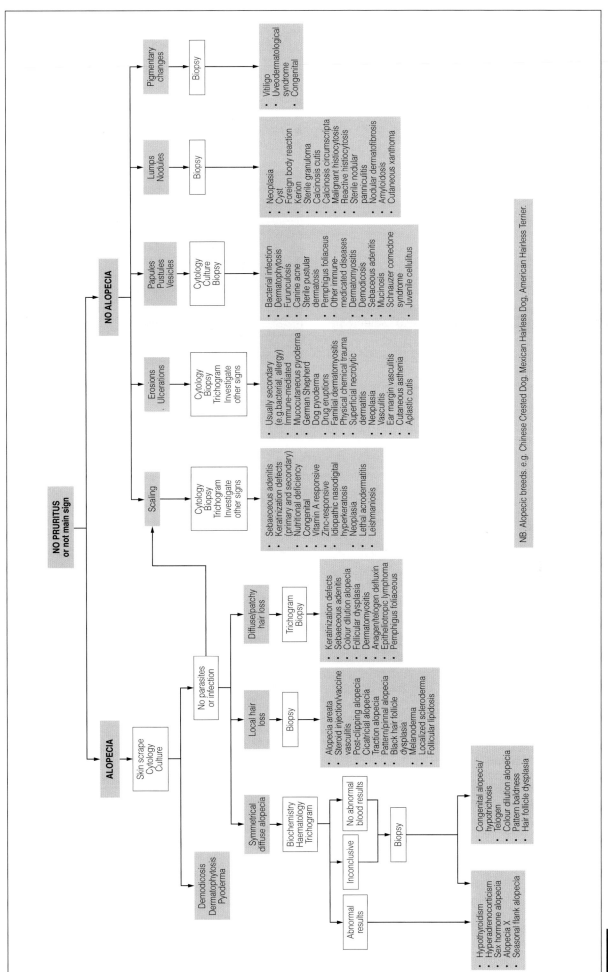

27.10 An approach to the dog with non-pruritic skin disease. Prior to embarking on using the chart, a thorough clinical history should be taken and physical examination carried out.

- **Hyperadrenocorticism**
- **Hypothyroidism**
- **Alopecia X**
- **Seasonal flank alopecia**
- Sex hormone-related alopecia
- Colour dilution alopecia
- Hair follicle dysplasia (most breed associated)
- Pattern baldness
- Congenital alopecia/hypotrichosis

27.11 Causes of symmetrical hair loss. The most common causes are in **bold**.

Dermatological signs include:

- Alopecia
- Hyperpigmentation
- Skin thinning
- Comedones
- Calcinosis cutis
- Phlebectasia (macular to papular erythematous lesions).

PRACTICAL TIP

While dogs with HAC are normally non-pruritic, the presence of secondary pyoderma or demodicosis may cause pruritus

Non-dermatological signs include:

- Polydipsia and polyuria (90% of cases)
- Polyphagia
- Swollen abdomen
- Muscle weakness
- Anoestrus/testicular atrophy.

Typical changes are seen in: biochemistry (raised cholesterol, alanine aminotransferase, alkaline phosphatase and glucose; decreased blood urea nitrogen); haematology (leucocytosis, neutrophilia, lymphopenia, eosinopenia); and urinalysis (low specific gravity and sometimes proteinuria). Radiography and ultrasonography can be used to assess the adrenal glands. Specific screening tests include the adrenocorticotrophic hormone (ACTH) stimulation test, dexamethasone suppression test and urine cortisol:creatinine ratio (the latter used only to rule out cases).

Trilostane is the treatment of choice (see Chapter 17). Alternatives are ketoconazole or mitotane (not available in the UK). Surgery is indicated in some cases, especially with adrenal neoplasia. More details on HAC can be found in the *BSAVA Manual of Canine and Feline Endocrinology.*

Hypothyroidism: Hypothyroidism is a relatively common endocrine disease. Certain breeds seem predisposed: Beagle, Great Dane, Golden Retriever, Dobermann, Irish Setter, Miniature Schnauzer, Cocker Spaniel, Shar Pei and Chow Chow. The peak age of onset is 5 years, and there is typically a slow progression. Dermatological signs include:

- Initially, a patchy alopecia at frictional sites (e.g. bridge of nose, tail)
- Later diffuse alopecia
- Hyperpigmentation
- Scaling and dry brittle hair
- Occasionally pyoderma and otitis externa.

The condition can present with a variety of these signs (Figure 27.12).

Non-dermatological signs include:

- Lethargy
- Weight gain
- Poor tolerance of cold and exercise
- Bradycardia
- Neurological and myopathy signs
- Corneal lipidosis.

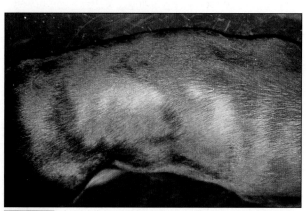

27.12 A middle-aged hypothyroid Dobermann bitch with hair loss, brittle hairs and hyperpigmentation.

Blood samples may show raised cholesterol and mild anaemia. Measuring total thyroxine and thyroid stimulating hormone is the diagnostic approach of choice. Other parameters that can be measured are free thyroxine and anti-thyroglobulin autoantibodies. The thyroid stimulation test (see *BSAVA Manual of Canine and Feline Endocrinology*) is regarded as the best available definitive test.

PRACTICAL TIPS

- Concurrent disease and certain medications can alter thyroid testing
- Euthyroid syndrome can give false-positive results

Treatment is through supplementation with thyroid medication (levothyroxine at 22 µg/kg orally q12h). After 8 weeks, post-pill screening allows dose adjustment. Therapy is lifelong.

Alopecia X: This denotes a broad group of conditions encompassing many that were previously referred to by various names, including growth hormone abnormalities, adrenal disease and follicular dysplasia in Nordic breeds. The cause in most cases has not been ascertained, but is likely a hormonal dysfunction. There is primary hair loss initially, especially on frictional areas (neck, thighs and tail), followed by the rest of the hairs in this region and the primary hairs on the trunk. The coat has a puppy-like appearance, which gradually thins, and hyperpigmentation develops. The head and legs are generally unaffected. Breeds affected are the Nordic breeds and poodles.

Careful history-taking and physical examination are used to rule out other diseases. Biopsy can be performed to rule conditions in or out. Interestingly, hair often regrows at biopsy sites.

Treatments that have been tried include castration, mitotane and trilostane (1–2 mg/kg q12h). It must be noted, however, that these are benign conditions, and consideration should be given as to whether the treatment might be worse than the condition. Melatonin (3–6 mg/dog q8–12h) has caused some cases to respond after several months (Paradis, 1999) and is tolerated well.

Seasonal flank alopecia: There is episodic hair loss, often seasonal, involving the trunk, especially the flanks. The condition is possibly related to photoperiod but has a genetic component, as there is a higher incidence in the Boxer, Bulldog and Airedale Terrier. There is a fairly rapid onset of benign alopecia of the thoracolumbar region, which lasts a few months and then resolves. Relapses often occur at the same time each year. Hyperpigmentation occurs and remains. History, clinical signs and biopsy results are used to rule out other diseases. This is a cosmetic disease, and the coat will regrow seasonally in most cases. Melatonin has been used with success when given before the onset.

Sex hormone-related alopecia: Several conditions have been associated with hormone abnormalities but, with the exception of hyperoestrogenism, most are probably due to other conditions. Hyperoestrogenism can be caused by testicular neoplasia, cystic ovaries and ovarian tumours. There is a symmetrical alopecia of the perineum and genital region that can extend along the ventrum to the neck, with hyperpigmentation. In males, nipple enlargement and a pendulous prepuce are seen, and an erythematous line is seen running along the median raphe of the prepuce. In females, nipple and vulvar enlargement along with oestrous cycle abnormalities are seen. Radiography and ultrasonography, and skin biopsy, can be performed to detect underlying causes. Treatment is by neutering.

Colour dilution alopecia: This is due to an abnormality in melanosomes, causing clumping and distortion of hair shafts. Several breeds have diluted variants in coat colour (e.g. Dobermann, Weimaraner, Yorkshire Terrier) and the alopecia only affects the diluted areas (Figure 27.13). Pyoderma can complicate the dry skin. Biopsy of the skin in diluted coat regions, along with trichograms, will demonstrate

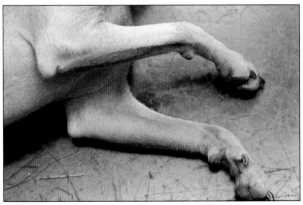

27.13 Colour dilution alopecia. This Dobermann has hair loss in the darker-haired regions but not in the lighter coloured hair regions. Note the clear demarcation between the areas.

melanin clumping. Oral treatments that have been tried include melatonin, retinoids, essential fatty acids and antibiotics (with variable to poor responses). Topical therapy with shampoos and emollients for dry skin have also been used to help improve skin condition.

Localized alopecia
Causes of localized alopecia are listed in Figure 27.14.

- **Black hair follicle dysplasia**
- **Post-clipping/traction/cicatricial alopecia**
- Alopecia areata
- Pattern and pinnal alopecia
- Melanoderma
- Follicular lipidosis
- Steroid injection or vaccine vasculitis
- Localized scleroderma (rare)

27.14 Causes of localized alopecia. The most common causes are in **bold**.

Black hair follicle dysplasia: This is an alopecia that affects only the black coated regions. Several breeds are affected (e.g. Bearded and Border Collies, Basset Hound, Beagle, Cavalier King Charles Spaniel). On biopsy, black-haired regions show melanin clumping while other areas are unaffected. Symptomatic therapy is used for the dry skin. There is no treatment for the hair loss.

Post-clipping, tractional and cicatricial alopecia: There is arrest of follicular growth following hair clipping, and the hair can take a long time to regrow. Tractional alopecia is usually associated with application of bands to tie hair up. No treatment is required other than checking for underlying endocrinopathies.

Alopecia areata: This is an uncommon focal or multifocal asymptomatic alopecia. It is an immune-mediated disease of anagen hair follicles. Biopsy of affected regions shows a lymphocyte accumulation around the hair follicle, among other changes. Occasionally microscopic examination of the hair will show shafts with suddenly tapered ends. Most cases recover with time, either spontaneously or after steroid treatment, albeit with lighter coloured hair. Topical and intralesional steroids are used.

Pattern and pinnal alopecia: This is a symmetrical localized hair loss associated with several fine-coated breeds (e.g. Dachshund). A ventral variant affects the perineum, thighs, ventrum including the neck, and behind the ears. A pinnal variant involves the outer surface of the pinnae. No treatment is necessary.

Melanoderma and alopecia in Yorkshire Terriers: Alopecia and hyperpigmentation affect the bridge of the nose and pinnae, and occasionally the tail and feet, in Yorkshire Terriers.

Follicular lipidosis: This occurs in Rottweilers, causing alopecia of the mahogany areas of the face and nose only; the black and other mahogany areas are unaffected.

Diffuse/patchy alopecia
Causes of diffuse or patchy alopecia are listed in Figure 27.15. Epitheliotropic lymphoma is discussed

- **Demodicosis**
- **Dermatophytosis**
- **Keratinization defects**
- **Sebaceous adenitis**
- Colour dilution alopecia
- Follicular dysplasias
- Dermatomyositis
- Anagen/telogen defluxion
- Epitheliotropic lymphoma
- Pemphigus foliaceus

27.15 Causes of diffuse/patchy alopecia. The most common causes are in **bold**.

under Lumps and nodules; pemphigus foliaceus is discussed under Papules, pustules and vesicles; primary and secondary keratinization abnormalities and sebaceous adenitis are discussed under Scaling and crusting; and colour dilution alopecia is discussed under Symmetrical alopecia.

PRACTICAL TIP

It is important to be aware of breeds that are naturally hairless, e.g. Chinese Crested Dog, Mexican Hairless Dog and American Hairless Terrier (Figure 27.16)

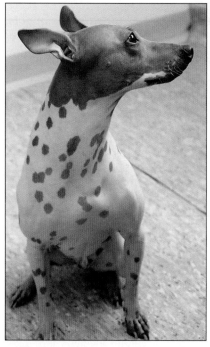

27.16

American Hairless Terrier. Note the lack of hair on the body that is normal for this breed.

Demodicosis: Increased numbers of *Demodex* mites (part of the normal skin 'flora') cause an inflammatory dermatosis when an immunological disorder allows proliferation. Lesions include alopecia, scaling, follicular casts, crusts, erythema, hyperpigmentation and lichenification. Ceruminous otitis can occur. Secondary bacterial infection occurs. Pruritus can occur, especially with *D. cornei*.

- *Localized* demodicosis is the most common form, with mild erythema and scale, mainly affecting the face (Figure 27.17), periorbital and periocular areas. This form usually resolves spontaneously.

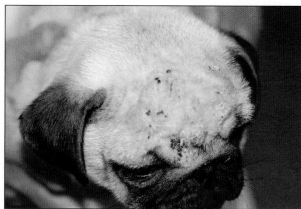

27.17 Patchy alopecia and associated self-trauma on the head of a 12-week-old Pug with localized demodicosis.

- *Generalized* demodicosis has more severe signs, with secondary infection that can lead to furunculosis, severe inflammation, exudation and a granulomatous reaction. It is important to look for underlying reasons.

Skin scrapings from affected areas (follicles should be squeezed prior to taking samples) and hair plucks may demonstrate the mites (see QRG 27.1). Biopsy may be necessary, especially with Shar Pei or foot lesions. There are several species (e.g. *D. canis*, *D. injai*, *D. cornei*).

Treatments include amitraz, ivermectin (200–600 µg/kg q24h) and milbemycin (1–2 mg/kg q24h). It is important to treat until two negative skin scrapings are achieved 2 weeks apart and then stop. A further skin scrape should be obtained 1 month after cessation of therapy to ensure remission.

Dermatophytosis: Dermatophyte fungi include *Microsporum canis* (often contracted from a cat), *Trichophyton mentagrophytes* (often from rodents) and *M. gypseum* (from the soil). Contact does not always result in infection. A variety of signs are seen, including alopecia, scales (Figure 27.18a), erythema, hyperpigmentation and pruritus. An uncommon presentation is a fungal nodule called a kerion. Dermatophytosis is mainly seen in young or older animals. *It is important to note that it is a zoonosis.* Diagnostic investigations include Wood's lamp investigation, microscopy, fungal culture and biopsy. Systemic antifungal treatment is used (e.g. ketoconazole at 10 mg/kg q24h; itraconazole at 5–10 mg/kg q24h). Topical antifungal therapy can be used with systemic therapy or, less effectively, as a sole treatment.

PRACTICAL TIP

Bacterial epidermal collarettes (Figure 27.18b) are commonly misdiagnosed as dermatophytosis

Follicular dysplasia: This is a non-colour-linked interruption of the normal hair cycle; both cyclical and structural interruption can occur. It is seen in various breeds with different presentations:

- Siberian Husky and Malamute: Onset is usually at 3–4 weeks but can be at 3–4 years. There is a

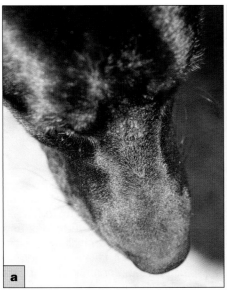

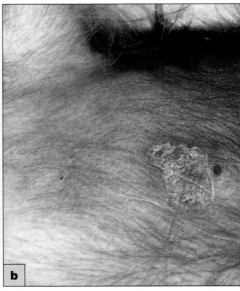

27.18

(a) Dermatophytosis with the usual presentation of alopecia and scaling in a cross-bred dog. **(b)** Circular lesions (epidermal collarettes) on a terrier with pyoderma. These are commonly mistakenly thought to be due to dermatophyte 'ringworm lesions', but nearly always represent a post pustular lesion.

change in colour and loss of guard hairs. The head and distal limbs are spared
- Dobermann, Miniature Pinscher and Manchester Terrier: Onset is at 1–4 years and the condition is cyclical
- Airedale Terrier, Boxer, Bulldog, Staffordshire Terrier, Wirehaired Griffon and Affenpinscher: Onset is at 2–4 years. There is flank and saddle region cyclical alopecia
- Irish Water Spaniel, Portuguese Water Dog and Curly Coated Retriever: Onset is at 2–4 years. There are fractured hairs. Initially the owner notices excess shedding when the coat is brushed, then there is partial thinning. Regrowth with weak hairs can occur but ultimately there is loss of the coat
- Other breeds reported include the Labrador Retriever and Sheltie.

Biopsy of affected areas is required for diagnosis. There is no specific treatment, but gentle grooming and skin care can help to minimize clinical signs.

Dermatomyositis: This is a hereditary inflammatory disease of the skin and muscles seen in collies, Shetland Sheepdogs and Baucerons and occasionally in other breeds. The condition is uncommon, but should be suspected if skin and muscle lesions are seen starting at an early age. Affected dogs can have difficulty eating and swallowing. Biopsy of skin and muscle are required for diagnosis. Treatment is difficult, but prednisolone (1–2 mg/kg q24h), vitamin E (200–500 IU q24h) and pentoxifylline (15 mg/kg q12h) have been used. Dermatomyositis carries a poor prognosis. Consult specialized texts for further details.

Anagen/telogen defluxion:
- Anagen defluxion is an abnormality of the hair follicle and shaft following an insult (e.g. drug, infection, endocrine, metabolic); it causes a sudden loss of hair but resolves with the next hair cycle.
- Telogen defluxion is an abrupt cessation of hair growth following an insult (e.g. high fever, pregnancy, shock, severe illness, surgery or anaesthesia) with hair loss 1–3 months later.

Diagnosis is via a trichogram (see QRG 27.3). Spontaneous resolution occurs in the next hair cycle.

Scaling and crusting
Causes of scaling and crusting are listed in Figure 27.19. Many dermatoses can result in secondary scaling and crusting, including allergic skin disease, skin infections, parasitic disease, endocrine and metabolic disorders and autoimmune disease. In such secondary cases, the underlying disease and seborrhoea need to be treated.

- **Sebaceous adenitis**
- **Primary keratinization disorders**
- **Secondary seborrhoea**
- Idiopathic nasodigital hyperkeratosis
- Zinc-responsive dermatosis
- Neoplasia
- Congenital disease (e.g. ichthyosis)
- Nutritional deficiency (e.g. generic dog food)
- Vitamin A-responsive (rare, adult onset in Cocker Spaniel)
- Epidermal dysplasia (rare, West Highland White Terrier)
- Lethal acrodermatitis (see Chapter 29)
- Leishmaniosis

27.19 Causes of scaling and crusting. The most common causes are in **bold**.

Sebaceous adenitis
This is caused by sebaceous gland inflammation, and affects young to middle-aged dogs. There is partial alopecia.

- Long-coated variant (e.g. Standard Poodle, Akita, Samoyed, German Shepherd Dog): Affected dogs have dull brittle hair with tightly adherent silvery white scale and follicular casts (Figure 27.20), initially occurring on the dorsum. Secondary infections can occur, resulting in pruritus and a smell. The Akita develops a more severe form with systemic illness. The German Shepherd Dog often has lesions starting on the tail and extending cranially.
- Short-coated variant (e.g. Vizsla, Dachshund): There is a 'moth-eaten' alopecia (serpiginous or circular) with mild scaling of the trunk, head and ears. Secondary infection is uncommon.

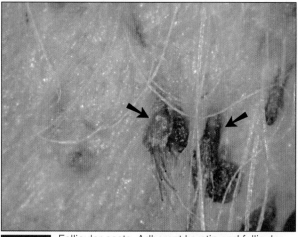

27.20 Follicular casts. Adherent keratin and follicular material on hair shafts (arrowed).

Diagnosis is via biopsy of affected areas; a granulomatous reaction is seen around the sebaceous glands.

The condition waxes and wanes naturally. Topical therapy involves spraying the affected areas with propylene glycol (50–70% in water) daily or the use of baby oil soaks. The preferred treatment is systemic therapy with ciclosporin (5 mg/kg orally q12h). Other therapies include tetracycline (250–500 mg/dog) + niacinamide (250–500 mg/kg) given in combination three times a day, essential fatty acids and retinoids. Secondary infections require antibiotics.

Primary keratinization disorders
Lesions vary from focal, thickly crusted plaques to diffuse and generalized scaling/crusting. There is also alopecia, erythema, lichenification and hyperpigmentation. The skin can be dry, greasy or a combination of both. Lesions are mainly truncal, though a ceruminous otitis can occur. Secondary infection is common (bacterial and *Malassezia*), especially in body folds, causing a malodorous change. The condition is exacerbated by inadequate diet, parasites, and by endocrine and metabolic disorders.

Various breeds can be affected, including the Cocker Spaniel, English Springer Spaniel, West Highland White Terrier, Basset Hound, Bulldog, German Shepherd Dog, Dobermann, Irish Setter, Shar Pei, Miniature Schnauzer, Cavalier King Charles Spaniel, Dachshund and Labrador Retriever. Biopsy of affected areas is helpful for diagnosis.

It is important to explain to the owner that the disease cannot be cured and the aim is to manage the clinical signs. Antiseborrhoeic shampoos and moisturizers are used:

- For dry skin, a shampoo containing salicylic acid and sulphur two or three times per week, followed by a moisturizer
- For greasy skin, shampoos containing benzoyl peroxidase or selenium sulphide are preferred, and more frequent applications.

Retinoids help in some cases. Secondary infections (a common reason for a sudden deterioration) should be treated.

Idiopathic nasodigital hyperkeratosis
Excess scale and crusting of the nasal planum and/or footpad is regarded as a senile change in breeds such as the Cocker Spaniel, Beagle, Bulldog and Basset Hound. The condition is generally asymptomatic but cracking can occur, with secondary infection resulting in pain. Footpad hyperkeratosis is seen in young dogs of certain breeds (see Chapter 29). Diagnosis is via biopsy of an affected region. Topical moisturizers can be helpful.

Epitheliotropic lymphoma
Epitheliotropic lymphoma (sometimes called mycosis fungoides) is a primary neoplastic cause of scaling, but is often missed. Scaling occurs in middle-aged to older animals. There are various syndromes and there is often a chronic history, often initially mimicking other diseases. There is exfoliative erythroderma, with erythema, scaling, depigmentation, alopecia and crusting (Figure 27.21), often involving allergic skin disease sites, mucocutaneous and oral sites. Most cases develop nodules or tumours within 3 months to 4 years. Pruritus is uncommon, except in the rare Sézary syndrome, where it can be severe and accompanied by lymphadenopathy. Diagnosis is via biopsy and cytology of lesions. Treatment is with lomustine (60–70 mg/m² orally q3–4wk for an average of 3–5 weeks), high doses of linoleic acid (3 ml/kg twice weekly), corticosteroids, retinoids or imiquimod. Advice should be sought from an oncologist. Prognosis is guarded to poor.

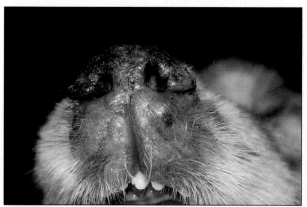

27.21 Cross-bred dog with alopecia, depigmentation, erythema and epidermal thickening of the nasal philtrum due to epitheliotropic lymphoma.

Zinc-responsive dermatosis
Alopecia, scaling, crusting and erythema of the eyelids (Figure 27.22), ears, feet, lips and external orifices is seen. One form occurs in young adult Siberian Huskies and Alaskan Malamutes; a second form is seen in rapidly growing large breeds, especially those fed on dry diets high in phytates. Diagnosis is via biopsy of affected lesions. Therapy includes oral zinc supplementation, with dietary change if indicated.

Erosions and ulceration
Conditions specifically associated with erosions or ulceration are listed in Figure 27.23. Dermatoses involving pruritus or self-damage, and rupture of pustules or vesicles, can also result in erosions or ulceration. Anal furunculosis is discussed in Chapter 30.

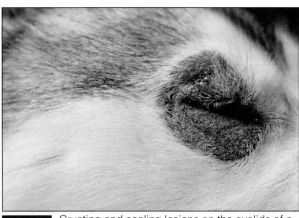

27.22 Crusting and scaling lesions on the eyelids of a young Siberian husky with zinc-responsive dermatosis.

- **Physical/chemical damage**
- **Mucocutaneous pyoderma**
- **German Shepherd Dog folliculitis, furunculosis, cellulitis**
- Drug-induced eruptions: erythema multiforme, toxic epidermal necrolysis
- Familial dermatophytosis
- Superficial necrolytic dermatitis
- Discoid and systemic lupus erythematosus
- Pemphigus foliaceus and bullous pemphigoid
- Neoplasia
- Vasculitis
- Cutaneous asthenia (collagen abnormality)
- Aplasia cutis

27.23 Conditions specifically associated with erosions or ulceration. The most common conditions are in **bold**.

Physical/chemical damage
Damage to the overlying epithelium (e.g. from chemical burns) should be treated with cleaning and the use of topical antibacterial ointments to deter secondary infection.

Mucocutaneous pyoderma
This is a relatively common condition but of unknown aetiology. It occurs in German Shepherd Dogs and crosses. There is swelling and erythema, with crusting and fissures of the mucocutaneous junctions, especially the lips. Diagnosis is via biopsy and cytology of the affected areas. Topical and systemic antimicrobials are used for a minimum of 4 weeks, but relapses occur.

German Shepherd Dog folliculitis, furunculosis and cellulitis
This is an immunologically mediated disease and is often severe. It affects middle-aged German Shepherd Dogs. Lesions include ulceration, fistulas, furunculosis, alopecia and hyperpigmentation, involving the rump, dorsum, ventral abdomen and thighs. Cellulitis can develop, along with pain. Diagnosis is via biopsy, cytology and culture of lesions.

It is essential to clip affected areas and to apply topical antimicrobial washes about twice a week. Long courses of systemic antibiotics are required. Relapses are not uncommon.

Drug-induced eruptions
Various drugs have been implicated (e.g. potentiated sulphonamides, cefalexin).

- Erythema multiforme (EM) can also have a viral, bacterial, neoplastic or idiopathic aetiology. Lesions include mucocutaneous vesicles leading to ulceration and erosion, oral lesions, and involvement of the footpads (lameness) and pinnae. Macular papular rashes occur (can be pruritic), as well as exfoliative erythroderma, with scaling. Urticaria and neuroangioedema can occur. Types of lesion include serpiginous, polycyclic and bull's eye lesions.
- Toxic epidermal necrolysis (TEN) is probably a more severe form of EM. Affected animals can have depression, fever and anorexia.

Diagnosis is via biochemistry, haematology, serology for antinuclear antibody (ANA) and skin biopsy, and reviewing the drug history. Any implicated medication should be stopped. Ciclosporin or pentoxifylline may help to reduce clinical signs. Corticosteroid use is controversial.

> **WARNING**
>
> TEN is a severe disease. Referral should be considered as it usually requires intensive care. Prognosis is poor

Superficial necrolytic dermatitis
This is a rare and severe skin disease. There is mucocutaneous erosion and ulceration of the lips, eyelids and anus, later developing crusts. Hyperpigmentation and lichenification of the skin are seen. Footpad lesions are prominent and fissures can develop, leading to pain. Pruritus can occur. Lesions involve pressure points, pinnae and genitalia. Secondary infection is common. Skin signs often precede systemic signs of lethargy, anorexia and weight loss. Polydipsia and polyuria can develop. Blood analysis can show liver enzyme changes and hypoalbuminaemia. Skin biopsy of lesions shows characteristic histopathological changes. The prognosis is guarded to poor, and therapy is aimed at treating secondary infections and supportive therapy for the systemic disease.

Discoid and systemic lupus erythematosus
- Discoid lupus erythematosus (DLE) is a relatively common immune-mediated disease and is relatively mild. Certain breeds are over-represented: collies, German Shepherd Dog, Siberian Husky, Sheltie, Alaskan Malamute, Chow Chow. Possible causes include drug reaction, UV light exposure and viral infection. Depigmentation and erosion or ulceration of the nasal planum is seen. The face, ears and mucous membranes are less often affected.
- Systemic lupus erythematosus (SLE) can be associated with some or all of a range of systemic signs, such as swollen joints, oral lesions, fever, lymphadenopathy, splenomegaly, hepatomegaly, and cardiac and pleural disease.

Diagnosis is through biopsy of lesional areas. Further tests include serology for ANA, the lupus erythematosus test and the Coombs' test; abnormal results are mostly seen in SLE but not DLE.

Treatments include tetracycline/niacinamide, vitamin E, topical steroids, prednisolone ± azathioprine or chlorambucil, pentoxifylline, ciclosporin and tacrolimus ointment. Exposure to UV light should be avoided. Prognosis is good for DLE but guarded for SLE.

Pemphigus complex and bullous pemphigoid

Pemphigus complex is uncommon to rare but may be seen in middle-aged to older dogs. Bullous pemphigoid is very rare.

Pemphigus foliaceus is the commonest condition in the group and is seen in the Akita, Bearded Collie, Chow Chow, Dachshund, Dobermann, Cocker Spaniel and Shar Pei amongst others. Often it is a reaction to medications (e.g. sulphonamides, cephalosporins). Vesicles, pustules leading to crusts (Figure 27.24), scaling, epidermal collarettes, erosions and alopecia are seen. Hyperkeratosis of the footpads, with fissuring can occur. Various nail abnormalities may also be seen. Lesions are located on the nasal planum, muzzle, periorbital area, pinnae and trunk and may also be found on the paws. Lymphadenopathy, depression and fever may occur, with variable pain and pruritus. Cytology of the pustules may show acantholytic cells (see QRG 27.2); biopsy of intact pustules is usually diagnostic. Various treatments are used, including corticosteroids, azathioprine, chlorambucil, ciclosporin, dapsone, cyclophosphamide and chrysotherapy. See specialist texts for therapeutic details and other syndromes in the pemphigus complex.

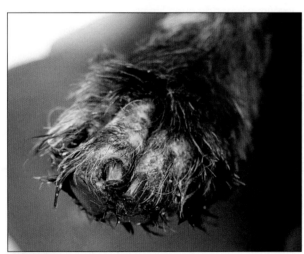

27.24 Pustules and crusting on the paw of a Cocker Spaniel with pemphigus foliaceus.

Vasculitis

Vasculitis is an inflammation of blood vessels. Causes include SLE, cold agglutinin, frostbite, disseminated intravascular coagulopathy, lymphoreticular tumours, drugs, vaccines, tick bite and staphylococcal/food hypersensitivity, but about 50% of cases are idiopathic. There is palpable purpura, haemorrhagic bullae, necrosis and 'punched out' ulcers involving the extremities, paws, pinnae, lips, tail and oral cavity. The skin can be painful when touched. Systemic signs include lethargy, lymphadenopathy, fever and weight loss; hepatic, renal or central nervous system involvement can occur. Various types of vasculitis are seen, including: nasal

arteritis (St Bernard, Schnauzer); juvenile polyarteritis (Beagle); ear margin vasculitis (Dachshund); familial cutaneous vasculopathy (German Shepherd Dog); and cutaneous and renal vasculopathy (Greyhound). Diagnosis is via biopsy of ulcerated areas. Further tests to perform may include ANA serology, Coombs' test and cold agglutinin assay. The underlying disease needs to be treated in addition to immunosuppressive therapy. Prognosis is guarded.

Papules, pustules and vesicles

Conditions that present primarily with papules, pustules or vesicles are listed in Figure 27.25. Bacterial infections are the primary cause of papule/pustule presentations and are discussed under Pruritic conditions (see Superficial pyoderma). Dermatophytosis, demodicosis and dermatomyositis are discussed under Alopecia; pemphigus foliaceus is discussed under Erosions and ulceration; sebaceous adenitis is discussed under Scaling and crusting.

- **Bacterial infection** (see Pruritus)
- **Furunculosis**
- **Demodicosis**
- **Dermatophytosis**
- Canine acne
- Juvenile cellulitis
- Pemphigus foliaceus and other autoimmune diseases
- Schnauzer comedone syndrome
- Sebaceous adenitis
- Mucinosis
- Dermatomyositis
- Sterile pustular dermatosis

27.25 Conditions presenting primarily with papules, pustules or vesicles. The most common conditions are in **bold**.

Furunculosis

This is a deep follicular bacterial infection, requiring prolonged antibiotic therapy. It has been discussed previously. It is often pruritic, and discharging.

Canine acne

Canine acne is a deep folliculitis and furunculosis involving the chin and lip of young dogs. It occurs almost exclusively in short-haired breeds (e.g. Boxer, Bulldog, Great Dane, Rottweiler, Mastiff). Initially it presents as erythematous papules or pustules, progressing to furunculosis with repeated trauma. It is pruritic, but can be painful. Skin scrapes and cytology are used to rule out demodicosis and dermatophytosis. Chronic lesions may be cultured. Mild lesions are treated with a benzoyl peroxidase shampoo and topical fucidin or mupirocin. More severe cases will require an appropriate course of antibiotics (3–6 weeks). Scarring can occur with chronic cases.

Juvenile cellulitis

Juvenile cellulitis ('puppy strangles') is an uncommon granulomatous/pustular dermatosis of the face and pinnae of puppies aged 3 weeks to 4 months. Various breeds can be affected but the Golden Retriever, Dachshund and Gordon Setter are more susceptible. Initial swelling occurs on the eyelids, lip and muzzle, with enlarged submandibular lymph nodes. There is progression to pustules all over the face and ears, especially the pinnae; these are often painful. There may also be lethargy and pyrexia. Some cases have lesions on the genitals and perianal region. Cytology shows pyogranulomatous inflammation but no microorganisms. Culture of lesions is usually sterile. Biopsy of lesions can be done if required. Aggressive and early therapy with steroids is necessary to prevent severe scarring.

Schnauzer comedone syndrome
Multiple comedones appear along the back in Miniature Schnauzers. There are palpable papules which can become infected. Biopsy can aid diagnosis. Topical antiseborrhoeic therapy is helpful. Human acne wipes, benzoyl peroxidase gels and shampoos can also be used and, if there is no response, selenium sulphide shampoo. The condition can be controlled but not cured.

Mucinosis
This condition can occur secondary to other conditions but an idiopathic form occurs in the Shar Pei. Excessive skin folding and vesicles are seen, with an abnormal accumulation of mucin in the skin. Biopsy is helpful, and a sticky very viscous liquid can be expressed (Figure 27.26). Corticosteroid therapy can help if the condition is problematic.

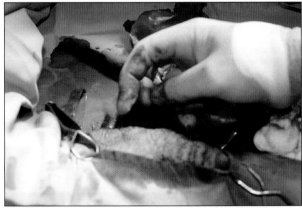

27.26 A young Shar Pei with mucinosis undergoing excessive skin fold removal. Sticky tenacious fluid can be seen coming from the resection site.

Lumps and nodules
Causes of lumps and nodules are listed in Figure 27.27. Skin tumours and cysts are discussed in Chapter 28.

- **Neoplasia/cysts**
- **Foreign body reaction**
- **Callus**
- Calcinosis cutis
- Calcinosis circumscripta
- Idiopathic sterile granuloma and pyogranuloma
- Sterile nodular panniculitis
- Kerion (dermatophyte nodule, uncommon)
- Amyloidosis
- Nodular dermatofibrosis
- Cutaneous xanthoma
- Malignant histiocytosis
- Reactive histiocytosis

27.27 Causes of lumps and nodules. The most common causes are in **bold**.

Foreign body reaction
Various items can be involved, e.g. grass awns, thorns, sticks, gun pellets. The reaction appears as a localized lesion with draining tracts and/or nodules. Surgical resection of the lesion and removal of the foreign body is required. Antibiotics are prescribed to clear associated infections.

Callus
This is a very common problem of older dogs, especially in large breeds and overweight animals. The elbow and hock are most commonly affected, but calluses may also occur on the sternum. They are a normal response to pressure and friction, but can become excessively thickened and infected, with erosion and ulceration. Diagnosis is through visual inspection. Protective bandaging, topical skin softeners and antimicrobial creams can be helpful. Some cases may require surgical resection, but there is a risk of wound breakdown.

Calcinosis cutis
Lesions develop secondary to iatrogenic hyperglucocorticoidism. Firm gritty papules, plaques and nodules with yellow/white contents are seen on the dorsum, axillae and groin. The condition is often mistaken for pyoderma in the early stages. Biopsy of affected skin can demonstrate calcium deposits, which along with the history, establishes the diagnosis. Weaning the dog off steroids over 2–12 months will usually cause lesions to resolve.

Calcinosis circumscripta
This is an uncommon condition of young large-breed dogs, especially the German Shepherd Dog. Lesions appear as firm white deposits, progressing to ulceration with a white discharge. They often occur at pressure points, but can occur on the tongue and palate. Diagnosis is from the physical appearance and lesion biopsy. Treatment is surgical excision of the lesions.

Idiopathic sterile granuloma or pyogranuloma
This is an uncommon inflammatory reaction, with collies, Weimaraners, Great Danes, Boxers and Golden Retrievers over-represented. Usually there are multiple lesions on the bridge of the nose, muzzle, periocular area, pinnae and paws. The lesions appear as firm papules, plaques or nodules, which are painless and non-pruritic. Ulceration and alopecia can develop. Diagnosis is via biopsy of the lesions; culture is usually negative for infection. Surgery is indicated for solitary lesions. If there are multiple lesions then systemic therapy is required, e.g. prednisolone (2–4 mg/kg q24h, then tapered) possibly with the addition of azathioprine (2 mg/kg q24h, tapering after response). There have been reports of response to tetracycline + niacinamide in combination.

Sterile nodular panniculitis
This is an uncommon condition. Affected dogs have deep nodules with ulceration and discharge, and can be systemically ill. There are various causes. Diagnosis is via biopsy of affected areas and cytology. Culture is used to rule out infectious causes. Surgical resection of small lesions can be performed and/or treatment with prednisolone (provided there is no infection).

Pigmentation disorders

Some causes of pigmentation disorders are listed in Figure 27.28.

- ■ **Inflammatory hyperpigmentation**
- ■ **Vitiligo**
- ■ Uveodermatological syndrome
- ■ Congenital conditions
- ■ Canine acanthosis nigricans (Dachshund)

27.28 Some causes of pigmentation disorders. The most common causes are in **bold**.

Inflammatory hyperpigmentation

This is the commonest cause of pigment being deposited in the skin. It occurs following an inflammatory reaction in the skin and is a useful indicator of previous inflammatory lesions, for example in atopic dogs.

Vitiligo

Vitiligo is a loss of pigmentation in the skin and hair. The cause is unknown. It is found in young dogs, and breeds affected include the Belgian Tervuren, Rottweiler (Figure 27.29), German Shepherd Dog and Dobermann. There is no treatment. The condition can wax and wane, which may lead people to presume a response to supplements.

Uveodermatological syndrome

The skin lesions of depigmentation usually follow uveitis. There is ulceration and crusting late on in disease. Certain breeds are over-represented, including the Akita, Chow Chow, Samoyed and Siberian Husky. It is recommended to consult an ophthalmic practitioner, as the uveitis can be difficult to resolve.

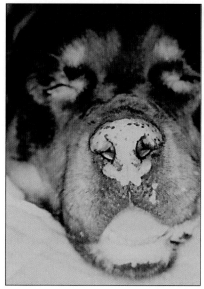

27.29

Vitiligo in a 5-year-old female Rottweiler, showing loss of pigmentation of the nasal planum, eyelids and oral mucosa.

References and further reading

Favrot C, Steffan J, Seewald W *et al.* (2010) A prospective study on the clinical features of chronic canine atopic dermatitis and its diagnosis. *Veterinary Dermatology* 21, 23–31

Guaguère E, Prélaud P and Craig M (2008) *A Practical Guide to Canine Dermatology*, Mérial–Kalianxis, Paris

Jackson H and Marsella R (2007) *BSAVA Manual of Canine and Feline Dermatology, 3rd edn*. BSAVA Publications, Gloucester

Miller WH, Griffin CE and Campbell KL (2013) *Muller and Kirk's Small Animal Dermatology, 7th edn*. Saunders Elsevier, St. Louis

Mooney C and Peterson M (2012) *BSAVA Manual of Canine and Feline Endocrinology, 4th edn*. BSAVA Publications, Gloucester

Paradis M (1999) Melatonin therapy in canine alopecia. In: *Kirk's Current Veterinary Therapy XIII*, ed. ED Bonagura, pp. 546–549. WB Saunders, Philadelphia

Rhodes KH and Werner AH (2002) *Blackwell's Five-Minute Veterinary Consult Clinical Companion: Small Animal Dermatology, 2nd edn*. Wiley-Blackwell, Oxford

QRG 27.1 Skin scraping for parasites

Equipment

- ■ Microscope slides
- ■ Coverslips
- ■ Scalpel blades (No. 15/21, blunted by rubbing sharp edge on metal)
- ■ Dental spatula
- ■ Liquid paraffin
- ■ Potassium hydroxide 10% (KOH)

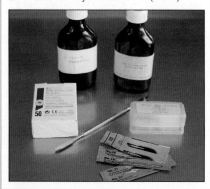

Technique

1 Identify representative lesions on the skin; fresh lesions are best.

2 Carefully clip hair from the area, avoiding losing any surface features such as scale and crust.

3 Apply a small amount of liquid paraffin or KOH to the scalpel blade or spatula (this helps collection of scraped material on to the instrument).

- ■ If looking for *Sarcoptes* mites it is useful to use potassium hydroxide as this helps clear the debris.

4 Scrape at a 45 degree angle to the skin, along the line of hair growth, and deep enough that blood can be seen seeping from capillaries.

- ■ A dental spatula is preferable where skin is delicate, e.g. eyelids.
- ■ Squeezing the skin prior to skin scraping can aid recovery of certain mites, e.g. *Demodex*.

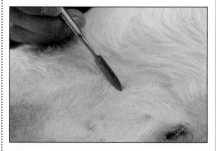

5 Transfer the accumulated scraped material from the instrument to a slide, and apply a coverslip. This last point is essential for successful viewing of samples. ▶

QRG 27.1 *continued*

6 Place the slide on the microscope stage and examine using the low power objective lens (X4 or X10).

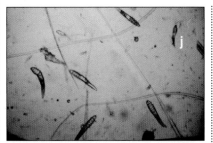

Demodex canis mites: note the characteristic cigar shape of the adults. j = juvenile. (Original magnification X100)

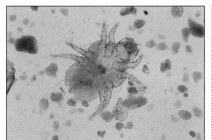

Cheyletiella mite from a skin scrape. (Original magnification X200)

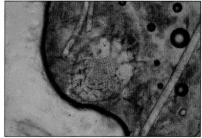

Sarcoptes scabiei mite from a deep skin scrape. (Original magnification X200; examined using potassium hydroxide)

QRG 27.2 Skin cytology

Equipment

- Clear adhesive tape
- Dental spatula
- Microscope slides
- Romanowsky-type stain (e.g. Diff-Quik)

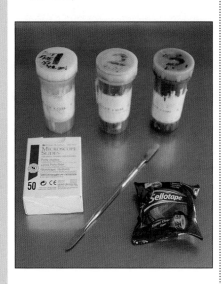

Tape strip technique

1 Take a piece of adhesive tape, approximately one and a half times the length of a microscope slide, holding it by the ends and not touching the central portion. Apply the tape to lesional skin, pressing it several times against the same area to obtain a good sample.

2 Attach the tape to one end of a microscope slide and fold the tape over on itself to leave the sticky surface, containing the sample, uppermost. Then fold the other end round to stick on the slide.

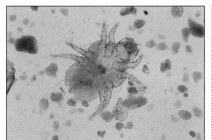

3 Stain the sample. If using Diff-Quik:

i. Dip the slide in the first stain (light blue) for only a couple of seconds; this avoids the tape clouding.
ii. Dip the slide into the red stain for five to ten 1-second dips.
iii. Dip the slide into the dark blue stain for five to ten 1-second dips.
iv. Rinse the slide with water.

4 Undo one end of the tape. Wrap the tape around the slide so that the stained material is sandwiched between the tape and the slide, and reapply the free end to the slide.

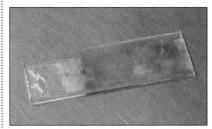

5 Dry the slide and examine under the microscope, initially with the low power objective to identify significant areas, then in more detail using the high power objective (usually X1000, with oil emersion).

Direct smear technique

1 Apply a microscope slide directly to a lesion that is moist, discharging or ulcerated.

- Alternatively, a dental spatula, with a small amount of water applied, can be used to scrape even dry or greasy areas, and obtain samples that can be smeared on to a microscope slide.

2 Air-dry the slide and stain (see above).

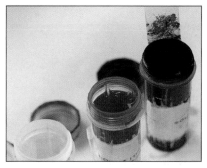

3 When rinsing, it is advisable to run the water on the non-stained back of the slide, letting the water flow around it, to avoid washing off material.

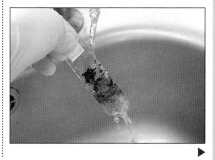

▶

QRG 27.2 *continued*

4 Allow the slide to dry, and examine as described above.

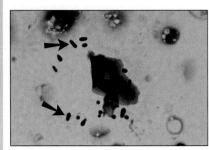

Cytology sample showing characteristic peanut-shaped *Malassezia* organisms (arrowed). (Diff-Quik; original magnification X1000, examined under oil emersion)

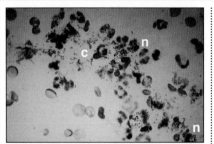

Cytology sample from a pyoderma lesion showing bacterial cocci (c) and active phagocytosis by neutrophils (n). (Diff-Quik; original magnification X1000, examined under oil emersion)

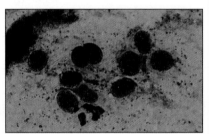

Mast cells containing granules, including a dividing cell, in a sample from a mastocytoma. (Diff-Quik; original magnification X1000, examined under oil emersion)

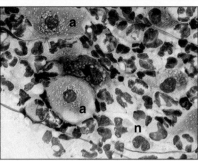

Sample from a pustule in a case of pemphigus foliaceous showing epithelial cells (acantholytic (a) cells), that have lost their adhesion to adjacent cells, giving them a rounded appearance. Neutrophils (n) are also present. (Diff-Quik; original magnification X1000, examined under oil emersion)

QRG 27.3 Obtaining a trichogram

Equipment

- Microscope slides
- Coverslips
- Liquid paraffin
- Artery forceps

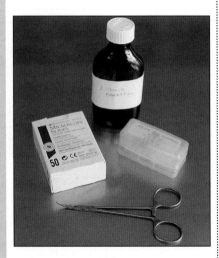

Technique

1 Apply a small amount of liquid paraffin to a slide.

2 Select a representative group of hairs and pluck using artery forceps.

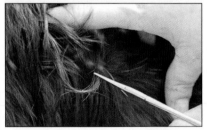

PRACTICAL TIPS

- Do not pluck using fingers, as anagen hairs will likely not be removed
- Note how easily the hair is removed: dead hairs epilate easily (e.g. as seen in endocrine or immune-mediated disease)

3 Align the hairs on the slide in the liquid paraffin, trying to keep the roots together, and apply a coverslip.

4 Examine the shafts, tips and roots of the hairs, using the X4 or X10 objective lens. Look for:

- Telogen and anagen hairs
- Shaft pathology
- Fractured hair (broken tips may indicate pruritus)
- Parasites
- Infection.

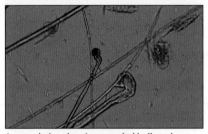

Anagen hairs, showing rounded bulb ends. (Original magnification X100)

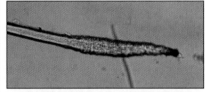

Telogen hair showing a tapered end. (Original magnification X200)

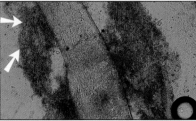

Dermatophytosis: arthroconidia can be seen surrounding the hair shaft (arrowed). (Original magnification X400)

QRG 27.4 Skin biopsy

Equipment

- Small surgical kit:
  - Scalpel handle and No. 15 blade
  - Small scissors
  - Tissue forceps
  - Artery forceps
  - Needle-holders
- Biopsy hook
- Biopsy punch 4–8 mm
- 2 metric (3/0 USP) suture material (e.g. polyglactin 910)
- Pots of formalin
- Plain pot

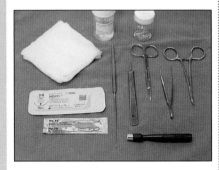

Patient preparation

- Biopsy may be performed with the dog sedated and with local anaesthesia, or under general anaesthesia, depending on the location of the lesion, how painful the area is, and the dog's temperament and health.
- For local anaesthesia, lidocaine without adrenaline should be used to avoid altering the pathology. The solution is infiltrated around the lesion, avoiding iatrogenic damage. After 10–15 minutes the area is checked for numbness.

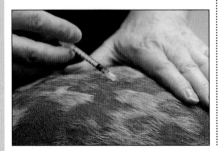

- Haired areas are clipped gently, avoiding removing surface features such as scale and crusts.
- Aseptic surgical preparation is not performed, to avoid removing surface features.

Technique

> **PRACTICAL TIPS**
>
> Lesion selection is very important and will affect the result:
> - Ulcerated lesions should be sampled at the edge, including both sides of the ulcer's periphery
> - Samples should be obtained from both primary and secondary lesions
> - Avoid self-traumatized lesions, which contain misleading changes

1 Make an elliptical incision with the scalpel around the sample area.

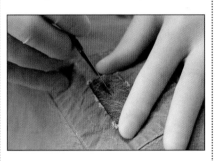

- If a biopsy punch is used, pressure is applied with the punch perpendicular to the skin and rotated in one direction only.

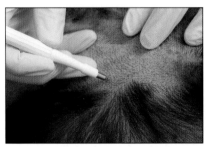

2 Lift the sample, ideally using a biopsy hook (atraumatic forceps can be used to grasp the deep fat).

3 Cut the sample free and transfer it to a sample pot (formalin for histopathology; plain for culture).

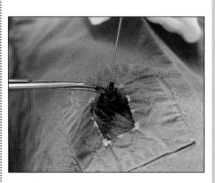

4 Close the wound using two or three sutures.

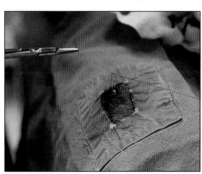

5 Send the samples to a recognized dermatohistopathologist.

> **PRACTICAL TIPS**
>
> - As many representative samples as is practical should be submitted, to ensure a good return
> - The submission form should contain a detailed history
> - Discuss the case with the pathologist

Pet's name: .... **Owner's name:** ....

Breed: .... **Sex:** .... **Age:** ....

Vaccination status: .... **Last worming:** ....

Current medications: ....

Describe the skin complaint ....
....

Circle the signs you have noticed: Scratching   Biting   Chewing   Licking   Rubbing   Dry skin   Dandruff   Reddened skin
Greasy skin   Smell

At what age did it begin? ....

Where on the body did it begin? ....

What did it look like initially? ....

How did it progress from there? ....

Circle 1 or 2 for each lesion if involved (1 for initially and 2 for now): Nose 1 2 Around eyes 1 2 Ears 1 2 Neck 1 2 Back 1 2
Hindend 1 2 Chest 1 2 Abdomen 1 2 Armpits 1 2 Groin 1 2 Forelegs 1 2 Forepaws 1 2 Hindlegs 1 2 Hindpaws 1 2

Rate the severity of the problem, 1 for mild to 5 for severe: ....

How itchy is the problem? 0 for not to 10 for severe: ....

Has the condition worsened with time? ....

Is the problem worse at any time of year, and if so when? ....

Does the condition alter with travelling to different areas? ....

If so, does your dog travel abroad and to where? ....

Describe where your pet sleeps and on what: ....

Are there any other pets and are they affected? ....

Do any of your dog's relatives have skin problems? ....

Do any in-contact people have skin problems? ....

List the percentage of time your dog spends Indoors   Outdoors

What medications have been prescribed for the problem? ....

Did any medications help? ....

Have steroids been prescribed? If so, what was the response? ....

Do you treat your pets for fleas? If so, with what and how often? ....

Do you treat the house for fleas? If so, with what and how often? ....

List all the foods fed to your dog, including all treats: ....
....

Does your pet have any of these signs? Cough Sneeze Runny eyes Vomiting Diarrhoea Excessive thirst Excessive appetite
Limp Lethargy Poor exercise tolerance Ear infections (please circle)

Have you any observations you would like to note? ....
....
....

An example of a questionnaire for a dog with a skin problem.

Lumps and bumps

Robert Williams

Owners will often present a dog having noticed one of the following:

- Lump
- Swelling
- Nodule
- Bump
- Tumour
- Boil
- Abscess
- Mass.

These terms are, colloquially, often used interchangeably to refer to cutaneous or subcutaneous accumulations of tissue that form a noticeable lesion either visually or on palpation. For simplicity, the term 'mass' will be used throughout this chapter.

Broadly, masses can be thought of in three ways:

- Simple masses (e.g. a small injection site reaction)
- Tumours (benign or malignant)
- Other masses (e.g. perineal hernia).

There are numerous possible explanations for the finding of a mass, from the 'simple' (e.g. a small subcutaneous lipoma in the flank) to the 'complex' (e.g. a grade III mast cell tumour affecting the prepuce). This chapter will describe a simple approach to dealing with the presentation of a mass as the chief complaint.

History

Pertinent questions might include the following:

- How long has the mass been present?
- Has it changed in size, appearance or colour recently?
- Has the animal had recent surgery?
- Has the dog been involved in a fight or any other traumatic experience?
- Where does the owner walk the dog; is the dog on or off the lead?
- Is the dog a working dog?
- Has the dog had any recent injections?
- Has the dog had any previous masses; if so, what were they?

- Has the dog been licking or chewing the mass?
- Has there been any discharge from the mass?

Some history findings and possible interpretations are noted in Figure 28.1.

Characteristic	Comment	Interpretation
Size	Constant size for a long duration	Suggests benignity or low grade of malignancy
	Small then suddenly large (or *vice versa*); or rapid growth	Rapid alteration in size may suggest: a change to malignancy; degranulation of mast cells; haemorrhage; or a burst abscess
Time present	Short duration: days to 1–2 weeks Long duration: >2 weeks to months to years	A mass present for a long time suggests benignity
Pruritus	Some owners will be alerted to the presence of a mass by the dog licking or chewing an area	Masses may be itchy, due to: release of histamine (e.g. mast cell tumour, urticaria); or inflammation (e.g. ulcerated carcinoma, interdigital granuloma)
Discharge	An obvious discharge may alert an owner to a problem	A burst abscess, infected ulcerated tumour or a seroma may all produce or leak fluid
Recent surgery	Several possible masses can be associated with recent surgery	Examples: seroma; incisional dehiscence; wound infection; suture reaction; failure of surgery
Recent injection	A soft non-painful pea- to bean-sized swelling at the site of a subcutaneous injection	Sterile granulomas occur occasionally following subcutaneous injection
Previous history	Seasonal problem	Interdigital granuloma; urticaria
	History of lipoma/wart, etc.	Warts/lipomas can be multiple
	Previous malignancy	Recurrence of tumour

28.1 History findings and how they can relate to the mass.

Clinical examination

A thorough clinical examination is very important.

PRACTICAL TIP

Try to avoid specific examination of the mass until the end of the examination. This will help prevent overlooking anything else that is pertinent

---

General points to consider are as follows:

- Is the mass solitary or are there multiple sites affected?
- Are there any signs of systemic illness? Malignant tumours can produce a variety of systemic signs. For example: hypercalcaemia in anal gland adenocarcinoma; vomiting/melaena due to histamine release from mast cell tumours; coughing associated with pulmonary metastases. It is important to note all systemic signs at the time of examination of a mass as they may be helpful in clinical staging once a diagnosis has been reached
- Are there more pressing medical problems affecting the dog than the mass, e.g. an elderly dog presented with a lipoma that is in obvious congestive heart failure?
- Is there any lymph node involvement, especially of the local draining lymph node?

It is important to record specific details of the mass, for example:

- Size
- Cutaneous *versus* subcutaneous
- Intact or ulcerated
- Hairy or hairless
- Sessile or pedunculated
- Red, hot or swollen
- Painful or not.

Diagnostic tests

On completion of the clinical examination, further information as to the type of mass can be acquired by examination of tissue samples obtained via fine-needle aspiration (FNA; see QRG 28.1) or biopsy (see QRG 28.2). The choice of sampling technique often depends on circumstance (such as owner finances, owner interest, temperament of the dog); however, there are several points to bear in mind.

- Making FNA a routine procedure as part of the examination of any mass, and the default tissue sampling technique, is good practice. The benefits are:
  - An appreciation by clients of an efficient and economic in-house test
  - The ability to identify benign lesions not requiring treatment, e.g. injection reaction
  - Avoiding the 'keep your eye on it' approach that risks missing a potentially serious problem.
- Whichever technique is employed, it should be remembered that the mass may be malignant and that a planned excision of the mass may be required, including a wide and deep margin.

- With FNA and incisional biopsy, the needle tract (or surgical approach) should pass only through tissue that would be excised in any future surgical treatment of the mass, and should not add to the area that would need to be excised.
- It is important to avoid seeding tumour cells into what may well be the tumour-free margin.
- Excisional biopsy should not be used in cases where there is a suspicion of a malignant mass, especially of a tissue type that requires a large tumour-free margin, such as a mast cell tumour (MCT) or a sarcoma.
  - Excisional biopsy could be employed when there is a likelihood of a mammary gland tumour (MGT) or lipoma, where the aim is to treat the mass and obtain tissue simultaneously and large tumour-free margins will not be required.

Tissue sampling options for suspected mass types are summarized in Figure 28.2. Cytological features of malignancy are described in Figure 28.3.

Mass type suspected	FNA	Incisional biopsy	Excisional biopsy
Simple			
Abscess	✓	✗	✗
Granuloma	✓	✗	✓
Sebaceous cyst	✓	✗	✓
Interdigital granuloma	✓	✗	✓
Seroma	✓*	✗	✗
Benign			
Lipoma	✓	✗	✓
Mammary gland tumour	✓	✓	✓
Histiocytoma	✓	✓	✓
Sebaceous adenoma	✓	✓	✓
Trichoepithelioma	✓	✓	✓
Malignant			
Mast cell tumour	✓	✓	✗
Mammary gland tumour	✓	✓	✓
Carcinoma	✓	✓	✓
Sarcoma	✓	✓	✗
Lymphoma	✓	✓	✗
Melanoma	✓	✓	✗

28.2 Tissue sampling options for suspected mass types. *Try to avoid sampling seromas; a healing surgical wound that develops a fluid-filled swelling should give a high index of suspicion that a seroma is present.

Nucleus
Variable/increased nucleus:cytoplasm ratio
Clumped chromatin
Large multiple and irregular nucleoli
Multinucleate cells

Cytoplasm
Increased basophilia
Vacuolation

Cells
Larger than typical cells for that cell type
Heterogeneous populations of the same cell type
Large sheets of attached cells (especially epithelial tumours); clumping of cells
Actively dividing cells, mitotic figures

28.3 Cytological features of malignancy.

Common conditions

This section deals with simple masses, benign and malignant masses in turn. This is not intended to be an exhaustive discussion but shows an approach that could be adopted for each type, along with a brief synopsis of the more common presentations. For more details on diagnosis, staging and treatment see the *BSAVA Manual of Canine and Feline Oncology* and the *BSAVA Manual of Canine and Feline Rehabilitation, Supportive and Palliative Care: Case Studies in Patient Management.*

Simple masses

There are numerous simple non-tumour masses that present regularly in first-opinion practice, often requiring minimal intervention. A lot of these masses are associated with younger or very active animals or those that have recently had veterinary treatment. It is appropriate to use FNA for most of these masses. Some of the more common simple masses are listed in Figure 28.4. Urticaria is discussed in Chapter 27; interdigital granuloma/abscess/foreign body is discussed in Chapter 29; impacted anal gland is discussed in Chapter 30; and mastitis is discussed in Chapter 26.

- Urticaria
- Injection site reaction (sterile granuloma)
- Granuloma (lick, tick bite)
- Haematoma
- Sebaceous cyst
- Abscess
- Seroma
- Interdigital granuloma/abscess/foreign body
- Impacted anal gland
- Mastitis
- Reactive lymph node
- Residual fat at the site of a sealed umbilical hernia

28.4 Some common simple superficial non-tumorous masses.

Injection site reaction

It is quite common to find a small, soft-to-firm, pea/bean-sized mass in the subcutaneous space at sites of injection such as the scruff. These masses are non-painful and the animals show no systemic signs of illness. The mass is a sterile granuloma and is usually a reaction to the drug carrier or adjuvant. The reaction is usually self-limiting and does not require treatment.

Granuloma

Other types of granuloma are described in Figure 28.5.

Abscess

Abscesses can be a variety of shapes and sizes, and can affect any part of the body. There are many causes, including penetrating trauma, foreign body, dog fights and post-surgical reactions. Abscesses produce typical clinical signs of heat, pain and swelling; as they mature, they will become soft to the touch, giving the impression that there is some fluid within the swelling. Dogs can be pyrexic and may display general signs of illness. FNA yields purulent material, which is pathognomonic. Treatment involves drainage, lavage, appropriate antibiosis and pain relief. The prognosis is generally excellent.

In severe cases, especially those affecting the limbs, the infection may be dissipated within the subcutaneous space (i.e. cellulitis). This can be a very debilitating condition, which may require hospitalization and aggressive treatment to manage.

Haematoma

Haematomas are the result of traumatic rupture of blood vessels and are acute in onset. There is often evidence of blunt trauma, such as a bruise on the overlying skin. FNA will yield blood (or serous fluid if the haematoma is chronic).

PRACTICAL TIP

It is worth bearing in mind that animals with a coagulopathy may well present with a haematoma and no other signs, so it is always worth considering the coagulation status of any animal presenting with a haematoma, particularly if the lesion is unexplained

---

Seroma

Seromas are fluid accumulations within the subcutaneous space of a surgical wound; formation occurs following surgery with poor haemostasis and failure to close dead space. Prevention is better than cure: particular attention should be paid to Halsted's principles of surgery, notably good haemostasis, accurate apposition of tissues and elimination of dead space; also, as little as possible foreign material (e.g. suture material) should be placed into the wound.

Seromas tend to be non-painful with minimal signs of inflammation. For the most part they require little in the way of treatment. The majority will resolve in 10–14 days. If the seroma is particularly large, re-operating to close dead space may be necessary. The prognosis is excellent.

Granuloma type	Examples	Treatment
Bacterial	Canine furunculosis caused by *Staphylococcus intermedius*	Appropriate medical therapy
Endogenous foreign body	Hair/keratin leading to bacterial furunculosis	Appropriate medical therapy ± surgical excision
Exogenous foreign body	Sutures, grass awns, thorns, glass splinters	Surgical excision
Parasitic	Tick bite	No treatment usually required. Excision if causing problems
Acral lick dermatosis	Deep bacterial folliculitis/furunculosis caused by repeated licking due to behaviour or immune-mediated problems (see Chapters 12 and 27)	Surgical excision. Treat underlying cause. Acupuncture
Idiopathic	Sterile pyogranulomatous dermatosis. Juvenile cellulitis	Appropriate medical therapy

28.5 Granuloma types and treatment.

> **WARNING**
>
> Do not be tempted to drain a seroma; it will refill and there is a risk of introducing bacteria into an otherwise sterile environment

Reactive lymph node

This is a reasonably common finding, particularly if there is skin disease affecting the distal limb. FNA and cytology should be performed on all lymph nodes that appear enlarged, particularly if there is no obvious reason for the enlargement.

Benign tumours

Common benign tumours are listed in Figure 28.6 and breed predispositions are considered in Figure 28.7. Most are amenable to FNA or simple excision. It is also possible to leave a benign mass *in situ* and monitor its behaviour.

> **PRACTICAL TIP**
>
> If choosing to leave a benign mass as it is, measure the dimensions, note the gross appearance and/or take a digital photograph of the mass and record this data in the dog's clinical notes. This will act as a baseline measure against which to judge the future behaviour of the mass

- Histiocytoma
- Lipoma
- Meibomian adenoma
- Papilloma
- Perianal gland adenoma
- Sebaceous gland tumour
- Trichoepithelioma

28.6 Common benign tumours.

Tumour	Breeds
Histiocytoma	Staffordshire Bull Terrier, Boxer, Cocker Spaniel, Dobermann, English Springer Spaniel, Labrador Retriever, West Highland White Terrier, Rottweiler, Shetland Sheepdog
Lipoma	Labrador Retriever, Dobermann, Cocker Spaniel, Weimaraner
Meibomian adenoma	Retriever breeds
Papilloma	Cocker Spaniel, Kerry Blue, Yorkshire Terrier, Poodle
Perianal adenoma	German Shepherd Dog, Lhasa Apso, Shih Tzu, English Bulldog, Cocker Spaniel, Samoyed, terriers
Sebaceous gland tumour	Beagle, spaniels, Lhasa Apso, Dachshund, Shih Tzu, Poodle
Trichoepithelioma	Cocker Spaniel, English Springer Spaniel, Basset Hound, German Shepherd Dog, Miniature Schnauzer

28.7 Breed predispositions for some common benign tumours.

Histiocytoma

These tumours are common in young dogs, with more than half of cases occurring before 2 years of age (hence their colloquial name of 'juvenile wart').

Although sometimes multiple, they usually present as solitary lesions on the head, pinnae or limbs especially and appear as raised, firm, well circumscribed dermal masses (Figure 28.8). The majority will regress spontaneously (though may be excised if traumatized). They often become quite inflamed immediately prior to regression.

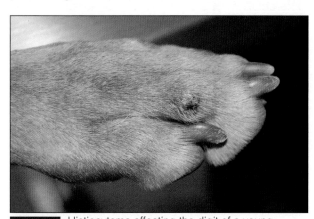

28.8 Histiocytoma affecting the digit of a young Labrador Retriever. The tumour was excised and the diagnosis confirmed histologically. Excision was curative.

Lipoma

These benign tumours of adipose tissue are a common finding in the subcutaneous tissues, or between muscle bellies in older dogs. They may be left *in situ* unless they are interfering with function (e.g. a large lipoma in the axilla or between limb muscles), in which case excision is recommended. Liposarcomas (malignant) are rare.

Meibomian gland tumour

These are the most common tumours of the eyelid (see also Chapter 21). They often appear like raised cauliflower-like lesions (Figure 28.9). Excision is indicated if they cause irritation.

Papilloma

These sessile or pedunculated cauliflower-like growths (Figure 28.10) are common in dogs and are often multiple. They are caused by the papillomavirus and can therefore be contagious. They rarely require treatment, though may be excised if traumatized. *They may undergo malignant change to squamous cell carcinoma.*

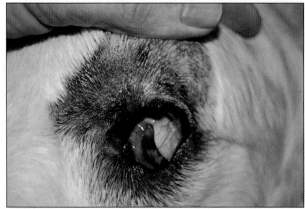

28.9 Meibomian gland tumour affecting the upper eyelid of a 10-year-old Labrador Retriever. Excision was curative.

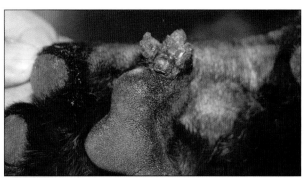

28.10 Papilloma affecting the foot of a young Labrador Retriever.

Perianal gland adenoma

These common tumours of the perianal glands (which are modified sebaceous glands) are usually seen in older, intact male dogs. They can also be seen in bitches, when it is important to check adrenal function as there is the suggestion of an underlying endocrinopathy. The tumours are ovoid masses that may be solitary or multiple and become ulcerated due to the stretching of the overlying skin as they enlarge. Castration alone will lead to regression of the majority, so excision combined with castration carries an excellent prognosis. In the bitch, excision should be curative.

Sebaceous gland tumour

These tumours are common and present as solitary, well circumscribed, raised, smooth, cutaneous masses. They may also be greasy, hyperkeratotic or wart-like. Ulceration is common, which may result in the discharge of thick creamy to caseous material. Excision is curative.

Trichoepithelioma

These cutaneous masses are common in middle-aged and older dogs, especially on the trunk (Figure 28.11). They may be solid or cystic and are well circumscribed. Excision is curative.

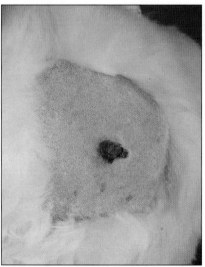

28.11

Trichoepithelioma affecting the flank of a Belgian Shepherd Dog.

Malignant tumours

The approach to a suspected malignancy is described in Figure 28.12. Once the tumour has been fully described, judgments can be made regarding treatment options and prognosis. Some of the more common presentations are outlined below.

1. History.
2. Clinical examination.
3. FNA of mass(es).
4. FNA of local lymph nodes, especially if enlarged.
5. Haematology, biochemistry and urinalysis, to help further define the health status of the dog and highlight any underlying illness or paraneoplastic syndrome (e.g. hypercalcaemia of malignancy).
6. Other appropriate tests (e.g. a coagulation profile in cases of haemorrhage or where haemorrhage can be expected; gastroscopy in dogs with mast cell tumours that show melaena ± vomiting).
7. If FNA cytology is non-diagnostic, or a tissue sample is required to define the tumour, then surgical biopsy is indicated.
    - It is often worthwhile performing a biopsy on a lymph node in cases of lymphoma to characterize which cell line is involved, as this gives information regarding prognosis and likely response to chemotherapy.
    - Biopsy can also aid in surgical planning, e.g. histological grading of mast cell tumour.
8. Tumour staging using the TMN (tumour, metastasis, node) system.
    - It is always worth using imaging to search for metastasis: three inflated views of the thorax (or CT if easily available), and abdominal ultrasonography. As previously mentioned, FNA of draining lymph nodes is also good practice.

28.12 Approach to a suspected malignant tumour. Further information on TMN staging can be found in the *BSAVA Manual of Canine and Feline Oncology*.

Malignant histiocytosis

Malignant histiocytosis, though rare, is possible and is most commonly seen in older Bernese Mountain Dogs and Retriever breeds. Cutaneous lesions are not common and signs include lethargy, weight loss, lymphadenopathy, hepatomegaly and pancytopenia, with a rapid progression to fatality.

Mammary gland tumour

MGTs are common in older (median age 11–12 years), predominantly entire bitches. Neutering prior to the first season will almost completely prevent their occurrence; neutering after the first season will decrease the occurrence, whereas after the second season there is little preventive effect (see also Chapter 5).

Tumours may be benign or malignant, and there may be mixed tissue types within the same mass so cytology can often be unreliable.

Treatment is by:

- Excision of the mass (for small solitary tumours or excisional biopsy)
- Mastectomy of a gland (for larger masses)
- Mastectomy of an entire mammary strip (for multiple masses or where propensity to metastasis is anticipated).

PRACTICAL TIPS

- Thoracic radiographs are *mandatory* prior to surgery, as approximately 25% of bitches with malignant tumours will have pulmonary metastases at the time of diagnosis
- If both chains of mammary glands are affected, it is better to stage excisions a few weeks apart to prevent the risk of wound dehiscence
- Ovariohysterectomy may be performed at the same time, and is often advocated, though it will not affect the prognosis or the likelihood of developing additional tumours in the remaining glands

Mast cell tumour

Mast cell tumours are the most common malignant cutaneous tumours of dogs and can affect dogs of any age. Although many MCTs appear as well defined, raised, red, hairless lesions, they can also mimic other lesions (including lipomas) or appear as soft fluctuant masses, which may appear bruised and contain sanguineous fluid (Figure 28.13). This illustrates the importance of FNA and cytology for all masses.

Manipulation of MCTs may cause histamine release and result in a wheal or flare reaction ('Darier's sign'). Histamine release may also cause vomiting and gastrointestinal ulceration, and these systemic signs are an important consideration in staging.

MCTs are easily diagnosed on cytology, due to the small to medium-sized round cells with abundant pink/red-staining cytoplasmic granules (when stained with Diff-Quik). Histology is useful, as the histological grade is an accurate prognostic indicator, with MCTs classed as low, intermediate or high grade depending on how well differentiated the cells are.

Surgery is the treatment of choice, with a wide excision. This may be combined with radiotherapy for aggressive tumours or where sufficient margins will be hard to achieve; early discussion with an oncologist may be helpful. There are two chemotherapy drugs for cases in which surgery is not possible, or where adequate margins cannot be guaranteed: masitinib and toceranib. Owners should always be given a cautious prognosis, even when excision appears to have been complete.

Soft tissue sarcoma

Soft tissue sarcomas originate from mesenchymal connective tissue and the exact tumour type is dependent on the tissue of origin, e.g. fibrosarcoma, haemangiopericytoma, peripheral nerve sheath tumour, haemangiosarcoma, leiomyosarcoma.

These are usually solitary tumours (Figure 28.14) and are most common in middle-aged and older dogs. The tumours may be soft or firm. They have poorly defined margins (even if pressure on surrounding tissues creates a pseudocapsule), such that they will infiltrate normal tissue and along fascial planes. Distant metastasis is via the haematogenous route and local lymph node involvement is rare.

Treatment is by wide surgical excision, including a fascial plane deep to the tumour. If 'clean' tumour-free margins are seen histologically, then prognosis is often good; 'dirty' margins, i.e. containing tumour cells, may indicate a need for wider excision or radiotherapy or chemotherapy. The first surgery gives the best chance of a cure, so it is always worth discussing these cases with a more-experienced colleague.

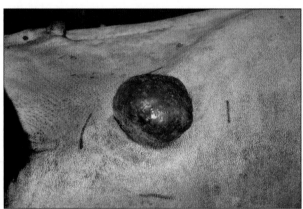

28.14 A soft tissue sarcoma affecting the left ventrolateral abdominal wall just caudoventral to the last rib. The black lines drawn on the skin indicate 3 cm lateral margins.

Lymphoma

Lymphoma can occur at any age, though it is more common in middle-aged and older dogs. Because it arises in lymphoid tissue, it can affect any part of the body (including skin and gastrointestinal tract), though typical sites are the lymph nodes, spleen and bone marrow; 85% of cases have multicentric disease.

Lymphoma is most commonly suspected following identification of generalized lymphadenopathy on clinical examination, as the submandibular, prescapular and popliteal nodes are readily palpable. Other non-specific signs that may alert the clinician include weight loss, lethargy and anorexia. Paraneoplastic hypercalcaemia is possible and so cases may

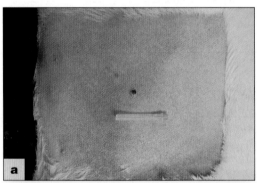

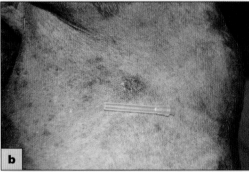

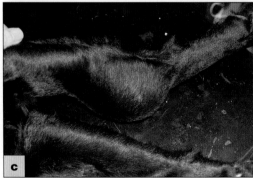

28.13 Mast cell tumours can present in a wide variety of ways: **(a)** small (3 mm diameter) nodule; **(b)** moderately sized (approximately 1 cm) mass; **(c)** large (8 cm diameter) fluid-filled mass affecting the antebrachium of a Labrador Retriever.

present with polyuria/polydipsia. Diagnosis is by cytology: FNA is adequate to confirm the diagnosis, but if the owner is amenable to chemotherapy then biopsy should be performed to enable immunophenotyping, which will facilitate the choice of chemotherapy protocol (and help determine the prognosis).

PRACTICAL TIP

It is worth avoiding taking samples from the submandibular nodes, as inadvertent sampling of salivary tissue is frustratingly common

---

Chemotherapy for lymphoma is commonly used in many veterinary practices and can give good rates of remission. If chemotherapy is declined, systemic steroid therapy may give palliative care, but progression of the disease will be rapid and euthanasia will be inevitable.

Paraneoplastic syndromes

Tumours often exert metabolic, endocrine and haematological effects on the body. These effects are known as 'paraneoplastic syndromes'. They are important factors to bear in mind, as they may be the reason for presentation or may complicate ▶

the management of an existing neoplastic disease. Common syndromes include:

- Haematological: anaemia, haemolysis, thrombocytopenia, disseminated intravascular coagulopathy
- Metabolic: cancer cachexia, fever
- Endocrine: hypercalcaemia, hypoglycaemia, hyperhistaminaemia
- Neurological: myasthenia gravis, hypertrophic pulmonary osteopathy
- Dermatological: hepatocutaneous syndrome

References and further reading

Carlotti DN (2005) Cutaneous and subcutaneous lumps, bumps and masses. In: *Textbook of Veterinary Internal Medicine, 6th edn*, ed. SJ Ettinger and EC Feldman, pp.43–46. Elsevier Saunders, St. Louis

Dobson JM and Lascelles BDX (2011) *BSAVA Manual of Canine and Feline Oncology, 3rd edn*. BSAVA Publications, Gloucester

Polton G (2010) Patients with neoplastic diseases. In: *BSAVA Manual of Canine and Feline Rehabilitation, Supportive and Palliative Care: Case Studies in Patient Management*, ed. S Lindley and PJ Watson, pp.232–267. BSAVA Publications, Gloucester

Miller WH, Griffin CE and Campbell KL (2013) Neoplastic and non-neoplastic tumours. In: *Muller & Kirk's Small Animal Dermatology, 7th edn*, ed. WH Miller *et al.*, pp.774–843. Elsevier Saunders, St. Louis

Van Nimwegen S and Kirpensteijn J (2012) Specific disorders (Skin). In: *Veterinary Surgery: Small Animal*, ed. KM Tobias and SA Johnston, pp.1303–1340. Elsevier Saunders, St. Louis

Withrow SJ and Vail DM (2007) *Withrow & MacEwen's Small Animal Clinical Oncology, 4th edn*. Elsevier Saunders, St. Louis

QRG 28.1 Fine-needle aspiration of a superficial mass

Equipment

- 23 G needle
- 5 ml syringe
- Several clean microscope slides
- Cytology stain, such as Diff-Quik
- Microscope

Needle-only method

1 Firmly secure the mass with the non-dominant hand.

2 Introduce the needle into the mass and move it forwards and backwards within the mass several times before completely withdrawing it.

- Don't spend too much time within the mass and don't push through and out of the mass (potentially seeding a tumour).

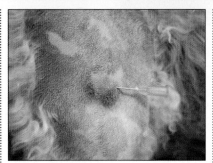

Position of the needle within the mass.

3 Fill a syringe with air, attach the needle and gently express the sample on to a glass slide.

4 Make a smear, stain and examine it with the microscope.

Needle and syringe method

1 Firmly secure the mass with the non-dominant hand.

2 Introduce the needle into the mass, moving it forwards and backwards within the mass, while simultaneously applying negative pressure with the attached syringe.

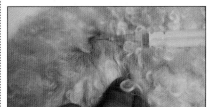

Position of the needle within the mass.

3 Once the sample has been collected into the syringe, stop applying negative pressure and then remove the needle from the mass.

4 Remove the needle from the syringe and fill the syringe with air. Re-attach the needle and gently express the sample on to a glass slide.

5 Make a smear, stain and examine it with the microscope.

QRG 28.2 Biopsy of a superficial mass

Equipment

- Routine equipment to prepare for aseptic surgery
- Basic surgical kit
- Sterile drape and swabs
- No. 10 scalpel blade
- Biopsy punch
- Suture for skin closure
- Histology pot containing formalin solution

Incisional biopsy

1 With the dog under general anaesthesia, prepare the mass for sterile surgery.

2 Using a scalpel blade, make a wedge-shaped incision into the mass, keeping within the confines of the mass.

- This sampling technique is analogous to taking a wedge-shaped slice from a pie.
- It is important not to disturb the surrounding tissue. If the mass is in a subcutaneous position, then make as

small a skin incision as possible directly over the mass.
- It is also possible to use a skin biopsy punch to harvest the sample.
- Try to ensure the sample is representative of the mass as a whole.

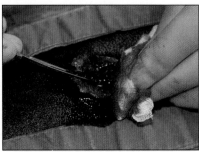

Wedge biopsy of an ulcerated skin mass on a 7-year-old female neutered Dobermann. Histology showed this to be an ulcerated melanoma.

3 Remove the wedge and place it in formalin.

4 Close the biopsy site routinely.

Excisional biopsy

1 Under general anaesthesia prepare the mass for sterile surgery.

2 Excise the entire mass with a small rim of unaffected skin.

- An elliptical incision is best.
- For very small masses it is possible to use a skin biopsy punch.

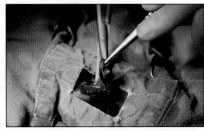

Complete excisional biopsy of a papillomatous mass in the same patient. Histology showed this to be a fibroepithelial polyp.

3 Place the sample in formalin.

4 Close the resultant wound.

Disorders of the paw

Ken Robinson

While it is possible for skin lesions to affect the paws exclusively, it is more common to have involvement of other areas as well. An approach to pruritic and non-pruritic skin disorders is given in Chapter 27. This chapter concentrates on those conditions that affect the feet and nails predominantly or exclusively. The paws, being weight-bearing, are also vulnerable to injury, e.g. lacerations, fractures. As with any other area of the body, paws can show congenital malformations but these are generally not common in practice.

Foot and footpad injuries

The canine footpad is designed to withstand shock, standing and abrasive forces. The stratum corneum is pigmented, thick and keratinized, with a rough surface composed of conical papillae. Despite this toughness, injuries can occur. More detail on wound management can be found in Chapter 10.

Physical problems that can affect the paw

- Foot and footpad lacerations (Figure 29.1)
- Abrasions (Figure 29.2), erosions and degloving injuries (Figure 29.3)
- Foreign bodies (Figure 29.4)
- Thermal and chemical injuries

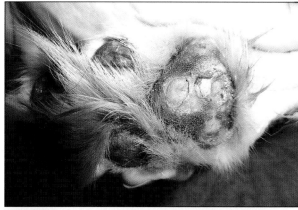

29.2 Vigorous exercise on hard surfaces (especially if protruding flints) can lead to shaving injuries to the pads, as in this collie cross. Healing is by the pad growing out to provide a new layer of dead surface. Clients should be warned that this is a slow process. (Courtesy of Helen Redfern)

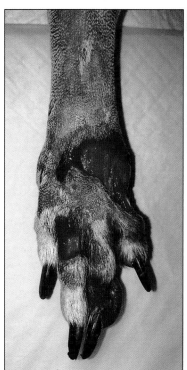

29.3

Road traffic accidents often lead to degloving injuries, as in this Whippet. With careful bandaging even large deficits can heal well by second intention. (Courtesy of Emma Hall)

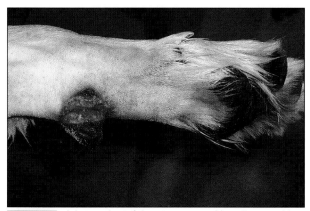

29.1 A laceration of the stopper pad in a 3-year-old cross-breed dog. (Courtesy of Rebecca Bailey)

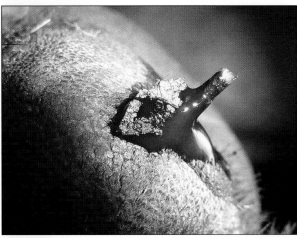

29.4 Penetrating foreign bodies, such as this thorn in the pad of a young German Shepherd Dog, are common in practice. (Courtesy of Helen Redfern)

Laceration

Superficial cuts to the foot and footpad can be treated by cleaning and bandaging (see QRG 29.1).

Lacerations in the skin are sutured as for other areas of the body (Figure 29.5).

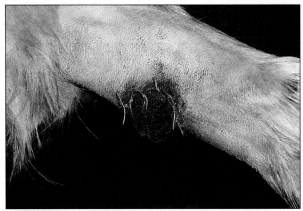

29.5 The same dog as in Figure 29.1. Following prompt cleaning, the wound was closed and left to heal by first intention. (Courtesy of Rebecca Bailey)

Where there is a deep laceration of the footpad this will require surgery to avoid a chronic non-healing deficit. Walking on such a lesion flattens and spreads the pad, thus separating the wound edges. A subcuticular support suture is used to reduce tension, followed by far–far–near–near sutures using 2 or 3 metric (3/0 or 2/0 USP) monofilament polypropylene, with the initial placement coursing below the base of the laceration (Figure 29.6). Postoperative antibiotics are advised, and a well padded support dressing to relieve the negative forces of the wound when weight-bearing. Sutures are removed after 10–14 days. It is important to warn the owner that there is a risk of wound breakdown.

Web resection may be required for interdigital web injuries that are not healing by secondary intention, or for neoplasms:

- An incision is made along the axial and abaxial edges of adjacent digits, on the dorsal and palmar/plantar surfaces and the web dissected free

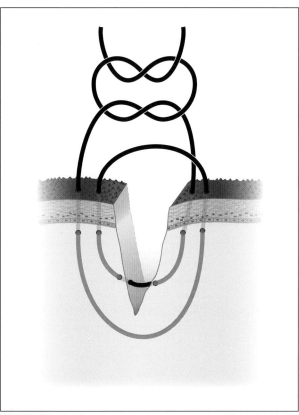

29.6 Far–far–near–near suture pattern. Note that the initial course of the suture material is below the base of the laceration.

- The wound edges are closed in a routine fashion and the foot protected with frequently changed dressings
- Sutures are removed after 10 days.

Fusion podoplasty may be considered where there are severed flexor tendons, or in cases of severe refractory interdigital pyoderma. It is strongly advised that these cases are referred to a specialist in this field.

Abrasions, erosions and degloving injuries

These wounds are best treated by allowing healing by secondary intention with contraction and epithelialization. A non-adherent absorbent/semi-absorbent dressing (see Chapter 10) is used, with antibiotic cover. Splinting can help healing, counteracting wound contraction antagonism, as weight-bearing pushes the wound edges apart. Acemannan hydrogel wound dressing containing aloe vera is useful. It is advisable to restrict exercise.

Digit amputation may be required in cases of severe trauma, or for tumours or chronic bacterial/fungal infection. The primary weight-bearing digits are the 3rd and 4th and should be preserved if possible. Lameness postoperatively is more likely if more than two digits are removed, or the 3rd or 4th digit is lost. The basic technique is described in QRG 29.2.

Thermal injuries

The paws are susceptible to burns and frostbite. Lesions should be debrided of all necrotic tissue and then can be treated in the same way as abrasions (see above). These cases often have extensive damage. More detail on burns can be found in Chapter 10.

Dew claw removal

Dew claw removal is carried out because of injury to, or from, the dew claws, especially on the hindlegs.

While legally allowed until puppies' eyes are open, the author prefers an age of 7 days as the upper limit for performing dew claw removal without general anaesthesia. Care should be taken in weak or ill puppies, delaying the procedure until they are strong enough. The area is sterilized, the digit removed with scissors and any bleeding cauterized. The area is kept clean for the next few days but does not need to be bandaged.

In dogs older than this, general anaesthesia is required. The procedure (see QRG 29.3) is then performed after 3 months of age and is often performed at the same time as neutering.

WARNING

It is important to note that some breeds have specific breed standards involving dew claws, e.g. Pyrenean Mountain Dog and Briard, which require double dew claws to be present on the hindlegs

---

Skin disorders affecting the paws

It is useful to divide cases according to their presenting signs. Algorithms for addressing pruritic and non-pruritic skin conditions are provided in Chapter 27.

Pruritus and erythema

Licking, chewing and biting of the feet is a relatively common presenting sign. There may be associated erythema, coat staining and hair loss. Causes of pruritus and erythema include (most common in **bold**):

- **Atopic dermatitis:**
  - Pedal lesions involve the interdigital areas (dorsal, palmar and plantar), and the carpal (Figure 29.7) and tarsal areas
  - While most dogs will have other areas affected, some may present with predominantly pedal signs. In treated cases, the feet may remain difficult to control.
- **Demodicosis:**
  - Does not always present with pruritus. Secondary lesions include pigmentation, scaling, crusting, exudation, nodules and draining tracts, and can be associated with pain. Secondary pyoderma is common
  - Can be restricted to just the feet (e.g. in Old English Sheepdog)
  - *Skin scrapings should be performed on ALL pododermatitis cases.* While skin scrapings and hair plucks should yield mites, chronic cases and some breeds (e.g. Shar Pei) may require biopsy
  - Pedal lesions are difficult to treat and may be resistant to therapy. As well as systemic therapy, localized treatment using amitraz mixed 1:9 with mineral oil or propylene glycol, applied once or twice weekly, may help (though this is an unauthorized use).

- **Bacteria or *Malassezia*:**
  - These cases are usually secondary, and require further investigation to establish the underlying cause
  - Various bacteria can be involved, especially *Staphylococcus pseudintermedius*, *Pseudomonas* and *Proteus*. Mixed infections can occur
  - *Malassezia* infection often presents as a brown exudate around the nailbed (see Figure 29.16) and on the nails
  - Cytology can be used to show whether cocci, rods or *Malassezia* are involved (see QRG 27.2)
  - Recurrent cases, with more than one foot involved and where the dog is non-pruritic between episodes, may indicate an underlying immune deficiency disorder, hypothyroidism or non-pruritic demodicosis.
- Contact dermatitis:
  - The ventral (Figure 29.8) and interdigital surfaces are usually the most severely affected, though less commonly it can involve the whole paw
  - Pruritus is often severe and difficult to control
  - Where only the feet are affected, attention should be directed towards finding out the main areas where the dog walks. *Covering one foot with a sock for 2–3 days and checking for improvement on that foot may justify further investigation.*
- Food hypersensitivity (see Chapter 27)
- Trombiculosis (see below).

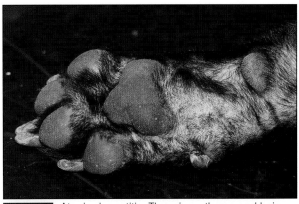

29.7 Atopic dermatitis. There is erythema and hair loss affecting the carpus and foot.

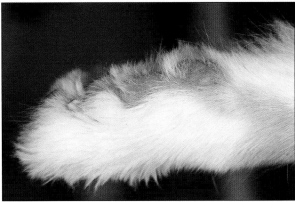

29.8 Contact dermatitis. There is erythema on the ventral surface of the paw and there was moderate pruritus. The signs were reduced by avoiding some grass areas.

Trombiculosis

This is a seasonal dermatitis, occurring from late summer to mid autumn, caused by the orange larval stages of the harvest mite *Trombicula* (subgen. *Neotrombicula*) *autumnalis*, which are visible to the naked eye (Figure 29.9). Infestation is predominantly pedal, but other areas of the skin can be affected, such as the ventral abdomen and pinnae (Henry's pocket). Papular lesions, some with crusting, are seen. The larvae, with 3 pairs of legs, can be identified microscopically. While infection is self-limiting, most animals find the mites irritating, and topical fipronil spray can be used once or twice weekly.

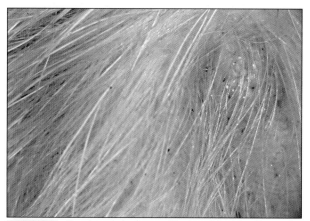

29.9   *Trombicula* (subgen. *Neotrombicula*) *autumnalis* mites visible in the interdigital area.

Non-pruritic alopecia

Alopecic lesions without evidence of pruritus (e.g. fractured hair shafts or hair staining) are not a common presentation for the feet. Causes of non-pruritic alopecia include (most common in **bold**):

- **Demodicosis:** Pedal lesions include scale and alopecia (Figure 29.10)
- **Dermatophytosis:** This may occasionally affect the feet exclusively, with scale, crust, follicular papules and pustules. Rarely, it can involve the nails (onychomycosis)
- Bacterial overgrowth (see Chapter 27)
- Ischaemic folliculopathy: Uncommon but warrants consideration in refractory cases. Causes include dermatomyositis and post-vaccination vasculitis.

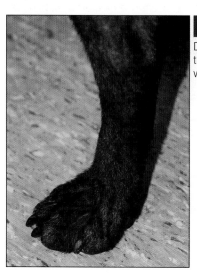

29.10

Demodicosis. Note the alopecic areas with scaling.

Nodules

A number of conditions may present with nodules, with or without draining tracts. Some of these conditions are very painful, and dogs may present with lameness.

Causes of nodules include (most common in **bold**):

- **Foreign bodies**
- **Bacterial furunculosis and pyogranulomas**
- **Demodicosis** (see above and Chapter 27)
- **Neoplasia**
- Fungal granulomas (see Chapter 27)
- Ruptured follicular cysts: Draining cysts requiring surgical resection and antibiotics
- Sterile pyogranulomas (see Chapter 27)
- Calcinosis cutis/circumscripta (see Chapter 27)
- Nodular dermatofibrosis of German Shepherd Dogs: Rare condition associated with renal or uterine tumours
- Xanthomatosis: yellowish/white nodules associated with dietary or metabolic causes.

Foreign body reaction

Common foreign bodies include splinters, thorns (see Figure 29.4) and interdigital grass awns (especially in long-coated breeds; Figure 29.11a). They often present as a discharging sinus. Diagnosis is by surgical exploration of the tract. Short-haired breeds (Figure 29.11b) can develop nodular lesions as a result of broken bristle-like hairs enclosed in a granuloma.

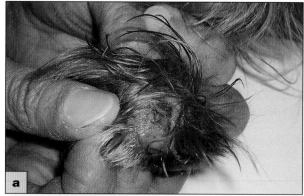

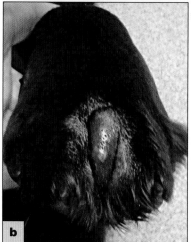

29.11   Interdigital spaces are common sites for foreign bodies, especially grass awns. **(a)** Long hair will trap the awn, which can migrate into the foot and lead to abscessation, as in this 4-year-old terrier. **(b)** Alternatively, penetration may be from the palmar aspect and present as an interdigital swelling, as in this 6-year-old Labrador Retriever. (Courtesy of Rebecca Bailey)

Treatment involves opening the nodule and removing the foreign body, or surgical resection of the granulomatous nodule. Where removal of the whole lesion is not achieved, it is important to leave the wound open to drain and heal by granulation. Bandaging should ideally be avoided, unless a poultice is applied; daily changing of the dressing is then required. The majority of cases require a course of antibiotics.

The footpad can be affected, with thorns and glass being common perforating foreign bodies; lesions appear as small draining openings on the pad, and the dog is often lame.

In footpad lesions, lateral pressure on the pad can isolate pain to the area and can extrude a foreign body such as a thorn. Glass can be more difficult to find but may show up on radiography of the pad and can be dug out using a hypodermic needle; if it is deeply embedded this will require general anaesthesia. All footpad cases require a course of antibiotics.

Bacterial furunculosis and pyogranulomas

These present as nodular lesions, often discharging, which can be painful and cause lameness. They are often secondary (e.g. to demodicosis, foreign body, chronic allergy), but no underlying cause can be found in some cases. Certain breeds are overrepresented, including English Bulldog, Great Dane, Basset Hound, Mastiff, Bull Terrier, Boxer, Dachshund, Dalmatian, German Shepherd Dog, Labrador and Golden Retrievers, setters and Pekingese. In shorthaired breeds, excessive pressure on the foot, especially as a result of being overweight, causes fracture of the hair shafts, with release of keratin into the dermis to act as a nidus for infection.

Affected paws are red and oedematous with nodules, ulcers, fistulas and haemorrhagic bullae with discharge. Nailbed involvement can occur. Diagnosis involves cytology, bacterial culture and sensitivity testing, and biopsy.

Treatment is difficult and includes: prolonged courses (8–12 weeks) of appropriate antibiotics; foot soaks with Epsom salts (magnesium sulphate) for 10–15 minutes; and topical antimicrobial ointments.

It is very important to treat until there is total resolution. Following surface healing, regular palpation of the interdigital region facilitates the decision to continue treatment if deep lesions (often painful) can still be palpated. Chronic cases may result in sterile nodules following treatment and may require steroids. Severe cases may require surgical debridement or even podoplasty.

Neoplasia

Cases can present with varying sizes of nodular masses, which can be ulcerated. Other signs can include erythema, scale, sometimes depigmented footpads, and variable pruritus. Nailbed carcinoma or keratoacanthoma usually involves a single digit. Neoplasms affecting the foot include mast cell tumour, histiocytoma (Figure 29.12), squamous cell carcinoma, melanoma, epitheliotropic lymphoma, inverted papilloma and eccrine adenocarcinoma. Diagnosis is via biopsy and cytology. Surgical management should be carried out where appropriate, with survey radiographs if any malignancy is suspected.

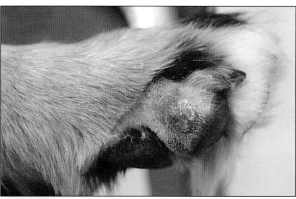

29.12 Histiocytoma in a young cross-breed dog. A raised dome-shaped lesion with some surface trauma is present on the paw. Surgery to remove this was successful.

Hyperkeratosis, crusting or fissures of the footpad

Dogs may be presented with footpads that have thickened skin, crusts or fissures. If the condition is severe, the dog may be lame.

Causes of footpad problems include (most common in **bold**):

- **Idiopathic or age-related hyperkeratosis**
- **Keratoma (corn)**
- Pemphigus foliaceus:
  - Can involve the feet exclusively but most cases involve other areas (see Chapter 27)
  - Nail lesions also occur (see later).
- Superficial necrolytic dermatitis (hepatocutaneous syndrome) (see Chapter 27)
- Zinc-responsive dermatosis (see Chapter 27)
- Breed-specific hyperkeratosis
- Lethal acrodermatitis (see Chapter 27)
- Erythema multiforme (see Chapter 27)
- Drug eruption (see Chapter 27)
- Dermatophytosis (see Chapter 27)
- Viral: Hyperkeratosis is commonly associated with canine distemper infection, but this is rarely seen due to effective vaccination
- Hookworm infestation.

Idiopathic or age-related hyperkeratosis

Excess keratin production with age is commonly seen in spaniels (especially Cocker; Figure 29.13.), Beagles and Basset Hounds. It is often associated with nasal lesions. Diagnosis is via clinical signs and biopsy. Symptomatic treatment is given daily with topical mineral oil or 50% propylene glycol.

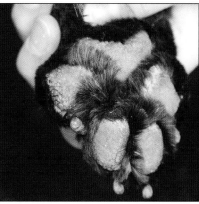

29.13

Hyperkeratosis of the footpad in an 11-year-old Cocker Spaniel.

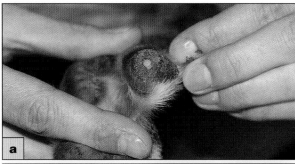

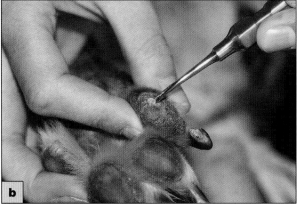

29.14 **(a)** A corn is visible as a pale mass in the centre of the pad of this Lurcher. **(b)** Hulling was carried out using a dental elevator.

Keratoma (corn)
Hard hyperkeratotic nodules that enlarge with time occur on the pad surface of Greyhounds and Lurchers (Figure 29.14a). There are various theories as to the cause, including foreign body injury, trauma, viral or anatomical problems. Lesions are painful, causing lameness. Diagnosis is from clinical signs.

The pad should first be cleaned. Hulling out of corns involves using a scalpel or, as the author prefers, a dental elevator (Figure 29.14b) to pare out the dead tissue. The crevice is cleaned and the pad kept covered for 1–2 weeks with dressings and antiseptic ointment. Recurrence is not uncommon. Some success in preventing recurrence has been claimed when using antiviral ointments after hulling.

Breed-specific hyperkeratosis
A severe hyperkeratosis develops by 6 months of age in certain breeds, including Golden and Labrador Retrievers, Irish, Norfolk and Kerry Blue Terriers, and Dogue de Bordeaux. Diagnosis is by breed and biopsy. Symptomatic therapy, similar to that for idiopathic hyperkeratosis, is appropriate.

Hookworm infestation
Hyperkeratotic paws that are painful and pruritic are associated with migration of hookworm larvae through the palmar/plantar aspect of the paws. This is not commonly seen, as most dogs are regularly wormed.

Ulcerative/sloughing footpads
While various lesions of the footpads can progress to ulceration, the following conditions, all described in Chapter 27, involve ulceration/sloughing as primary signs:

- Epitheliotropic lymphoma (other lesions include hyperkeratosis, depigmentation and crusting)

- Drug eruption
- Immune-mediated diseases (e.g. discoid/systemic lupus erythematosus, dermatomyositis, erythema multiforme, toxic epidermal necrolysis, pemphigus vulgaris, bullous pemphigoid, cold agglutinin disease)
- Ischaemic vasculopathy/vasculitis
- Uveodermatological syndrome
- Squamous cell carcinoma.

Depigmentation
Depigmentation of the skin, hair and nails of the feet occurs in vitiligo (see Chapter 27). This is a hereditary hypopigmentation disorder, which is merely cosmetic and requires no treatment.

Nail disorders

Terminology

- Onychodystrophy: deformity due to abnormal growth
- Onychorrhexis: brittle nails (splitting/breaking)
- Onychomadesis: sloughing of nail
- Onychomalacia: softening of nail
- Onychoclasis: breaking of nail
- Onychoschizia: splitting (± lamination) of nail
- Onychogryphosis: hypertrophy and abnormal nail curvature
- Onychomycosis: fungal infection of nail
- Onychocryptosis: ingrowing nail
- Paronychia: inflammation of soft tissue around nail
- Pyonychia: purulent infection of nail

Nail disorders may involve just one foot and only a few nails ('asymmetrical') or can affect all feet ('symmetrical')

Overgrown nails are a common presentation in practice. Care should be taken to try to ascertain whether there is a pathological cause rather than just being due to a lack of exercise. Overweight and certain orthopaedic conditions affecting the flexor tendons can result in overgrown nails; merely clipping the nails will not solve the problem in such cases.

Nail clipping: hints and tips

- Learn the correct anatomy of the nail
- Ensure good quality nail clippers are used
- Cut 3–4 millimetres distal to the visible vasculature of the nail

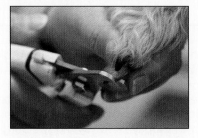

- Pigmented nails are best compared with non-pigmented nails as a guide ▶

- If all nails are pigmented, a useful tip is to extend a line parallel to the base of the pad and try to cut below where this intersects on the nail
- If unsure, always try to cut small amounts at a time from the tip, until the dog starts to show resentment
- At any sign of pain STOP!
- If cutting results in bleeding then apply pressure and cauterize with a silver nitrate stick or ferric chloride solution. NB This is intended to cauterize the vessel to prevent bleeding, not to produce a messy clot that will dislodge easily and lead to further haemorrhage

Asymmetrical nail disorders

Causes of asymmetrical nail disorders include (most common in **bold**):

- **Trauma**
- **Infections**
- Neoplasia (e.g. squamous cell carcinoma, melanoma, mast cell tumour, keratoacanthoma)
- Vascular occlusion/ischaemia (uncommon).

Trauma

Trauma is the most common nail problem seen in practice, usually affecting one or a few nails, and showing asymmetry (Figure 29.15). An apparent symmetrical presentation, with all feet involved, can occur if there has been an association with excessive running on hard surfaces, like asphalt, concrete or gravel. There may be secondary bacterial infection. Dogs are often profoundly lame.

Broken nails can be avulsed if they are loose, by grasping with forceps and pulling swiftly. Sedation is often required, especially if the nail is damaged proximally. The exposed quick usually heals, but may occasionally require resection of the nail or, rarely, the nail and 3rd phalanx (see QRG 29.4) under general anaesthesia.

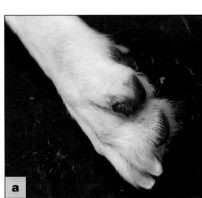
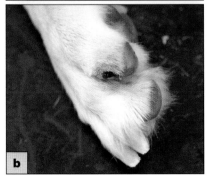

29.15

(a) Traumatic nail injury following a car accident. The outer nail shell has been lost, exposing the sensitive 'quick'. **(b)** Appearance following removal of the quick with bone cutters.

Infections

Infections of the nail often occur following trauma but can also be secondary to hypothyroidism, hyperadrenocorticism, diabetes mellitus, atopy or immune-mediated disease. Onychodystrophy and other conditions can lead to scarring or damage of the coronary band, with resultant defective nail growth and infection. In many cases there is a visible exudate below the nail.

- Fungal infections can occur, with dermatophytes growing into the nail keratin, but other areas of the skin are usually also affected. Nails are brittle, easily broken and powdered.
- *Malassezia* may affect the nail only, with brown, dry staining of the nail fold and nail (Figure 29.16). Atopy is often an underlying condition in these cases.
- Rarely, parasitic infections can affect the nails; e.g. demodicosis (causing paronychia), hookworm infestation (rapid nail growth), leishmaniosis (onychogryphosis).

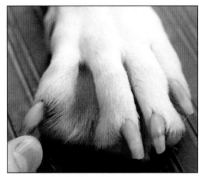

29.16

Early *Malassezia* infection of the nail and nailbed. Notice the brown discoloration at the base of the nail.

Diagnosis: Cytology and culture of the exudate can be performed. Scrapings from the nail can also be cultured for dermatophytes.

Treatment: Detached or loose nails are removed with forceps under general anaesthesia. Antimicrobial medication is prescribed, often for prolonged periods.

Onychectomy

- Indications for nail removal are broken nails, nailbed infections and tumours involving the nail

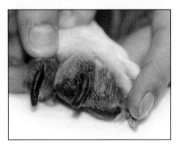

- If only the nail is to be removed, then the use of bone cutters to section the nail at the level of the nailbed can be employed under general anaesthesia. Digital pressure is applied with a swab following cutting, to slow the bleeding and the area subsequently thermocauterized
- For more extensive lesions, removal of the nail and distal phalangeal bone is required (see QRG 29.4)

Symmetrical nail disorders
Causes of symmetrical nail disorders include:

- Infections (see above for details)
- Immune-mediated disorders (see also Chapter 27):
  - Cases often involve the nail fold, leading to paronychia or onychomadesis
  - Where only the nails are involved, the most likely cause is symmetrical lupoid onychodystrophy (see below), lupus erythematosus, bullous pemphigoid or pemphigus vulgaris
  - If there is paronychia and footpad involvement, pemphigus foliaceus is more likely; affected nails can show onychodystrophy, onychorrhexis and onychogryphosis
  - Cryoglobulinaemia, drug reactions and vasculitis can also cause nail disorders.
- Idiopathic onychodystrophy
- Idiopathic onychomadesis
- Epidermolysis bullosa
- Dermatomyositis
- Ergotism
- Thallotoxicosis
- Linear epidermal nevi
- Nutritional deficiencies (e.g. zinc)
- Necrolytic migratory erythema
- Disseminated intravascular coagulopathy.

Symmetrical lupoid onychodystrophy
This is the most common immune-mediated condition of the nails, affecting dogs between 3 and 8 years of age. The German Shepherd Dog is predisposed, but cases have been reported in Rottweilers and Schnauzers. Initially there may be a single nail affected on two or more paws, but within 2–9 weeks all nails are affected. There is sloughing of nails, with poor and brittle nail regrowth. Affected dogs are lame. Bacterial secondary infection can occur. The condition is regarded as a reaction pattern with several possible causes (e.g. food hypersensitivity, drug toxicity). Biopsy is required for diagnosis.

Some response has been reported to an elimination diet and antibiotics. Most cases require immunomodulating drugs, e.g. glucocorticoids or the tetracycline/niacinamide combination. Response usually takes 3–4 months, but most cases relapse on cessation of therapy.

Idiopathic onychodystrophy
This features multiple nail and paw involvement but is not secondary to other conditions such as onychomadesis and onycholysis. Secondary infection is seen but there is poor response to antibiotics. Breeds associated with the condition include the Siberian Husky, Dachshund, Rhodesian Ridgeback, Rottweiler and Cocker Spaniel (spaniels can have seborrhoea). Older dogs are more prone. Diagnosis involves biopsy. Some response has been reported to oral treatment with gelatin or biotin; retinoids have also been tried, with variable response.

Idiopathic onychomadesis
This condition is seen in German Shepherd Dogs, Whippets and English Springer Spaniels, and possibly in the Rottweiler. Onychomadesis with secondary infection under the nail plate, onychoschiziasis and onychorrhexis are seen. Changes in the mineral composition of the nail may also occur. Diagnosis involves biopsy. Some cases respond to pentoxifylline (15 mg/kg q8–12h).

References and further reading

Carlotti DN, Prélaud P and Guaguère E (2008) Diagnostic approach to nail disorders, In: *A Practical Guide to Canine Dermatology*, ed. E Guaguère, P Prélaud and M Craig, pp. 535–540, Merial, Kalianxis

Ghubash R (2007) An approach to diseases of the nasal planum and footpads. In: *BSAVA Manual of Canine and Feline Dermatology, 3rd edn*, ed. H Jackson and R Marsella, pp. 103–109. BSAVA Publications, Gloucester

Miller WH, Griffin CE and Campbell KL (2013) *Muller and Kirk's Small Animal Dermatology, 7th edn*. WB Saunders, Philadelphia

Pin D, Prélaud P and Guaguère E (2008) Diagnostic approach to pododermatitis. In: *A Practical Guide to Canine Dermatology*, ed. E Guaguère, P Prélaud and M Craig, pp. 525–533. Mérial, Kalianxis

Rhodes KH and Werner AH (2002) *Blackwell's Five-Minute Veterinary Consult, Clinical Companion, Small Animal Dermatology, 2nd edn*, Wiley-Blackwell, Oxford

Santoro D (2007) An approach to diseases of the claws and claw folds. In: *BSAVA Manual of Canine and Feline Dermatology, 3rd edn*, ed. H Jackson and R Marsella, pp. 121–124. BSAVA Publications, Gloucester

QRG 29.1 Applying a foot bandage

1 Trim the nails if overgrown.

2 Apply padding between the toes, and also under the stopper pad and dew claw if present.

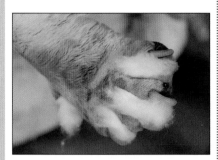

Using a layer of cotton wool bandage, commence at the dorsal aspect of the paw and roll the bandage down over the distal aspect of the paw and up to the palmar/plantar aspect. Then roll the bandage back on itself down to the distal aspect of the paw and back up to the dorsal aspect. Continue by wrapping the bandage around the paw in a spiral fashion from the distal aspect to the top, with the bandage overlapping by about half to two-thirds of its width, covering the whole paw.

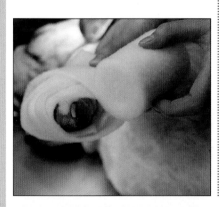

3 Apply a conforming bandage on top in a similar fashion and secure with tape.

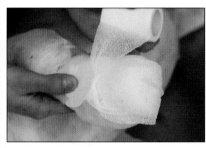

4 Cover again, this time using adhesive bandage.

1. Apply two strips, crossed at right angles, over the distal end and secure them up the sides.

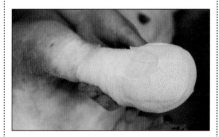

2. Cover the whole foot with the bandage, in a spiral fashion as above, finishing with the adhesive bandage applied to the dog's hair at the top.

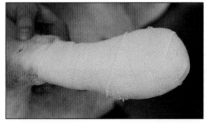

Bandage care

- A plastic bag can be used (e.g. re-used intravenous drip bags, which are very strong) to protect the bandage when the dog is walking outside. The bag should be removed when indoors to prevent condensation.

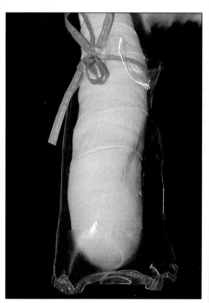

- Some dogs may require bitter sprays applied to the dressing to prevent chewing, or in some cases an Elizabethan collar may be necessary.

QRG 29.2 Toe amputation

Patient positioning and preparation

- Positioning of the dog can vary depending on size and limb shape: dorsal or ventral recumbency may be suitable but often, particularly with long thin legs, it is easier to place the dog in lateral recumbency and use an assistant to support the leg.
- Hair is clipped from the foot and the toe to be removed and the skin prepared aseptically for surgery. It is often helpful to soak the foot in a bath of the chlorhexidine scrub solution.

Equipment

A basic surgical kit is required.

Technique

1 Make an incision in the interdigital webbing on either side of the digit to be removed, on both the dorsal and plantar/palmar surfaces. The author prefers to make joining incisions at the proximal end of the digit, a few millimetres distal to the metacarpophalangeal or metatarsophalangeal joint, resulting in a skin flap.

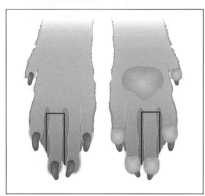

Diagrammatic representation of dorsal and plantar/palmar incisions for digit amputation. For ease of interpretation this shows removal of the 3rd digit. It should be noted, however, that the possibility of a degree of lameness must be explained to the owner if either the 3rd or 4th digit is to be removed.

2 Dissect free the flexor and extensor tendons, ligaments and joint capsule.

3 Haemorrhage is usually profuse but easily controlled with haemostats, though the digital vessels at the proximal end of the toe usually need ligation.

4 Incise through the metacarpophalangeal or metatarsophalangeal joint with the scalpel blade and dissect the digit free. Wherever possible, the metacarpophalangeal joint should be preserved as removal would compromise support of the foot and lead to chronic lameness. Scrape the joint surface with a scalpel blade to remove any remaining tissue.

5 Draw the upper and lower skin flaps over the end of the remaining bone and suture in place. Suture the wound edges of the remaining digits as shown, using far–far–near–near sutures (see Figure 29.6) of 2 metric (3/0 USP) polypropylene, creating a U-shaped suture line between the toes.

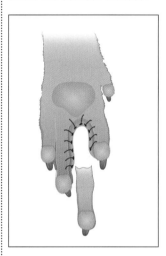

Postoperative care

Dressings are applied and changed every 3 days until the sutures are removed after 10 days. It is important to stress that dressings must be kept dry and clean.

QRG 29.3 Dew claw removal under general anaesthesia

Patient preparation

- The region around the dew claw is clipped and prepared aseptically.

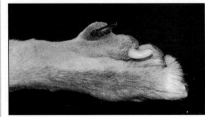

This cross-bred dog has double dew claws on its hindleg.

- A surgical drape is applied over the dew claw to be removed.

Equipment

A basic surgical kit is required.

Procedure

1 An elliptical incision is made around the base of the dew claw.

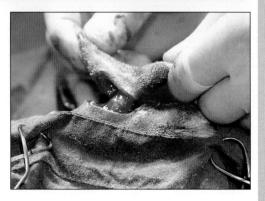

▶

QRG 29.3 continued

2

- Many hindleg dew claws do not possess a proximal phalanx. In this case the digit can be removed by severing the soft tissue attachments with scissors. The blood vessel is then ligated.

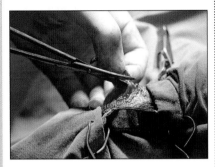

- Where this is not the case, the digit is abducted to dissect down to the metacarpophalangeal or metatarsophalangeal joint, and the dorsal common and axial palmar digital blood vessels are ligated. A scalpel blade is used to cut through the tendons, ligaments and joint capsule, and then to disarticulate the joint. The digit is then removed.

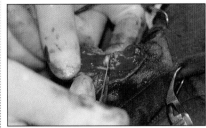

3 The dead space is closed using 2 metric (3/0 USP) polyglactin 910.

4 Skin closure is routine, using an intradermal suture or skin sutures.

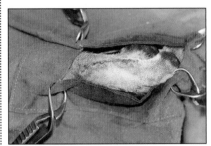

Postoperative care

- A soft padded dressing is applied for 3–5 days. It should be stressed to the owner that this must be kept dry.

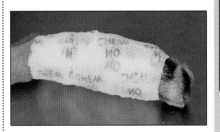

- This is a clean elective surgical procedure and should not require antibiotic cover.
- Strict rest is advised.
- Where external skin sutures have been used, they are removed after 10 days.

QRG 29.4 Removal of a nail and distal phalanx

This is indicated where the nail and/or nailbed has been badly traumatized, or where biopsy is required for investigation of nail disease.

Patient preparation and positioning

The toe is shaved, prepared aseptically and draped for surgery.

WARNING

Where histopathology is required, care must be taken not to remove important pathological changes

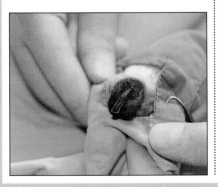

Equipment

A basic surgical kit is required.

Technique

1 Make an elliptical incision around the nailbed.

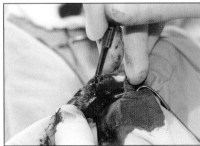

2 Dissect the distal phalangeal bone free, preserving the footpad.

3 Ligate the digital blood vessels.

4 Disarticulate the joint with a scalpel blade.

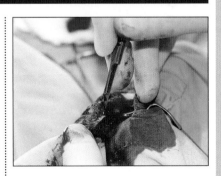

5 Remove the nail and phalangeal bone.

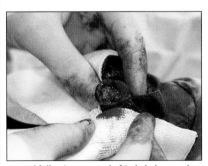

Wound following removal of 3rd phalanx and nail, showing the end of the 2nd phalangeal bone and the footpad flap. ▶

QRG 29.4 *continued*

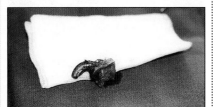

Removed nail and 3rd phalanx. These can be sent for histology.

6 Draw the pad over the distal segment of the 2nd phalangeal bone and suture it to the skin to close the defect.

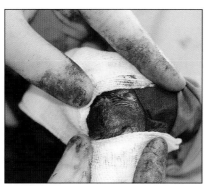

Coaptation of wound edges with subcuticular sutures of 2 metric (3/0 USP) polyglactin 910.

7 Skin sutures (2 metric (3/0 USP) polypropylene) are placed for added security.

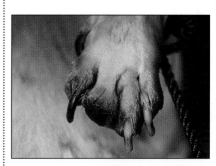

Postoperative care

A foot bandage is applied and changed every 3 days until the skin sutures are removed 10 days after the operation. It is very important to stress to the owner that the dressing must be kept clean and dry.

Conditions of the anus, perineum and tail

Julian Hoad

There is method in the seeming madness of dealing with the anus and tail in one chapter:

- Similar clinical signs may be seen with disorders of the two structures
- Surgery of the tail is occasionally performed to improve conditions of the anus
- Problems with the tail may occasionally lead to anal problems.

Thus, the two are inextricably linked.

Common presenting signs

- Many dogs with diseases of the tail or anus present with tenesmus and chewing or licking of the tail base, perineum, inguinum or hindlimbs. These signs are not exclusive to specifically anal or tail problems (Figure 30.1); they can also be caused by skin infections or irritations (with fleas being the number one suspect; see Chapter 27), urinary disorders (see Chapter 26) or behavioural problems (see Chapter 12). While many clients will attribute anal irritation to worms, in the majority of cases worms are the least likely cause.
- Irritation of the tail may cause dyschezia and may even result in the passage of faeces, which the owner may perceive as faecal incontinence or a breakdown in house training.
- Pain on sitting or walking may reflect disease in the tail or perineum but could also indicate a locomotory problem (see Chapter 15).

- Parasitism of the gastrointestinal tract
- Colitis
- Anal sac disease
- Prostatic disease
- Inflammation or pain of the tail base
- Colorectal or anal tumours
- Perineal hernia
- Urolithiasis
- Cystitis
- Anal fistula
- Large bowel intussusception
- Rectal foreign bodies

30.1 Conditions that may cause faecal straining or tenesmus.

- A reluctance to wag the tail, or miscarriage of the tail, may be due to anal or perineal problems.
- Impacted anal sacs or perineal hernias may present as lumps in the perineal area.
- Owners may have noticed an unusual or unpleasant smell emanating from their dog's rectum. This may be due to flatulence caused by fermentative processes, or may be a sign of infection of the perineum or impaction of the anal sacs.
- Blood may be present in the faeces: digested blood from the upper gastrointestinal tract makes the faeces dark and tarry (melaena); or fresh blood may be produced either at the end of defecation or mixed in with the faeces (haematochezia).
- Fresh blood coming from the rectum unassociated with defecation is termed rectorrhagia.

History

On initial presentation, a full history should be taken, including signalment. Very young puppies are more likely to have a developmental problem, such as atresia ani; whereas older or mature dogs may have neoplasia or chronic diseases. The duration of signs is important, and whether any particular seasonal or diurnal aspect to the condition has been noticed.

It is important to keep an open mind. For example: the presence of faecal staining around the anus may indicate diarrhoea, or it may be secondary to straining due to anal sac impaction, congenital abnormalities, or tail base pain. Older male dogs may have hyperplasia of the perianal glands that causes the anus to become thickened and irregular and may predispose to perineal faecal soiling.

Physical examination

The skin and fur of the perineum should be examined initially for signs of fur loss, wounds, self-trauma or masses. A gloved hand should be used to examine the anus gently and to gain an appreciation of the level of pain or discomfort the patient may be experiencing. Many dogs find rectal examination threatening and may become aggressive: this is more likely to happen if they are in pain.

1. A lubricant such as K-Y jelly or Vaseline should be used to facilitate insertion of a gloved first finger into the anal ring.
2. If the right hand is used, the thumb may be rotated around the finger on the outside to enable any masses to be palpated.
3. The anal sacs should be felt and assessed for fullness and the presence of any masses. At this stage, light pressure can be used to attempt to empty the sacs (see later). Any discharge should be examined for blood and other abnormal secretions.
4. Progressing the finger deeper, the rectal mucosa should be palpated for any masses or strictures. Strictures will feel like tight bands and may be very painful.
5. The rectum should feel like a symmetrical tube; any deeper recesses laterally may indicate rectal diverticula or perineal hernias.
6. In a male dog, the prostate gland should be palpated on the ventral floor of the pelvis, and assessed for size, symmetry and discomfort.
7. Finally, the dorsal pelvic canal should be palpated carefully to feel for any enlargement of the sublumbar lymph nodes. This is especially important if any masses have been palpated in the anal sacs.
8. Having removed the finger, the glove should be very carefully examined for the presence of blood.

Common disorders of the anus

The disorders below are described in approximate order of commonness.

Anal sac disease

Anal sac disease is probably the most common perineal problem seen in first-opinion practice, and should be at the top of the differential list for any dog presented for biting the tail base or 'scooting'. Most cases involve anal sac impaction, although abscessation and neoplasia are also common. Anal sac neoplasia is discussed later.

Diagnosis of the presence of anal sac disease is often evident from the history; however, a careful rectal examination should reveal enlargement of one or both anal sacs, presence of blood in the discharge, or a mass lesion.

Anal sac impaction

The anal sacs lie between the external and internal anal sphincter muscles. As the sacs have no muscles themselves, emptying relies on the glands being squeezed between the external sphincter and faeces during defecation, or on sudden firm contraction of the external sphincter (e.g. in a fear response). Although how the sacs become impacted is not completely understood, there are several predisposing factors (Figure 30.2).

In most cases, emptying the sacs is simple and curative. The sacs may be emptied by external or internal compression.

- **External compression** involves placing a gloved hand over the anus, coming up from below, so that the thumb is placed at about the 8 o'clock position

- Anal conformation
- Breed
- Diarrhoea
- Inflammatory skin disease
- Lax anal sphincter
- Low-fibre diet
- Neutering status (increased frequency after oestrus)
- Obesity
- Reduced exercise

30.2 Factors predisposing to anal sac impaction.

and the third finger at about the 4 o'clock position. The fingers and thumb are firmly but gently squeezed together with a slight upwards movement.
  - It is prudent to have some cotton wool or tissue in the hand to catch any fluid.
  - Although better tolerated by most patients, the external method may fail to empty the sacs sufficiently, and does not allow for palpation of the sacs, which may reveal additional disease (e.g. thickening of the sac lining or masses).
- **Internal compression** involves inserting a lubricated and gloved index finger just within the anus, coming up from below; the thumb is then brought towards this on the outside, at around the 8 o'clock position. The sac should be easily palpable. Using moderate pressure, the sac is squeezed from the outer margin towards the anal ring. The process is repeated for the other sac, this time inserting the thumb and using a finger to squeeze from the outside.
  - Provided the digit is inserted gently and relatively slowly, there is rarely a problem with the size of the digit: after all, the faecal girth of even a small dog is usually greater than the thumb.

> **PRACTICAL TIP**
>
> Always position the dog with its anus pointing away from the client – and from yourself. Occasionally, the secretion can fire quite a distance!

Depending on the duration of impaction, and the presence of other sac disease, the secretion may appear clear or cloudy and yellow, grey or brown in colour; the consistency may be watery or creamy, have flocculent material within it, or can even be a thick paste. Figure 30.3 demonstrates the variety of anal sac contents that may be found.

> **WARNING**
>
> The presence of blood indicates inflammation. Unless a mass is palpable, it is almost certainly indicative of sacculitis

In some instances it can be difficult to evacuate the sacs; this may be due to the presence of a thickened, inspissated (dried out) secretion, or due to inflammation at the sac opening. Repeating the compression in a day or so may help: if not, flushing the sac under sedation may be necessary (see later). If an individual dog requires its anal sacs emptying frequently, or the process is not well tolerated, then it may be worth considering an anal sacculectomy.

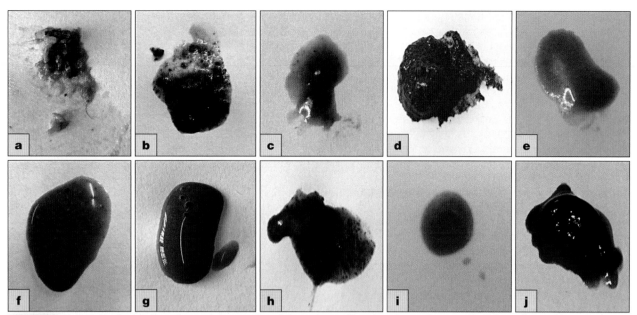

30.3 A variety of secretions from anal sacs: **(a–g)** from dogs without anal sac disease; **(h–j)** from dogs with anal sacculitis. In (h) the secretion appears grossly normal but the sac was inflamed and painful. In (i) and (j) the presence of blood is highly suggestive of inflammation.

Anal sacculitis

Sacculitis may be a sequel to chronic impaction, or may appear acutely. Sedation or anaesthesia is often required to express the sacs, as they may be extremely painful. Having emptied the sacs, they should be cannulated and flushed with enough sterile Hartmann's (lactated Ringer's) solution to result in a clear fluid being expressed (usually flushing with 3–5 ml eight to ten times). Antibiotics may be instilled into the sac, or administered systemically (the latter is generally recommended). There is no clear consensus as to whether steroids are beneficial.

Anal sac abscess

Anal sac abscesses are most likely progressions of anal sacculitis. They are often associated with a marked degree of malaise and discomfort: affected dogs may be reluctant to sit down, and often really resent examination of the perineum and anus. A burst abscess is relatively easy to spot: there is usually a purulent discharge (which may or may not be blood-tinged) lateral to the anus, and the overlying skin is invariably reddened and inflamed. It may be more difficult to identify an anal sac abscess that has not burst, although a painful fluctuant mass adjacent to the anus is strongly suggestive.

Treatment involves lancing and flushing the abscess under sedation or general anaesthetic. Isotonic saline or dilute chlorhexidine solution may be used: however, if the latter is used then it is important to take a swab of the lanced abscess discharge *before* flushing. A bacteriological swab may be used; or a small nip of anal sac tissue may be placed in a sterile glass bottle and sent for culture. Whilst awaiting the results, a broad-spectrum antibiotic (the author's preference is either potentiated amoxicillin or clindamycin) should be commenced and non-steroidal anti-inflammatory drugs (NSAIDs) given. If the condition fails to clear completely, or recurs, anal sacculectomy should be performed (Figure 30.4). This procedure is described and illustrated in the *BSAVA Manual of Canine and Feline Wound Management and Reconstruction*.

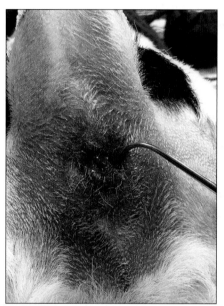

30.4 A 5-year-old male neutered cross-breed dog with recurrent anal sac impaction, prepared for anal sacculectomy. The dog has been placed in sternal recumbency with its tail elevated and tied. A probe has been inserted into the right anal sac, to demonstrate the position of the opening.

Trauma

As with any injury, the rest of the animal should be carefully examined for the presence of other injury or illness (see Chapter 10).

Perineal wounds should be flushed with copious amounts of sterile isotonic fluid, and meticulously examined for any tears in the mucosa of the anus or rectum.

- Simple wounds to the rectal mucosa (those not involving the submucosa) may be repaired using absorbable monofilament suture material such as poliglecaprone. Although continuous suture patterns may be used, interrupted sutures may be easier to place and will not cause distortion of the mucosa if they are not tied too tightly.

- The skin of the perineum may be sutured with absorbable or non-absorbable monofilament material; monofilament is preferred as there is less risk of capillary tracking of infection. If non-absorbable material is used, the temperament of the patient must be borne in mind: how easy will removal of the sutures be?
- Deep wounds to the perineum may warrant the placement of surgical drains.
- Antibiotics are generally advised for 5 days after repair.
- Analgesics must be used: lack of adequate analgesia may well lead to tenesmus or self-trauma.

Complications such as anal stricture or faecal incontinence can occur with even relatively minor wounds, and clients should therefore be warned as to the potential seriousness. For detailed advice on the management of anal wounds see the *BSAVA Manual of Canine and Feline Wound Management and Reconstruction*.

Neoplasia

Tumours of the anus and tail may cause many of the clinical signs described above (straining; biting at the rear end; scooting; and tending to sit down suddenly, as if stung).

Owners may notice a mass or swelling, or blood in the faeces or bleeding from the anus; they may also notice changes in shape of the faeces, e.g. ribbon-like faeces due to compression from a tumour. Whilst anal sacculitis or abscessation may also present as bulges or perineal swellings, most of these cases are fairly easy to diagnose due to: the presence of blood or pus within the anal sacs; erythema and pain over the swelling; and pyrexia in many cases. Any type of soft tissue tumour may be found in the perineal region, and it is also possible for osteosarcoma of the ischial tuberosity to present as a bulging mass in this area. Another potential differential would be a perineal hernia (see later).

To help distinguish between types of 'lump', a careful history should be taken; this should include the signalment and perineal signs, and whether any other clinical signs have been noticed, such as polyuria/polydipsia (PU/PD), weight loss or weakness.

Rectal examination should be carried out to assess the presence of any masses, integrity of the pelvic wall (see Perineal hernia, later) and whether there is any enlargement of the sublumbar lymph nodes.

> **WARNING**
>
> Care should be taken during rectal examination, especially if there is a history of straining. Insertion of a finger may cause considerable pain and trigger tenesmus, or even defecation. It may be wise to mention this to the owner prior to the examination, and to withdraw and consider sedation if there are signs of pain

Fine-needle aspiration (FNA) of the mass and cytology may be carried out (see Chapter 28), although it may be wise to examine the area first using radiography or ultrasonography if a perineal hernia is suspected, to avoid the risk of leakage of bowel flora or of damage to the urinary tract.

Rectal polyps

Rectal polyps may occasionally protrude from the anus during straining. They often bleed and may resemble dark cherries or strawberries (Figure 30.5).

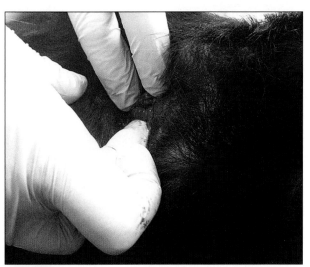

30.5 This 9-year-old neutered Labrador Retriever bitch presented with a history of tenesmus and haematochezia, passing fresh blood from the anus. A rectal polyp was palpable via a rectal examination. The patient has been anaesthetized to allow exteriorization of the polyp, which may be seen as a small, strawberry-like lesion.

Rectal examination should reveal the presence of a pedunculated mass, although care should be taken as many dogs will find the examination uncomfortable and may try to strain. It is usually possible to remove polyps near the anus by 'pull-through' surgical techniques (Figure 30.6; see also *BSAVA Manual of Canine and Feline Abdominal Surgery*); this is usually curative, although some polyps may undergo malignant transformation (see *BSAVA Manual of Canine and Feline Oncology*).

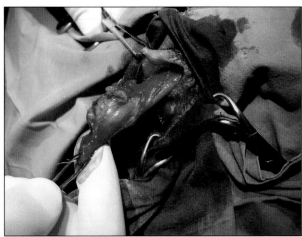

30.6 Rectal pull-through procedure in a 10-year-old male neutered cross-breed dog with a circumferential mass within the rectal wall. A circumferential incision has been made around the anal ring, and the rectum has been drawn caudally through the anal ring, exteriorizing the mass. The mass was then excised and the rectal mucosa sutured to the anal ring, thus recreating the rectal stoma. In this case, the mass was found to be a leiomyoma. The patient went on to survive for a further 18 months before being euthanased for an unrelated problem.

Anal sac neoplasia

The presence of an obvious mass within the region of the anal sac should always alert the clinician to the possibility of apocrine gland adenocarcinoma. These highly malignant tumours, which are over-represented in Cocker Spaniels, may present as an obvious mass, noticed by the owners, or as a perineal problem, with scooting, chewing of the rear end or dyschezia. Alternatively, cases may present with PU/PD, due to the production of a protein (similar to parathyroid hormone) that causes hypercalcaemia. Although anal sac adenocarcinoma was previously felt to be more common in bitches, recently it has been found that there is no sex predisposition.

If a mass is felt, blood samples should be taken for a routine biochemical and haematology profile; calcium measurement should be included. Rectal examination should be carried out to check for the presence of enlarged sublumbar or iliac lymph nodes: these may be palpated dorsal to the rectum, as far cranially as possible, although radiography and ultrasonography should be used to investigate the pelvic canal fully.

Lymphadenopathy indicates a poor prognosis, although dogs may have extended survival times after removal of the primary mass and the lymph nodes together with chemotherapy. For a detailed discussion of the stabilization of hypercalcaemia prior to surgery, and of the techniques for excision and chemotherapy for apocrine gland adenocarcinoma, the reader is directed to the BSAVA Manual of Canine and Feline Oncology.

Perianal adenoma

Also known as circumanal adenoma or hepatoid gland adenoma, this is the most common perineal tumour of the dog. Since hepatoid adenomas are predominately androgen-dependent, they tend to occur much more frequently in intact male dogs.

Perianal adenomas can present as rounded or pedunculated masses (Figure 30.7) of variable size, usually on the anal ring, although they can originate from the ventral tail base. They can also present, however, as thickened, irregular tissue, often with bluish inclusions, diffusely spread around the perineal area. These latter lesions may be difficult to remove, although if present in intact males will usually respond to castration.

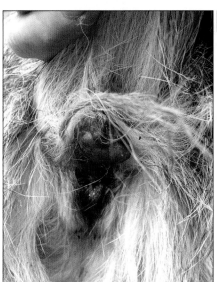

30.7

A perianal adenoma on the dorsal anal ring of a 10-year-old entire male Border Terrier. The mass was debulked at surgery and the dog was castrated. The adenoma regressed completely and no recurrence was seen.

Although malignant variations exist (perianal adenocarcinoma), these are by far a minority and on the whole the prognosis is good for perianal adenomas. Cytology (e.g. of a fine-needle aspirate) prior to surgery will allow a decision to be made regarding the necessary margin of excision:

- A benign adenoma may be removed with minimal margins
- Adenocarcinomas will require wide margins, with consideration of removal of draining lymph nodes and adjunct chemotherapy.

Castration at the time of mass removal tends to prevent or reduce recurrence. If castration is performed prior to lump removal, even quite large masses may shrink, allowing for easier surgical removal at a later date.

External blockage

Long-haired dogs may develop matting of the hair over the anus (pseudocoprostasis). In the author's experience, Yorkshire Terriers, Bearded Collies, Shetland Sheepdogs and Cavalier King Charles Spaniels seem to be relatively more prone. The condition tends to occur in these breeds following bouts of diarrhoea. If left unnoticed, severe constipation or obstipation can result. The condition also predisposes to fly strike. Treatment involves clipping the matted hair away and ensuring that no hardened faeces remain in the rectum.

Anal prolapse

Anal prolapse may occur after repeated or prolonged tenesmus. It is more common in young or immature dogs, following gastrointestinal disease, although it can be seen in dogs of any age as a sequel to cystitis, colitis, rectoanal tumours, or other conditions causing straining. The mucosa of the anus is seen to protrude through the anal orifice. Rectal prolapse is a more severe presentation, involving part or all of the rectum.

Diagnosis of anal prolapse is straightforward, based on appearance, although it is important to rule out the presence of anal or rectal tumours, or of intussusception (although that is very uncommon). The anal prolapse is replaced under sedation or general anaesthesia, usually requiring a little lubrication. A purse-string suture may be required to prevent recurrence. Treatment of the inciting cause is required.

Faecal incontinence

Faecal incontinence may occur after surgery of the anus, although it is uncommon (unless surgery is ventral to the anus and risks damaging the pudendal nerve); up to 50% of the external anal sphincter may be removed with no long-term ill effects, although temporary incontinence (lasting several weeks) may be seen. It is more common to see faecal incontinence with neurological disease, or after bilateral perineal hernia repair. Whatever the cause, the prognosis for faecal incontinence is grave. Owners should be carefully counselled on the unlikely chances of recovery, and euthanasia should be offered. It can be a very emotive decision for the client to make, and they may feel that they are being selfish by contemplating euthanasia for a dog that may otherwise be well. The hygiene and public health implications of a faecally incontinent dog may be useful considerations in coming to a decision.

Anal strictures

Strictures are formed by scar tissue and fibrosis replacing the normal mucosa or submucosal layers of the anus or distal rectum. This may be due to neoplasia, or wounds (surgical or otherwise) affecting the anal ring. The usual signs of straining and dyschezia may be seen, with thin stools typically being produced. Diagnosis is by rectal examination, and treatment is by repeated bougienage of the anus under general anaesthesia. If the stricture fails to improve, or recurs, then surgery such as a rectal pull-through (see above) may be required (see *BSAVA Manual of Canine and Feline Abdominal Surgery*).

Perianal fistula

Also termed anal furunculosis, this is a condition typically seen in middle-aged German Shepherd Dogs, although it has been reported in other breeds (especially collies and Irish Setters). The clinical signs are of ulcerated wounds and discharging sinuses in the perianal region (Figure 30.8). Detailed discussion of the aetiology and various treatment options are beyond the scope of this chapter, and the reader is recommended to see the *BSAVA Manual of Canine and Feline Gastroenterology* and the *BSAVA Manual of Canine and Feline Abdominal Surgery* for more information. It seems likely that there is an immune-mediated basis to the disease, possibly akin to Crohn's disease in humans; certainly most cases will respond to a combination of dietary management and immunosuppressive medication, such as ciclosporin. Surgical excision of recalcitrant lesions may be required, but there is no rationale for performing a high amputation of the tail, which has historically been proposed.

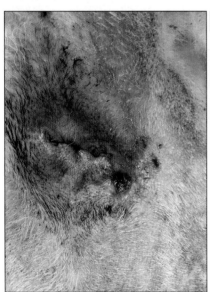

30.8

Anal fistula in a 6-year-old male neutered German Shepherd Dog. The condition cleared up completely after a dietary change.

Perineal hernia

The pelvic diaphragm essentially supports the rectum and separates the abdominal contents from the pelvic canal. It consists of the levator ani and coccygeus muscles, the external anal sphincter and the perineal fascia. Atrophy of elements of the pelvic diaphragm,

under the influence of testosterone, allows the rectum to deviate and dilate into the potential space created; it may also allow caudal abdominal viscera to enter the perineal area.

Affected dogs may present in obvious pain, with a unilateral or bilateral perineal swelling, though more often the presentation revolves around tenesmus and disturbance of normal defecation. If the bladder or prostate gland is involved in the hernia, stranguria may also be present (see Chapter 26). With few exceptions, intact male dogs are affected. Breed predispositions are at present uncertain: historically, docked breeds seemed to be more prone, suggesting a potential aetiology for the condition; however, data are lacking for the incidence of perineal hernias since the ban on docking came into force in the UK in 2007.

Diagnosis of perineal hernia is from clinical presentation and by rectal examination, which will confirm a lack of rectal support on one or both sides, and of dilatation or sacculation of the rectum. Ultrasonography may be useful to look for retroflexion of the bladder or prostate gland. Surgical reconstruction of the pelvic diaphragm through muscle transposition is the treatment of choice (see *BSAVA Manual of Canine and Feline Abdominal Surgery*) and castration is mandatory.

Disorders of the tail

The disorders below are described in approximate order of commonness.

Trauma

As with any injury, the rest of the animal should be carefully examined for the presence of other injury or illness (see Chapter 10). For detailed advice on the management of tail wounds see the *BSAVA Manual of Canine and Feline Wound Management and Reconstruction*.

Assessment should be made as to the nature and age of the wound, as this will affect the management of the wound and the consideration for antibiosis. The tail should be examined to see whether there is any loss of sensation, or whether any bumps, suggesting fracture, can be palpated. If so, radiographic examination should be performed.

> **PRACTICAL TIP**
>
> Tail chasing may occur in some breeds (particularly Staffordshire Bull Terriers) as part of a central neurological dysfunction. Owners may interpret this as a response to pain. There is also a risk of self-trauma

It is worth noting that even minor lacerations to the tail can be notoriously frustrating to treat: bandaging is difficult; self-trauma is common; and wagging of the tail leads to further haemorrhage and dehiscence. Owners of dogs with tail injuries should be made aware of this at the outset, as many seemingly trivial wounds can result in the need for amputation of all or part of the tail.

Initial wound treatment involves copious flushing to remove as much debris as possible. A fresh wound may then be closed primarily if enough skin is present: however, tension on the wound is to be avoided, as this will lead to poor wound healing and may result in necrosis of the tail skin. If it is not possible to close a tail wound without tension, management of the wound with dressings to encourage healing by secondary intention (granulation tissue formation) should be performed. Such wounds often heal surprisingly well on the tail, though it is worthwhile mentioning to the owner that it may take 3–4 weeks for healing to occur.

If the tail tip shows signs of chronic trauma (usually evidenced by dried necrotic skin, though in severe cases bone may be visible), it is best to perform an amputation of the tail tip as such wounds rarely heal and are subject to repeated self-trauma. The amount of tail that needs to be removed will depend on the extent of the injury and also on the behaviour of the dog. Removal to a level one to two vertebrae proximal to the injured portion will usually suffice: however, in breeds that wag the tail excessively it may be wiser to remove more to prevent future injury.

Tail gland hypertrophy

Tail gland hypertrophy ('stud tail') is a common presentation of older intact male dogs, although it can also be seen in castrated males and occasionally in bitches. The proximal third of the dorsal tail is well imbued with modified sweat glands known as supracaudal glands. Hypertrophy of these glands may occur due to idiopathic causes or hypothyroidism, but the condition is most commonly due to hyperandrogenism and is commonly linked to testicular neoplasia. Dogs present with a chronic history of hair loss along the dorsal base of the tail, and the appearance is typically that of scabby, thickened, irregular skin. There may be secondary inflammation or infection from self-trauma, although any irritation is usually of low grade. An intact male should be carefully examined for testicular tumours. Castration will often improve the condition, although in many cases the alopecia and hyperplasia will persist. Antibiotics and regular use of a degreasing shampoo may help improve the condition in idiopathic cases. If no improvement is seen, it may be necessary to perform a biopsy (preferably surgically) to distinguish the condition from hepatoid adenoma or (rarely) adenocarcinoma.

Tail fold intertrigo (corkscrew tail, ingrowing tail)

The foreshortened deformed tail characteristic of certain breeds (English and French Bulldogs, Boston Terrier, Pug) may in some individuals be so deviated that a considerable skin fold exists at the tail base. As with skin folds elsewhere around the body, these are prone to irritation, inflammation and infection. Affected individuals may present with typical signs of anal and tail disease (scooting, biting at the rear, discomfort whilst sitting). Diagnosis is by careful examination of the tail base to find the sore skin fold. There will frequently be a malodorous discharge and there may be a build up of waxy secretions from the supracaudal glands. Treatment involving attention to hygiene (bathing) and topical corticosteroid application may ameliorate mild cases, but definitive treatment of severe cases relies on resection of the skin fold (see *BSAVA Manual of Canine and Feline Wound Management and Reconstruction*).

Tail paralysis or paresis

There are various potential causes for lowered tail carriage in dogs (Figure 30.9). By far the most common cause in general practice is 'swimmer's tail'; a muscular paresis often seen in Labrador Retrievers (whether they have been swimming or not).

Neurological
- Lumbosacral stenosis
- Degenerative myelopathy
- Disc disease
- Meningitis
- Spinal neoplasia
- Spinal trauma

Pain
- Tail trauma
- Infection
- Neoplasia
- Perineal and anal disease

Miscellaneous
- 'Swimmer's tail': primarily in Labrador Retrievers, though can affect Golden and Flat-Coated Retrievers, English Pointers and setters
- 'Cold bathing': hypothermic neuropraxia
- Conformation

30.9 Causes of poor tail carriage.

A full clinical examination should include obtaining a detailed history regarding any lameness or ataxia. Proprioceptive deficits in the hindlimbs (see Chapter 16) makes a neurological cause more likely. Neurological testing should assess the presence or absence of superficial pain perception; if this is absent, then deep pain perception should be assessed, and the tail should be examined for evidence of perfusion injury (a pulse oximeter is invaluable for this purpose).

WARNING

Never test for deep pain sensation if superficial pain is present

Treatment will depend on the underlying cause. 'Swimmer's tail' usually responds to NSAIDs, although it may take 2 weeks to improve.

References and further reading

Aronson L (2003) Rectum and anus. In: *Textbook of Small Animal Surgery, 3rd edn,* ed. D Slatter, pp.682–707. Saunders, Philadelphia.
Aronson LR (2012) Rectum, anus and perineum. In: *Veterinary Surgery: Small Animal,* ed. KM Tobias and SA Johnston, pp.1564–1601. Elsevier Saunders, St. Louis
Dobson JM and Lascelles BDX (2011) *BSAVA Manual of Canine and Feline Oncology, 3rd edn.* BSAVA Publications, Gloucester
Evans HE and de Lahunta A (1988) *Miller's Guide to the Dissection of the Dog, 3rd edn.* WB Saunders, Philadelphia
Hall E, Simpson J and Williams D (2005) *BSAVA Manual of Canine and Feline Gastroenterology, 2nd edn,* BSAVA Publications, Gloucester
Hedlund CS (2002) Surgery of the perineum, rectum and anus. In: *Small Animal Surgery, 2nd edn,* ed. TW Fossum, pp.415–449. Mosby, St. Louis
Niles JD and Williams JM (2005) The large intestine and rectum. In: *BSAVA Manual of Canine and Feline Abdominal Surgery,* ed. JM Williams and JD Niles, pp.125–167. BSAVA Publications, Gloucester
Williams J and Moores A (2012) *BSAVA Manual of Canine and Feline Wound Management and Reconstruction, 2nd edn.* BSAVA Publications, Gloucester

Index